OHIO UNIVERSITY
LIBRARY
WITHDRAWN

ANNALS OF
THE NEW YORK ACADEMY
OF SCIENCES

Volume 850

EDITORIAL STAFF

Executive Editor
BILL M. BOLAND

Managing Editor
JUSTINE CULLINAN

Associate Editors
JOYCE HITCHCOCK
MARY KATHERINE BRENNAN

The New York Academy of Sciences
2 East 63rd Street
New York, New York 10021

THE NEW YORK ACADEMY OF SCIENCES
(Founded in 1817)

BOARD OF GOVERNORS, October 1997–September 1998

RICHARD A. RIFKIND, *Chairman of the Board*
ELEANOR BAUM, *Vice Chairman of the Board*
RODNEY W. NICHOLS, *President and CEO* [ex officio]

Honorary Life Governors
WILLIAM T. GOLDEN   JOSHUA LEDERBERG
JOHN T. MORGAN, *Treasurer*

Governors

D. ALLAN BROMLEY	LAWRENCE B. BUTTENWIESER	PRAVEEN CHAUDHARI
RONALD L. GRAHAM	BILL GREEN	HENRY M. GREENBERG
JACQUELINE LEO	WILLIAM J. McDONOUGH	KATHLEEN P. MULLINIX
SANDRA PANEM	CHARLES RAMOND	SARA LEE SCHUPF
JAMES H. SIMONS	WILLIAM C. STEERE, JR.	TORSTEN N. WIESEL

MARTIN L. LEIBOWITZ, *Past Chairman of the Board*

HELENE L. KAPLAN, *Counsel* [ex officio]   CRAIG PURINTON, *Secretary* [ex officio]

COOLEY'S ANEMIA
SEVENTH SYMPOSIUM

ANNALS OF THE NEW YORK ACADEMY OF SCIENCES
Volume 850

COOLEY'S ANEMIA
SEVENTH SYMPOSIUM

Edited by Alan R. Cohen

The New York Academy of Sciences
New York, New York
1998

Copyright © 1998 by the New York Academy of Sciences. All rights reserved. Under the provisions of the United States Copyright Act of 1976, individual readers of the Annals are permitted to make fair use of the material in them for teaching or research. Permission is granted to quote from the Annals provided that the customary acknowledgment is made of the source. Material in the Annals may be republished only by permission of the Academy. Address inquiries to the Executive Editor at the New York Academy of Sciences.

Copying fees: For each copy of an article made beyond the free copying permitted under Section 107 or 108 of the 1976 Copyright Act, a fee should be paid through the Copyright Clearance Center, 222 Rosewood Drive, Danvers, MA 01923. The fee for copying an article is $3.00 for nonacademic use; for use in the classroom, it is $0.07 per page.

∞ The paper used in this publication meets the minimum requirements of American National Standard for Information Sciences—Permanence of Paper for Printed Library Materials, ANSI Z39.48-1984.

COVER ART: *Expression of globin genes. The flow of genetic information from the DNA sequence to the final protein product involves several discrete steps. First, the coding strand is copied into RNA by a process called transcription. Processing of the RNA species includes modifications of the 5' end, referred to as capping, addition of adenosines on the 3' end, and splicing to remove intron sequences. The final mRNA species is transported to the cytoplasm where it is translated into protein. The α- and β-like chains assemble spontaneously to form hemoglobin molecules. Mutations that cause thalassemia may interfere with any one of these major processes, namely transcription, processing, transport, or translation. (From National Heart, Lung, and Blood Institute/NIH report, Cooley's Anemia: Progress in Biology and Medicine 1995)* Spacecraft photograph Most of Africa and portions of Europe and Asia can be seen in this spectacular photograph taken from the Apollo II spacecraft during its translunar coast toward the moon. Apollo II, with Astronauts Neil A. Armstrong, Michael Collins, and Edwin E. Aldrin, Jr. aboard, was already 98,000 nautical miles from Earth when this picture was taken (courtesy of NASA).

Library of Congress Cataloging-in-Publication Data

Cooley's anemia : seventh symposium / edited by Alan R. Cohen.
    p. cm. — (Annals of the New York Academy of Sciences, ISSN 0077-8923 ; v. 850)
    "Seventh Cooley's Anemia Symposium . . . held in Cambridge, Massachusetts on May 30–June 2, 1997" — Contents p.
    ISBN 1-57331-121-9 (cloth : alk. paper). — ISBN 1-57331-122-7 (paper : alk. paper)
    1. Thalassemia—Congresses. I. Cohen, Alan, 1946–
II. Cooley's Anemia Symposium (7th : 1997 : Cambridge, Mass.)
III. Series.
    [DNLM: 1. beta-Thalassemia congresses. 2. Fetal Hemoglobin congresses. WH 170 C774 1998]
Q11.N5 vol. 850
[RC641.7.T5]
500 s—dc21
[616.1'52]
DNLM/DLC
for Library of Congress   98-17791
                                                                                           CIP

CDP/PCP
Printed in the United States of America
ISBN 1-57331-121-9 (cloth)
ISBN 1-57331-122-7 (paper)
ISSN 0077-8923

ANNALS OF THE NEW YORK ACADEMY OF SCIENCES

Volume 850
June 30, 1998

COOLEY'S ANEMIA
Seventh Symposium[a]

Editor and Symposium Chairman
ALAN R. COHEN

Organizing Committee
ARTHUR BANK, FRANK G. GROSVELD, GUIDO LUCARELLI, DAVID G. NATHAN,
ARTHUR W. NIENHUIS, NANCY F. OLIVIERI, AND GEORGE STAMATOYANNOPOULOS

CONTENTS

Preface. *By* A. R. COHEN xiii

Thalassemia in the Next Millennium: Keynote Address.
  By D. J. WEATHERALL 1

Part I. Globin Gene Expression and Regulation
A. *Cis* Control

Developmental Control of ε- and γ- Globin Genes.
  By G. STAMATOYANNOPOULOS 10

The Dynamics of β-Globin Gene Transcription. *By* F. F. GROSVELD, E. DE BOER,
  J. GRIBNAU, T. TRIMBORN, M. WIJGERDE, and P. FRASER 18

β-YAC Transgenic Mice for Studying LCR Function. *By* K. R. PETERSON,
  P. A. NAVAS, and G. STAMATOYANNOPOULOS 28

Molecular Basis of Hereditary Persistence of Fetal Hemoglobin.
  By B. G. FORGET 38

Reduced β -Globin Gene Expression in Adult Mice Containing Deletions of
  Locus Control Region 5' HS-2 or 5' HS-3. *By* T. J. LEY, B. HUG,
  S. FIERING, E. EPNER, M. A. BENDER, and M. GROUDINE 45

Expression and Developmental Control of the Human α-Globin Gene Cluster.
  By S. A. LIEBHABER and J. E. RUSSELL 54

[a]This volume is the result of a conference entitled **Seventh Cooley's Anemia Symposium** sponsored jointly by the New York Academy of Sciences and the Cooley's Anemia Foundation, held in Cambridge, Massachusetts on May 30–June 2, 1997.

B. Transcriptional Control

Transcriptional Factors for Specific Globin Genes.
  By J. J. BIEKER .... .64

Silencing and Activation of Embryonic Globin Gene Expression. *By* G. D.
  GINDER, R. SINGAL, J. A. LITTLE, N. DEMPSEY, R. FERRIS, and S. Z. WANG . . 70

C. Pharmacologic Induction of Fetal Hemoglobin

Hemoglobin Switching Protocols in Thalassemia: Experience with Sodium
  Phenylbutyrate and Hydroxyurea. *By* G. J. DOVER .... .80

Cellular and Molecular Effects of a Pulse Butyrate Regimen and New Inducers
  of Globin Gene Expression and Hematopoiesis. *By* T. IKUTA, G. ATWEH,
  V. BOOSALIS, G. L. WHITE, S. DA FONSECA, M. BOOSALIS, D. V. FALLER,
  and S. P. PERRINE .... .87

Elimination of Transfusions through Induction of Fetal Hemoglobin Synthesis in
  Cooley's Anemia. *By* N. F. OLIVIERI, D. C. REES, G. D. GINDER, S. L. THEIN,
  J. S. WAYE, L. CHANG, G. M. BRITTENHAM, and D. J. WEATHERALL ..... .100

Butyrate Trials. *By* M. D. CAPPELLINI, G. GRAZIADEI, L. CICERI, A. COMINO,
  P. BIANCHI, M. POMATI, and G. FIORELLI 110

Hydroxyurea Therapy in Thalassemia. *By* D. LOUKOPOULOS, E. VOSKARIDOU, A.
  STAMOULAKATOU, Y. PAPASSOTIRIOU, V. KALOTYCHOU, A. LOUTRADI, G. COZMA,
  H. TSIARTA, and N. PAVLIDES 120

The Role of Recombinant Human Erythropoietin in the Treatment of
  Thalassemia. *By* E. A. RACHMILEWITZ and M. AKER .... .129

Part II. Gene Transfer

Improved Amphotropic Retrovirus-mediated Gene Transfer into Hematopoietic
  Stem Cells. *By* D. M. BODINE, C. E. DUNBAR, L. J. GIRARD, N. E. SEIDEL,
  A. P. CLINE, R. E. DONAHUE, and D. ORLIC .... .139

Retroviral Vectors Aimed at the Gene Therapy of Human β-Globin Gene Disorders.
  By R. PAWLIUK, T. BACHELOT, H. RAFTOPOULOS, C. KALBERER, R. K. HUMPHRIES,
  A. BANK, and P. LEBOULCH 151

Targeted Integration of a Recombinant Adeno-Associated Viral Globin Gene
  Vector into Human Chromosome 19. *By* J. BERTRAN, Y. YANG, P. HARGROVE,
  E. F. VANIN, and A. W. NIENHUIS .... .163

High-Level Transfer and Long-Term Expression of the Human β-Globin Gene in a
  Mouse Transplant Model. *By* H. RAFTOPOULOS, M. WARD, and A. BANK . . 178

Part III. Clinical Management of Cooley's Anemia and Its Complications

Pathophysiology of Iron Overload. *By* C. HERSHKO, G. LINK, and
  I. CABANTCHIK .... .191

The Origin of the Differences in (*R*)- and (*S*)-Desmethyldesferrithiocin: Iron
Clearing Properties. *By* R. J. BERGERON, J. WIEGAND, K. RATLIFF-THOMPSON,
and W. R. WEIMAR 202

Long-term Trials of Deferiprone in Cooley's Anemia. *By* N. F. OLIVIERI and
G. M. BRITTENHAM 217

A Multi-Center Safety Trial of the Oral Iron Chelator Deferiprone. *By* A. COHEN,
R. GALANELLO, A. PIGA, and C. VULLO 223

Survival and Disease Complications in Thalassemia Major. *By* C. BORGNA-PIGNATTI,
S. RUGOLOTTO, P. DE STEFANO, A. PIGA, F. DI GREGORIO, M. R. GAMBERINI,
V. SABATO, C. MELEVENDI, M. D. CAPPELLINI, and G. VERLATO 227

New Approaches to the Management of Hepatitis and Endocrine Disorders in
Cooley's Anemia. *By* B. WONKE, A. V. HOFFBRAND, P. BOULOUX, C. JENSEN,
and P. TELFER 232

Diagnosis and Management of Iron-induced Heart Disease in Cooley's Anemia.
By M. JESSUP and C. S. MANNO 242

Global Epidemiology of Hemoglobin Disorders *By* M. ANGASTINIOTIS
and B. MODELL 251

Part IV. Transplantation for Thalassemia

Bone Marrow Transplantation in Thalassemia: The Experience of Pesaro
By G. LUCARELLI, M. GALIMBERTI, C. GIARDINI, C. POLCHI, E. ANGELUCCI,
D. BARONCIANI, B. ERER, and D. GAZIEV 270

Current and Future Preparative Regimens for Bone Marrow Transplantation in
Thalassemia. *By* R. STORB, C. YU, H. J. DEEG, G. GEORGES, H.-P. KIEM,
P. A. MCSWEENEY, R. A. NASH, B. M. SANDMAIER, K. M. SULLIVAN,
J. L. WAGNER, and M. C. WALTERS 276

Treatment of Iron Overload in the "Ex-Thalassemic": Report from the Phlebotomy
Program. *By* E. ANGELUCCI, P. MURETTO, G. LUCARELLI, M. RIPALTI,
D. BARONCIANI, B. ERER, M. GALIMBERTI, M. ANNIBALI, C. GIARDINI,
D. GAZIEV, S. RAPA, and P. POLCHI 288

Late Effects of Bone Marrow Transplantation for Thalassemia. *By* A. PIGA,
F. LONGO, V. VOI, S. FACELLO, R. MINIERO, and B. DRESOW 294

In Utero Transplantation for Thalassemia. *By* A. W. FLAKE and
E. D. ZANJANI 300

Unrelated and HLA-Nonidentical Related Donor Marrow Transplantation for
Thalassemia and Leukemia: A Combined Report from the Seattle Marrow
Transplant Team and the International Bone Marrow Transplant Registry.
By K. M. SULLIVAN, C. ANASETTI, M. HOROWITZ, P. A. ROWLINGS, E. W.
PETERSDORF, P. J. MARTIN, R. A. CLIFT, M. C. WALTERS, T. GOOLEY, J. SIERRA,
J. E. ANDERSON, J. BJERKE, M. SIADAK, M. E. D. FLOWERS, R. A. NASH, J. E.
SANDERS, F. R. APPELBAUM, R. STORB, and J. A. HANSEN 312

Part V. Thalassemia Intermedia

Relationship between Genotype and Phenotype: Thalassemia Intermedia.
    By R. GALANELLO and A. CAO .... .325

The Hemoglobin E Syndromes. *By* D. C. REES, L. STYLES, E. P. VICHINSKY,
    J. B. CLEGG, and D. J. WEATHERALL .... .334

The Morbidity of Bone Disease in Thalassemia. *By* E. P. VICHINSKY .... .344

Part VI. Psychosocial Aspects of Thalassemia

The Psychosocial Impact of Chronic Disease. *By* C. POLITIS .... .349

Psychosocial Integration of Adolescents and Young Adults with Thalassemia
    Major. *By* A. DI PALMA, C. VULLO, B. ZANI, and A. FACCHINI .... .355

Future Orientation and Life Expectations of Adolescents and Young Adults with
    Thalassemia Major. *By* S. BUSH, F. S. MANDEL, and P.-J. GIARDINA ...... .361

Patient Psychosocial Perspectives. *By* G. POTENZA and R. CAZZETTA .... .370

✢

Summary of the Seventh Cooley's Anemia Symposium. *By* D. G. NATHAN ..... .374

Poster Presentations

Molecular Biology

5′ HS1 and the Distal β-Globin Promoter Functionally Interact in Single Copy
    β-Globin Transgenic Mice. *By* P. PASCERI, D. PANNELL, X. WU,
    and J. ELLIS .... .377

An *in Vitro* Model of Human Erythropoiesis for the Study of
    Hemoglobinopathies. *By* P. MALIK, L. W. BARSKY, and T. C. FISHER ..... .382

Full Developmental Silencing of the Embryonic ζ-Globin Gene Reflects
    Instability of Its mRNA. *By* J. E. RUSSELL, A. E. LEE,
    and S. A. LIEBHABER .... .386

Red Blood Cells

RBC Adhesion to Cremaster Endothelium in Mice with Abnormal Hemoglobin
    Is Increased by Topical Endotoxin. *By* X-W. LIU, S. S. PIERANGELI, J. BARKER,
    T. M. WICK, and L. L. HSU .... .391

Enhancement by Ubiquitin Aldehyde of Proteolysis of Hemoglobin α-Subunits
    in β-Thalassemic Hemolysates. *By* J. R. SHAEFFER and R. E. COHEN ..... .394

Genotype/Phenotype, Screening, and Diagnostic Considerations

An α-2 Globin Gene Initiation Codon Mutation in a Vietnamese Patient with
  Hb H Disease. *By* F. KUTLAR, T. V. ADAMKIEWICZ, R. B. MARKOWITZ,
  L. HOLLEY, and A. KUTLAR 398

The Montreal Thalassemia Screening Program: Response of the High School
  Students. *By* A. CAPUA 401

Spectrum of β-Thalassemia Mutations in Oman. *By* S. DAAR, H. M. HUSSEIN,
  T. MERGHOUB, and R. KRISHNAMOORTHY 404

Molecular Basis of β-Thalassemia in Bahrain: An Epicenter for a Middle East
  Specific Mutation. *By* N. JASSIM, T. MERGHOUB, O. PASCAUD,
  H. AL MUKHARRAQ, R. DUCROCQ, D. LABIE, J. ELION, R. KRISHNAMOORTHY,
  and S. AL ARRAYED 407

Hemoglobin E/β Thalassemia: The Canadian Experience. *By* M. FOULADI,
  M. L. MACMILLAN, E. NISBET-BROWN, N. KLEIN, J. BARLAS, J. S. WAYE,
  and N. F. OLIVIERI 410

α- And β-Thalassemia in Thailand. *By* S. FUCHAROEN, P. WINICHAGOON,
  N. SIRITANARATKUL, J. CHOWTHAWORN, and P. POOTRAKUL 412

Homozygous Hemoglobin Constant Spring with Normal Electrophoresis:
  A Possible Cause for Under Diagnosis. *By* L. KRISHNAMURTI
  and J. A. LITTLE 415

Audit of Prenatal Diagnosis for Hemoglobin Disorders in the United Kingdom:
  The First Twenty Years. *By* B. MODELL, M. PETROU, M. LAYTON, L. VARNAVIDES,
  C. MOISELY, R. H. T. WARD, C. RODECK, K. NICOLAIDES, A. FITCHES,
  and J. OLD 420

Spectrum of β-Thalassemia Mutations in Guadeloupe (French West Indies) and
  Interactions with Other Hemoglobinopathies. *By* M. ROMANA, L. KÉCLARD,
  A. FROGER, C. BERCHEL, and G. MÉRAULT 423

α-Globin Mutations and Rearrangements in Israel: PCR-Based Analysis Reveals
  Ethnic Diversity. *By* D. RUND, V. ORON-KARNI, D. FILON,
  and A. OPPENHEIM 426

Correlation of ζ-Globin ELISA with PCR for (– –^{SEA}) Deletion and Clinical
  Diagnosis for α- Thal-1 Trait. *By* R. A. SIMKINS, K.-A. THAN, B. SCHAPIRO,
  E. S. CHOI, and P. R. DAOUST 429

The Diverse Molecular Basis and Mild Clinical Picture of HbH Disease in Israel.
  By H. TAMARY, G. KLINGER, L. SHALMON, H. KIRSCHMANN, A. KOREN,
  M. BENNET, and R. ZAIZOV 432

Phenotypic Prediction in β-Thalassemia. *By* P. J. Ho, G. W. Hall,
L. Y. Luo, D. J. Weatherall, and S. L. Thein 436

The Impact of Asian Immigration on Thalassemia in California.
By F. Lorey and G. Cunningham 442

Fetal Hemoglobin

Detection of Fetal Hemoglobin in Erythrocytes by Flow Cytometry. *By*
T. A. Campbell, R. E. Ware, and M. Mason 446

Hydroxyurea and Hemin Affect Both the Transcriptional and Post-Transcriptional
Mechanisms of Some Globin Genes in Human Adult Erythroid Cells.
By P. Kollia, E. Fibach, M. Politou, C. T. Noguchi, A. N. Schechter,
and D. Loukopoulos 449

Treatment of Two Infants with Cooley's Anemia with Sodium Phenylbutyrate.
By M. L. MacMillan, M. Fouladi, E. Nisbet-Brown, J. S. Waye, and
N. F. Olivieri 452

Erythropoietin Level and Effect of rHuEPO in β-Thalassemic Mice. *By* R. A. Popp,
S. G. Shinpock, D. M. Popp, G. K. Clemons, and D. B. Van Wyck 455

Increase in Hemoglobin Concentration during Therapy with Hydroxyurea in
Cooley's Anemia. *By* B. R. Saxon, J. S. Waye, and N. F. Olivieri 459

Preliminary Report: Hydroxyurea Produces Significant Clinical Response in
Thalassemia Intermedia. *By* L. Styles, B. Lewis, D. Foote, L. Cuda,
and E. Vichinsky 461

Clinical Issues

Iron Overload and Antioxidant Status in Patients with β-Thalassemia Major.
By K. Reller, B. Dresow, M. Collell, R. Fischer, R. Engelhardt, P. Nielsen,
M. Dürken, C. Politis, and A. Piga 463

Effect of Iron Chelator L1 on Iron Absorption in Man. *By* B. Dresow, R. Fischer,
P. Nielsen, E. E. Gabbe, and A. Piga 466

Survival and Morbidity in Transfusion-dependent Thalassemic Patients on
Subcutaneous Desferrioxamine Chelation: Nearly Two Decades of
Experience. *By* E. M. Calleja, J. Y. Chen, M. Lesser, R. W. Grady,
M. I. New, and P. J. Giardina 469

Regulation of Glucose Disturbances with Glibenclamide in Patients with
Thalassemia. *By* V. Ladis, C. Theodorides, F. Palamidou, S. Frissiras,
H. Berdousi, and C. Kattamis 471

Bone Metabolism in Thalassemia. *By* F. Garofalo, A. Piga, R. Lala, S. Chiabotto,
M. Di Stefano, and G. C. Isaia 475

Selective Loss of Anterior Pituitary Volume with Severe Pituitary-Gonadal Insufficiency in Poorly Compliant Male Thalassemic Patients with Pubertal Arrest. *By* R. CHATTERJEE, M. KATZ, A. OATRIDGE, G. M. BYDDER, and J. B. PORTER 479

A Trial to Investigate the Relationship between DFO Pharmacokinetics and Metabolism and DFO-Related Toxicity. *By* J. B. PORTER and A. FAHERTY 483

Deferoxamine Stability in Intravenous Solution. *By* C. ROSE, C. CAMBIÉ, G. FORZY, M. MAHIEU, P. FENAUX, and F. BAUTERS 488

Nontransfusional Iron Overload in Thalassemia: Association with Hereditary Hemochromatosis. *By* D. C. REES, B. M. SINGH, L. Y. LUO, S. WICKRAMASINGHE, and S. L. THEIN 490

Stem Cell Transplantation

Mixed Chimerism after Bone Marrow Transplantation in Thalassemia. *By* S. NESCI. M. MANNA, G. LUCARELLI, P. TONUCCI, M. DONATI, O. BUFFI, F. AGOSTINELLI, and M. ANDREANI 495

Bone Marrow Transplantation for Homozygous β-Thalassemia—The Memorial Sloan-Kettering Cancer Center Experience. *By* F. BOULAD, P. GIARDINA, A. GILLIO, N. KERNAN, T. SMALL, J. BROCHSTEIN, K. VAN SYCKLE, D. GEORGE, P. SZABOLCS, and R. J. O'REILLY 498

Bone Marrow Transplantation in Thalassemia: A Role for Radiation? *By* Y. S. LEE, K. M. KRISTOVICH, J. M. DUCORE, E. VICHINSKY, V. L. CROUSE, B. E. GLADER, and M. D. AMYLON 503

Psychosocial Issues and Health Care Delivery

Patient-Oriented Research Facilitated through the Establishment of the Nurses Network for Cooley's Anemia (CANNA). *By* S. M. CARSON and L. QUILL 506

The Social Impact of Migration on Disease: Cooley's Anemia, Thalassemia, and New Asian Immigrants. *By* N. HEER, J. CHOY, and E. P. VICHINSKY 509

The Psychosocial Burden of Cooley's Anemia in Affected Children and Their Parents. *By* N. KLEIN, A. SEN, J. RUSBY, S. RATIP, B. MODELL, and N. F. OLIVIERI 512

Outreach Strategies for Asian Pacific Island Communities. *By* J. CHOY, R. C. YAMASHITA, D. FOOTE, N. HEER, and E. P. VICHINSKY 514

Approaches to Working with Adult Thalassemia Patients in Pediatric Settings. *By* L. WEISSMAN, M. TREADWELL, D. FOOTE, N. HEER, and E. P. VICHINSKY 516

From a Distance: Using Information Technologies to Overcome Geographic
  Boundaries in Thalassemia Service Delivery. *By* R. C. YAMASHITA,
  K. QUIROLO, J. CHOY, and D. FOOTE 518

Patient Cultures: Thalassemia Service Delivery and Patient Compliance.
  By R. C. YAMASHITA, D. FOOTE, and L. WEISSMAN 521

Index of Contributors 523

Financial assistance was received from:

Major Funders

- NATIONAL HEART, LUNG, AND BLOOD INSTITUTE/NIH
- NATIONAL INSTITUTE OF DIABETES AND DIGESTIVE AND KIDNEY DISEASES/NIH

Contributor

- APOTEX RESEARCH, INC.
- NATIONAL INSTITUTE OF CHILD HEALTH AND HUMAN DEVELOPMENT/NIH

The New York Academy of Sciences believes it has a responsibility to provide an open forum for discussion of scientific questions. The positions taken by the participants in the reported conferences are their own and not necessarily those of the Academy. The Academy has no intent to influence legislation by providing such forums.

PREFACE

ALAN R. COHEN

The Seventh Cooley's Anemia Symposium, held in Cambridge, Massachusetts in June, 1997, continued the fine tradition begun more than 30 years ago of providing a forum for the presentation of new and exciting research related to thalassemia. While scientific directions and clinical care have changed dramatically in three decades, the goals of this meeting have remained remarkably constant. The Symposium is the international focal point for the presentation of new advances in the understanding of Cooley's anemia. Moreover, it provides a unique opportunity for basic scientists, clinical researchers, clinicians and patients to learn from one another and to explore the very important crossroads between basic and applied research. The importance of this interaction was well illustrated in the Seventh Symposium by the discussion of the molecular biology of hemoglobin switching, followed by the presentation of the results of trials of fetal hemoglobin enhancing agents. Similarly, the discussion of the pathophysiology of iron overload and the pharmacologic and biochemical characteristics of an ideal iron chelator was followed by presentations on the clinical assessment of iron stores and the results of clinical trials of an orally active chelating agent.

It is particularly pleasing to note that subjects that were grouped together under the heading of *Future Research in Thalassemia* at the Sixth Symposium, such as stem cell transplantation and gene transfer, now had their own full sessions to reflect their remarkable progress. For example, transplantation in thalassemia has moved into new areas of research such as the use of alternative donors, transplantation *in utero*, and the optimal management of iron overload after stem cell transplant. The field of gene transfer has seen an acceleration in the development of animal models of thalassemia, effective vectors and successful murine expression, all represented in the Seventh Symposium.

Two other aspects of the Symposium and these proceedings deserve special emphasis. First, thalassemia intermedia has been given the more extensive attention it deserves in light of its importance worldwide and its increasing frequency in the United States. Second, the longer life expectancy of patients with Cooley's anemia has created a new set of issues such as osteoporosis and fertility that are now being addressed in clinical research studies that hold the promise of matching increasing length of life with a parallel improvement in the quality of life.

I would like to extend my deep appreciation to the Cooley's Anemia Foundation for their support for the Symposium and their long-standing, extraordinary commitment to scientific investigation, clinical care and education related to thalassemia. Peter Chieco, President of the Foundation, Gina Cioffi, National Executive Director, and members of the Medical Advisory Board were instrumental in the development of the Symposium. I would also like to thank Dr. Rashid Shaikh and Ms. Sherryl Usmani of the New York Academy of Sciences for their assistance, responsiveness, and insight in planning and implementing the Symposium. I am grateful to Doctors Claude Lenfant, Clarisse Reid, Helena Mishoe and Alan Levine of the NHLBI, Drs. David Badman and Philip Gorden of the NIDDK, and Dr. Yvonne Maddox of NICHHD for their support of the Symposium and their dedication to Cooley's anemia. Ms. Joyce Hitchcock has expertly performed the unenviable task of transforming the Symposium talks into the papers in this volume, and Ms. Minerva Barayuga has managed many of the administrative details since the planning for the Symposium began three years ago.

I would like to express particular gratitude to Dr. Elias Schwartz who took me to my first Cooley's Anemia Symposium in 1980 and Nunzio Cazzetta whom I first met on that occasion. Both of these men have been wise and judicious mentors and colleagues who have constantly reminded me that good science and good patient care must never lose sight of one another.

Thalassemia in the Next Millennium

Keynote Address[a]

D. J. WEATHERALL[b]

MRC Molecular Haematology Unit, Institute of Molecular Medicine, University of Oxford, John Radcliffe Hospital, Oxford, OX3 9DS United Kingdom

ABSTRACT: Over the next decade it will be essential to make the thalassemia problem more visible to governments and international health agencies that are involved in health care in the emerging countries. This will require detailed population surveys to determine the gene frequencies of the important forms of thalassemia, together with a better understanding of their natural history and of the factors that modify their clinical phenotypes. In particular, more needs to be learnt about the natural history and ways of managing the intermediate forms of β thalassemia. While research should continue towards definitive forms of treatment it is important, in the meantime, to pursue the development of cheap and safe oral chelating agents and to carry out clinical trials of drugs that may interact one with another to elevate the level of fetal hemoglobin, particularly in patients with different types of β thalassemia intermedia. The partial control of the disease by carrier detection and prenatal diagnosis will only be feasible in emerging countries if it is possible to obtain the financial support of the major international agencies and the cooperation of their governments and communities; the remarkable success of this approach in some of the Mediterranean islands is a good example of what can be achieved.

Since the first of this series of conferences on Cooley's Anemia, held in December 1963, enormous progress has been made in thalassemia research. Although many questions remain unanswered, we have a reasonable understanding of the molecular pathology and pathophysiology of most of the common forms of the disease and this information has led to remarkable advances in its control by screening and prenatal diagnosis, and in its symptomatic management.

Paradoxically, however, the thalassemias are likely to pose an increasing world health problem in the immediate future. In introducing what will presumably be the last Cooley's Anemia Conference of the present millennium it is important, therefore, to try to define our priorities for thalassemia research in the future and, in particular, to ask whether it will be possible to apply its results to the control and management of the disease on the scale required.

THALASSEMIA AS A WORLD HEALTH PROBLEM

Over the second half of the present century there has been a remarkable transition in the demography of common illness.[1,2] With the exception of sub-Saharan Africa there has been a major decline in childhood mortality, reflecting a reduction in the so-called "first

---

[a]The studies carried out in Oxford which are described in this review were supported by the Medical Research Council and Wellcome Trust.
[b]Tel: +1865 222359; Fax: +1865 222501; E-mail: janet.watt%mailgate.JR2@ox.ac.uk

generation diseases," that is childhood infection, malnutrition and reproductive risks. Hence, in emerging countries babies with serious genetic diseases like thalassemia now survive the early months of life. Throughout the Middle East, the Indian sub-continent and Southeast Asia, thousands of children will be born annually with thalassemia, many of whom will live long enough to require treatment.[3] The results of demographic changes of this kind were graphically illustrated in Cyprus, a country that underwent this transition shortly after World War II.

Thalassemia was not identified in Cyprus until 1944 when, after a major malarial eradication program and related improvements in public health measures, it became clear that among the children of the island population there was a common form of anemia which was not due to infection.[4] By the early 1970s it was estimated that, if no steps were taken to control the disease, in about 40 years the blood required to treat all the severely affected children would amount to 78 000 units per annum, 40% of the population would be donors, and the total cost to the health services would equal or exceed the island's health budget.[5]

In recent projections of the changing pattern of disease burden for the next millennium, published by the World Bank and WHO, as assessed by DALYs (Disability-Adjusted Life Years), congenital anomalies rank thirteenth for the disease burden for demographically developing countries.[1,2] Thalassemia and the sickling disorders are not mentioned in these reports and, though it is difficult to determine how this figure has been arrived at, there is no evidence that the diseases have been included in these estimations.

Unfortunately, although much progress has been made towards determining the different thalassemia mutations in small population samples, a review of the thalassemia literature over recent years indicates that the important task of collecting good population data on the frequency of the disease has been seriously neglected. If the major international health agencies are to be made aware of the thalassemia problem it is vital that information of this type is obtained, together with an assessment of the health burden cause by the different types of thalassemia, in terms of DALY's.

Despite these uncertainties enough is known to give some indication of the magnitude of the problem that will be faced by the emerging countries in the near future. At this meeting in 1969 it was estimated that there were more than 60 different varieties of thalassemia in Thailand and over a quarter of a million symptomatic children.[6] It has been estimated recently that, over the next 30 years, approximately 100,000 new cases of hemoglobin E thalassemia alone will be added to the Thai population; the World Bank's estimate of a population increase in this country between 1991 and 2025 of 57 to close to 100 million is correct,[2] this figure may be a gross underestimate. In Indonesia, in which the Bank estimates a population increase from 180 to close to 300 million, the situation may be even more serious, although recent studies have shown that there is an uneven distribution of β-thalassemia and hemoglobin E among the different island populations, preliminary surveys indicate that, in some, up to 10 percent of the population are carriers for either hemoglobin E or β thalassemia.[7] Similar gene frequencies for these variants are found in parts of India, which could double its population of around 860 million by 2025, and from what is known of the figures for Sri Lanka, Malaysia and Vietnam it is clear that there will also be a massive increase in the population of children requiring expensive treatment for thalassemia (FIG. 1). Thus although these figures offer only the broadest approximation of the truth, it is clear that hemoglobin E thalassemia, and to a lesser extent β-thalassemia, will pose a major world health problem over the next few years.

The α thalassemias achieve even higher gene frequencies than the β-thalassemias and hemoglobin E, and in some populations the α^+ thalassemias appear to be moving towards fixation.[7] However, they do not present a serious health problem and it is only the α^o thalassemias, which are restricted to parts of Southeast Asia and the Mediterranean, that are of importance in this respect (FIG. 2). However, the drain on health services produced by

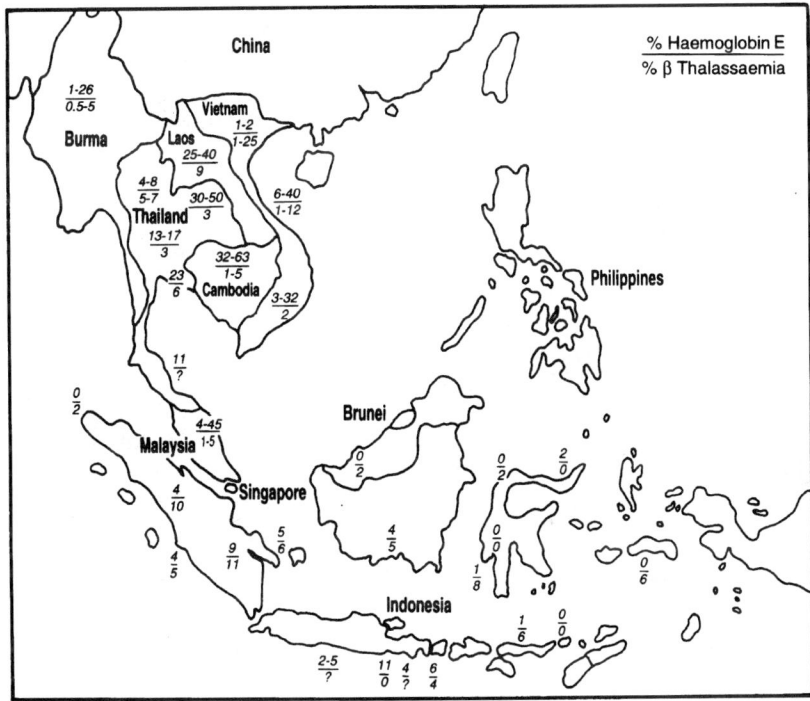

FIGURE 1. Distribution of β thalassemia and hemoglobin E in SE Asia.

the hemoglobin Bart's hydrops syndrome and more severe forms of hemoglobin H disease should not be underestimated.

POPULATION GENETICS AND DYNAMICS OF THE THALASSEMIAS

Although it was suggested by J.B.S. Haldane as early as 1948 that the high frequency of the thalassemias might reflect heterozygote advantage due to reduced susceptibility to malaria, it is only of recent years that the mechanisms whereby such protection might be mediated have been clarified. Research of this type has been extended to the study of other genetic polymorphisms related to present or past malaria and the results may have important implications for an understanding of the marked variation in response to intercurrent illness among the different populations in which thalassemia is common.

Thalassemia and Malaria

The discovery that in every population in which thalassemia is common there is a different pattern of mutation suggests that the disease must have arisen independently in different parts of the world and then reached its high frequency by locally acting factors such as drift and selection.[7] Although a variety of studies has hinted that the selective factor might be malaria,[7] it is only in recent years that it has been possible to put this hypothesis

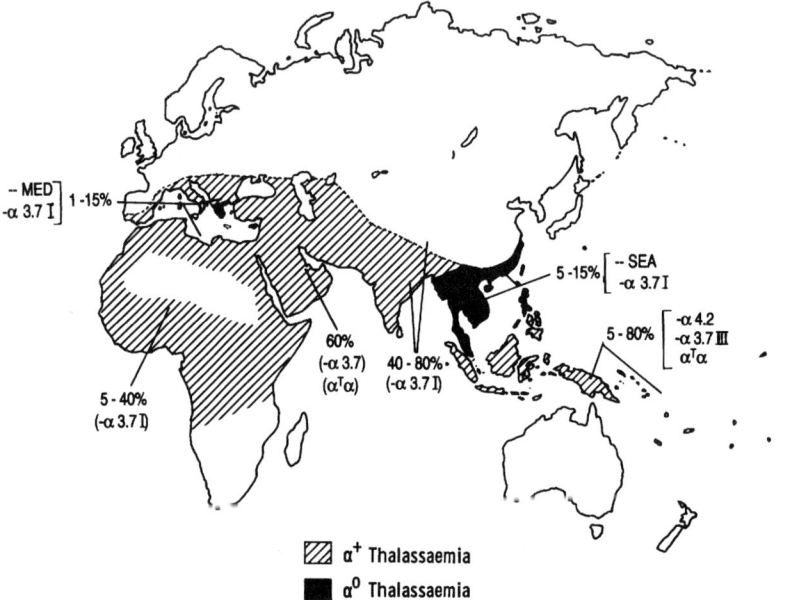

FIGURE 2. World distribution of α thalassemia.

onto a solid experimental footing. Much of this new information has come from studies of α thalassemia in Melanesia and Polynesia.

Surveys of malaria prevalence reveal that, before eradication campaigns, the disease was endemic below 2500m in Papua New Guinea and in parts of the Melanesian archipelago. In these malarious regions, α^+ thalassemia has a gene frequency proportional to the prevalence of malaria.[8] As the disease becomes less frequent in the interior of Papua New Guinea, so does α^+ thalassemia, and there is a gradual decline in the gene frequency across Vanuatu down to New Caledonia, where malaria does not occur. It is possible, of course, that this distribution simply reflects the fact that a⁺ thalassemia was transported to these island populations from the mainland and that the gene frequency was gradually diluted as populations moved south. However, this explanation was ruled out by the observation that the molecular forms of α^+ thalassemia in the island populations are completely different to those on the Asian mainland.[7,8] Thus there is a clear altitude and north-south correlation between α thalassemia and present or past malaria in this region.

Recently, a case-control study carried out in north Papua New Guinea has demonstrated a clear protective effect of the homozygous state for α^+ thalassemia against the serious complications of *P. falciparum* malaria.[9] Furthermore, some hints about the possible mechanisms involved have been obtained from studies in Vanuatu.[10] In a large cohort of babies of different a globin genotypes, followed carefully over the first years of life, it has been found that, quite unexpectedly, those homozygous for α^+ thalassemia have a higher frequency of both *P. vivax* and *P. falciparum* malaria in the first two years of life, after which this effect is not seen. This remarkable observation indicates that the interaction between α thalassemia and malaria may be extremely subtle. It suggests that α^+ thalassemia homozygotes are more susceptible to malaria at a time when the disease rarely kills; this may provide them with an immunizing dose of malaria which offers later protection. In areas in which both types of malaria occur, the earliest infections in life are usually due to *P. vivax*. Furthermore, there is a hint that there may be some cross-immunization between this form of malaria and that due to *P. falciparum*. These observations therefore offer a conceptual framework for an understanding of how α thalassemia may protect against malaria.[10]

If the homozygous state for α⁺ thalassemia has no effect on fitness, this may be an example of a transient rather than a balanced polymorphism, whereby if malaria persists α⁺ thalassemia will go to fixation. There is, however, insufficient information about the phenotype expression of α⁺ thalassemia to be absolutely certain that it has no deleterious effects.

It will now be important to repeat this type of study on populations in which β thalassemia or hemoglobins S and E are common. It may be that α thalassemia is a special case, but it is also possible that these other common variants have reached their high gene frequencies in a similar manner.

If the high gene frequencies for the thalassemias and common hemoglobin variants reflect protection against malaria it is difficult, at first sight, to understand why the different mutations have not become more widely distributed in the world population. Why is hemoglobin S not seen in Southeast Asia or hemoglobin E in Africa, and why don't the same β thalassemia mutations occur in different parts of the world? It seems likely that this reflects the fairly recent appearance of malaria as the principal agent that has maintained these polymorphisms, a notion that is strengthened by an analysis of the relationship between β thalassemia and β globin gene haplotypes.[7]

Other Genetic Changes in Thalassemic Populations Mediated through Malaria

It is now clear that other red cell polymorphisms, including glucose-6-phosphate dehydrogenase deficiency and variation in membrane structure and blood groups, have been shaped by malaria (TABLE 1).[11] However, recent studies indicate that genetic variability due to selection by malaria is not confined to erythrocytes.[11–13] It is now clear that certain polymorphisms of the HLA-DR system are associated with substantial protection against both cerebral malaria and severe malarial anemia. Another polymorphic system which has been uncovered, and which is clearly related to malaria, involves the gene encoding tumor necrosis factor-a (TNF-α). A single base change at position -308 of the promoter is associated with a markedly increased risk of cerebral malaria and death.[12] Subsequently, this polymorphism has been implicated in increased levels of TNF-α expression *in vitro*, an observation that is compatible with the clinical finding that higher plasma levels of TNF-α are observed in malarial patients who have a poor clinical outcome. Another promoter polymorphism, at -238, has also been related to susceptibility to malaria. As well as malaria, there is evidence that these polymorphisms alter susceptibility to leishmaniasis, leprosy and tuberculosis.[11]

Other forms of genetic variability, including iron loading, may also be related to differential susceptibility to malaria.[13]

These recent observations may be of profound importance in our understanding of the different responses to intercurrent illness in populations with a high frequency of thalassemia. Like the hemoglobinopathies these polymorphisms are turning out to have a patchy distribution, again probably due to the very recent appearance of malaria as the selection agent. Thus individual responses to intercurrent infection or iron loading may vary widely between thalassemic populations and have an important effect on the pattern of infectious illness and on other complications of the disease.

TABLE 1. Genetic Polymorphisms Associated with Susceptibility to Malaria

Hemoglobin
    Structural variants
    Thalassemia
Red Cell Membrane
    Band 3 deletion; ovalocytosis
    Blood groups; Duffy, ABO(H), Le(a), Kidd
    Glycophorins
Red Cell Metabolism
    G6PD. Na/K
HLA DR
Iron Transport
TNF α

PATHOPHYSIOLOGY AND GENOTYPE/PHENOTYPE RELATIONSHIPS

As we move to more extensive screening and counseling programs, followed by prenatal diagnosis, or to more experimental forms of therapy, it is becoming increasingly important to be able to anticipate the likely severity of thalassemic phenotypes by analysis of the genetic constitution of parents of potential children with the disease. Although there is some evidence for the molecular basis for the phenotypic variability of the more severe forms of α thalassemia, particularly hemoglobin H disease, globally the most important questions relate to the variable phenotypes of β thalassemia and hemoglobin E thalassemia.

Although there is some broad understanding of the mechanisms that may modify the phenotype of the β thalassemias and their interactions,[14,15] many questions remain unanswered (TABLE 2). It is clear that important factors include the severity of the particular β thalassemia allele, or alleles in compound heterozygotes, the co-inheritance of different forms of α thalassemia, and varying ability to produce hemoglobin F. However, when all these factors have been taken into consideration there is considerable, unexplained variability in the clinical phenotypes in both homozygous β thalassemia and hemoglobin E thalassemia. It seems likely that at least some of this unexplained phenotypic heterogeneity may be related to the capacity to produce γ chains after the neonatal period. While persistent γ chain synthesis and the production of hemoglobin F probably reflect the pattern of ineffective erythropoiesis, erythroid expansion, and cell selection in the marrow and the blood, it is clear that genetic factors are also involved. Some of these may be *trans*-acting, including the nature of the β thalassemic mutation itself, polymorphisms related to the γ globin gene promoters, and others. However, recent studies suggest that there are at least two loci unlinked to the β globin gene cluster that may play a major role in setting the level of fetal hemoglobin production, now assigned to the X chromosome[16] and chromosome 6.[17] Family studies indicate that other loci which presumably encode for *cis*-acting regulatory molecules may also be involved.

These observations raise the issue of whether other important factors that can modify the phenotype of the β chain hemoglobinopathies remain to be discovered. Topics that still

TABLE 2. Modifiers of β Thalassemia Phenotype

β Globin Loci
    β thalassemia mutations
    Compound heterozygosity
    Dominant mutations
    Differential splicing of RNA products
α Globin Loci
    α thalassemias
γ Globin Loci
    Cis acting
    Trans acting
Other Genetic Polymorphisms
Non-Genetic Factors

warrant further research include genetic variability in the rate of proteolytic destruction of excess α chains and the possibility that variation in splicing mechanisms may play a role in setting the phenotype of β thalassemias due to splice site mutations. While further studies of these mechanisms may throw some light on the heterogeneity of the β thalassemias, it is likely that there may be other and completely unexplored factors involved. This is a subject that requires urgent investigation.

PRIORITIES FOR FUTURE RESEARCH IN THE THALASSEMIAS

If it is accepted that the thalassemias will present a major health problem to the emerging countries over the next few decades it is important that, as the richer countries pursue research into their control and management, they keep in mind the needs of the emerging countries and try to develop technologies which are cheaper and more adaptable to large, relatively poor rural populations.

Screening

If we are to be able to anticipate the burden that the thalassemias will pose for the provision of health care in the emerging countries it is essential that adequate population surveys are carried out to determine their frequency. Our priorities should be the β thalassemias and their interactions with β chain variants, particularly hemoglobin E and hemoglobin S β thalassemia. In every population in which these conditions are common their distribution is uneven and we must therefore carry out regional surveys combined with forward predictions about the likely increase in the size of the communities under study. Although simple and rapid electrophoretic and chromatographic techniques are available that will identify the important structural hemoglobin variants and β thalassemia they are all tedious to apply in large population studies. Even when applied scrupulously, single-tube osmotic fragility tests are relatively unreliable and do not identify the important structural hemoglobin variants. While research to develop cheaper and rapid screening methods should continue it is now clear that large population surveys are feasible using blood spotted onto filter paper and analyzed by HPLC.[18] While the basic equipment is expensive, one or two facilities of this type held in centers in the developing countries could enable major population surveys to be initiated at a relatively low cost.

Natural History and Phenotype/Genotype Relationship Studies

While the clinical burden and methods of management of the severe, transfusion-dependent forms of β thalassemia are well understood it is becoming clear that some of the intermediate forms of β thalassemia, particularly hemoglobin E thalassemia, will pose a major problem for the emerging countries over the next few years. As well as carrying out research directed at trying to understand the reasons for the wide phenotypic diversity of these conditions, as outlined earlier, it is vitally important that studies are initiated to analyze their natural history. From recent observations in the emerging countries it is clear that many patients with these disorders are being treated by rote, and are receiving unnecessary blood transfusions. It is vital, therefore, that some guidelines are established for the better management of these intermediate forms of β thalassemia. In particular, we need to understand the indications for transfusion, and more about the rates of iron loading and the complications of later life.

Counselling and Prenatal Diagnosis

Once having established the magnitude of the problem and having set up adequate screening programs, and knowing more about the intermediate forms of the disease, individual countries will have to decide whether they want to establish prenatal diagnosis programs. Overall, the technology is well developed[19] and the major problem will be to establish centers with the obstetric and technical expertise to carry out these programs. Currently, this approach offers the best hope of controlling the important forms of β thalassemia in those emerging countries in which it is acceptable on religious and other grounds.

Towards Better Forms of Treatment

Given the current limitations of bone marrow transplantation, and the slow speed of progress towards definitive gene therapy, we may be left with transfusion and iron chelation as the mainstays of treatment for the foreseeable future. And even if gene therapy does become a reality it is likely to be prohibitively expensive. Although current approaches to augmenting fetal hemoglobin production have proved disappointing in the case of transfusion-dependent β thalassemia, there are hints that some of the agents that have been investigated might, if used in combination, have the ability to raise the fetal hemoglobin by one or two grams in at least some patients with the intermediate forms of β thalassemia.[20,21] It is quite clear that many patients with hemoglobin E thalassemia would benefit enormously from this approach and therefore clinical trials should be established to find the optimal drug combinations. It is important to pursue this road because, although there are major efforts being made to identify more effective agents of this kind, there is no guarantee that they will be found. And, since there are hints that individual responses to agents that stimulate hemoglobin F production may be related to the molecular pathology of particular forms of thalassemia, or to other genetic factors,[21] it is important to determine if this is the case as a prelude to further trials of the therapeutic use of these agents.

Probing the Genetic Constitution of Thalassemic Populations

As mentioned earlier, it is now clear that many genetic polymorphisms other than those involving the red cell have come under selection pressures in thalassemic populations. It will be particularly important, therefore, to try to determine the patterns of infection that involve thalassemic children and to try to relate these to the increasingly broad range of polymorphic systems that are being unearthed in relationship to present or past malaria.

REFERENCES

1. AD HOC COMMITTEE ON HEALTH RESEARCH RELATING TO FUTURE INTEVENTION OPTIONS. 1996 World Health Organization, Geneva.
2. THE WORLD BANK. 1993 World Development Report. Investing in Health. Oxford University Press, Oxford.
3. WEATHERALL, D. J. & J. B. CLEGG. 1996. Thalassemia—A global public health problem. Nature Med. **2:** 847–849.
4. FAWDRY, A. L. 1944 Erythroblastic anaemia of childhood (Cooley's) anaemia in Cyprus. Lancet **i:** 171–176
5. WHO WORKING GROUP ON THE COMMUNITY CONTROL OF HEREDITARY ANAEMIAS. 1983. Bull. World Health Organ. **61:** 63–80
6. WASI, P., S. NA-NAKORN, S. POOTRAKUL, M. SOOKANEK et al. 1969. Alpha- and beta-thalassemia in Thailand. Ann. N.Y. Acad. Sci **165:** 60–82.
7. FLINT, J., R. M. HARDING, A. J. BOYCE & J. B. CLEGG. 1993. The population genetics of the haemoglobinopathies. Clin. Haematol. **6:** 215–262.
8. FLINT, J., A. V. S. HILL, D. K. BOWDEN, S. J. OPPENHEIMER et al. 1986. High frequencies of α thalassaemia are the result of natural selection by malaria. Nature **321:** 744–750.
9. ALLEN, S. J., A. O'DONNELL, N. D. E. ALEXANDER, M. P. ALPERS et al. 1997. α thalassemia protects children against disease due to malaria and other infections. Proc. Natl. Acad. Sci. USA **94:** 14736–14741.
10. WILLIAMS, T. N., K. MAITLAND, S. BENNETT, M. GANCZAKOWSKI et al. 1996. High incidence of malaria in a-thalassaemia children. Nature **383:** 522–525.
11. HILL, A. V. S. 1996. Genetics of infectious disease resistance. Curr. Opin. Genet. Dev. **6:** 348–353.
12. MCGUIRE, W., A. V. S. HILL, C. E. M. ALLSOPP, B. M. GREENWOOD et al. 1994. Variation in the TNF-alpha promoter region associated with susceptibility to cerebral malaria. Nature **371:** 508–511.
13. MILLER, L. H. 1994. Impact of malaria on genetic polymorphism and genetic diseases in Adricans and African Americans. Proc. Natl. Acad. Sci. USA. **91:** 2415–2419.
14. WEATHERALL, D. J. 1995. The molecular basis for phenotypic variability of the common thalassaemias. Mol. Med. Today **1:** 15–20.
15. WEATHERALL, D. J. 1994. Thalassemia. *In* The Molecular Basis of Blood Diseases, 2nd edit. S. STAMATOYANNOPOULOS, A. W. NIENHUIS, P. W. MAJERUS & H. VARMUS, Eds.: 157–206. W.B. Saunders Company, Philadelphia.
16. DOVER, G. J., K. D. SMITH, Y. C. CHANG, S. PURVIS et al. 1992 Fetal hemoglobin levels in sickle cell disease and normal individuals are partially controlled by an X-linked gene located at Xp22.2. Blood **80:** 816–824.
17. CRAIG, J. E., J. ROCHETTE, C. A. FISHER, D. J. WEATHERALL et al. 1996. Dissecting the loci controlling fetal haemoglobin production on chromosomes 11p and 6q by the regressive approach. Nature Genet. **12:** 58–64.
18. HUISMAN, T. H. J. 1993. The structure and function of normal and abnormal haemoglobins. Clin. Haematol. **6:** 1–30.
19. Cao, A. & Rosatelli, M. C. 1993. Screening and prenatal diagnosis of the haemoglobinmopathies. Semin. Hematol. **33:** 263–286.
20. OLIVIERI, N. F. 1995. Clinical experience with reactivation of fetal hemoglobin in the beta hemoglobinopathies. Semin. Hematol. **33:** 24–42.
21. OLIVIERI, N. F., D. C. REES, G. D. GINDER, S. L. THEIN et al. 1997. Treatment of thalassaemia major with phenylbutyrate and hydroxyurea. Lancet **350:** 491–492.

Developmental Control of ε- and γ- Globin Genes[a]

Q. LI,[b] K. R. PETERSON,[b,c] AND G. STAMATOYANNOPOULOS[b-d]

[b]*Division of Medical Genetics, Department of Medicine, and*
[c]*Department of Genetics, University of Washington, Seattle,
Washington 98195, USA*

ABSTRACT: In the last few years there have been considerable advances in the understanding of the molecular control of globin genes during development. Several insights have been obtained with studies using transgenic mice. The 5′ to 3′ order of the genes in the β locus, the proximity of the genes to the locus control region and the availability of transcriptional factors have been implicated in the developmental activation of globin genes. Globin genes are turned off by two general mechanisms, autonomous gene silencing involving sequences located in the proximal and distal promoters and competition between genes for interaction with the locus control region. The current understanding of the control of embryonic (ε) and fetal (γ) globin genes is reviewed.

The purpose of this review is to summarize the current understanding of the molecular control of human β-like globin gene switching. Globin gene switching provides a prototypical system for studying the control of gene activity in eukaryotes. An understanding of this phenomenon will be of potential importance for the development of molecular therapies for β-thalassemia and sickle cell disease. Below we summarize what is known about the control of ε- and γ-globin genes with emphasis on the studies done the last few years in our laboratories.

CONTROL OF THE ε-GLOBIN GENE

Very little is known about the activation of ε-globin gene expression in the embryonic stage of development. Presumably two factors play a dominant role, proximity to the LCR and embryonic stage-specific transcriptional factors. More is known about the mechanism whereby the ε-globin gene is turned off when the definitive stage of erythropoiesis starts in the fetal liver.

Early studies in transgenic mice used μLCR-ε or 5′HS2-ε constructs and demonstrated that all sequences required for ε gene silencing are located in a 3.7 kb *Eco*RI ε gene fragment containing about 2 kb of sequence upstream of the ε-globin gene cap site.[1,2] This upstream region contains a sequence located between positions -182 and -467 of the ε gene promoter, that has been shown to act as a silencer in transient expression assays.[3] Raich *et al.* have shown that deletion of this sequence results in continued ε gene expression in adult life, thus providing direct evidence that this sequence contains a silencer that acts *in vivo*.[4] Several studies[5–10] identified erythroid lineage-specific and constitutive transcription factors that bind within the -182 to -467 sequence (FIG. 1). A GATA-1 site is located around position -208. A YY1 site that overlaps two GATA-1 sites in opposite orientation is located around position -269. At position -379, there is a CACCC sequence, presumably

---

[a]Work reported here was supported by: NIH Grants DK 45365, HL 80899, HL 53750.
[d]Address correspondence to G. Stamatoyannopoulos at the Division of Medical Genetics.

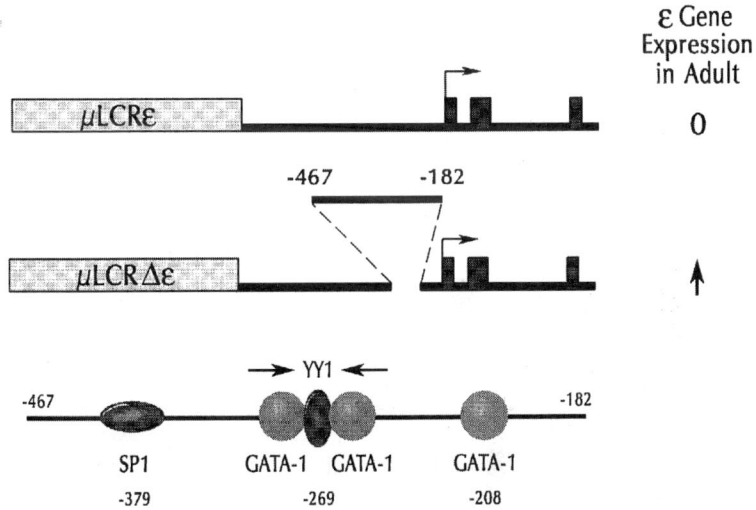

FIGURE 1. Summary of the evidence indicating that the developmental control of ε-globin gene is autonomous and all sequences required for ε-gene silencing are located in the ε gene promoter (see text).

the binding site of SP1 or another related CACCC binding protein. Raich et al.[9] mutated these sites to abolish binding of the respective transcription factors, individually or in combination. Mutation of GATA-1 at -208 resulted in continued ε gene expression in the adult, demonstrating that GATA-1 acts as repressor of ε gene expression when it binds that site. In contrast, when GATA-1 binds at position -165, it acts as an ε gene activator.[5] Disruption of YY1 binding at -269 results in continued ε gene expression in the adult, indicating that like GATA-1 at position -208, YY1 is an ε gene repressor.[9] ε-globin gene expression is reduced, but not abolished, in adult mice when the binding of SP1 (or another related protein) to the -379 CACCC motif is disrupted. These results suggest that multiple factors, both erythroid-specific and ubiquitous, participate in the formation of the the repressor complex that turns off the ε-globin gene in the liver stage of erythropoiesis. The two GATA-1 sites tandemly arranged around position -269 do not participate in ε gene silencing because disruption of GATA-1 binding at these sites is not associated with continued ε gene expression in the adult stage of development. Recently, Liu et al.[11] have suggested that the -179 to -304 region contains another element; deletion of this sequence results in reduction of both ε- and γ-globin gene expression. Confirmation of these results (based on the use of β-globin locus YAC transgenics) is highly warranted.

Recent studies using a binary transgenic mouse system confirmed that GATA-1 acts as an ε gene repressor.[12] A human GATA-1 (hGATA-1) construct was synthesized that restricts increased GATA-1 expression to erythroid lineages. In this construct, hGATA-1 was driven by the β-globin promoter linked to a μLCR sequence.[12] Human β-globin locus YAC transgenic mice were produced that expressed hGATA-1 in the embryonic, fetal and adult stages of development. In these mice, there was a striking decline in human ε-globin gene expression in the embryonic stage of development, while there was no effect on γ- or β-globin gene expression (FIG. 2) This data provide direct evidence that GATA-1 is a specific repressor of the human ε-globin gene. Significantly, there was no repression of the murine ε^y gene, which is the orthologue of the human ε gene. This finding can be explained

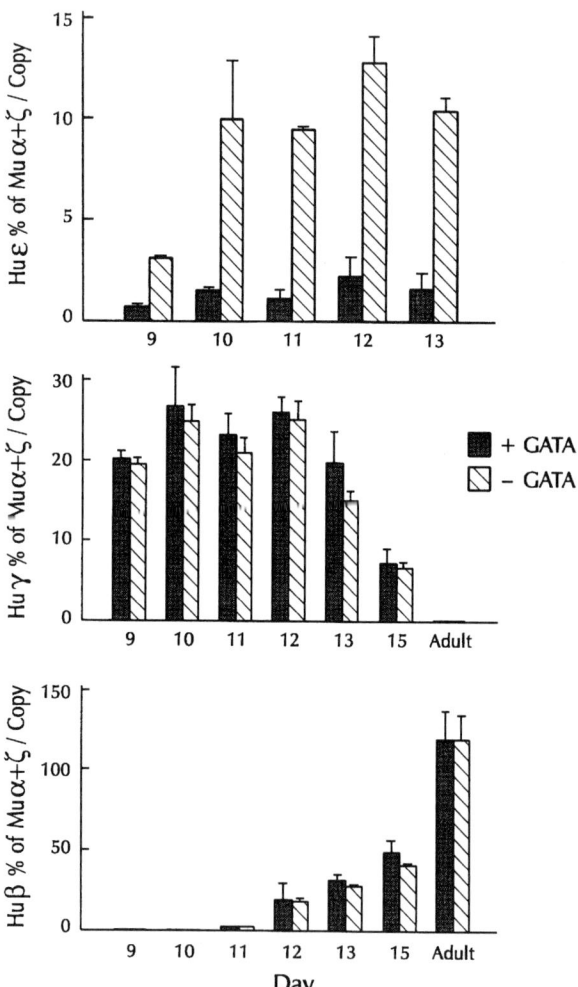

FIGURE 2. Human ε, γ, β gene expression in + or − hGATA-1 mice. GATA-1 overexpression suppresses human ε gene expression in β-YAC transgenic mice (see text and Li et al.[12]).

by the fact that the murine ε^y gene lacks the GATA-1 site at position -208, the position at which the repressor effect of GATA-1 is mediated.[12]

Additional negative and positive elements have been detected in the upstream ε gene promoter using transient expression assays.[13] The relevance of these elements to the *in vivo* control of ε gene expression should be confirmed with studies in transgenic mice. More recently, we have focused on the proximal ε gene promoter by producing transgenic mice in which the uLCR was linked to an ε gene with a minimal promoter extending to position -179. In these mice, ε gene expression in embryonic cells was as high as in control mice carrying a μLCR ε transgene with a 1.9 kb promoter, indicating that all the sequences required for ε gene activation are located in the proximal ε gene promoter. ε gene expression in the μLCR -179 ε mice declines during development indicating that the minimal ε gene promoter contains sequences required for ε gene silencing (Li et al., in press).

CONTROL OF γ-GLOBIN GENE EXPRESSION

It has been postulated that γ-globin gene expression is activated in the fetal stage of development by the action of fetal stage-specific transcription factors. Evidence to support this hypothesis is found in experiments where the fetal globin genes have been transactivated following fusion with cells expressing a fetal or an embryonic globin program.[14,15] Direct evidence for the existence of γ-globin gene-specific transcription factors is, however, still lacking.

The involvement of the proximal γ-globin gene promoter in γ gene silencing or activation has been shown by the existence of naturally occurring mutations that cause non-deletional hereditary persistence of fetal hemoglobin (HPFH). Studies in transgenic mice have also disclosed certain positive and negative regulatory elements located in the γ gene promoter.[16]

To investigate the role of *cis*-acting elements in the γ gene promoter, we produced several γ gene promoter truncations and studied their effects in transgenic mice. Three elements have been identified through these studies; a negative element located distal to position -141, a positive element located between positions -141 and -201, and a negative element located between positions -378 and -730. This last element behaves like a position-dependent γ gene silencer.[16]

Studies in transgenic mice have also clarified the contribution of sequences placed 3′ to the γ-globin genes on the control of γ-globin gene expression. The differences in the phenotypes of deletion HPFH and deletion δβ thalassemia syndromes have been known for about 30 years. In HPFH there is high γ-globin expression which is pancellularly distributed in the red blood cells, while in δβ thalassemia there is significantly less γ gene expression and the fetal hemoglobin is heterocellularly distributed in the red cells. The difference between the two phenotypes has been attributed to a regulatory element between the γ and δ genes. It has been suggested that the deletion of this element results in the phenotype of HPFH; while its retention results in the phenotype of the δβ thalassemia.[17] Transgenic mice carrying β-globin locus YACS with 3′ deletions of varying length have been produced.[18] Although these deletions mimicked the 5′ breakpoints of HPFH and δβ thalassemia mutants none caused continued γ expression in the adult mice raising doubts about the existence of the postulated regulatory sequence between the γ and δ genes.[18] More recently, Arcasoy et al. demonstrated that transgenic mice in which sequences placed downstream of the 3′ breakpoint of HPFH-1 were juxtaposed to the ^Aγ-globin gene have high γ-globin gene expression in the adult stage[19] providing evidence that "imported enhancers"[20,21] underlie the high γ-globin gene expression in HPFH.

THE ROLE OF LCR SEQUENCES IN γ AND ε GENE SILENCING

In addition to the globin gene promoters, LCR sequences appear to play a role in globin gene regulation during development. Evidence for the contribution of the LCR was first provided by Fraser et al.[22] by linking each individual 5′HS of the LCR with a construct containing the ε, γ, and β genes. Their experiments provided evidence that 5′HS3 and 5′HS4 are involved in the developmental control of γ- and β-globin gene expression. A detailed analysis of the development regulation of the γ- and β-globin genes under the control of 5′HS2 or 5′HS3 demonstrated that 5′HS3 and 5′HS2 confer different developmental profiles on γ and β gene expression.[23]

The role of LCR sequences in ε gene regulation is supported by the effect of a deletion of 5'HS3 in the context of the β-locus YAC. Peterson et al.[24] have shown that a 2.3 kb 5'HS3 deletion results in a decline in expression of the ε-globin gene. Recently, we have produced transgenic mice carrying a 300 bp deletion of the 5'HS3 core (Navas et al., in press). In contrast to a previous report in which a similar deletion has catastrophic effects on the expression of all globin genes,[25] a very specific phenotype was produced by the 5'HS3 core deletion: ε-globin expression was essentially absent in the yolk sac cells and, in contrast, there was a significant increase in γ-globin mRNA in these embryonic erythroblasts. Surprisingly, γ-globin gene expression was totally absent at the onset of the fetal liver stage of erythropoiesis. These data suggest that the 5'HS3 core is necessary for the interaction of the LCR with the ε gene promoter in embryonic cells and the γ gene promoter during the fetal stage of erythropoiesis.

Involvement of LCR sequences in the developmental control of the γ-globin gene has also been implicated from studies of the control of γ-globin gene expression in transgenic mice. Enver et al. used a 3.3 kb HindIII γ-globin gene fragment linked to 2.5 kb μLCR to study the control of γ-globin expression and found continued γ-globin expression in the adult stage of development.[26] Thus, this γ gene escapes developmental control. On the other hand, Dillon and Grosveld reported that mice carrying a 5.7 kb γ-globin gene fragment linked to a 20 kb LCR displayed normal developmental control; i.e., they lack γ gene expression in the adult stage.[27] The difference in expression between the 2.5 μLCR-3.3 kb γ and the 20 kb LCR-5.9 kb γ mice could be attributed either to the extra sequences 3' of the γ-globin gene or the extra LCR sequences contained in the 20 kb LCR. It was recently found[28] that transgenic mice carrying a 2.5 kb μLCR linked to a 5.9 kb γ-globin gene continue to express high levels of γ-globin in the adult stage development (FIG. 3), suggesting that the sequences 3' to the ^{A}γ globin gene are not responsible for the phenotypes of the transgenic mice reported in the studies of Enver et al.[26] and Dillon and Grosveld[27] These data suggest that sequences located within the LCR complex are involved in γ gene silencing.[28]

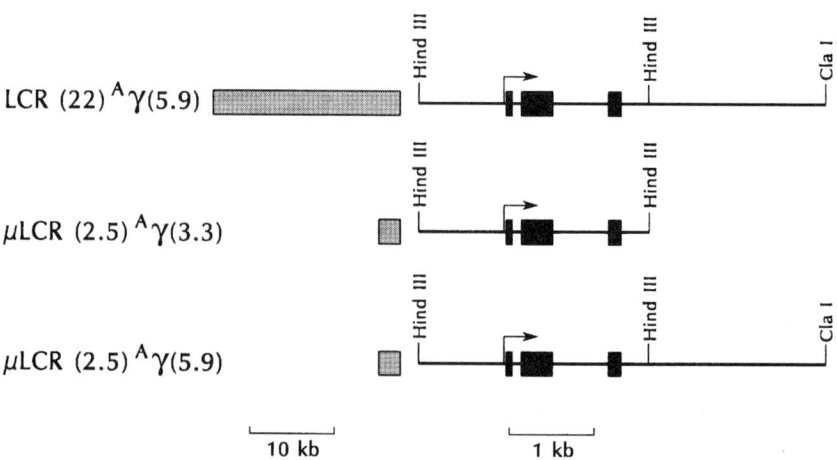

FIGURE 3. Evidence that LCR sequences play a role in γ gene downregulation (see text and Stamatoyannopoulos et al.[28]).

THE ROLE OF COMPETITION

Competition between globin genes for interaction with the LCR has been suggested to be a major mechanism of globin gene switching.[29,30] It is unlikely that competition plays a role in ε gene silencing since repression of the ε-globin gene expression appears to be autonomous.[1,2] Competition could be the reason that differences exist in ε and γ gene expression levels in human versus murine embryonic cells. The murine yolk sac environment favors the expression of the human γ-globin genes and typically in the yolk sac of the β-YAC transgenic mice there is about twofold higher γ than ε gene expression. In humans, the opposite situation exists; ε gene expression is about 10-fold higher than γ gene expression in the red cells of the human embryos. These differences in expression pattern clearly distinguish between the effects of proximity to the LCR and the effects of environment on ε gene expression. The distance of the ε gene from the LCR is the same in the β-locus YAC mice and in the human embryo. The difference in the level of expression of the ε- and γ-globin genes must be attributed to the differences in the transcriptional environment of the embryonic erythroblasts between the two species. In murine yolk sac cells, the environment favors the interaction of the γ gene with the LCR and ε gene expression is decreased. In human yolk sac erythroblasts, ε gene interaction with the LCR is favored.

When the liver stage of erythropoiesis starts in the mouse, there is exclusive murine β major and β minor globin gene expression and total absence of murine embryonic $ε^y$ and βh1 expression. In contrast to the mouse, there is almost exclusive γ-globin expression early in human fetal liver erythropoiesis. In β-locus YAC transgenic mice, γ-globin expression occurs mostly in the yolk sac and to only a small degree in fetal liver cells. The already low level of γ-globin expression further declines during fetal development and is totally silenced after birth. This pattern of human γ-globin expression in the murine fetus can be attributed either to the very limited presence, early in the liver stage of erythropoiesis, of a transcriptional environment that activates γ-globin gene, or to the appearance of an environment that represses the γ-globin gene later, as the liver stage of erythropoiesis progresses. Only limited information can be obtained regarding the competitive control of human γ and β gene switching by measuring human γ-globin and β-globin expression during the liver stage of erythropoiesis of the β-locus YAC fetuses. The main evidence for competition between the γ and β genes comes from the experiments of Enver et al.[27] and Behringer et al.[28] comparing γ and β gene expression when the γ and β genes were individually or tandemly linked to the LCR. These studies have shown that the γ and β genes lose their developmental regulation when they are linked individually to the LCR, while they undergo normal developmental control when they are in their normal tandem arrangement. Such results can be best interpreted by a competition mechanism of γ and β gene switching.

REFERENCES

1. RAICH, N. *et al.* 1990. Autonomous development control of human embryonic globin gene switching in transgenic mice. Science **250:** 1147–1149.
2. SHIH, D. M., R. J. WALL & G. SHAPIRO. 1990. Developmentally regulated and erythroid-specific expression of the human embryonic β-globin gene in transgenic mice. Nucleic Acids Res. **18:** 5465–5472.
3. XIAN CAO, S. *et al.* 1989. Identification of a transcriptional silencer in the 5′-flanking region of the human ε-globin gene. Proc. Natl. Acad. Sci USA **86:** 5306–5309.
4. RAICH, N. *et al.* 1992. Demonstration of a human ε-globin gene silencer with studies in transgenic mice. Blood **79:** 861–864.
5. GONG, Q., J. STERN & A. DEAN. 1991. Transcriptional role of a conserved GATA-1 site in the human ε-globin gene promoter. Mol. Cell. Biol. **2:** 2558–2566.
6. YU, C. Y. *et al.* 1991. The CACC box upstream of human embryonic epsilon globin gene binds Sp1 and is a functional promoter element in vitro and in vivo. J. Biol. Chem. **266:** 8907–8915.

7. GUMUCIO, D. L. *et al.* 1992. Phylogenetic footprinting reveals a nuclear protein which binds to silencer sequences in the human γ and ε globin genes. Mol. Cell. Biol. **12:** 4919–4929.
8. GUMUCIO, D. L. *et al.* 1993. Phylogenetic footprinting reveals unexpected complexity in transfactor binding upstream from the ε-globin gene. Proc. Natl. Acad. Sci. USA **90:** 6018–6022.
9. RAICH, N. *et al.* 1995. GATA-1 and YY1 are developmental repressors of the human ε-globin gene. EMBO J. **14:** 801–809.
10. PETERS, B. *et al.* 1993. Protein-DNA interactions in the ε-globin gene silencer. J. Biol. Chem. **268:** 3430–3437.
11. LIU, Q., J. BUNGERT & J. D. ENGEL. 1997. Mutation of gene-proximal regulatory elements disrupts human ε-, γ-, and β-globin expression in yeast artificial chromosome transgenic mice. Proc. Natl. Acad. Sci. USA **94:** 169–174.
12. LI, Q. *et al.* 1997. Binary transgenic mouse model for studying the trans control of globin gene switching: Evidence that GATA-1 is an *in vivo* repressor of human ε gene expression. Proc. Natl. Acad. Sci. USA **94:** 2444–2448.
13. TREPICCHIO, W. L., M. A. DYER & M. H. BARON. 1993. Developmental regulation of the human embryogenic β-like globin gene is mediated by synergistic interactions among multiple tissue- and stage-specific elements. Mol. Cell. Biol. **13:** 7457–7468.
14. BARON, M. H. & T. MANIATIS. 1986. Rapid reprogramming of globin gene expression in transient heterokaryons. Cell **46:** 591–602.
15. ZITNIK, G., P. HINES, G. STAMATOYANNOPOULOS & T. PAPAYANNOPOULOU. 1991. Murine erythroleukemia cell line GM979 contains factors that can activate silent chromosomal human γ-globin genes. Proc. Natl. Acad. Sci. USA **88:** 2530–2534.
16. STAMATOYANNOPOULOS, G. *et al.* 1993. Developmental regulation of human γ-globin genes in transgenic mice. Mol. Cell. Biol. **13:** 7636–7644.
17. HUISMAN, T., W. SCHROEDER, G. EFREMOV, H. DUMA, B. MLADENOVSKI, C. HYMAN, E. RACHMILEWITZ, N. VOUVER, A. MILLER, A. BRODIE, J. R. SHELTON, J. B. SHELTON & G. APPEL. 1974. The present status of the heterogeneity of fetal hemoglobin in beta-thalassemia: An attempt to unify some observations in thalassemia and related conditions. Ann. N. Y. Acad. Sci. **232:** 107–124.
18. PETERSON, K. R. *et al.* 1995. Use of yeast artificial chromosomes (YACs) in studies of mammalian development: production of β-globin locus YAC mice carrying human globin developmental mutants. Proc. Natl. Acad. Sci. USA **92:** 5655-5659.
19. ARKASOY, M. O. *et al.* 1997. High levels of human γ-globin gene expression in adult mice carrying a transgene of deletion-type hereditary persistence of fetal hemoglobin. Mol. Cell. Biol. **17:** 2076–2089.
20. FEINGOLD, E. A. & B. G. FORGET. 1989. The breakpoint of a large deletion causing hereditary persistence of fetal hemoglobin occurs within an erythroid DNA domain remote from the β-globin gene cluster. Blood **74:** 2178–2186.
21. ANAGNOU, N. P., C. PEREZ-STABLE, R. GELINAS, F. CONSTANTINI, K. LIAPAKI, M. CONSTANTOPOULOU, T. KOSTEAS, N. K. MOSCHONAS & G. STAMATOYANNOPOULOS. 1995. Sequences located 3' to the breakpoint of the hereditary persistence of fetal hemoglobin (HPFH) -3 deletion exhibit enhancer activity and can modify the developmental expression of the human fetal ^Aγ-globin gene in transgenic mice. J. Biol. Chem. **270:** 1–8.
22. FRASER, P., S. PRUZINA, M. ANTONIOU & F. GROSVELD. 1993. Each hypersensitive site of the human β-globin locus control region confers a different developmental pattern of expression on the globin genes. Genes & Dev. **7:** 106–113.
23. LI, Q. & J. A. STAMATOYANNOPOULOS. 1994. Position independence and proper developmental control of γ-globin gene expression require both a 5' locus control region and a downstream sequence element. Mol. Cell. Biol. **14:** 6087–6096.
24. PETERSON, K. R. *et al.* 1996. Effect of deletion of 5'HS3 or 5'HS2 of the human β-globin locus control region on the developmental regulation of globin gene expression in β-globin locus yeast artificial chromosome transgenic mice. Proc. Natl. Acad. Sci. USA **93:** 6605–6609.
25. BUNGERT, J. *et al.* 1995. Synergistic regulation of human β-globin gene switching by locus control region elements HS3 and HS4. Genes & Dev. **9:** 3083–3096.
26. ENVER, T. *et al.* 1989. The human β-globin locus activation region alters the developmental fate of a human fetal globin gene in transgenic mice. Proc. Natl. Acad. Sci. USA **86:** 7033–7037.

27. DILLON, N. & F. GROSVELD. 1991. Human γ-globin genes silenced independently of other genes in the β-globin locus. Nature **350:** 252–254.
28. STAMATOYANNOPOULOS, J. A., C. H. CLEGG & Q. LI. 1997. Sheltering of γ-globin expression from position effects requires both an upstream locus control region and a regulatory element 3′ to the ^{A}γ globin gene. Mol. Cell. Biol. **17:** 240–247.
29. ENVER, T. *et al.* 1990. Developmental regulation of human fetal-to-adult globin gene switching in transgenic mice. Nature **344:** 309–313.
30. BEHRINGER, R. R. *et al.* 1990. Human γ- to β-globin gene switching in transgenic mice. Genes & Dev. **4:** 380–389.

The Dynamics of Globin Gene Expression and Gene Therapy Vectors

FRANK GROSVELD,[a,c] ERNIE DE BOER,[a] NIALL DILLON,[b] JOOST GRIBNAU,[a] ERIC MILOT,[a] TOLLEIV TRIMBORN,[a] MARK WIJGERDE,[a] AND PETER FRASER[a]

[a]*MGC-Department of Cell Biology and Genetics, Erasmus University, P.O. Box 1738, 3000 DR, Rotterdam, the Netherlands*

[b]*Gene Regulation and Chromatin Group, MRC Clinical Sciences Center, Hammersmith Hospital, DuCane Road, London W12 0NN, United Kingdom*

ABSTRACT: The most important level of regulation of the β-globin genes is by activation of all of the genes by the Locus Control Region (LCR) and repression of the early genes by an as yet unknown factor acting on sequences flanking the genes. Superimposed on this is a mechanism in which the early genes (ε and γ) suppress the late genes (δ and β) by competition for the interaction with the LCR. Although this extra level of gene regulation is quantitatively of less importance than the direct repression mechanism, it has important implications and has provided an excellent assay system to probe the regulation of transcription at the single cell level.

These studies indicate that the LCR interacts with individual globin genes and that LCR/gene interactions are dynamic with complexes forming and dissociating continually. The levels of expression of each of the genes appear to depend on: 1) the frequency of interaction which is itself dependednt on the distance of the gene to the LCR, 2) the affinity of the LCR for the gene and 3) the stability of the LCR/gene complex. The latter two are dependent on the balance of transcription factors. We conclude that transcription only appears to take place while the LCR and gene interact and that the level of transcription is determined by the frequency and duration of such interaction rather than by changes in the rate of transcription of promoters.

The β globin locus consists of five developmentally regulated genes that are activated at different stages of erythroid development (FIG. 1). The genes are arranged in the order in which they are activated during development with ε expressed first in the embryonic yolk sac. Between six and ten weeks gestation, there is a gradual switch to expression of the γ genes which predominate during the fetal liver stage. In the later fetal liver and neonatal stages, there is a further transition to expression of the β gene and the γ genes are almost completely silenced during adult life. Defects in the locus are responsible for the various forms of β thalassaemia and sickle cell anaemia (for review see Weatherall, 1993[1]).

The locus has been characterized in detail over a number of years, and this results in the identification of the principal functional elements involved in its regulation. The entire locus is activated by the locus control region (LCR) contained within a 15 kb region located 5′ of the ε gene[2] and the presence of this region is an absolute requirement for the

[c]Corresponding author: Tel: +31 10 4087593; Fax: +31 10 4360225.

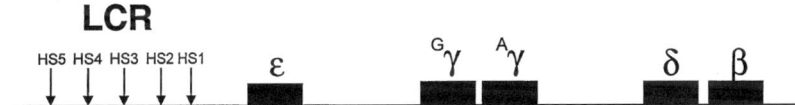

FIGURE 1. Structure of the human β-globin locus. The LCR is indicated by five arrows representing the individual hypersensitive sites.

expression of all of the genes in the locus. Many groups have studied the protein factors that bind to the individual hypersensitive regions of the LCR and tested their use in functional expression experiments. However this paper will focus on basic mechanisms involved in long range interactions in chromatin *in vivo*.

A number of effects on gene expression are known to be the result of long range action by regions of DNA on one or more target sequences. Such effects include transcriptional activation by distal control elements, heterochromatinization of translocated genes to give position effect variegation, and phenomena such as silencing and insulation. The phenomenon of transcriptional regulation by sequences that are located at long distances from the promoter has been known for many years, but it is still not clear how such regulation takes place. Two models have been proposed for the activation of gene transcription after chromatin activation of a locus. In one model the sole function of distal elements is to generate a favorable chromatin structure which allows the promoter to bind transcription factors in a stochastic fashion.[3–5] In contrast with this are the looping models which propose that distally located sequences are brought into direct contact with promoters.[6–8]

The basic property that we have exploited to test these models comes from genetic studies that showed that the expression of one gene in the locus can reduce that of the others.[9] This competitive effect has been studied extensively in transgenic mice,[10–12] and there is clear evidence that it operates in a polar manner with the genes located proximally to the LCR having a stronger suppressive effect on the more distally located genes.[11] The simplest explanation for the observed downregulation would be that activation is achieved through direct interaction between the genes and the LCR and that only one gene can interact with the LCR at any one time. In contrast the binary model[4] excludes direct interaction and proposes transcriptional interference by downstream topological changes or compartmentalization to explain the downregulation of distal genes.[5]

Thus we describe the use of competition between globin genes to probe the mechanism of gene activation and we conclude that regulation takes place via a direct interaction between the LCR and the genes and that such interactions can only take place with one gene at any time. The implication of these studies is manyfold. The presence of other genes near a newly integrated globin locus or expression cassette can negatively influence the expression of the globin genes. Such neighboring genes could be influenced by the presence of the LCR and become activated or be enhanced in their expression in red blood cells. Likewise the presence of neighboring regulatory regions could lead to the expression of globin genes in cells other than red cells and lead to the reduction of expression of neighbouring genes in non red cells. Finally, disturbance of this LCR/gene complex by small deletions of hypersensitive regions from the LCR leads to two different types of position effects when the globin locus is integrated in a heterochromatic region of the genome. The majority of these effects have been described for many different situations and genes. However we will not attempt to summarize all these studies, but merely provide a basic explanation based on our studies with the globin system.

SINGLE GENE TRANSCRIPTION

The study of the dynamics of globin gene competition were based on the ability to introduce a single β globin gene locus in transgenic mice[13] and analysis of the primary transcripts on a single cell basis at the time that the locus switches from the γ to the β gene in a competitive manner. In order to detect short-lived events at the site of transcription in the nucleus, we used fluorescence *in situ* hybridization (FISH) to the introns of the globin genes. These are known to have a half life of three minutes *in vivo*.[14] Most of the transcription signals in fetal liver cells that are homozygous for the transgenic locus are in fact single gene transcription signals (γ red or β green) with a minority of double gene signals (red plus green gives yellow). Moreover the proportion of switching cells (red and green signals in the same cell) is constant while the balance of transcription is changing on day 11.5 to day 12.5 from γ to β. Thus the switch is not occurring in a progressive manner from γ only signals to double signals to β signals only. Instead the double gene signals (yellow) result from the decay of the primary transcript signal from one gene (7 minutes, Gribnau *et al.*, submitted) and the ongoing transcription signal from the other gene.[14] Thus we suggest that the transcription of the genes is a dynamic process with the LCR interacting with only one of the genes to give transcriptionally competent complex at any given moment. When such a complex dissociates transcription initiation stops until the LCR forms a new complex with the same gene or one of the other genes. This was confirmed by the presence of many cells present in transgenic mice that are heterozygous for the human locus, that have the β globin mRNA (the late gene product) in the cytoplasm, but which are synthezising only γ globin (the early gene) product at the time of analysis.[14] Hence the LCR appears to switch back and forth between the genes (flip-flop), resulting in single gene transcription but producing both mRNA's in the same cell.

This mechanism can be probed differently by the inhibition and release of transcriptional elongation through the use of DRB (Gribnau *et al.*, submitted). When fetal liver cells that are heterozygous for the human β globin locus are incubated with DRB and examined by FISH for primary transcription signals from the first or second intron, they show the normal presence of γ- and β-globin first intron signals but an absence of second intron signals. This result indicates that trancription initiation still takes place, but that elongation is abrogated after few hundred nucleotides.[15] When the DRB is subsequently washed out, a different result would be expected for a mechanism that operates via a single gene transcription mechanism than for one that can transcribe two genes at the same time. In the first case the appearance of double gene signals (transcription of one gene and decay of the primary transcript of the other gene after a flip-flop) should lag behind the appearance of single gene signals (γ or β). In the case of co-transcription the double gene signal should appear at the same rate as the single gene signals. Counting of the signals after the release of the DRB block shows that the single (second intron) signals are re-established before the double gene signals, favoring a mechanism of single gene transcription (FIG. 2). Thus the results strongly argue against the model of stochastic access of transcription factors after activation of the locus. It also argues against the type of mechanisms that propose that distal regulatory sequences act as entry sites for polymerase complexes which would scan the locus in search of a promoter, the so-called "scanning model" (for example, Picard, 1985[16]). Such a mechanism would not result in alternate gene transcription without postulating additional parameters and constraints.

THE KINETICS OF FLIP-FLOP TRANSCRIPTION: FREQUENCY OF INTERACTION

The single gene transcription model with the LCR alternately associating and dissociating with the genes predicts that the level of gene transcription is determined by the product of the frequency of complex formation and the lifetime of the complex.[17] The frequency of interaction via looping would be dependent on the relative distance of the genes from the promoter, while the stability and lifetime of the complex would depend on the balance of transcription factors in the nucleus. Together these parameters would determine the competitive ability of each of the genes in the locus. However, it is not possible to examine frequency and duration as independent variables in the experiments described above, because γ and β are different genes whose levels of expression change during the process of switching from γ to β. These factors introduce unknown variables into the analysis which limit the precision with which the kinetics of transcriptional competition can be measured.[14] In order to eliminate these variables we generated mutant loci that contain a second functionally equivalent β gene at two different positions in the locus to allow the study of only the frequency of interaction.[18] Two modified loci were constructed, each containing a second β-globin gene (βm) which was marked so that its transcript could be distinguished from that of the wild-type gene. In mutant locus 1 (ML1), the βm replaced the ε gene while in mutant locus 2 (ML2) it was inserted close to the cap site of the δ gene (FIG. 3A). Marking of the gene was achieved by replacing part of exon 1 and 2 and all of intron 1 with the equivalent sequences from the Aγ gene, which are not known to have any regulatory sequences.[19–21]

Since a multi-copy tandem array would place an LCR close to the 3' end of the wild-type β-globin gene it was necessary to analyze animals that carried only a single copy of the modified loci.

mRNA analysis showed that the steady state RNA levels of the two β globin genes are dependent on their relative distance from the LCR. Additional measurement of primary transcripts showed that the number of transcriptional periods of each gene correlate with the levels of steady state RNA (FIG. 3B). This provides independent evidence for direct interaction between the LCR and individual promoters and excludes transcriptional interference as a mechanism for the polarity of gene activation and silencing observed in the locus.[5] If the latter were the case it would not be expected that an increase in distance between the β-globin genes (from ML2 to ML1) would result in a more severe repression of the distal gene. If anything the opposite (or no effect of distance) would be expected.

Hence we conclude that the LCR appears to interact with the genes via looping and that the frequency of the interaction is dependent on the relative distance of a gene to the LCR. Interestingly it can also be calculated from the RNA *in situ* analysis that the lifetime of a β-globin transcription period is approximately 8 minutes.[18] Analysis of the transcription of these genes in the embryonic period of development show that the β-globin gene is normally kept silent at the early stages through competition with the ε- and γ-globin genes. These results have obvious implications for gene therapy vectors. If multiple genes driven by a single regulator were to be introduced, this would lead to competitive expression of the genes with an advantage for the proximal genes determined by the distances between the genes and the regulator. Such proximal advantages may be amplified by transcriptional interference if the genes are very close to each other.

THE KINETICS OF FLIP-FLOP TRANSCRIPTION: STABILITY OF INTERACTION

The second parameter in addition to distance in the transcriptional mechanism described above is the stability of the interaction, which is presumably dependent on the balance of transcription factors in the nucleus. If this were the case than the alteration of the level of a critical transcription factor should influence the kinetics of flip-flop transcription. To test this hypothesis we changed the level of the transcription factor EKLF, which specifically binds to the β-globin, but not the γ-globin CAC box in the proximal part of the promoters of the respective genes.[22] Reducing the level of EKLF was achieved

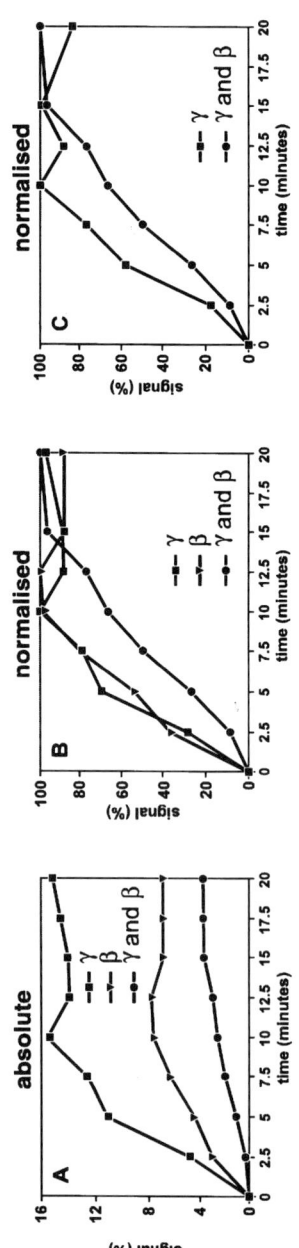

FIGURE 2. Kinetics of reappearance of single versus double primary transcription signals. **Panel A**: γ- and β primary transcript signals were scored after release of the DRB block to transcription elongation in 11.5 day fetal liver cells plotted versus time. *Squares*, γ single signals; *Triangles*, β single signals; *Circles*, γ and β double signals. **Panel B**: The curves in panel A were normalized to their maximum values. The results show the early appearance of foci having single γ- or β- globin signals and a clear lag in reappearance of double (γ and β) signals. **Panel C**: *Circles*, reappearance of double signals in *cis* (as in panel B), *Squares*, reappearance of double γ signals in *trans* (*i.e.* both alleles expressing in the same cell). The latter curve approximates the single signal curves in panel B and shows a random appearance.

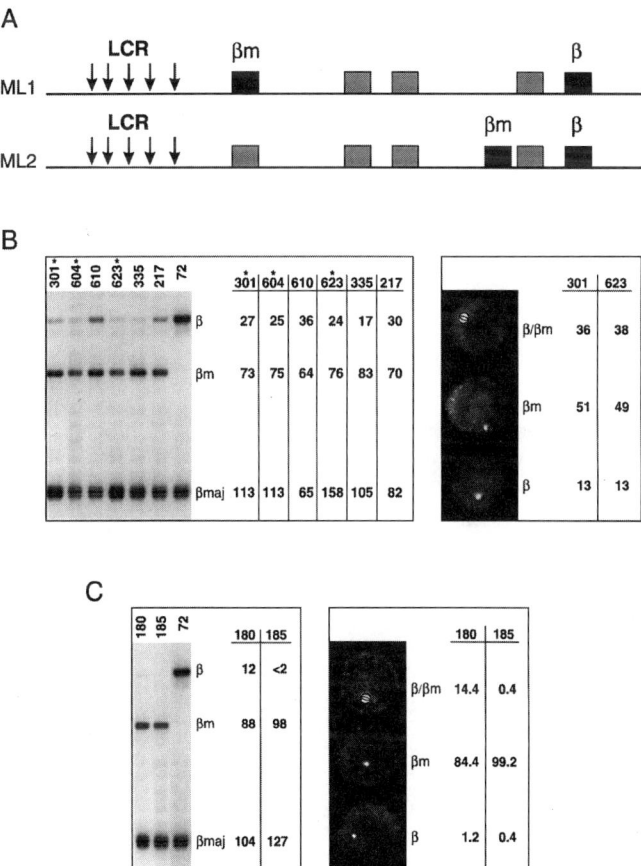

FIGURE 3. A: The ML1 and ML2 construct with the βm and β genes. **B**: *Left bottom panel.* S1 analysis of adult blood RNA from lines transgenic for ML2 and the wild-type β-globin locus.[13] The protected fragments are indicated on the right. The bands were quantitated by phosphorimage analysis. The numbers were normalized to 100% total human β and are shown on the right. *Top row*: β/β+βm; *middle row*: βm/β+βm; *bottom row*: βmaj/β+βm. An asterisk indicates the single copy lines. *Right hand panel. In situ* hybridization of two of the ML2 lines with the percentages of cells showing βm/β double, βm single and β single signals. **C**: Wild-type and mutant loci span a distance of 70 kb. In the ML1 locus the β- and βm-genes are 50 kb and 6.8 kb respectively from the 3′ end (HS1) of the LCR (56.7 and 13.6 from the middle of the LCR), while the equivalent distance for the Gγ gene is 28 kb. In ML2 the distances of the β and βm genes from the 3′ end of the LCR are 53.7 kb and 42.8 kb respectively (60.5 kb and 49.4 kb from the middle of the LCR).

through homologous recombination in embryonic stem cells and the generation of heterozygous or homozygous EKLF null mice.[22] As expected homozygous null mice die early after the onset of fetal erythropoiesis through the lack of β-globin synthesis.[23,24] When the EKLF null mice also carry a transgenic human β-globin locus their lifetime is slightly extended through the synthesis of γ globin, which is independent of EKLF.[17,25] More interesting are the heterozygous mice which contain half the normal amount of EKLF. When the γ- versus β-globin synthesis in these mice is measured during the switching process in the fetal liver, it shows that the balance of the competition between these genes is changed in favor of the γ-globin genes,[17] although the γ-globin genes are still suppressed at the normal time of development. These altered levels of transcription are completely accounted for by the number of primary transcription signals of the two genes when examined by RNA FISH analysis. Conversely, when EKLF is overexpressed, the balance of transcription is changed in favor of the β-globin gene (Philipsen, submitted). Hence we conclude that the stability of the LCR/β gene complex has been affected by the change in levels of EKLF, which strongly suggests that the changes in the levels of gene transcription are due to an alteration in the lifetime of the complex rather than a change in the rate of initiation during any given transcription period.

POSITION EFFECTS

In general distal genes in single copy integrations show some sensitivity to the position of integration in the mouse genome,[13] in particular when the LCR interacts predominantly with a proximal gene. In that situation the distal gene is not engaged by the LCR for most of the time and would therefore be available for an interaction with neighboring mouse sequences and this is for example visible when the two ML1 transgenic lines are compared to each other and the other transgenic lines from which we conclude that the distal β gene in ML1 line 185 is influenced by a negative position effect.[23] This could be the result from an integration event of the ML1 locus close to a negative regulatory sequence at the distal end of the locus. Owing to proximity this would only have a measurable effect on the distal b gene in ML1. A similar result would be obtained, if an endogenous gene were present near the distal end of the locus at the site of integration. Such a gene would in effect become part of the globin locus and take part in the competitive equilibrium in the locus. Owing to proximity to the distal gene and its long distance from the LCR this negative effect due to competition would readily be a measurable on the expression of the distal gene, which is closest and already expressed at low levels.

The implication of this result is that it would be advantageous to place the gene close to the regulatory regions in a gene therapy vectors to minimize the chance of such a position effect, unless some form of insulator sequence could be added to the vector.[26-28]

More dramatic position effects are observed when the transgenic locus is integrated in a heterochromatic region of the mouse genome. However this only occurs when individual hypersensitive sites are deleted from the globin locus.[29] Similar effects were observed with the CD2 gene.[30] In the case of the β-globin locus two types of position effects were observed. The first (also observed by Festenstein *et al.*[30] for CD2) is position effect variegation (PEV) and results in a subpopulation of erythroid cells which express the human globin genes. As a consequence both the level of mRNA and DNase sensitivity have been severely decreased in the total population of cells. Analysis of globin precursor RNA however that the transgene in the expressing subpopulation of cells is continuously transcribed at a level that is comparable to that observed in lines which have the same deletion, but where the locus has been integrated in a euchromatic region of the genome. It is thought that the decision to become active versus inactive is determined stochastically at the locus rather cellular level, since expressing subpopulation size is maintained through successive generations and homozygous PEV transgenics[29] show an increase in the expressing subpopulation size (for example, Elliot *et al.*, 1995).

The second type of position effect exhibits low levels of transgene expression in all erythroid cells as evidenced by the S1 and mRNA *in situ* analysis.[29] However, this low level of expression appears not to be caused by a decrease in the transcription rate of the individual genes and DNase hypersensitivity is maintained. Precursor RNA analysis reveals that only a fraction of the erythroid cells are transcribing the transgene at any moment, suggesting that low expression in these lines is caused by a decrease in the amount of time that the transgene is transcriptionally active in a particular cell. Thus the transgenes in these erythroid cells are switching on and off, while the full LCR single copy transgenics appear constitutively active. The on and off transcription is also seen to a lesser extent in non-heterochromatic LCR deletion transgenes. Transcription *in situ* analysis of these lines shows that the percentage of erythroid cells which are transcriptionally positive for human b-globin is lower than the single copy full LCR lines. This suggests that the LCR in the deletion lines spends a considerable amount of time uncoupled from the genes.[14] The length of time that the LCR remains uncoupled appears to be exaggerated in the pericentromeric lines which suggests that heterochromatin formation is somehow interfering with LCR activation leading to a severe reduction in expression. Clearly this process is very different from PEV and has not been described previously. Preliminary analysis indicates that the β globin in one of these lines is expressed in a period during the replication phase of the cell cycle (Milot, unpublished).

Previous results had shown that the individual HS of the LCR appeared additive, as most or all were necessary for full expression.[32] The data with the HS deletion loci suggest that this additive effect is not accomplished through an increase in the density of polymerases on an individual gene, but (at least in part) through an increase in the stability of the LCR/gene complex leading to increased frequency and duration of transcription periods.

DISCUSSION

Our results have important implications on the proposed mechanisms of LCR activation of gene expression and by inference for the design of gene therapy constructs. Perhaps the most interesting implication of the studies described above is that the initiation of transcription from a competent gene in the "open" chromatin domain of the globin locus originates only through direct complex formation with the LCR via a looping process and that the maintainence of transcription initiation requires continued association of the LCR to load the polymerase onto the template and provide the necessary co-factors such as acetylases and kinases for initiation and elongation. Our results show that deletions which decrease the stability of LCR/gene interactions shorten the duration of such associations thereby reducing the transcriptional output from a given gene by decreasing the period of activity. This effect is most obvious in heterochromatic regions of the genome where the LCR spends a significant amount of time uncoupled ie. not activating any globin gene. Hence we conclude that the LCR determines the level of gene expression by determining the frequency and the duration of transcription periods rather than only controlling the rate of transcription.

REFERENCES

1. WEATHERALL, D. 1993. Bailliere's Clin. Haematol. **6**:
2. GROSVELD, F., G. BLOM VAN ASSENDELFT, D. GREAVES & G. KOLLIAS. 1987. Position-independent, high-level expression of the human β-globin gene. Cell **51**: 975–985.
3. WEINTRAUB, H. 1988. Formation of stable transcription complexes as assayed by analysis of individual templates. Proc. Natl. Acad. Sci. USA **85**: 5819–5823.
4. WALTERS, M. C., W. MAGIS, S. FIERING, J. EIDEMILLER, D. SCALZO, M. GROUDINE & D. I. MARTIN. 1996. Transcriptional enhancers act in cis to suppress position-effect variegation. Genes Dev. **10**: 185–195.
5. MARTIN, D. I., S. FIERING & M. GROUDINE. 1996. Regulation of beta-globin gene expression: straightening out the locus. Curr. Opin. Genet. Dev. **4**: 488–495.

6. BICKEL, S. & V. PIROTTA. 1992. Self association of the Drosophila zeste protein is responsible for transvection effects. EMBO J. **9**: 2959–2967.
7. MULLER, H., J. SOGO & W. SCHAFFNER. 1989. An enhancer stimulates transcription in trans when attached to the promoter via a protein bridge. Cell **58**: 767–777.
8. PTASHNE, M. 1988. How eukaryotic transcriptional activators work. Nature. **335**: 683–689.
9. GIGLIONI, B., C. CASINI, R. MANTOVANI, S. MERLI, P. COMI, S. OTTOLENGHI, G. SAGLIO, C. CAMASCHELLA & U. MAZZA. 1984. A molecular study of a family with Greek hereditary persistence of fetal hemoglobin and beta-thalassemia. EMBO J. **11**: 2641–2645.
10. ENVER, T., N. RAICH, A. J. EBENS, T. PAPAYANNOPOULOU, F. COSTANTINI & G. STAMATOYANNOPOULOS. 1990. Developmental regulation of human fetal-to-adult globin gene switching in transgenic mice. Nature **344**: 309–313.
11. HANSCOMBE, O., D. WHYATT, P. FRASER, N. YANNOUTSOS, D. GREAVES, N. DILLON & F. GROSVELD. 1991. Importance of globin gene order for correct developmental expression. Genes & Dev. **5**: 1387–1394.
12. PETERSON, K. R., C. H. CLEGG, C. HUXLEY, B. M. JOSEPHSON, H. S. HAUGEN, T. FURUKAWA & G. STAMATOYANNOPOULOS. 1993. Transgenic mice containing a 248-kb yeast artificial chromosome carrying the human beta-globin locus display proper developmental control of human globin genes. Proc. Natl. Acad. Sci. USA **90**: 7593–7597.
13. STROUBOULIS, J., N. DILLON & F. GROSVELD. 1992. Developmental regulation of a complete 70-kb human β-globin locus in transgenic mice. Genes & Dev. **6**: 1857–1864.
14. WIJGERDE, M., F. GROSVELD & P. FRASER. 1995. Transcription complex stability and chromatin dynamics in vivo. Nature **377**: 209–213.
15. MARSHALL, N. F. & D. H. PRICE. 1992. Control of formation of two distinct classes of RNA polymerase II elongation complexes. Mol. Cell. Biol. **12**: 2078–2090.
16. PICARD, D. 1985. Viral and cellullar enhancers. *In* Oxford Surveys on Eukaryotic Genes 2. N. Maclean, Ed.: 24–48. Oxford University Press. Oxford.
17. WIJGERDE, M., J. GRIBNAU, T. TRIMBORN, B. NUEZ, S. PHILIPSEN, F. GROSVELD & P. FRASER. 1996. The role of EKLF in human beta-globin gene competition. Genes Dev. **10**: 2894–2902.
18. DILLON, N., T. TRIMBORN, J. STROUBOULIS, P. FRASER & F. GROSVELD. 1997. The effect of distance on long range chromatin interactions. Cell.
19. BODINE, D. & T. LEY. 1987. An enhancer element lies 3' to the human Aγ-globin gene. EMBO J. **6**: 2997–3004.
20. BEHRINGER, R., R. HAMMER, R. BRINSTER & R. D. PALMITER. 1987. Two 3' sequences direct adult erythroid specific expression of human β-globin genes in transgenic mice. Proc. Natl. Acad. Sci. USA **84**: 7056–7059.
21. ANTONIOU, M., E. DE BOER, G. HABETS & F. GROSVELD. 1988. The human β-globin gene contains multiple regulatory regions: identification of one promoter and two downstream enhancers. EMBO J. **7**: 377–384.
22. BIEKER, J. J. & C. M. SOUTHWOOD. 1995. The erythroid Krüppel-like factor transactivation is a critical component for cell specific inducibility of a β-globin promoter. Mol. Cell. Biol. **15**: 852–860.
23. NUEZ, B., D. MICHALOVICH, A. BYGRAVE, R. PLOEMACHER & F. GROSVELD. 1995. Defective haematopoiesis in fetal liver resulting from inactivation of the EKLF gene. Nature **375**: 6529: 316–318.
24. PERKINS, A. C., A. H. SHARPE & S. H. ORKIN. 1995. Lethal β-thalassaemia in mice lacking the erythroid CACCC-transcription factor EKLF. Nature **375**: 318–222.
25. PERKINS, A. C., K. M. GAENSLER & S. H. ORKIN. 1996. Silencing of fetal globin expression is impaired in the absence of the adult β-globin gene activator protein EKLF. Proc. Natl. Acad. Sci. USA **93**: 12267–12271.
26. KELLUM, R. & P. SCHEDL. 1991. A position effect assay for boundaries of higher order chromatin domains. Cell **64**: 941–951.
27. KELLUM, R. & P. SCHEDL. 1992. A group of scs elements function as domain boundaries in an enhancer blocking assay. Mol. Cell. Biol. **12**: 2424–2430.
28. CHUNG, J., M. WHITELEY & G. FELSENFELD. 1993. A 5' element of the chicken β-globin domain serves as an insulator in human erythroid cells and protects against position effect in Drosophila. Cell **74**: 505–514.

29. MILOT, E., J. STROUBOULIS, T. TRIMBORN, M. WIJGERDE, E. DE BOER, A. LANGEVELD, K. TAN-UN, W. VERGEER, N. YANNOUTSOS, F. GROSVELD & P. FRASER. 1996. Heterochromatin effects on the frequency and duration of LCR-mediated gene transcription. Cell **87**: 105–114.
30. FESTENSTEIN, R., M. TOLAINI, P. CORBELLA, C. MAMALAKI, J. PARRINGTON, M. FOX, A. MILIOU, M. JONES & D. KIOUSSIS. 1996. Locus control region function and heterochromatin-induced position effect variegation. Science **271**: 1123.
31. ELLIOTT, J. I., R. FESTENSTEIN, M. TOLAINI & D. KIOUSSIS. 1995. Random activation of a transgene under the control of a hybrid hCD2 locus control region/Iq enhancer regulatory element. EMBO J. **14**: 575–584.
32. GROSVELD, F., N. DILLON & D. HIGGS. 1993. The regulation of human globin gene expression. Baillieres Clin. Haematol. **6**: 31–55.
33. SCHEDL, P. & F. GROSVELD. 1995. Domains and boundaries. *In* Chromatin Structure and Expression: Frontiers in Molecular Biology. Oxford University Press, pp. 172–196.

β-YAC Transgenic Mice for Studying LCR Function[a]

KENNETH R. PETERSON,[b,c,d] PATRICK A. NAVAS,[b] AND GEORGE STAMATOYANNOPOULOS[b,c]

[b]Division of Medical Genetics, Department of Medicine, and
[c]Department of Genetics, University of Washington, Seattle, Washington 98195, USA

ABSTRACT: We have developed methods to produce transgenic mice using yeast artificial chromosomes (YACs) and have applied these methods to the analysis of globin gene regulation using 248 kb β-globin locus YACs (β-YACs). The advantages of YAC transgenics are: 1) developmental regulation can be studied in the context of the whole locus, 2) mutations may be readily introduced into the YAC, and 3) the effect of these mutations on gene expression can be analyzed. Mice containing the wild-type β-YAC show proper regulation of globin gene expression during development. Transgenics carrying a β-YAC bearing a –117 $^A\gamma$ mutation showed the anticipated phenotype of Greek HPFH, demonstrating that mutant β-YACs can be used to generate mice that recreate human globin developmental mutants. Transgenic mice with YACs have also been used to examine the function of the LCR. Transgenic mice were generated with a β-YAC containing a deletion of LCR DNAse I-hypersensitive site 3 (5′HS3). Our results suggest that: 1) the LCR contains functionally redundant elements, 2) the formation of a LCR complex does not require all of the HSs, 3) the individual HSs may modulate the interaction of the LCR with specific globin genes during development, and 4) that most of the HS activity is confined to the core region.

Transgenic mouse technology has been essential to the elucidation of regulatory mechanisms that control human β-like globin gene expression during development. Current models of globin gene switching, including both silencing and competition, were largely defined using mice produced from constructs that linked globin gene sequences to various cis-acting regulatory motifs. However, these simple recombinant constructs suffer from several drawbacks due to the upper size limit of the DNA molecule that can be manipulated in vitro without shear or denaturation. Decisions must be made in the design of these transgene constructs that result in distortion of the organization of the locus, elimination of normal distances between genes and control elements, and omission of sequences with unknown regulatory relevance. To circumvent these problems, we developed methodology to generate transgenic mice using human β-globin locus yeast artificial chromosomes (β-YACs) as transgenes.[1] Using YACs, the regulation of globin genes can be studied without affecting the organization of the locus.

YACs offer several advantages (TABLE 1). First, long DNA sequences can be manipulated in vitro without degradation. Second, β-like globin gene expression can be studied in the context of the entire locus. Third, a wide spectrum of mutations can be introduced using homologous recombination in yeast. β-YAC transgenic mice show normal regulation of the human β-globin genes, have been used to recreate phenotypes of human mutants and appear to exhibit site-of-integration-independent and copy number-dependent gene expression.[1–5]

[a]National Institutes of Health Grants DK45365 and HL53750 supported this work.
[d]Corresponding Author: Division of Medical Genetics, Department of Medicine, Mailbox 357720, 1705 N.E. Pacific Street, University of Washington, Seattle, WA 98195-7720; Tel: Office, (206) 616-4527; Lab, (206) 616-3332; Fax: (206) 543-3050; E-mail: krpete@u.washington.edu

TABLE 1. Advantages of YAC Transgenics

- β-YAC transgenic mice:
  1. Normal regulation of the human β-globin genes.
  2. Recreate phenotypes of human mutants.
- YAC transgenics offer several advantages:
  1. Manipulation of long DNA sequences *in vitro*.
  2. Study of genes in the context of the entire locus.
  3. Introduction of mutations using yeast homologous recombination.

GENERATION OF TRANSGENIC MICE WITH β-YACS

Several technical hurdles had to be overcome before YACs could be successfully and reproducibly used as transgenes (TABLE 2). These problems are summarized here. One potential recurrent problem is that single yeast clones often contain both wild-type and mutant YACs after mutagenesis of the target YAC.[4] The yeast host may carry two or more copies of the wild-type YAC prior to introduction of a mutation. If only one copy integrates the incoming mutant sequence and selectable marker by homologous recombination, the yeast cell will survive selection. After counter-selection for yeast that have lost the selectable marker, the YAC population may be mixed, comprised of both wild-type and mutant YACs. Multiple YACs may be segregated into individual cells by mating the haploid yeast to form diploid yeast, followed by sporulation of the diploids and germination of the spores into new haploid cells.[6] Alternately, YAC-containing yeast may be crossed with *kar* mutant strains,[7–9] which are defective in nuclear fusion. Thus, in crosses between a YAC-containing strain and a *kar* mutant strain, karyogamy does not occur and a heterokaryon is formed with two nuclei. Haploid progeny derived from a heterokaryon share parental cytoplasm, but contain the nucleus from one parent or the other. Occasionally, the YAC will be transferred from one nucleus to the other in a heterokaryon. Selection is for the YAC and against the donor nucleus; thus, multiple copies of the YAC may be segregated from one another.

After manipulation in yeast, extensive handling of YAC DNA *in vitro* becomes problematic. The goal is to purify and microinject intact YAC DNA without shear or degradation, while preparing a concentrated solution free of insoluble particles that may clog the injection needle. High molecular weight DNA can be isolated and maintained in the presence of high ionic strength buffer during purification and microinjection.[1,10] Methods for purification, concentration of the DNA solution into a range acceptable for microinjection and removal of particulates are published in detail elsewhere.[11,12]

Finally, the presence of deleted YAC copies *in vivo* is a continuing problem that occasionally occurs regardless of the best precautions. Much of this problem has been alleviated by recent improvements in YAC purification and microinjection procedures and by using β-YACs that are smaller and/or more amenable to structural analysis *in vivo*.

TABLE 2. Generation of Transgenic Mice with YACs

- **Problem**: Presence of wild-type and mutant YACs in a single yeast clone after mutagenesis.
- *Solution*: Segregate multiple YACs by yeast mating and sporulation or transfer by *kar* crossing.
- **Problem:** Purification and injection of intact YAC DNA without shear or denaturation.
- *Solution*: Isolate and maintain YAC in presence of high ionic strength buffer during purification and injection.
- **Problem:** Deleted YAC copies *in vivo*.
- *Solution*: Improvements in YAC purification and injection techniques, YAC vector and identification of mouse lines containing deleted YACs.

However, identification of mouse lines containing deleted YACs remains the best defense against utilizing aberrant transgenics that might yield misleading data. This aspect of YAC transgenesis will be described in greater detail below.

MUTAGENESIS OF YAC DNA SEQUENCES

Perhaps the most attractive aspect of using YACs as transgenes is the ability to introduce mutations and analyze their effect on gene expression within an intact, otherwise unaltered, locus. Point mutations, deletions, or insertions can all be targeted to a YAC using either the "pop-in," "pop-out" or gene replacement methods of homologous recombination.[13-15] "Pop-in," "pop-out" mutagenesis requires the transfection of only one construct followed by a two-step selection process, whereas gene replacement utilizes two constructs in a series of transfections. In most cases, the former method is preferred and all classes of mutations can be introduced using this method.

Yeast integrating plasmids (YIPs) containing a selectable marker and the mutated sequence of interest are used in "pop-in," "pop-out" recombination (FIG. 1). One prerequisite for this method is the availability of a unique restriction site within the cloned fragment, located asymmetrically relative to the mutation. In the first step (FIG. 1A), the linearized YIP construct is transformed into yeast. YIPs cannot autonomously replicate; thus, the only way the selectable marker can be maintained is if the YIP is integrated by homologous recombination between the target YAC sequence and the incoming mutated sequence. The host yeast is URA⁻ in this example; recombinants are selected for URA⁺ prototrophy. The resulting YAC carries a duplication of the target sequence, one wild-type and one mutant, with the YIP vector and selectable marker sequences in between.

In the second step (FIG. 1B), selection for URA⁺ is removed by the addition of uracil. The reverse recombination event between the duplicated wild-type and mutant sequences occurs spontaneously at a frequency of 10^{-4} to 10^{-5}. These events may be selected for using 5-fluoroorotic acid (5-FOA). Yeast that are URA⁺ metabolize 5-FOA to a toxic product, but recombinants that have lost the URA⁺ selectable marker become 5-FOA^R. This second recombination event results in either conversion to the mutant sequence or reversion to the wild-type sequence. Southern blot hybridization of restriction enzyme digests, PCR, DNA sequence analysis or a combination of these methods identifies mutant versus wild-type YACs. If the yeast contain a mix of wild-type and mutant YACs, they are segregated as described above, prior to purification and microinjection of the YAC.

The utility of YAC mutagenesis for studying globin gene regulation was demonstrated by introducing a point mutation at –117 relative to the $^A\gamma$-globin gene mRNA start site.[3] In humans, this G to A transition causes the Greek form of hereditary persistence of fetal hemoglobin (HPFH[16-18]). Adult transgenic mice bearing the –117 β-YAC expressed γ-globin mRNA at a level of 5% of total human globin mRNA; transgenics carrying wild-type β-YACs have less than 0.5% γ-globin mRNA in the adult stage of development. Thus, the mutant transgenics displayed an HPFH phenotype, demonstrating that human developmental phenotypes associated with mutations in the β-globin locus could be re-created in mice.

To better understand the role of the individual DNAse I-hypersensitive sites (HSs) in locus control region (LCR) function, deletions of the individual sites were made using the methodology described above.[5] The effect of a 5'HS3 deletion is described here. The deletion in the ΔHS3 β-YAC is 2.3 kb and encompasses conserved regions of sequence determined by alignment of available LCR 5'HS3 sequences from different species (FIG. 2).

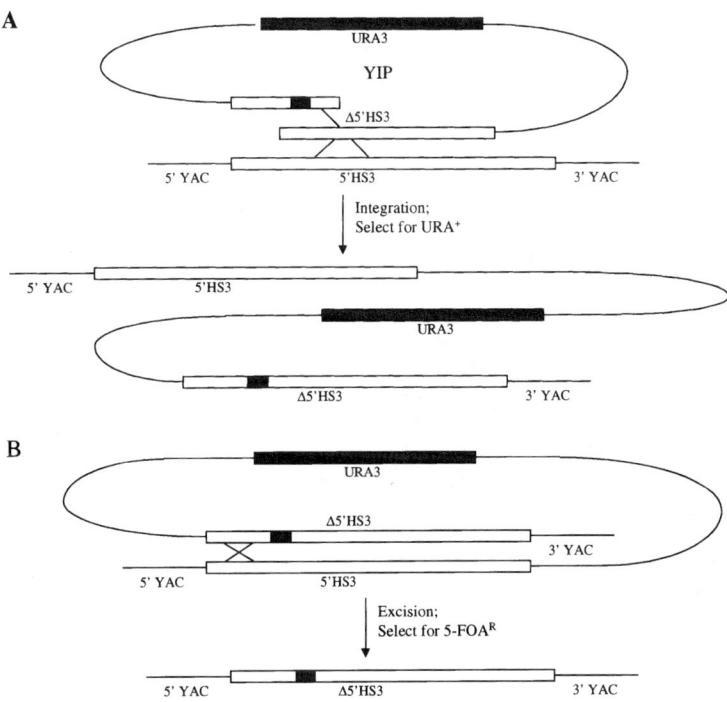

FIGURE 1. "Pop-in", "pop-out" method of homologous recombination in yeast used to introduce mutations into YACs. **A)** "Pop-in" step. **B)** "Pop-out" step. Introduction of a 5′HS3 deletion into the human β-globin locus YAC is illustrated here. Details of the method are described in the text.

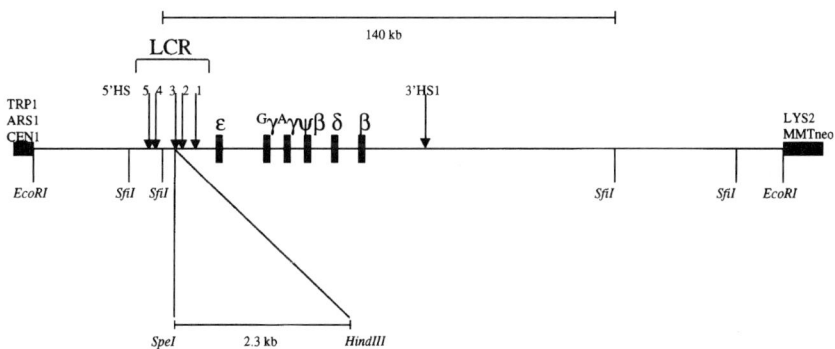

FIGURE 2. Location and extent of a 5′HS3 deletion in the β-YAC LCR. Shown at the top is the organization of the β-YAC. The locations of the LCR and its 5 HSs (HS1-5), the globin genes and 3′HS1 are indicated above the diagram. *Sfi*I restriction enzyme sites utilized in structural analysis are shown below the line. The bar above the locus indicates the 140 kb *Sfi*I fragment used diagnostically to determine locus integrity in transgene copies. Yeast chromosomal elements and selectable markers are indicated above the vector arms (*black boxes*). ARS1, replication origin; CEN1, centromere; TRP1, tryptophan biosynthesis; LYS2, lysine biosynthesis; MMTneo, G418^R.

THE PROBLEM OF STRUCTURAL ANALYSIS IN β-YAC TRANSGENIC MICE

As mentioned above, one of the problems with YAC transgenics is the occurrence of deletions in integrated YAC copies. Deletions are located at the 5' and 3' ends of the transgenes; internal deletions have not been detected. This observation suggests that deletions are caused by breakage during handling of the DNA *in vitro* between yeast and mouse, rather than as a result of recombination processes *in vivo* following microinjection. Regardless of the cause, it is imperative that only mice with intact transgenes be used for functional studies, since deletions may remove essential regulatory sequences or genes that would skew an analysis of the site-directed mutation. The identified β-YACs are 248 and 150 kb in size.[19] Both lack unique restriction sites that flank the entire locus, but the 248 kb β-YAC has *Sfi*I sites located between 5'HS4 and 5'HS3 of the LCR and downstream from 3'HS1 (FIG. 2). Thus, most of the locus is contained on this 140 kb *Sfi*I fragment and its presence serves as a good indicator that the locus is intact.

Standard Southern blot analysis of transgenic DNA to detect globin locus fragments of less than 10 kb may demonstrate that all locus sequences are present, but does not indicate whether they are linked in one or more contiguous complete locus copies. We have developed an assay for the structural integrity of the 248 kb β-YAC that allows us to screen individual copies of the locus for intactness (FIG. 3). Agarose blocks containing high mass DNA are prepared from single-cell liver suspensions of transgenic animals (FIG. 3A). Portions of the block are digested with *Sfi*I, the digested blocks are loaded in individual wells of an agarose gel and the DNA is fractionated by pulsed-field gel electrophoresis (PFGE). The gel is Southern-blotted, individual lanes are cut from the membrane, and these membrane strips are hybridized to a series of probes spanning the locus within the 140 kb *Sfi*I fragment (FIG. 3B). The membrane is then re-assembled and autoradiography is performed. A picture of each copy emerges, showing if and where deletions have occurred and how much of the locus is present. Occasionally, one or both of the *Sfi*I sites may be deleted, but the locus is intact. When this occurs, the transgene copy will appear larger or smaller than 140 kb, depending upon the location of the nearest *Sfi*I site in the murine genome. Mice with intact loci are used for further analysis.

Two Δ5'HS3 β-YAC lines were established.[5] A diagram showing the structures of the transgene copies and the location of deletions within each copy is shown in FIGURE 4. Both lines lacked 5'HS3 and contained copies that minimally extended from 5'HS2 through the β-globin gene enhancer 3' of the gene (data not shown). Other analyses demonstrated the presence of 5'HS5 and 5'HS4 (data not shown).

EFFECT OF THE 5'HS3 DELETION ON β-LIKE GLOBIN GENE EXPRESSION

Deletion of 5'HS3 resulted in a significant decrease of ε-globin gene expression and an increase of γ-globin gene expression in embryonic cells (TABLE 3).[5] β-globin gene expression was reduced in the fetal liver, but was unaffected in the adult. The deletion did not affect the temporal pattern of globin gene switching. These data indicate that 5'HS3 may have some specificity for interaction with the ε-globin gene and enhancement of its expression. Similarly, a 2.3 kb deletion of the mouse LCR 5'HS3 minimally reduced embryonic $ε^y$ and βh1 gene expression in yolk sac-derived erythroid cells and adult $β^{maj}/β^{min}$ gene expression in adult erythrocytes.[20] Thus, deletion of the entire HS produced only modest effects on globin gene expression. In contrast, deletion of the 225 bp 5'HS3 core element in the context of a β-YAC resulted in a major disruption of globin gene expression at all stages of development.[21]

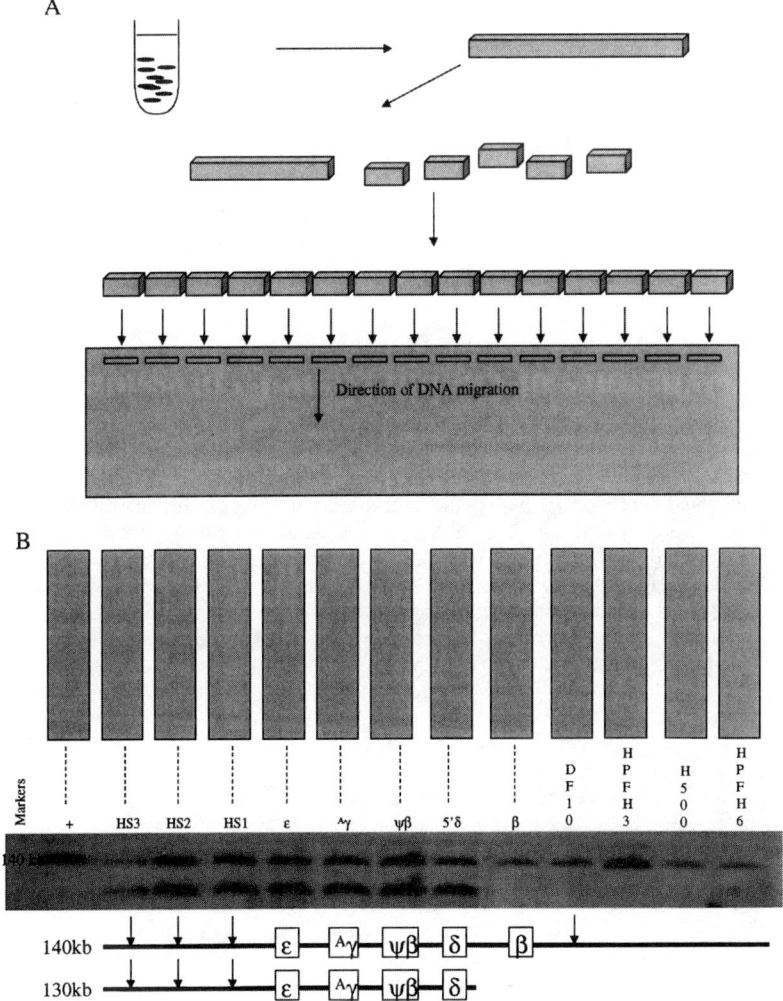

FIGURE 3. Structural analysis of β-YAC transgene integrity. Panels **A** and **B** depict a flow chart of the steps involved in screening for intact human β-globin loci in β-YAC transgenic mice. **A**) Single cell liver suspensions are prepared and used to prepare high mass DNA in agarose plugs. The plug is sliced and the slices are digested with *Sfi*I. Digested slices are loaded in separate lanes of an agarose gel and the DNA is fractionated by pulsed-field gel electrophoresis. **B**) The pulsed-field gel is blotted and cut into strips and the strips are hybridized individually with probes spanning the β-globin locus. The strips are then pieced together and autoradiography is performed. A picture of each transgene copy emerges; the location of the 140 kb *Sfi*I fragment is indicated on the left next to a positive control (+). A schematic diagram of each copy is shown below the autoradiogram. See text for more details.

A model, which may reconcile these seemingly conflicting data, is presented in FIGURE 5. The individual HSs of the LCR may interact with each other to form a holocomplex that may, in turn, interact with the globin genes by a looping mechanism.[22,23] The structure of

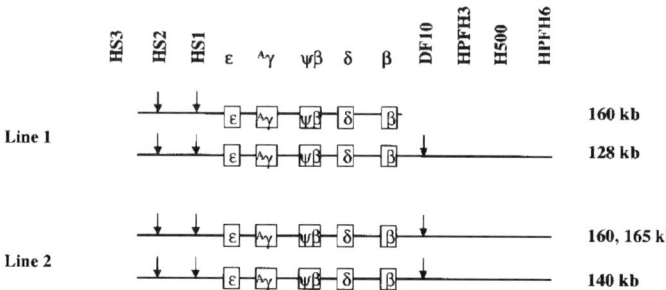

FIGURE 4. Schematic diagram of individual ΔHS3 β-YAC copies in the two established transgenic lines.

the holocomplex may be determined and constrained by the sequences flanking the HS core elements, with the core elements forming an active site that interacts with the globin gene promoters (FIG. 5A). Individual HSs within the holocomplex active site may have some predilection for enhancement of expression of a specific globin gene (i.e., 5'HS3 for ε-globin gene expression). When an entire HS is deleted (core and flanking regions), the remaining HSs may form an alternate holocomplex conformation with a modified active center that functions, but less efficiently and with some alteration of specificity (FIG. 5B). The HS core region deletions may function as *cis*-acting dominant negative mutations. These mutations may not affect the conformation of the holocomplex, but disrupt the function of the LCR active center (FIG. 5C), resulting in a holocomplex that cannot effectively enhance globin gene expression.

SUMMARY

Deletion of 5'HS3 sequences in the context of an otherwise intact locus provides information regarding LCR function that contrasts to that obtained using constructs in which individual globin genes are linked to individual HSs. For example, 5'HS3 was shown to be the most active site during the embryonic stage of development and was the only site capable of directing high level γ-globin gene expression during fetal hematopoiesis.[22,24] Deletion of the entire 5'HS3 in the β-YAC did not cause a decrease in γ-globin gene expression; instead we observed a decrease in ε-globin gene expression and a slight increase in γ-globin gene expression.[5] Our results show that analysis of LCR function is best accomplished in the context of an intact β-globin locus. YACs provide the proper tool for the analysis of these LCR structure-function relationships. Questions such as the structural requirements for the formation of the LCR complex, the minimum number or combinations of HSs that are essential for LCR holocomplex formation, and the functional

TABLE 3. Phenotypes of 5'HS3 Deletions

Size of Deletion	System Used	Phenotype	Reference
2.3 kb	248 kb β-YAC	Small changes in ε and γ expression. Essentially normal β expression.	5
2.3 kb	Knockout mice	Minor decrease in expression of all murine globin genes.	20
225 bp	155 kb β-YAC	Major decrease in expression of all globin genes of the YAC.	21

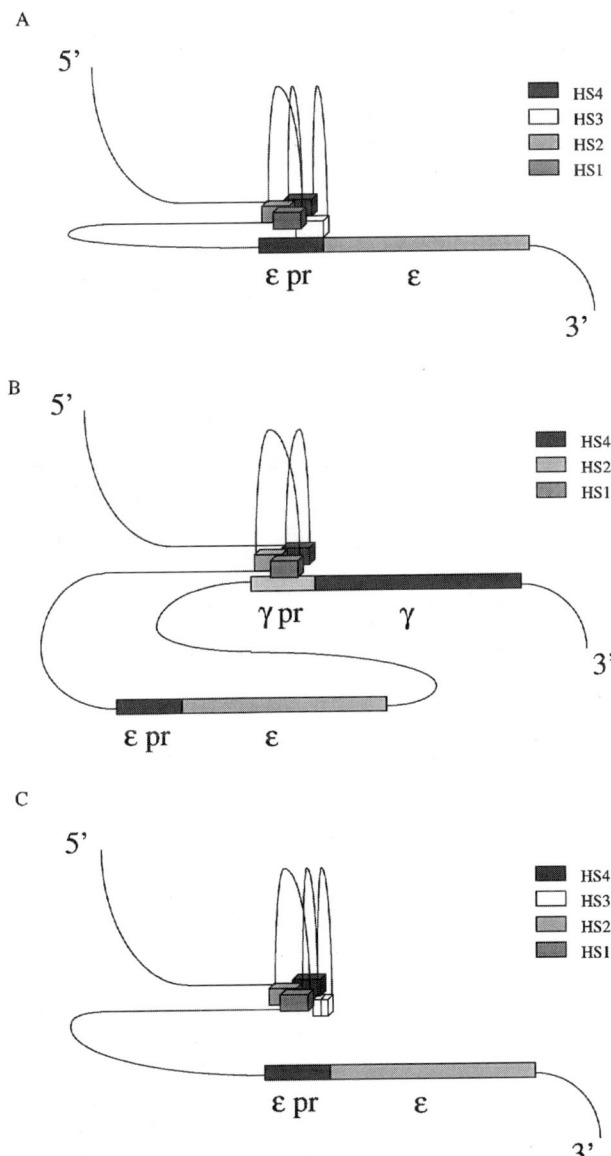

FIGURE 5. Model of the LCR holocomplex and the effect of 5'HS3 deletions on its structure and function in the embryonic yolk sac. **A)** The core-flanking sequences (indicated as loops) determine the conformation of the holocomplex and constrain the HSs (indicated as variously shaded blocks) to form an active site that interacts with the globin genes. 5'HS3 is shown here to have a preference for interaction with the ε-globin gene. **B)** An alternate, less functional, holocomplex conformation with a modified active center is adapted when the entire 5'HS3 (core and flanking sequences) is deleted. This holocomplex favors interaction with the γ-globin gene. **C)** The 5'HS3 core-flanking sequences maintain the normal holocomplex conformation when only the 5'HS3 core is deleted, but the active site is disrupted. The LCR does not effectively enhance globin gene expression.

significance of the order in which the HSs are arrayed within the LCR can be addressed using YAC technology.

ACKNOWLEDGMENTS

We thank Tony Blau for critically reviewing this manuscript.

REFERENCES

1. PETERSON, K. R., C. H. CLEGG, C. HUXLEY, B. M. JOSEPHSON, H. S. HAUGEN, T. FURUKAWA & G. STAMATOYANNOPOULOS. 1993. Transgenic mice containing a 248 kb human β locus yeast artificial chromosome display proper developmental control of human globin genes. Proc. Natl. Acad. Sci. USA **90**: 7593–7597.
2. GAENSLER, K. M., M. KITAMURA & Y. W. KAN. 1993. Germ-line transmission and developmental regulation of a 150-kb yeast artificial chromosome containing the human β-globin locus in transgenic mice. Proc. Natl. Acad. Sci. USA **90**: 11,381–11,385.
3. PETERSON, K. R., Q. LI, C. H. CLEGG, T. FURUKAWA, P. A. NAVAS, E. J. NORTON, T. G. KIMBROUGH & G. STAMATOYANNOPOULOS. 1995. Use of yeast artificial chromosomes (YACs) in studies of mammalian development: Production of β-globin locus YAC mice carrying human globin developmental mutants. Proc. Natl. Acad. Sci. USA **92**: 5655–5659.
4. PETERSON, K. R., C. H. CLEGG, Q. LI, P. A. NAVAS, E. J. NORTON, K. A. LEPPIG & G. STAMATOYANNOPOULOS. 1995. Analysis of hemoglobin switching in transgenic mice using β-globin locus yeast artificial chromosomes. *In* Hemoglobin Switching. G. Stamatoyannopoulos, Ed.: 45–58. Intercept, Ltd. Andover, U.K.
5. PETERSON, K. R., C. H. CLEGG, P. A. NAVAS, E. J. NORTON, T. G. KIMBROUGH & G. STAMATOYANNOPOULOS. 1996. Effect of deletion of 5'HS3 or 5'HS2 of the human β-globin locus control region on the developmental regulation of globin gene expression in β-globin locus yeast artificial chromosome transgenic mice. Proc. Natl. Acad. Sci. USA **93**: 6605–6609.
6. NEMETH, A. H., N. HUNTER, M. P. COLEMAN, R. H. BORTS, E. J. LOUIS & K. E. DAVIES. 1993. Rescue of a single yeast artificial chromosome from a cotransformation event utilizing segregation at meiosis. GATA **10**: 123–127.
7. HUGERAT, Y., F. SPENCER, D. ZENVIRTH & G. SIMCHEN. 1994. A versatile method for efficient YAC transfer between any two strains. Genomics **22**: 108–117.
8. SPENCER, F., Y. HUGERAT, G. SIMCHEM, O. HURKO, C. CONNELLY & P. HIETER. 1994. Yeast *kar1* mutants provide an effective method for YAC transfer to new hosts. Genomics **22**: 118–126.
9. SPENCER, F. & G. SIMCHEN. 1996. Transfer of YAC clones to new yeast hosts. *In* Methods in Molecular Biology, Vol. 54: YAC Protocols. D. Markie, Ed.: 239–252. Humana Press. Totowa, NJ.
10. GNIRKE, A., C. HUXLEY, K. PETERSON & M. V. OLSON. 1993. Microinjection of intact 200- to 500-kb fragments of YAC DNA into mammalian cells. Genomics **15**: 659–667.
11. PETERSON, K. R., C. H. CLEGG, Q. LI & G. STAMATOYANNOPOULOS. 1997. Production of transgenic mice with yeast artificial chromosomes. Trends Genet. **13**: 61–66.
12. PETERSON, K. R. 1997. Production and analysis of transgenic mice containing yeast artificial chromosomes. *In* Genetic Engineering, Principles and Methods, Vol. 19. J. K. Setlow, Ed.: 235–255. Plenum Press. New York, NY.
13. ROTHSTEIN, R. 1995. Targeting, disruption, replacement, and allele rescue: Integrative DNA transformation in yeast. *In* Methods in Enzymology, Vol. 194: Guide to Yeast Genetics and Molecular Biology. C. Guthrie & G. R. Fink, Eds.: 281–301. Academic Press. San Diego, CA.
14. DUFF, K. & C. HUXLEY. 1996. Targeting mutations to YACs by homologous recombination. *In* Methods in Molecular Biology, Vol. 54. YAC Protocols. D. Markie, Ed.: 187–198. Humana Press. Totowa, NJ.
15. MCCORMICK, S. P. A., K. R. PETERSON, R. E. HAMMER, C. H. CLEGG & S. G. YOUNG. 1996. Generation of transgenic mice from yeast artificial chromosome DNA modified by gene targeting. Trends Cardiovasc. Med. **6**: 16–24.

16. STAMATOYANNOPOULOS, G. & A. W. NIENHUIS. 1994. Hemoglobin switching. *In* Molecular Basis of Blood Diseases, 2nd edit. G. STAMATOYANNOPOULOS, A. W. NIENHUIS, P. MAJERUS & H. VARMUS, Eds.: 107–155. W. B. Saunders. Chicago, IL.
17. GELINAS, R., B. ENDLICH, C. PFEIFFER, M. YAGI & G. STAMATOYANNOPOULOS. 1985. G to A substitution in the distal CCAAT box of the $^A\gamma$-globin gene in Greek hereditary persistence of fetal hemoglobin. Nature **313**: 323–325.
18. COLLINS, F. S., J. E. METHERALL, M. YAMAKAWA, J. PAN, S. M. WEISSMAN & B. G. FORGET. 1985. A point mutation in the $^A\gamma$-globin gene promoter in Greek hereditary persistence of fetal hemoglobin. Nature **313**: 325–326.
19. GAENSLER, K. M. L., M. BURMEISTER, B. H. BROWNSTEIN, P. TAILLON-MILLER & R. M. MEYERS. 1991. Physical mapping of yeast artificial chromosomes containing sequences from the human β-globin gene region. Genomics **10**: 976–984.
20. HUG, B. A., R. L. WESSELSCHMIDT, S. FIERING, M. A. BENDER, E. EPNER, M. GROUDINE & T. J. LEY. 1996. Analysis of mice containing a targeted deletion of β-globin locus control region 5' hypersensitive site 3. Mol. Cell Biol. **16**: 2906–2912.
21. BUNGERT, J., U. DAVÉ, K.-C. LIM, K. H. LIEUW, J. A. SHAVIT, Q. LIU & J. D. ENGEL. 1995. Synergistic regulation of human β-globin gene switching by locus control region elements HS3 and HS4. Genes & Dev. **9**: 3083–3096.
22. FRASER, P., S. PRUZINA & F. GROSVELD. 1993. Each hypersensitive site of the human β-globin locus control region confers a different developmental pattern of expression to the globin genes. Genes & Dev. **7**: 106–113.
23. WIJGERDE, M., F. GROSVELD & P. FRASER. 1995. Transcription complex stability and chromatin dynamics *in vivo*. Nature **377**: 209–213.
24. LI, Q. & J. A. STAMATOYANNOPOULOS. 1994. Position independence and proper developmental control of γ-globin gene expression require both a 5' locus control region and a downstream sequence element. Mol. Cell. Biol. **14**: 6087–6096.

Molecular Basis of Hereditary Persistence of Fetal Hemoglobin

BERNARD G. FORGET[a]

*Department of Internal Medicine, Section of Hematology,
Yale University School of Medicine, 333 Cedar Street, Room 403 WWW,
New Haven, Connecticut 06520-8021, USA*

ABSTRACT: Increased levels of fetal hemoglobin (HbF) can ameliorate the clinical course of inherited disorders of β-globin gene expression, such as β thalassemia and sickle cell anemia. In a group of disorders called hereditary persistence of fetal hemoglobin (HPFH), expression of the γ-globin gene of HbF persists at high levels in adult erythroid cells. Molecular studies of the HPFH syndromes have identified several important regulatory elements for the normal pattern of γ-globin gene expression. Deletion as well as nondeletion types of HPFH have been identified. The nondeletion types of HPFH are characterized by the presence of point mutations, in the promoter region of one or another γ-globin gene, that are thought to alter interactions between various transcription factors and the promoter. The deletion types of HPFH are thought to deregulate the normal developmental pattern of γ-globin gene expression due to the juxtaposition of normally distant cis-acting factors into the vicinity of the γ genes. These findings have provided us with a more sophisticated understanding of the molecular basis for the persistent γ-gene expression in these syndromes and point to certain strategies for potential future attempts at gene therapy for β-globin gene disorders.

Hereditary persistence of fetal hemoglobin or HPFH is characterized by the presence of a substantial elevation of fetal hemoglobin (Hb F) in RBCs of heterozygotes, as well as in those of homozygotes and compound heterozygotes for HPFH and other hemoglobinopathies. HPFH is usually due to deletions of different sizes involving the β-globin gene cluster or to point mutations in the γ-globin gene promoters (reviewed in refs. 1–3). The precise molecular basis of certain forms of heterocellular HPFH remains unknown although some types are clearly not genetically linked to the β-globin gene cluster.

HPFH is generally described or referred to as a distinct disorder with a different phenotype from δβ thalassemia, but one should probably not consider the two disorders as being unambiguously separate entities but rather as a group of disorders with a variety of partially overlapping phenotypes that sometimes defy classification as one syndrome or the other. The following is a working definition that is generally applied to the classification of these disorders: δβ thalassemia usually refers to a group of disorders characterized in heterozygotes by a mild but definite thalassemia phenotype of hypochromia and microcytosis together with a modest elevation of Hb F that is heterogeneously distributed among red cells. In contrast, HPFH refers to a group of disorders with substantially higher levels of Hb F, and in which there is usually no associated phenotype of hypochromia and microcytosis in heterozygotes. In addition, the increased Hb F in heterozygotes with the typical forms of HPFH is distributed in a relatively uniform (pancellular) fashion among all of the red cells rather than being distributed in a heterogeneous (heterocellular) fashion among a

[a]Tel: (203) 785-4144; Fax: (203) 785-7232; E-mail: bernard.forget@yale.edu

subpopulation of so-called F cells, as in δβ thalassemia. Homozygotes for both conditions totally lack Hb A and Hb A$_2$, indicating absence of δ and β globin gene expression *in cis* to the typical forms of δβ thalassemia and HPFH determinants. The apparent striking qualitative difference in cellular distribution of Hb F between HPFH and δβ thalassemia may be due in great part to the quantitative differences in Hb F per cell and the sensitivity of the methods used to detect Hb F cytologically. However, it would appear that the increased amount of Hb F in HPFH is caused by a genetically determined failure to suppress γ globin gene activity postnatally in most if not all erythroid cells, rather than being due to selective survival of the normally occurring sub-population of F cells such as occurs in sickle cell anemia, β$^+$ and β^0 thalassemia. Nevertheless, heterocellular forms of HPFH, without a β-thalassemia phenotype, have been described. Therefore, in the final analysis, there is definitely some overlap between these two sets of syndromes at the level of their clinical and hematological phenotypes as well as at the level of their molecular basis.

DELETIONS ASSOCIATED WITH HB KENYA AND HEREDITARY PERSISTENCE OF FETAL HEMOGLOBIN

Hb Kenya is a structurally abnormal hemoglobin that, like Hb Lepore, contains a "hybrid" or fused β-like globin chain resulting from a non-homologous crossing-over event between two globin genes in the β cluster. However, whereas the Lepore crossover occurred between the δ- and β-globin genes, the Kenya gene resulted from crossover between the ^{A}γ- and β-globin genes (FIG. 1). The crossover occurred in the second exons of the ^{A}γ and β genes, between the codons for amino acids 80 to 87, and resulted in deletion of ~24 kb of DNA between the ^{A}γ and β genes. Unlike Hb Lepore, that is associated with a β-thalassemic phenotype, Hb Kenya is associated with a phenotype of pancellular ^{G}γ HPFH: erythrocytes of affected heterozygotes have normal red cell indices and contain 7-23% Hb Kenya as well as approximately 10% Hb F, all of which is of the ^{G}γ type and is distributed among the red cells in a relatively pancellular fashion.

The finding of Hb Kenya was initially thought to provide support for an early theory that proposed the existence of gene control elements in the DNA between the γ and δ genes, deletion of which in HPFH (and Hb Kenya) but not in δβ thalassemia, resulted in incomplete postnatal suppression of γ-gene activity in all erythroid cells. However, the most likely explanation for the HPFH phenotype associated with Hb Kenya is the influence on the ^{G}γ-and Kenya gene promoters of a well characterized enhancer element in the 3' flanking DNA of the β-globin gene that becomes translocated into closer proximity of the γ-globin gene promoters by the recombination/deletion event (FIG. 1). The Lepore crossover results in a β thalassemia rather than a HPFH phenotype presumably because the 3' β-globin gene enhancer is not translocated in close enough proximity to the γ-globin genes; other factors involved in the thalassemic phenotype of the Lepore mutation include instability of the δβ mRNA as well as decreased transcriptional activity of the δ gene promoter that drives expression of the δβ fusion gene.

A total of six deletions have been described in the β-globin gene cluster that are associated with a phenotype of pancellular HPFH (FIG. 1). HPFH-5, identified in an Italian family, is relatively short and extends from a point ~3 kb 5' to the δ gene to a point 0.7 kb 3' to the β gene, proximal to the position of its 3' enhancer (FIG. 1). The molecular basis of the HPFH phenotype associated with this deletion is presumably similar to that of Hb Kenya and due to the influence on the two γ-gene promoters of the 3' β-globin gene enhancer translocated into their vicinity by the deletion. The other five HPFH deletions are considerably more extensive in size and fall into two different size classes. HPFH-1 and HPFH-2, found in blacks, are the result of extensive deletions of nearly identical sizes, involving approximately 105 kb of DNA, with breakpoints staggered by only 5-6 kb (FIG. 1), whereas

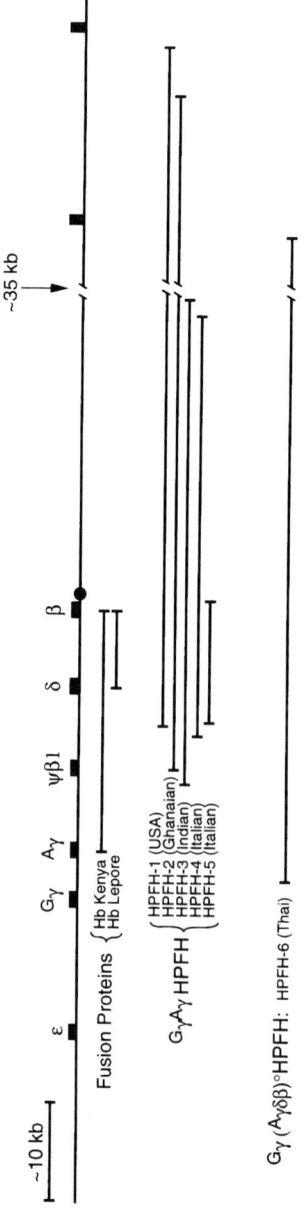

FIGURE 1. Deletions of the β-globin gene cluster associated with fusion proteins and HPFH. The circle 3' to the β-globin gene enhancer. The filled vertical boxes at the 3' breakpoints of the HPFH-1 and HPFH-6 deletions indicate the locations of DNA sequences with homology to olfactory receptor genes. The references for the individual mutations are cited in references 1, 2, and 4.

the HPFH-6 deletion (identified in Thais) is of a very similar size (~101 kb) but is shifted more in the 5′ direction and is associated with deletion of the $^A\gamma$-globin gene.[4] The deletions associated with HPFH-3 (in Asian Indians) and HPFH-4 (in Southern Italians) are less extensive, encompassing approximately 50 kb and 40 kb respectively; the 3′ breakpoints of these latter two deletions are separated by only ~2 kb, and are located ~30 kb downstream from the position of the β-globin gene, or ~50 to 60 kb more proximal than the 3′ breakpoints of HPFH-1 and HPFH-2 (FIG. 1).

The clustering of the 3′ breakpoints of the five largest deletions in three discrete regions has focused attention on the nature of the DNA sequences at these sites and their possible role in the generation of the HPFH phenotype. The DNA at the 3′ breakpoint of HPFH-1 has a number of interesting properties: it has gene enhancer activity in various assay systems[5]; it is specifically hypomethylated[5] and contains a DNase I hypersensitive site in erythroid cells[6]; and it contains a large open reading frame,[5] indicated by the vertical filled box in FIGURE 1, that encodes a protein homologous to members of the superfamily of G protein-coupled receptors,[5] and in particular the family of olfactory receptors (Forget, et al., unpublished). All of these properties suggest the presence in this DNA of a gene that is active in erythroid cells. The Spanish type of $^G\gamma^A\gamma$ (δβ)^0 thalassemia, that is associated with a thalassemic rather than a HPFH phenotype has a 5′ breakpoint that is very close to that of HPFH-1 but extends for an additional 6 to 7 kb in the 3′ direction, deleting the DNA at the HPFH-1 3′ breakpoint that has these interesting properties. This finding suggests a role for these sequences in the generation of the HPFH phenotype in HPFH-1 and HPFH-2. In fact, when a DNA fragment with a structure very similar to that of HPFH-2 (and containing the HPFH-1 3′ breakpoint DNA) is used to generate transgenic mice, the mice express the γ-globin transgene at a high level and in a virtually pancellular fashion in adult erythroid cells.[7] It is noteworthy that the DNA at the 3′ breakpoint of HPFH-6 has enhancer activity in transient expression systems and also contains a sequence that is homologous to a member of the olfactory receptor family (filled vertical box in FIG. 1).[4,8] The olfactory receptor sequences at the HPFH-1 and HPFH-6 breakpoints share approximately 55% identity with one another (Forget, et al., unpublished results). The 3′ breakpoints of HPFH-3 and HPFH-4 are located within a complex array of repetitive DNA sequences, and these DNA sequences have been shown to possess enhancer-like properties in different assay systems, including transgenic mice.[9]

The unifying theory that emerges from the study of the largest HPFH deletions is that the DNA sequences at the 3′ deletion breakpoints, that become juxtaposed to the γ genes as a result of the deletion events, may influence γ-gene expression, in a manner analogous to the presumed influence of the 3′ β-globin gene enhancer on γ-gene expression in Hb Kenya and HPFH-5. Mechanisms by which this could occur include the presence of enhancer-like sequences in the 3′ breakpoint DNA or the presence in this DNA of an active chromatin configuration that could have a spreading and activation effect on the expression of the neighboring γ-globin genes.

NONDELETION FORMS OF HPFH

In contrast to the deletional types of HPFH (except for HPFH-6) where both linked $^G\gamma$ and $^A\gamma$ genes are overexpressed, only one or the other γ gene is usually overexpressed in the best characterized nondeletion types of HPFH. However, there also exist less well characterized nondeletion forms of heterocellular HPFH in which there is overexpression of both $^G\gamma$ and $^A\gamma$-globin genes. Because of the restricted pattern of γ-globin gene expression in the more typical forms of $^G\gamma$ and $^A\gamma$ forms of nondeletion HPFH, it was assumed that the mutations in these syndromes were likely to be located near the affected gene. Therefore, molecular studies focused initially on the DNA sequence analysis of the overexpressed (presumably mutant) γ genes in these disorders.

The results of these structural analyses revealed a number of different point mutations in the promoter region of the overexpressed γ gene in individuals with different types of nondeletion HPFH (see TABLE 1). These point mutations have clustered in three distinct regions of the 5'-flanking DNA of the affected γ-globin genes. Five different mutations have been identified in the region located approximately 200 base pairs from the "cap site" or site of transcription initiation of the γ genes, specifically at position -202 (C→G) of the ^{G}γ gene and positions -202 (C→T), -198 (T→C), -196 (C→T), and -195 (C→G) of the ^{A}γ gene (TABLE 1). This region of DNA which had not previously been suspected of playing a role in the regulation of γ- gene expression, is very G+C rich and its sequence bears homology to that of known control elements of other genes such as the 21 bp repeat of the SV 40 virus promoter and the distal element of the thymidine kinase gene of *Herpes simplex virus*. It is noteworthy that the G+C rich sequence of the latter genes is known to be the binding site of a ubiquitous *trans*-acting protein factor called Sp1. Subsequent studies of the γ-gene promoters have demonstrated that the -200 region is also a binding site for Sp1 and at least one other ubiquitous DNA-binding protein. The -202 (C→G) mutation

TABLE 1. Nondeletion Forms of Hereditary Persistence of Fetal Hemoglobin (HPFH)

Type and Racial Group	Mutation in Globin Gene	Percentage of Hb F in Heterozygotes
Pancellular ^{G}γ HPFH		
Black	^{G}γ : -202 (C→G)	15–25
Black	^{G}γ-: 175 (T→C)	20–30
Sardinian	^{G}γ: -175 (T→C)	17–21
Japanese	^{G}γ: -114 (C→T)	11–14
Pancellular ^{A}γ HPFH		
Southern Italian	^{A}γ: -196 (C→T)	12–16
Chinese	^{A}γ: -196 (C→T)	14–21
Black	^{A}γ: -175 (T→C)	36–41[a]
Greek	^{A}γ: -117 (G→A)	10–20
Sardinian	^{A}γ: -117 (G→A)	12–16
Black	^{A}γ: -117 (G→A)	11–16
Black	^{A}γ: -114 to -102 deleted	30–32
Pancellular ^{G}γ^{A}γ HPFH		
Chinese	Unknown	20–25
Heterocellular ^{G}γ HPFH		
Black (Atlanta)	^{G}γ^{A}γ: -158 (C→T)	2.3–3.8
Japanese	^{G}γ: -114 (C→T)	11–14
Heterocellular ^{A}γ HPFH		
Black	^{A}γ: -202 (C→T)	1.6–3.9
British	^{A}γ: -198 (T→C)	3.5–10
Brazilian	^{A}γ: -195 (C→G)	4.5–7
Black (Georgia)	^{A}γ: -114 (C→T)	2.6–6
Heterocellular ^{G}γ^{A}γ HPFH		
Swiss	Unknown	1–4
Black (Seattle)	Normal γ-gene promoters	3–8

[a]The one patient studied was doubly heterozygous for Hb A and Hb C. About 20% of the Hb F (or 8% of the total Hb) was of the ^{G}γ type, and the ^{G}γ gene in *cis* to the -175 ^{A}γ mutation carried the -158 C→T change.

The references for the individual mutations are cited in references 1 and 2.

also creates a strong binding site for the stage selector protein (SSP), a complex of proteins (at least one of which is erythroid-specific) which normally binds to the proximal (−50) region of the γ-globin gene and is thought to be an important regulator of γ-globin gene expression.[10,11] The -202 (C→G) and -196 mutations are associated with high levels of Hb F (15-20%) expressed in a pancellular fashion whereas the -202 (C→T), -198, and -195 mutations are associated with lower levels of Hb F (3-10%) expressed in a heterocellular fashion (see TABLE 1) (reviewed in refs. 1-3).

The second region containing a mutation associated with nondeletion HPFH is located at position -175. A point mutation (T→C) at this position of either $^G\gamma$ or $^A\gamma$ gene is associated with a phenotype of pancellular HPFH with high levels of Hb F (15–25%). This region of DNA is noteworthy because it contains an octanucleotide sequence that is present in the promoter region of a number of genes and is the binding site of another ubiquitous *trans*-acting factor called OCT-1. In addition, the octamer consensus sequence of the γ-gene promoters is flanked on either side by a consensus sequence for the erythroid-specific factor GATA-1. The point mutation at position -175 affects the one nucleotide that is present in the partially overlapping binding sites of both OCT-1 and GATA-1.

The third region affected by a point mutation in nondeletion HPFH is in the area of a well known regulatory element of globin and other genes: the CCAAT box sequence. In the γ-globin genes, the CCAAT box is duplicated and the mutation associated with the Greek ($^A\gamma$) type of nondeletion HPFH is a G→A substitution at position -117, 2 bases upstream of the distal CCAAT box of the $^A\gamma$-globin gene promoter. The base change disrupts a pentanucleotide sequence, YYTTGA (Y=pyrimidine), that is highly conserved immediately upstream of the CCAAT sequence in all animal fetal and embryonic genes. Another mutation with a similar phenotype involves the deletion of 13 base pairs of DNA, from position -102 to -114, encompassing the distal CCAAT box and adjacent 3′ DNA of the $^A\gamma$-globin gene. The CCAAT box region is known to be the binding site of a number of *trans*-acting factors, including the ubiquitous factors CCAAT binding protein (CP1) and CCAAT displacement factor (CDP) as well as the erythroid-specific factor NF-E3. A third mutation has also been identified that consists of a C→T base substitution at position -114 of the $^G\gamma$ or $^A\gamma$ globin-gene, within the distal CCAAT consensus sequence.

The unifying model by which these various mutations are thought to affect hemoglobin switching proposes that these base changes alter the binding of a number of different *trans*-acting factors to critical regions of the γ-globin gene promoters and thereby prevent the normal postnatal suppression of γ-globin gene expression. The specific abnormalities of protein/DNA interactions that have been observed when nondeletion HPFH γ-globin gene promoter sequences have been compared to normal γ-gene promoter sequences have been previously reviewed and discussed.[1-3] The mutations could prevent the binding of negative regulatory factors or enhance the binding of positive regulatory factors. Either mechanism could be operative with one mutation or the other.

CONCLUSIONS

Significant insight into the normal regulation of expression of the human β-globin gene cluster has been gained in the last decade by a detailed analysis of the group of disorders called HPFH. On the basis of this information, several important regulatory elements have been identified for the normal functioning of the β-globin gene cluster as well as for the persistent expression of γ-globin genes in adults with HPFH. These results provide us with a more sophisticated understanding of the molecular basis of these syndromes and point to certain strategies for potential future attempts at gene therapy for globin gene disorders. For example, gene therapy vectors for the purpose of providing high levels of γ-globin gene expression in adult erythroid cells could be designed to contain γ-globin genes with mutant promoters, such as those found in certain forms of nondeletion HPFH, with or without enhancer-like elements such as those found at the 3' breakpoints of HPFH-1 and HPFH-6.

REFERENCES

1. BOLLEKENS, J. A. & B. G. FORGET. 1991. δβ Thalassemia and hereditary persistence of fetal hemoglobin. Hematol. Oncol. Clin. North Am. **5**: 399–422.
2. FORGET, B. G. & H. A. PEARSON. 1995. Hemoglobin synthesis and the thalassemias. *In* Blood: Principles and Practice of Hematology. R. I. Handin, S. E. Lux, T. P. Stossel, Eds.: 1525–1590. J. B. Lippincott, Philadelphia.
3. STAMATOYANNOPOULOS, G. & A. W. NIENHUIS. 1994. *In* Molecular Basis of Blood Diseases, 2nd edit. G. Stamatoyannopoulos A. W. Nienhuis, P. W. Majerus, H. E. Varmus, Eds.: 107–155. W. B. Saunders, Philadelphia.
4. KOSTEAS, T., A. PALENA & N. P. ANAGNOU. 1997. Molecular cloning of the breakpoints of the hereditary persistence of fetal hemoglobin Type-6 (HPFH-6) deletion and sequence analysis of the novel juxtaposed region from the 3' end of the β-globin gene cluster. Hum. Genet. **100**: 441–445.
5. FEINGOLD, E. A. & B. G. FORGET. 1989. The breakpoint of a large deletion causing hereditary persistence of fetal hemoglobin occurs within an erythroid DNA domain remote from the β-globin gene cluster. Blood **74**: 2178–2186.
6. ELDER, J. T., W. C. FORRESTER & C. THOMPSON, *et al.* 1990. Translocation of an erythroid-specific hypersensitive site in deletion-type hereditary persistence of fetal hemoglobin. Mol. Cell. Biol. **10**: 1382–1389.
7. ARCASOY, M. O. *et al.* 1997. High levels of human γ-globin gene expression in adult mice carrying a transgene of deletion-type hereditary persistence of fetal hemoglobin. Mol. Cell. Biol. **17**: 2076–2089.
8. KOSTEAS, T. *et al.* 1996. Complete sequencing and functional analysis of the HPFH-6 enhancer: detection of multiple motifs for transcription factors and identification of an open reading frame. Blood **88**(Suppl.1): 150a.
9. ANAGNOU, N. P. *et al.* 1995. Sequences located 3' to the breakpoint of the hereditary persistence of fetal hemoglobin-3 deletion exhibit enhancer activity and can modify the developmental expression of the human fetal Aγ-globin gene in transgenic mice. J. Biol. Chem. **270**: 10256–10263.
10. JANE, S. M., A. W. NIENHUIS & J. M. CUNNINGHAM. 1995. Hemoglobin switching in man and chicken is mediated by a heteromeric complex between the ubiquitous transcription factor CP2 and a developmentally specific protein. EMBO J. **14**: 97–105.
11. JANE, S. M. *et al.* 1993. Methylation enhanced binding of Sp1 to the stage selector element of the human γ-globin gene promoter may regulate developmental specificity of expression. Mol. Cell. Biol. **13**: 3272–3281.

Reduced β-Globin Gene Expression in Adult Mice Containing Deletions of Locus Control Region 5' HS-2 or 5' HS-3[a]

TIMOTHY J. LEY,[b,d] BRUCE HUG,[b] STEVEN FIERING,[c] ELLIOT EPNER,[c] M.A. BENDER,[c] AND MARK GROUDINE[c]

[b]Washington University School of Medicine, Departments of Internal Medicine and Genetics, Division of Bone Marrow Transplantation and Stem Cell Biology, St. Louis, Missouri 63110-1093, USA

[c]Fred Hutchinson Cancer Research Center, Seattle, Washington, USA

ABSTRACT: To gain insights into the functions of individual DNA'se hypersensitive sites within the β globin locus control region (LCR), we deleted the endogenous 5' HS-2 and HS-3 regions from the mouse germline using homologous recombination techniques. We demonstrated that the deletion of either murine 5' HS-2 or 5' HS-3 reduced the expression of the embryonic εy and βh1 globin genes minimally in yolk sac-derived erythrocytes, but that both knockouts reduced the output of the adult β (β-Major + β-Minor) globin genes by approximately 30% in adult erythrocytes. When the selectable marker PGK-Neo cassette was retained within either the HS-2 or HS-3 region, a much more severe reduction in globin gene expression was observed at all developmental stages. PGK-Neo was shown to be expressed in an erythroid-specific fashion when it was retained in the HS-3 position. These results show that neither 5' HS-2 nor HS-3 is required for the activity of embryonic globin genes, nor are these sites required for correct developmental switching. However, each site is required for approximately 30% of the total LCR activity associated with adult β-globin gene expression in adult red blood cells. Each site therefore contains some nonredundant information that contributes to adult globin gene function.

The human β-globin gene cluster contains five functional genes that are expressed during specific developmental stages.[1] Sequences within or near the individual globin genes are sufficient to direct developmental stage-specific and tissue-specific expression, but high-level globin gene expression in transgenic models requires distant regulatory sequences that are collectively called the locus control region (LCR).[2-7] This region is comprised of a series of several erythroid-specific, developmentally stable DNA'se hypersensitive sites that contain highly conserved sequences that are essential for LCR activity.[8-23] The hypersensitive sites have been tested individually in transient and stable transfection assays, in tissue culture cells and in transgenic mice. HS-2 and 4 seem to contain approximately 25% of the total LCR activity, and HS-3 contains approximately 50%

---

[a]This work was supported by NIH DK 38682, CA49712, and DK49786 (TJL) and HL48356 and DK44746 (MG).

[d]Corresponding author: Washington University School of Medicine; 660 South Euclid Ave., Box 8007; St. Louis, MO 63110-1093; Tel: (314) 362-8831; Fax: (314) 362-9333; E-mail: timley@im.wustl.edu

of the total LCR activity required to direct high level expression of linked globin genes in these model systems.[13]

Recent studies have focused on the activities of the individual hypersensitive sites within the context of the entire β-globin cluster.[24–32] These approaches have been used to avoid the complications of studying small DNA fragments in which distant or undefined regulatory sequences may be missing. Transgenic animals have been made using large DNA fragments derived from the human β-globin cluster, either as ligated cosmids, or as yeast artificial chromosomes. Although these transgenes are correctly regulated, the levels of expression from individual genes within the cluster are highly variable with different integration sites. Unfortunately, these integration site-specific effects can obscure quantitative differences in globin gene expression caused by the linked mutations. As an alternative, mutations have been made in the endogenous mouse β-globin cluster using homologous recombination and site-specific recombination technology. Kim et al.[33] and Fiering et al.[34] have shown that insertion of different selectable marker cassettes within the human LCR are capable of inactivating the linked human β-globin gene in the mouse erythroleukemia cell environment. This finding is consistent with a model in which the foreign marker gene competes with the β-globin gene for the activity of the LCR, as well as other models (see DISCUSSION). This phenomenon, now known as the "neighborhood effect", is a confounding variable in the interpretation of many homologous recombination experiments where the selectable marker cassette has been left within the mutant locus. Indeed, several recent experiments have shown that the retained PGK-Neo cassettes can alter the expression of linked genes nearby.[35,36]

Therefore, to study the functions of the highly conserved murine 5′ HS-2 and 5′ HS-3, we decided to delete the regions containing these conserved elements from the mouse genome using homologous recombination, and then remove the PGK-Neo selectable marker cassette from the mutant alleles using site-specific recombinases. Mutant mice were obtained and analyzed, and were shown to have minimal defects in embryonic globin gene expression and no defects in hemoglobin switching. However, the adult β-globin genes that were linked to the mutations demonstrated a 30–35% reduction in output. These results show that HS-2 and 3 have non-redundant functions that contribute to adult β-globin expression, but that these individual sites are not required for embryonic globin gene expression or hemoglobin switching.

MATERIALS AND METHODS

The materials and methods used to create the mutant mice described in these studies were completely described in recent publications.[37,38]

RESULTS

Retained PGK-Neo Cassettes in the 5′HS-2 or HS-3 Positions Reduce Embryonic and Adult Globin Gene Expression.

When the PGK-Neo cassette was left in either the 5′HS-2 or HS-3 position (ΔHS2/Neo$^+$, ΔHS3/Neo$^+$, see FIG. 1), we observed striking reductions in the output of the εy and βh1 globin genes at embryonic days 9.5 through 14.5 (see TABLE 1). Similarly, retention of PGK-Neo in the HS-2 or HS-3 positions led to striking reductions in the output of the linked adult β-globin genes in adult red cells. Removal of the PGK-Neo cassette from either position dramatically increased globin gene expression (TABLE 1).

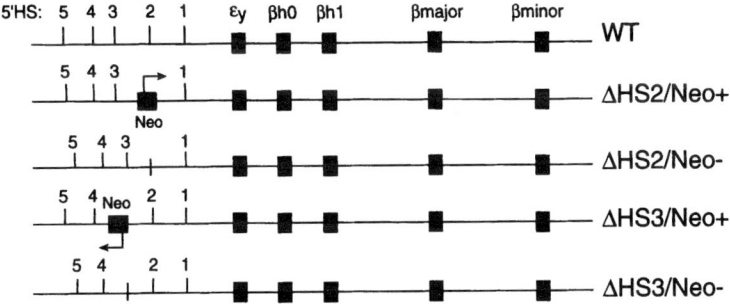

FIGURE 1. Diagrams of the mouse β-globin gene cluster and the mutations described in this report. The locations of the 5'HS within the β-globin locus control region are shown at the left, and the β-like globin genes in the cluster are shown as black boxes. The PGK-Neo cassettes are shown as black boxes within the HS-2 or HS-3 positions of the LCR. The removal of the Neo cassette by either FLP recombinase (for the HS-2 deletion) or Cre recombinase (for the HS-3 mutation) are shown as lines in the position of the deleted HS, to indicate the residual target sites for the recombinase that are left behind after site-directed recombination.

The mechanism responsible for the neighborhood effect described here is not yet clear. However, we have analyzed the expression of PGK-Neo itself in three different knockout mice in which the PGK-Neo cassette was inserted into three different hematopoietic loci. The results of these studies are shown in FIGURE 2. We designed a PGK-Neo probe for S1 nuclease protection assays so that correctly initiated PGK-Neo mRNA would protect a probe fragment of 291 nucleotides from S1 digestion. This probe, and probes for granzyme B, cathepsin G, and β2 microglobulin were simultaneously hybridized with test RNAs and subjected to S1 protection analysis. We analyzed RNA obtained from resting spleens, from spleens undergoing a one way mixed lymphocyte reaction (MLR) for five days, and from bone marrow obtained from animals containing either no PGK-Neo cassette (WT), a PGK-Neo cassette inserted into the murine granzyme B gene, a PGK-Neo cassette inserted into the cathepsin G gene, or a PGK-Neo cassette inserted into murine HS-3. Correctly initiated PGK-Neo was not detected in the tissues of wild-type mice (*lanes 1–3*). However, correctly initiated PGK-Neo mRNA was detected in the activated splenocytes from granzyme B deficient animals (*lane 5*); the activation of PGK-Neo parallels the activation of granzyme B during T cell activation.[36]

TABLE 1. Expression of Globin Genes Linked to Mutant β-Globin Locus Control Regions

Genotype	Globin Gene Expression (% of WT)		βmaj+min (Adult)	Homozygous (-/-) Embryonic Viability
	εy (E9.5/10.5)	βH1 (E9.5/10.5)		
WT	100/100	100/100	100	100%
ΔHS2/Neo+	11/25	43/30	35	0%
ΔHS2/Neo−	113/114	105/74	65	100%
ΔHS3/Neo+	30/45	34/20	45	50%
ΔHS3/Neo−	83/88	92/88	70	100%

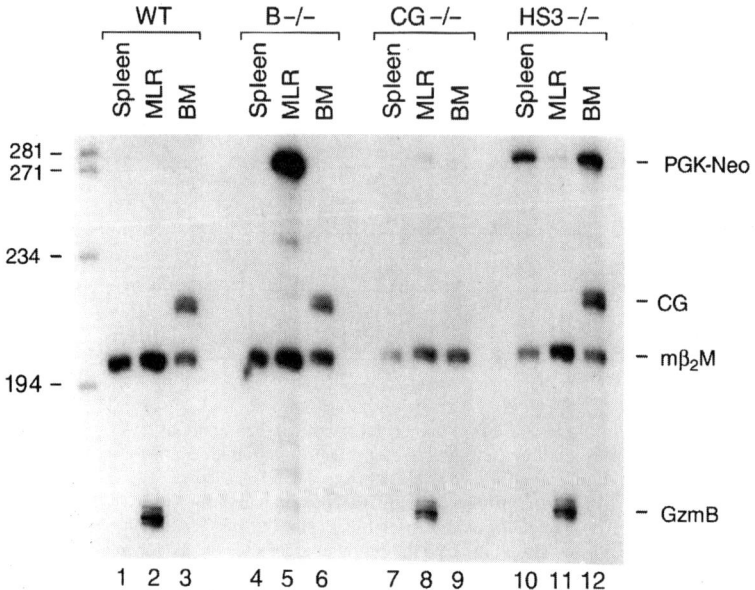

FIGURE 2. Expression of PGK-Neo in wild-type, granzyme B-/-, cathepsin G-/-, and ΔHS-3/Neo⁺ (HS3-/-) mice. RNA (15 μg) derived from resting spleen, MLR, and bone marrow from each animal was analyzed using S1 nuclease protection assays; each mRNA sample was cohybridized with probes for granzyme B, cathepsin G, PGK-Neo, and β_2-microglobulin. Note that abundant, correctly initiated PGK-Neo mRNA is detected in MLR lymphocytes only when the cassette is located within the granzyme B gene (*lane 5* versus *lane 8* and *lane 11*). PGK-Neo is detected in the spleen and bone marrow of mice containing the cassette in the murine β globin LCR (*lanes 10 and 12*); both of these organs contain erythroid precursors in adult mice (Reprinted with permission from the National Academy of Sciences).

Correctly initiated PGK-Neo mRNA was not detected in any of these compartments in mice containing the cathepsin G mutation, even though expression was expected in the bone marrow compartment. In contrast, mice containing the PGK-Neo cassette in the 5'HS-3 position revealed high-levels of correctly initiated PGK-Neo mRNA in the resting spleen and bone marrow, with minimal levels of PGK-Neo in activated splenocytes. Since the spleens and bone marrows of these young mice contain significant populations of erythroid precursors, these results suggest that expression of PGK-Neo is due to the location of the cassette within the β-globin LCR, which has converted this "housekeeping" gene to an erythroid-specific gene.[36] These results demonstrate that the PGK-Neo cassette disrupts LCR function in both the granzyme B locus and the human globin gene locus.

Minimally Altered Embryonic Globin Gene Expression, and a 30–35% Reduction in Adult Globin Gene Expression in Mice Containing Deleted 5'HS-2 or HS-3.

The PGK-Neo cassette was removed from the 5'HS-2 position using FLP recombinase mediated deletion, and from the 5'HS-3 position using CRE-recombinase.[37,38] The removal of the PGK-Neo cassettes was confirmed using standard Southern blotting methodology.

In heterozygous mice containing the deleted PGK-Neo cassette (Δ/neo-), the output of the linked εy, βh1, and adult β globin genes was substantially increased (to near wild-type levels) over mice containing the PGK-Neo cassette in the same position (see FIG. 1 and TABLE 1). These results show that the embryonic globin genes have nearly normal function in the absence of either 5'HS-2 or HS-3. In contrast, the linked adult β globin genes have a significant reduction in output (levels are 65-70% that of wild-type) when either HS site is missing (TABLE 1), suggesting that each site contains non-redundant information for the function of the adult β-like globin genes.

Embryonic Lethality in Mice Homozygous for ΔHS-2/neo+ and ΔHS-3/neo+ mutations

When heterozygous mice containing the ΔHS-2/neo$^+$ mutation are bred, no mice homozygous for the 5'HS-2 deletion are born. In contrast, heterozygous ΔHS-3/neo$^+$ matings yielded a ratio of wild-type to heterozygous to homozygous animals of 26:52:12. This finding suggests that at some time during development (perhaps E9-E10) the level of β-like globin chains in homozygous animals is below the threshold for survival for the 5'HS-2 mutation, and approximately at the threshold for survival for the 5'HS-3 mutation. Adult animals bearing the homozygous ΔHS-3/neo$^+$ mutation are viable and fertile, but have reduced mean cell volumes, hematocrits and mean cell hemoglobin concentration.[38] Reticulocyte counts are significantly elevated (10–15%) in these animals. These hematologic parameters are consistent with the mild thalassemia syndrome that would be predicted from a 55% reduction in the total adult β-globin gene output.

DISCUSSION

The goal of this study was to define the essential functions of murine β-globin 5' HS-2 and HS-3 within their native chromosomal contexts. We therefore removed each of these sites by homologous recombination, and then removed the selectable marker gene from the mutant LCR by site-specific recombination. These mutations did not significantly alter embryonic globin gene expression or hemoglobin switching, but reduced the expression from the linked β-globin genes by a moderate amount, demonstrating that each of these elements has non-redundant functions for adult globin gene expression.

The minimal alterations in globin gene expression obtained with deletions of 5' HS-2 or HS-3 strongly suggest that neither of these hypersensitive sites contains the dominant chromatin opening activity of the locus.[39] Although 5'HS-2 and HS-3 each has high levels of "LCR-activity" in transgenic mouse assays, the effects of their removal on murine globin gene expression are small. We cannot make conclusions about the redundancy of the hypersensitive sites until the remaining sites have been deleted; however, it appears that the loss of a single hypersensitive site can largely be compensated for by residual LCR activity in the remaining hypersensitive sites. Since 5'HS-2 and HS-3 deletions both cause an approximate 30% reduction in adult β-globin expression, our results suggest that neither site can fully compensate for the absence of the other, and that each contains unique motifs that are not redundant.

These results stand in contrast to those obtained in studies where ligated cosmids or YACs containing deletions of HS-2 or HS-3 are stably integrated into the mouse genome and then analyzed for human globin gene output. Peterson et al.[30] examined a 1.94 kb deletion encompassing human HS-2 within the context of a 248 kb YAC. In the single line that was examined, the output of ε, γ, and β globin were all reduced to about 50% compared with the expression expected from a wild-type YAC clone. Similarly, Milot et al.[31] examined the effects of a 2.4 kb HS-2 deletion on the expression of globin genes using a ligated 70 kb cosmid. Four founder lines containing one, one, three, or eight copies of the integrated transgene displayed highly variable outputs of the γ and β globin genes, suggesting that 5'HS-2 was required to minimize integration-site-specific variegation.

Similar studies have been done with deletions of 5'HS-3. Bungert et al.[29] examined the human globin gene expression patterns in transgenic mice containing a 155 kb YAC containing a small (0.225 kb) deletion of human 5'HS-3. In the two lines examined, there was a dramatic reduction in the output of ε, γ, and β globin gene expression, compared to wild-type YACs. Milot et al.[31] examined the effect of a 1.38 kb 5'HS-3 deletion on the output of linked globin genes using 70 kb ligated cosmids. Four founder lines, containing 3-12 copies of the integrated transgene, demonstrated 20-30% the levels of γ, and 10-50% the levels of β globin mRNA compared with the wild-type transgene. Finally, Peterson et al.[30] and Nayas et al.[32] have examined the consequences of a large (2.32 kb) and a small (0.23 kb) 5'HS-3 deletion on linked globin gene output in the context of a 248 kb YAC. The large deletion produced a reduction in the output of ε globin, with no reduction in γ or β globin gene expression; the small deletion had minimal consequences in four independent founder lines examined at embryonic day 15.5. Collectively, the variability in these studies suggests that LCR 5'HS deletions are difficult to study using large transgenes because of the inherent problem of variegation that accompanies these models. The mechanisms that cause this variegation may be integration-site dependent, or it may be due to frequent rearrangements of large DNA fragments.[27] Nonetheless, in these assays, the presence of 5'HS-2 and HS-3 within the large transgenes seems to reduce the integration site-specific variation in expression of the linked globin genes.

Regardless, the normal functions of the hypersensitive sites within the LCR must be defined within the context of the native chromosomal locus. The LCR does not exist to facilitate globin gene expression in aberrant genomic locations; it is important not to assign functions to the LCR based only on its behavior in random integration models. The deletion studies performed in the native chromosomal context strongly suggest that individual hypersensitive sites are either completely dispensable or redundant for normal globin gene switching and for embryonic globin gene function, a finding that recapitulates the observations that the LCR is not required for normal human γ→β globin switching in transgenic mice.[40] Nonetheless, 5'HS-2 and HS-3 each contains non-redundant functions that are critical for full output from the linked adult β-globin genes. These results support previous studies that suggest that the functions of 5'HS-2 and HS-3 are not entirely overlapping; for example, 5'HS-2 has classical enhancer function, while 5'HS-3 does not.[18] Additionally, single copies of 5'HS-3, but not 5'HS-2, are capable of directing high level β-globin gene expression in independent integration sites.[39] Even though both of these sites have high levels of LCR activity in transgenic mouse assays and stable-integration assays, they are clearly not functionally identical, and they cannot substitute for one another.

The mechanism by which PGK-Neo disrupts LCR function is not yet clear. The effects on LCR function are not due to sequences unique to PGK-Neo, since additional selectable marker cassettes have produced the same effects.[33,34] The orientation of PGK-Neo in the HS-2 and HS-3 mutations is different (see FIG. 1); therefore, there is not a strict orientation requirement for its ability to disrupt LCR function. Clearly, PGK-Neo is transcribed at high levels from its own promoter in an erythroid-specific fashion in mice that contain the HS-3 mutation.[36] Similarly, the PGK-Neo cassette is "captured" by a putative LCR in the granzyme B locus, so that this housekeeping gene becomes a T cell-inducible gene when it is placed within the body of the granzyme B gene. In that location, PGK-Neo disrupts the expression of multiple granzyme genes downstream from granzyme B. That result suggests that the LCR of that locus can influence multiple granzyme genes simultaneously, similar to that reported for the β-globin LCR with the duplicated γ-globin genes.[41] The disruption of LCR function by the PGK-Neo cassette could be explained by a direct interaction with the LCR, by alterations in the topology of the locus caused by the active PGK-Neo cassette, or by as yet undefined mechanisms.

The viabilities of homozygous HS-2/neo⁺ and DHS-3/neo⁺ mice differ substantially. Homozygous ΔHS-2/neo⁺ mice all die at embryonic days 10.5-11.5. Approximately 50% of homozygous ΔHS-3/neo⁺ mice survive to birth and then have no defects in adulthood, except for a mild thalassemia-like syndrome.[37,38] The reason for the difference in viability is probably explained by the levels of embryonic globin gene expression in these two mutant mice. The ΔHS-3/neo⁺ mutation reduced embryonic εy globin gene expression to 28% and βh1 expression to 30% to that of wild-type on E9.5, but the ΔHS-2/neo⁺ mutation reduced εy globin expression to 11% and βh1 to 43% that of wild-type on E9.5. The effect on survival is probably due to to very low levels of εy gene expression on day 9.5. Collectively, these data define the threshold of embryonic globin gene expression that is required for embryonic survival.

In summary, our data has helped to define the roles of individual hypersensitive sites for the function of linked globin genes within a native chromosomal context. The information that is obtained from studies of this kind is different from that obtained using transgenic approaches, where substantial variegation, even with wild-type globin gene clusters, is frequently observed. Additional loss-of-function mutations of hypersensitive sites are currently in being analyzed, including loss-of-function mutations that delete several hypersensitive sites (*e.g.* HS2+3 or HS2+3+4) within a single mutation. The information obtained from these studies should help to further define the mechanisms by which individual hypersensitive sites function within the LCR.

ACKNOWLEDGMENTS

We thank Pam Goda, Robin Wesselschmidt, and Agnes Telling for technical assistance. Nancy Reidelberger expertly prepared the manuscript.

REFERENCES

1. STAMATOYANNOPOULOS, G. & A. W. NIENHUIS. 1994. The Molecular Basis of Blood Diseases. Chapter 4: Hemoglobin Switching. G. Stamatoyannopoulos, A. W. Nienhuis, P. Leder, P. W. Majerus, Eds.: 107–155. W.B. Saunders, Philadelphia.
2. CHADA, K., J. MAGRAM, K. RAPHAEL, G. RADICE, E. LACY & F. COSTANTINI. 1985. Specific expression of a foreign β-globin gene in erythroid cells of transgenic mice. Nature **314**: 377–380.
3. CHADA, K., J. MAGRAM & F. COSTANTINI. 1986. An embryonic pattern of expression of a human fetal globin gene in transgenic mice. Nature **319**: 685–688.
4. DILLON, N. & F. GROSVELD. 1991. Human γ-globin genes silenced independently of other genes in the β-globin locus. Nature **350**: 252–254.
5. MAGRAM, J., K. CHADA & F. COSTANTINI. 1985. Development regulation of a cloned adult β-globin gene in transgenic mice. Nature **315**: 338–340.
6. TOWNES, T., J. LINGREL, H. CHEN, R. BRINSTER & R. PALMITER. 1985. Erythroid-specific expression of human β-globin genes in transgenic mice. EMBO J. **4**: 1715-1723.
7. TRUDEL, M., J. MAGRAM, L. BRUCKNER & F. COSTANTINI. 1987. Upstream Gγ-Globin and Downstream β-Globin sequences required for stage-specific expression in transgenic mice. Mol. and Cell. Biol. **7**: 4024–4029.
8. DHAR, V., A. NANDI, C. L. SCHILDKRAUT & A. SKOULTCHI. 1990. Erythroid-specific nuclease-hypersensitive sites flanking the human β-globin domain. Mol. Cell. Biol. **10**: 4324–4333.
9. FORRESTER, W., U. NOVAK, R. GELINAS & M. GROUDINE. 1989. Molecular analysis of the human β-globin locus activation region. Proc. Natl. Acad. Sci. USA **86**: 5439–5443.
10. TUAN, D., W. SOLOMON, Q. LI & I. LONDON. 1985. The "β-like globin" gene domain in human erythroid cells. Proc. Natl. Acad. Sci. USA **82**: 6384–6388.

11. DRISCOLL, M., C. DOBKIN & B. ALTER. 1989. γδβ-Thalassemia due to a *de novo* mutation deleting the 5' β-globin gene activation-region hypersensitive sites. Proc. Natl. Acad. Sci. USA **86**: 7470–7474.
12. FORRESTER, W. C., C. THOMPSON, J. T. ELDER & M. GROUDINE. 1986. A developmentally stable chromatin structure in the human β-globin gene cluster. Proc. Natl. Acad. Sci. USA **83**: 1359–1363.
13. FRASER, P., J. HURST, P. COLLIS & F. GROSVELD. 1990. DNase1 hypersensitive sites 1, 2, and 3 of the human β-globin dominant control region direct position-independent expression. Nucleic Acids Res. **18**: 3503–3507.
14. GROSVELD, F., G. VAN ASSENDELFT, D. GREAVES & G. KOLLIAS. 1987. Position-independent, high-level expression of the human β-globin gene in transgenic mice. Cell **51**: 975–985.
15. PHILIPSEN, S., D. TALBOT, P. FRASER & F. GROSVELD. 1990. The β-globin dominant control region: Hypersensitive site 2. EMBO J. **9**: 2159–2167.
16. TALBOT, D., P. COLLIS, M. ANTONIOU, M. VIDAL, F. GROSVELD & D. GREAVES. 1989. A dominant control region from the human β-globin locus conferring integration site-independent gene expression. Nature **338**: 352–355.
17. HARDISON, R., J. XU, J. JACKSON, J. MANSBERGER, O. SELIFONOVA, B. GROTCH, J. BIESECKER, H. PETRYOWSKA & W. MILLER. 1993. Comparative analysis of the locus control region of the rabbit β-like globin gene cluster: HS3 increases transient expression of an embryonic ε-globin gene. Nucl. Acids Res. **21**: 1265–1272.
18. HUG, B. A., A. M. MOON & T. J. LEY. 1992. Structure and function of the murine β-globin locus control region 5' HS-3. Nucl. Acids Res. **20**: 5771–5778.
19. JIMENEZ, G., K. B. GALE & T. ENVER. 1992. The mouse β-globin locus control region: hypersensitive sites 3 and 4. Nucl. Acids Res. **20**: 5797–5803.
20. LI, Q., B. ZHOU, P. POWERS, T. ENVER & G. STAMATOYANNOPOULOS. 1990. β-globin locus activation regions: Conservation of organization, structure, and function. Proc. Natl. Acad. Sci. USA **87**: 8207–8211.
21. LI, Q., B. ZHOU, P. POWERS, T. ENVER & G. STAMATOYANNOPOULOS. 1991. Primary structure of the goat β-globin locus control region. Genomics **9**: 488–499.
22. MOON, A. & T. J. LEY. 1990. Conservation of the primary structure, organization, and function of the human and mouse β-globin locus-activating regions. Proc. Natl. Acad. Sci. USA **87**: 7693–7697.
23. SHEHEE W., D. LOEB, N. ADEY, F. BURTON, N. CASAVANT, P. COLE, C. DAVIES, R. MCGRAW, S. SCHICHMAN, D. SEVERYNSE, C. VOLIVA, F. WEYTER, G. WISELY, M. EDGELL & C. HUTCHISON III. 1989. Nucleotide sequence of the BALB/c mouse β-globin complex. J. Mol. Biol. **205**: 41–62.
24. BEHRINGER, R. R., T. M. RYAN, R. D., PALMITER, R. L. BRINSTER & T. M. TOWNES. 1990. Human γ- to β-globin gene switching in transgenic mice. Genes & Dev. **4**: 380–389.
25. ENVER, T., N. RAICH, A. J. EBENS, T. PAPAYANNOPOULOU, F. COSTANTINI & G. STAMATOYANNOPOULOS. 1990. Developmental regulation of human fetal-to adult globin gene switching in transgenic mice. Nature **344**: 309–313.
26. GAENSLER, K., M. KITAMURA & Y. KAN. 1993. Germ-line transmission and developmental regulation of a 150-kb yeast artificial chromosome containing the human β-globin locus in transgenic mice. Proc. Natl. Acad. Sci. USA **90**: 11381–11385.
27. PETERSON, K., C. CLEGG, C. HUXLEY, B. JOSEPHSON, H. HAUGEN, T. FURUKAWA & G. STAMATOYANNOPOULOS. 1993. Transgenic mice containing a 248-kb yeast artificial chromosome carrying the human β-globin locus display proper developmental control of human globin genes. Proc. Natl. Acad. Sci. USA **90**: 7593–7597.
28. STROUBOULIS, J., N. DILLON & F. GROSVELD. 1992. Developmental regulation of a complete 70-kb human β-globin locus in transgenic mice. Genes & Dev. **6**: 1857–1864.
29. BUNGERT, J., U. DAVÉ, K-C. LIM, K.H. LIEUW, J.A. SHAVIT, Q. LIU & J. D. ENGLE. 1995. Synergistic regulation of human β-globin gene switching by locus control region elements HS3 and HS4. Genes & Dev. **9**: 3083–3096.
30. PETERSON, K. R., C. H. CLEGG, P. A. NAVAS, E. J. NORTON, T. G. KIMBROUGH & G. STAMATOYANNOPOULOS. 1996. Effect of deletion of 5'HS2 or 5'HS3 of the human β-globin locus control region on the developmental regulation of globin gene expression in β-globin

locus yeast artificial chromosome transgenic mice. Proc. Natl. Acad. Sci. USA **93**: 6605–6609.
31. MILOT, E., J. STROUBOULIS, T. TRIMBORN, M. WIJGERDE, E. DE BOER, A. LANGEVELD, K. TAN-UN, W. VERGEER, N. YANNOUTSOS, R. GROSVELD & P. FRASER. 1996. Heterochromatin effects on the frequency and duration of LCR-mediated gene transcription. Cell **87**: 105–114.
32. NAYAS, P.A., C.H. CLEGG, E. SKARPIDI, K.R. PETERSON & G. STAMATOYANNOPOULOS. 1997. β-YAC transgenic mice carrying a deletion of 234 bp core sequence of hypersensitive site 3: Relevance to function of the LCR. Blood **88**: 462a [abstract].
33. KIM, C., E. EPNER, W. FORRESTER & M. GROUDINE. 1992. Inactivation of the human β-globin gene by targeted insertion into the β-globin locus control region. Genes & Dev. **6**: 928–938.
34. FIERING, S., C. KIM, E. EPNER & M. GROUDINE. 1993. An "in-out" strategy using gene targeting and FLP recombinase for the functional dissection of complex DNA regulatory elements: analysis of the β-globin locus control region. Proc. Natl. Acad. Sci. USA **90**: 8469–8473.
35. OLSON, E. N., H.-H. ARNOLD, P. W. J. RIGBY & B. J. WOLD. 1996. Know your neighbors: Three phenotypes in null mutants of the myogenic bHLH gene MRF4. Cell **84**: 1–4.
36. PHAM, C. T. N., D. M. MACIVOR, B. A., HUG, J. W. HEUSEL & T. J. LEY. 1996. Long-range disruption of gene expression by a selectable marker cassette. Proc. Natl. Acad. Sci. USA **93**: 13090–13095.
37. FIERING S., E. EPNER, K. ROBINSON, Y. ZHUANG, A. TELLING, M. HU, D. I. K. MARTIN, T. ENVER, T. J. LEY & M. GROUDINE. 1995. Targeted deletion of 5′HS2 of the murine β-globin LCR reveals that it is not essential for proper regulation of the β -globin locus. Genes & Dev. **9**: 2203–2213.
38. HUG, B. A., R. L. WESSELSCHMIDT, S. FIERING, M. A. BENDER, E. EPNER, M. GROUDINE & T. J. LEY. 1996. Analysis of mice containing a targeted deletion of β-globin locus control region 5′ hypersensitive site 3. Mol. & Cell. Biol. **16**: 2906–2912.
39. ELLIS J., K. C. TAN-UN, A. HARPER, D. MICHALOVICH, N. YANNOUTSOS, S. PHILIPSEN & F. GROSVELD. 1996. A dominant chromatin-opening activity in 5' hypersensitive site 3 of the human β globin locus control region. EMBO J. **15**: 562–568.
40. STARCK J., R. SARKAR, M. ROMANA, A. BHARGAVA, A. SCARPA, M. TANAKA, J. CHAMBERLAIN, S. WEISSMAN & B. FORGET. 1994. Developmental regulation of human γ- and β-globin genes in the absence of the locus control region. Blood **84**: 1656–1665.
41. BRESNICK, E. H. & G. FELSENFELD. 1994. Dual promoter activation by the human β globin locus control region. Proc. Natl. Acad. Sci. USA **91**: 1314–1317.

Expression and Developmental Control of the Human α-Globin Gene Cluster

STEPHEN A. LIEBHABER[a] AND J. ERIC RUSSELL[b]

[a]*Howard Hughes Medical Institute and Departments of Genetics and Medicine, University of Pennsylvania School of Medicine, Clinical Research Building, Room 428, Philadelphia, Pennsylvania 19104-6148, USA*

[b]*Departments of Medicine and Genetics, University of Pennsylvania School of Medicine, Abramson Research Building, Room 316F, Children's Hospital of Philadelphia, 34th and Civic Center Boulevard, Philadelphia, Pennsylvania 19104, USA*

ABSTRACT: The human α-globin gene cluster contains three functional genes ζ, α2 and α1. The ζ globin gene is expressed exclusively in the primitive erythroblasts of the embryonic yolk sac and is selectively silenced during the transition from primitive to definitive erythropoesis. The two α-globin genes are expressed through development; they are expressed at equivalent levels in embryonic cells at a 2.6 : 1 ratio of α2 : α1 in fetal and adult cells. The dominant contribution of the α2-globin locus to overall expression of adult α-globin is reflected in the more severe phenotype resulting from mutations that affect this locus. Developmental silencing of the ζ-globin gene reflects both transcriptional and posttranscriptional mechanisms. Transcriptional silencing is mediated by an interaction between the ζ-globin gene promoter and a silencer located in the 3′ flanking region. This transcriptional silencing is only partial, and residual levels of ζ-globin mRNA are subject to subsequent degradation. This instability of ζ-globin mRNA relative to that of α-globin mRNA reflects differences in their respective 3′UTR segments; the ζ-globin mRNA 3′UTR has a lower affinity for a sequence-specific mRNP stability complex which assembles at this site. The α-globin mRNA assembles this complex at a higher efficiency and mutations which interfere with 3′UTR function result in corresponding loss of α-globin gene expression. These data outline a developmental pathway for the α-globin gene cluster which reflects transcriptional and posttranscriptional controls.

The α-globin gene cluster contains three loci of clear functional significance: ζ, α2 and α1.[1,2] The expression of ζ globin is limited to the primitive erythroblasts in the embryonic yolk sac. In contrast, α-globin is probably expressed at all developmental stages. Yolk sac erythroblasts express the two α-globin loci equally, while expression of the α2-globin gene is selectively induced concurrent with establishment of definitive erythropoiesis in the fetal liver. Induction of the α2-globin gene establishes its dominance: the ratio of α2 : α1-globin mRNAs and the ratio of their respective levels of protein synthesis in fetal and adult erythroid cells is approximately 2.6 : 1.[3] The two α-globin genes are identical for more than 600 bps 5′ to the transcription initiation site and through most of the transcribed region. The mechanism(s) which underlie the observed dominance of the α2-globin locus are not fully defined.

Two attributes of α-cluster genes which define their developmental stage-specific expression are the reciprocal silencing of ζ-globin expression and induction of α-globin

[a]Tel: (215) 898-7834; Fax (215) 898-1257; E-mail: Steve_L@hmivax.humgen.upenn.edu

expression at the embryonic-to-fetal transition, and the sustained high-level expression of the α-globin throughout fetal and adult life. Studies carried out in our laboratory indicate that these processes reflect combined transcriptional and posttranscriptional controls.[4] Normal adult levels of α-globin expression depend on high-level stability of α-globin mRNA.[5] Loss of this attribute results in the most frequent cause of nondeletional a-thalassemia, $\alpha^{Constant\ Spring}$ (α^{CS}). Our present understanding of α-globin mRNA stabilization is reviewed in the next section of this paper. Full silencing of the ζ-globin gene is dependent on both transcriptional inactivation and on destabilization of ζ-globin mRNA in fetal and adult erythroblasts. Our studies on the transcriptional and post-transcriptional aspects of ζ-globin gene silencing are summarized in the next two sections, respectively. This chapter concludes with a model which proposes that transcriptional induction of α-globin expression, transcriptional silencing of ζ-globin gene expression, and the destabilization of ζ-globin mRNA are related and interdependent processes.

HIGH-LEVEL STABILITY OF HUMAN α-GLOBIN mRNA REFLECTS THE ASSEMBLY OF A SEQUENCE-SPECIFIC RNA-PROTEIN COMPLEX ON ITS 3′UTR

Expression of α-globin is initiated by transcriptional activation of the two, co-expressed α-globin loci, α1 and α2. Transcriptional silencing occurs mid-way though erythropoesis in the bone marrow. Globin mRNAs remain translationally active for an additional 4-6 days. Final clearance of all mRNAs is then effected in the circulating reticulocytes. Thus, considering the biology of erythroid differentiation and function, mRNA stability is a crucial determinant of α-globin gene expression.[5] The long half-life of α-globin mRNA, in excess of 16-24 hours, contributes economy to the bulk synthesis of the highly abundant α-globin and allows its continued synthesis during a prolonged transcriptionally-silent period in marrow and circulating reticulocytes.

The importance of mRNA stability to α-globin gene function is highlighted by the impact upon red cell development when this property is lost (FIG. 1). The most common form of nondeletional α-thalassemia is a single base substitution in the translation termination codon: UAA→CAA. This α^{CS} mutation, carried by millions of individuals in Southeast Asia, results in loss of 98% of expression from the affected gene. As the α^{CS} mutation is located at the dominant α2 locus, the effect on α-globin synthesis is particularly deleterious.[6] The deficit in expression from the α^{CS} locus can be traced to destabilization of the α^{CS} mRNA,[7,8,9] which results from entry of the ribosome into the α-globin mRNA 3′UTR.[9] This observation suggested to us that migrating ribosomes might interfere

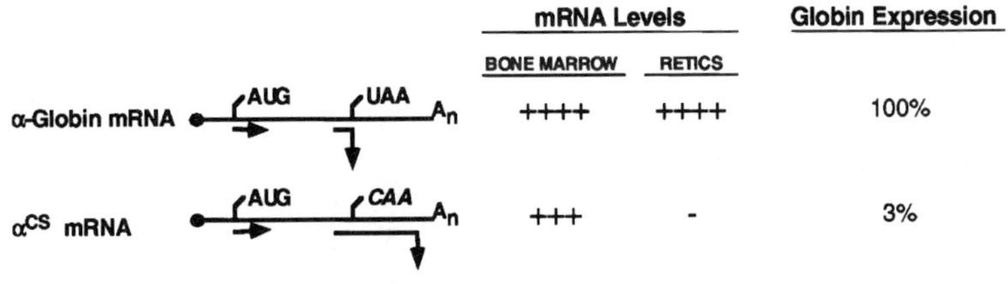

FIGURE 1. The Constant Spring mutation, α^{CS}, destabilizes α-globin mRNA. Levels of wild-type and CS mutant α-globin mRNA were measured in the transcriptionally active bone marrow and in reticulocytes which are several days posttranscriptional. The relative drop in concentration of the α^{CS} mRNA and the corresponding decrease in the level of α-globin gene expression from the α^{CS} locus reflects the instability of the α^{CS} mRNA.

with the structure and/or function of a stability determinant positioned in the normally ribosome-free 3′UTR.

We first attempted to map the borders and internal anatomy of the 3′UTR stability element using two technically independent approaches. In the first, a series of nonsense mutations were introduced into the 3′UTR of the α^{CS} mRNA which permitted ribosomes to enter defined distances into this region. Mutations positioned to permit the leading edge of the ribosome to disrupt the "stability determinant" should result in mRNA destabilization. This approach permitted clear demarcation of the 5′ border of the stability element.[9] A second experimental approach allowed a more detailed structural analysis of the stability element. Thirteen sets of base-substitutions ("linker scanning mutations") were introduced between the intact termination codon and the poly(A) addition site of wild-type α-globin mRNA. Each set of mutations was tested for its effect on mRNA stability.[10] These two mapping approaches gave mutually consistent results and identified a set of pyrimidine-pure, cytosine (C)-rich elements which appeared to be involved in stabilization of the α-globin mRNA.

We next asked whether the pyrimidine-rich stability element(s) within the 3′UTR functions *via* interaction with cytosolic protein factors.[11] Radioactive α-globin mRNA 3′UTRs were incubated in cytosolic extract from MEL cells and electrophoresed on a nondenaturing gel (electrophoretic mobility shift assay; EMSA). The UTRs were incorporated into an RNA-protein (RNP) complex which self-competed with α-3′UTR and was highly sensitive to competition by poly(C). In contrast, complex formation was not competed by high concentrations of a variety of unrelated mRNAs, tRNA, or the homoribopolymers poly(G), poly(A), and poly(U). These competition studies suggested that the mRNP complex, which we call the *α-complex*, is highly sequence-specific and contains one or more poly(C)-binding proteins.

The relevance of the α-complex to mRNA stability was tested using the set of linker-scanning mutations in the 3′UTR for which we knew the stability phenotype (see above). The stability of α-globin mRNA containing these mutations correlated perfectly with their ability to assemble an α-complex. From these data we concluded that the α-complex was relevant to α-globin mRNA stability.[11]

The protein composition of the α-complex was assessed by RNA affinity chromatography. The α-globin 3′UTR was fixed to a solid matrix and was incubated with metabolically labeled cytosolic proteins (S100 extract). After repeated washing, the retained proteins were eluted with a high-salt buffer and analyzed by SDS-PAGE. Three bands were identified, corresponding to proteins with apparent molecular weights of 39, 41, and 43 kDa.[11] The 39 kDa protein was identified as a poly(C) binding protein by its capacity to bind radioactive poly(C). This component was subsequently purified and its cognate full-length cDNAs were isolated based upon partial peptide sequence.[12] Characterization of the protein sequences and corresponding cDNAs indicated that the 39 kDa band contained two highly similar but distinct poly(C) binding proteins subsequently named αCP1 and αCP2. These proteins have an 87% structural identity and each contains three repeats of a 60 amino acid RNA-binding motif, the KH domain, found in a subset of RNA binding proteins (FIG. 2). To directly prove that αCP1 and αCP2 were involved in α-complex assembly, the cloned αCP cDNAs were expressed in transfected cultured cells, and S100 cytosolic extracts from these transfected cells were incubated with an α3′UTR probe. The αCP proteins were then specifically immunoprecipitated and the mRNAs which co-precipitated were analyzed. The αCP1 and αCP2 immunoprecipitations each brought down the α-globin mRNA probe in a sequence-specific manner.[12] These data demonstrated that both αCP proteins can incorporate into the α-complex. Whether both are present in the same α-complex or are mutually redundant in complex assembly is not known.

Since much of our work on human α-globin mRNA stability was carried out in mouse cells, we hypothesized that the mouse (m) α-globin mRNA should share the 3′UTR

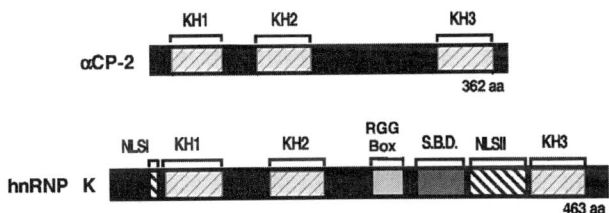

FIGURE 2. The αCP protein contains three repeats of the cannonical KH RNA-binding domain. The structure of the αCP-2 protein is shown.[12] The positions of the three repeats of the 50 amino acid KH domain are noted. Below this is a diagram of the index protein for which the KH domain was named; hnRNP K. The hnRNP K contains, in addition to the three KH domains, two separate nuclear localization signals, NLS I and II, a SH3-binding domain, and a second type of RNA interaction motif, the RGG box.[24,25]

polypyrimidine stability motif. The mα-globin mRNA 3'UTR contains a pyrimidine-rich region with remarkable structural conservation to the counterpart human sequence. Furthermore, these regions appear to subserve the same stability function: mutation of the mα-globin mRNA in this region results in its destabilization in transfected cells.[13] The mα-3'UTR also assembles an RNP complex when incubated with cytosolic S100 extract. Surprisingly, however, the mα-complex and the hα-complexes are distinct when compared by EMSA and by cross competition studies. In addition, the C-rich hα-globin 3'UTR (repeating motif of CCUCCC) is replaced in the mα-3'UTR by a more equal distribution of C and U. In parallel with these differences, αCP is replaced by a somewhat larger (45 kDa) poly(CT) binding protein in the mα-complex. Thus, a shift in the exact sequence of the 3'UTR polypyrimidine track between mouse and human is matched by a shift in the composition of the 3'UTR RNP complex. Remarkably, this parallel evolution of *cis* and *trans* components appears to have maintained stabilizing function.[13]

The proteins which form the α-complex are ubiquitous, suggesting that they may interact with a wide spectrum of mRNAs, affecting their stability and/or function. To test this possibility, we mapped the minimal binding domain for the α-complex within the α-globin 3'UTR and used this 20 base sequence to identify conserved sequences in other 3'UTRs.[14] This search revealed three additional, nonglobin mRNAs: 15-lipoxygenase, α1-collagen, and tyrosine hydroxylase. All three of these mRNAs are highly stable; moreover, pyrimidine rich motifs in the 3'UTR of each have been implicated in mRNA function or stability (FIG. 3). Remarkably, each of these 3' UTRs assembled an RNP complex which included the 39 kDa αCP. Thus, the α-complex, or a set of closely related complexes, appears to have a wide role in stabilization of mRNAs, including human α-globin.

THE EMBRYONIC HUMAN ζ-GLOBIN GENE UNDERGOES DEVELOPMENTAL SILENCING INITIATED BY AN ELEMENT IN THE 3' FLANKING REGION

In parallel with the migration of erythropoesis from the yolk sac to the fetal liver, the embryonic globin genes, ζ and ε, are selectively silenced. Expression from the embryonic genes is replaced by expression from the fetal/adult α-globin genes and the fetal γ-globin genes, respectively. We and others have demonstrated that ζ-globin gene silencing is gene-autonomous, *i.e.*, that downregulation of ζ-globin gene expression is independent of its location within the α-globin gene cluster and is not influenced by competition with adjacent α-globin genes.[15–19] This property permitted us to introduce the isolated human

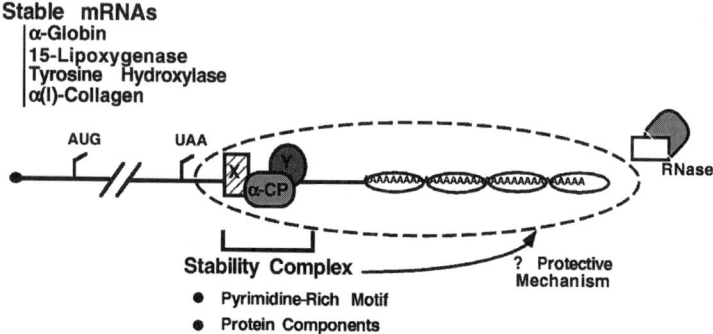

FIGURE 3. Four distinct mRNAs share common elements of a 3'UTR stabilizing RNP complex. The four stable mRNAs sharing a 3' UTR stability determinant are listed above the diagram. Below this is a diagram of a 3'UTR containing an assembled RNP complex. The 4 complexes all contain αCP protein. This complex is shown protecting the 3' polyA tail from a hypothetical RNase.

(h) ζ-globin gene, and potentially informative derivatives, into the mouse genome to study hζ-globin gene expression during development.[16] The intact hζ-globin gene, with 500 bp of 5' flanking sequences and 2.2 kb of 3' flanking sequences expresses ζ-globin mRNA at high levels in E9.5 yolk sac erythroblasts, but is downregulated more than 50-fold in definitive E16.5 fetal liver erythroblasts (FIG. 4). Thus silencing of the hζ-globin gene with limited 5' flanking sequences and an extended 3' flanking sequence is appropriate and gene-autonomous in the transgenic mouse.

To identify *cis* elements important to ζ-globin gene silencing, we introduced truncations into the 3' flanking region of the ζ-globin transgene, and synthesized additional chimeric transgenes comprising segments of the hζ-and hα2-globin genes.[16] The results of these

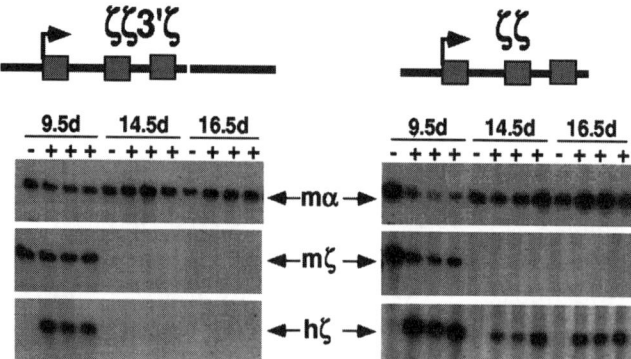

FIGURE 4. Developmental silencing of the human ζ-globin gene depends on a determinant within the 3' flanking region. The structure of the ζ-globin gene containing its promoter, transcribed region with three exons, and 2.2 kb of 3' flanking sequences, is shown to the left and the same gene lacking the 3' flanking sequences is shown to the right. The autoradiographs are of RNase protection studies using probes specific for the detection of mα-, hζ-, and hα-globin mRNAs. The RNA samples are harvested from the 9.5 day embryonic yolk sac and the 14.5 and 16.5d fetal liver. It is evident that both the endogenous mζ and the hζ-transgene silence at the embryonic/fetal juncture and that this silencing is lost for the hζ-transgene with the deletion of its 3' flanking sequences.

studies were unexpected. The developmental expression profile of hα- and hζ-globin transgenes containing reciprocal exchanges of their promoters paralleled the identity of the respective genes. However, this effect was limited, and could not fully account for the total silencing observed for the intact ζ-globin gene. Other chimeric α/ζ-globin transgenes identified two additional determinants that had a more substantial effect on ζ-globin gene silencing. Removal of the 3′ flanking region significantly blunted ζ-globin gene silencing during fetal development (FIG. 4). mRNA transcribed from this truncated ζ-globin gene was normally processed at its 3′ terminal, suggesting that continued expression of the ζ-globin gene in fetal liver and adult marrow reflected loss of a silencing element. The silencing activity of the 3′-flanking region determinant appears to depend upon the identity of the gene promoter: substitution of the α- for the ζ-globin gene promoter diminishes the activity of the ζ3′ silencing element.[16] These data suggest a productive interaction between the 5′ promoter and 3′ flanking regions of the ζ-globin gene that is of importance in mediating its transcriptional silencing.

The putative silencer element 3′ to the hζ-globin gene has been mapped in transgenic mice by expression of derivative ζ-globin genes containing site-specific mutations (Z. Wang and S. Liebhaber, unpublished data). These studies have identified a 108 bp element located 1.5 kb 3′ to the poly(A) addition site that appears to function as a developmental silencer of the ζ-globin gene. The mechanism through which this element mediates transcriptional silencing is now under investigation.

DEVELOPMENTAL SILENCING OF THE hζ-GLOBIN GENE REFLECTS INSTABILITY OF THE ζ-GLOBIN mRNA IN FETAL/ADULT ERYTHROID CELLS

A second major determinant of ζ-globin gene silencing is located within the transcribed region. When the ζ-globin transcribed region is replaced by the corresponding α-globin transcribed region (bracketed by the intact ζ-globin promoter and full ζ-globin 3′ flanking region) gene silencing is reduced nearly 8-fold[16] (FIG. 5). We have investigated the basis for this effect by studying the kinetics of hζ- and hα-globin mRNA decay.

To determine the stability of hζ-globin mRNA in the fetal/adult period it was necessary to dysregulate ζ-globin gene transcriptional control to permit expression during these post-embryonic developmental stages. This was done in two independent ways, both of which resulted in appreciable levels of ζ-globin mRNA synthesis in the adult bone marrow. The first approach was to link the ζ-globin transcribed region to the α-globin promoter. The second was to delete the 3′-flanking region silencer element from the ζ-globin gene (see above). Both methods resulted in levels of ζ-globin mRNA in the adult bone marrow which could be easily detected. To determine the stability of ζ-globin mRNA encoded by these two genes, we compared the levels of ζ-globin mRNA in the bone marrow, the site of active transcription, and in the reticulocytes, cells that are several days post-transcriptional. A parallel study was carried out for the hα-globin mRNA. Levels of transgene mRNA were compared to levels of endogenous highly stable, mα-globin mRNA. This analysis indicated that hα-globin mRNA is as stable as mα-globin mRNA, while hζ-globin mRNA is four-fold less stable. Thus silencing of ζ-globin gene at the level of transcription is partial and is completed by rapid turnover of the residually-transcribed ζ-globin mRNA.[20]

Why is ζ-globin mRNA less stable than α-globin mRNA? Considering the importance of the 3′UTR to α-globin mRNA stability, we posited that differences in this region might underlay the distinct differences in α- and ζ-globin mRNA stabilities. This was tested by measuring the stability of α- and ζ-globin mRNAs in which the 3′UTRs had been

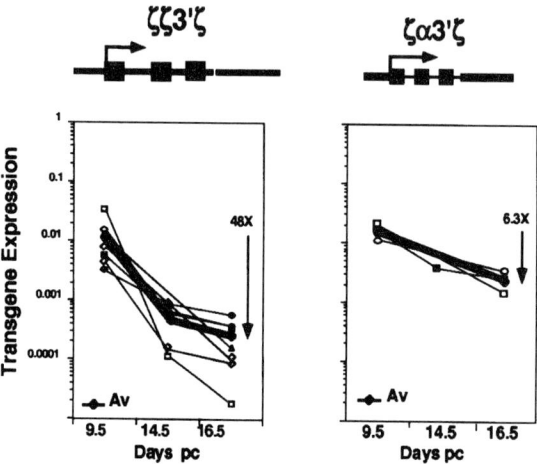

FIGURE 5. The developmental silencing of the ζ-globin gene is dependent on determinant(s) in the transcribed region. The structures of the ζ-globin gene (as in FIG. 4) and the same gene in which the transcribed region has been replaced with the corresponding region from the hα-globin gene. The developmental profiles of the two genes are shown in the graphs with the dates of RNA harvest shown at the bottom (as defined in FIG. 4). Each of several individual lines were studied and the mean of their values is shown by the heavy line. The fold silencing is shown to the right of each respective

exchanged. As predicted, substitution of the ζ-globin 3'UTR by the corresponding region of the hα-globin mRNA stabilized the ζ-globin mRNA. Reciprocally, substitution of the α-globin 3'UTR by the corresponding region of the ζ-globin mRNA was destabilizing. While the effect on mRNA stability was significant in both cases, it was not total, suggesting that additional unrecognized stability determinants may exist in one or both mRNAs.

The above data support the conclusion that the 3' UTR sequences are major determinants of α- and ζ-globin mRNA stability. We therefore asked whether the ζ-globin 3'UTR was able to assemble the α-complex. Considering its inability to exert a significant stabilizing function, we were surprised to observe by EMSA analysis that the ζ3'UTR could assemble an RNP complex with the identical mobility and sensitivity to poly(C) competition as the authentic α-complex. Nevertheless, the intensity of the complex was reproducibly less that of an α-complex assembled in parallel on the α-globin 3'UTR. To quantitate the abilities of the two 3'UTRs to assemble the α-complex, we measured their apparent dissociation constants. These data revealed a 6-fold lower apparent dissociation constant of the α-complex for the hα- than the hζ-globin 3'UTR. This was consistent with the relative intensities of the two reaction products on EMSA and was consistent with a greater effectiveness of the α-3'UTR to stabilize mRNA.

Alignment of the α- and ζ-globin 3'UTR sequences reveals a remarkable conservation in three polypyrimidine tracts encompassing the *cis* elements of the α-complex. There are, however, clear differences, including the relative position of the second tract, and a C→G transversion in the center of the major (third) tract of the ζ-globin 3'UTR. The relevance of this transversion to the observed difference in the stabilizing functions of the α- and ζ-globin 3'UTRs was tested by comparing the effect of this transverison on α-complex assembly. This substitution resulted in a major loss of complex activity on the α-3'UTR. These data suggest that the loss of stability of ζ-globin mRNA reflects one or more critical divergences from the sequence of the α-globin 3′UTR. The maintenance of the overall conservation in structure, however, suggests that this region may serve an unrecognized role, perhaps in the function or stability of the ζ-globin mRNA in the embryonic erythroid environment.

The mechanism of mRNA stabilization by the α-complex has been approached by asking whether there is a linkage to poly(A) tail kinetics.[21] In the case of the α^{CS} mutation we were able to demonstrate that destabilization of the α-globin mRNA was paralleled by an accelerated shortening of its poly(A) tail.[22] Similarly, comparison of the human α- and ζ-globin mRNAs revealed that the poly(A) tails on the less stable ζ-globin mRNA were significantly shorter than on the more stable α-globin mRNA.[20] These data suggest that the α-complex may mediate mRNA stabilization protection of the poly(A) tail. This finding is consistent with recent observations in yeast systems that poly(A) shortening can be the rate-limiting reaction in mRNA decay, triggering 5′ decapping and subsequent destabilization by 5′→3′ exonuclease digestion.[23] The mechanism through which the α-complex interacts with the poly(A) tail and controls the rate-limiting events in α-globin turnover is the subject of our current studies.

SUMMARY AND MODEL

The above studies suggest that the developmental control of the human α-globin gene cluster is a complex reaction involving mechanisms operating at both the transcriptional and posttranscriptional levels. The various components of this model are illustrated in FIGURE 6. Transcriptional silencing appears to be initiated soon after the ζ-globin gene is activated in the primitive erythroblasts in the embryonic yolk sac. This silencing is dependent on a developmentally regulated determinant located in the remote 3′ flanking region which interacts with the ζ-globin gene promoter. This transcriptional switch is incomplete, as ζ-globin gene transcription continues at low levels in the definitive fetal and adult ery-

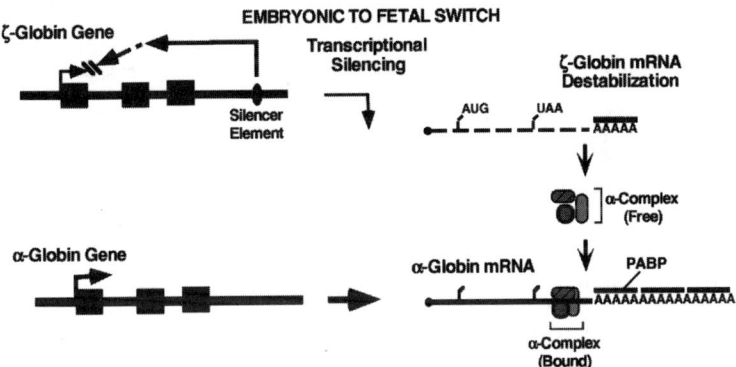

FIGURE 6. Model: Developmental silencing of the human ζ-globin gene is based on both transcriptional and post-transcriptional mechanisms. The ζ- and α-globin genes are diagrammed to the left. The promoter (*arrow*) and 3 exons (*filled boxes*) are indicated. The initial transcriptional silencing of the ζ-globin promoter is indicated by the interaction of the "Silencer Element" in the 3′ flanking region with the promoter. The ζ- and α-globin mRNAs are shown to the right of the diagram. Both mRNAs depend on the assembly of an RNP complex for their stability. The α-3′UTR has a higher affinity for this complex and hence "steals" the limiting cytosolic proteins from the ζ-globin mRNA. This "cross-talk" between the two mRNAs sets up a novel posttranscriptional mechanism for gene regulation (PABP = poly(A) binding protein).

throblasts. The ζ-globin mRNA transcribed during these later stages of development appears to be cleared post-transcriptionally. The accelerated clearance of ζ-globin mRNA reflects its relative instability, which is attributed to a minor sequence divergence in 3'UTR elements when compared to the corresponding region in the α-globin mRNA. This sequence difference permits the α-globin 3'UTR to compete more avidly for α-complex assembly and achieve a higher level of stability than ζ-globin mRNA. During the embryonic-to-fetal transition, induction of α-globin gene transcription and reciprocal down-regulation of ζ-globin gene transcription results in a dramatic switch in the cytoplasmic levels of the two mRNAs. This process presents the cytoplasm with elevated levels of the high affinity α3'UTR, which efficiently competes limiting α-complex components from the low-affinity ζ3'UTR. Hence, cross-talk between the two mRNAs serves as a reinforcing mechanism to complete the gene silencing which is transcriptionally initiated. Much of this model is hypothetical and will require further study for confirmation.

REFERENCES

1. LIEBHABER, S.A. 1989. α-Thalassemia: A review. Hemoglobin **13**: 685–731.
2. HIGGS, D. R., M. A. VICKERS, A. O. WILKIE, I. M. PRETORIOUS, A. P. JARMAN & D. J. WEATHERALL. 1989. A review of the molecular genetics of the human α-globin gene cluster Blood **73**: 1081–1104.
3. ALDITAR, M., F. E. CASH, C. PESCHLE & S. A. LIEBHABER. 1992. Developmental switch in the relative expression of the α1- and α2-globin genes in humans and in transgenic mice. Blood **79**: 2471–2474.
4. LIEBHABER, S. A., X. WANG, M. KILEDJIAN & I. M. WEISS. 1995. Cis and trans control of globin mRNA stability. In Proceedings of the 9th Conference on Hemoglobin Switching **31**: 375–389.
5. RUSSELL, J. E., J. MORALES & S. A. LIEBHABER. 1997. The role of mRNA stability in human globin gene expression. In Nucleic Acid Research and Molecular Biology. **57**: 259–287.
6. LIEBHABER, S. A., F. E. CASH, & S. K. BALLAS. 1986. Human α-globin gene expression: the dominant role of the α2-locus in mRNA and protein synthesis. J. Biol. Chem. **261**: 15327–15333.
7. LIEBHABER, S. A. & Y. W. KAN. 1981. Differentiation of the mRNA transcripts originating from the α1- and α2-globin genes in normals and alpha-thalassemics. J. Clin. Invest. **68**: 439–446.
8. HUNT, D. M., D. R. HIGG, P. WINICHAGOON, J. B. CLEGG & D. J. WEATHERALL. 1982. Haemoglobin Constant Spring has an unstable alpha chain messenger RNA. Brit. J. Haem. **51**: 405–413.
9. WEISS, I. M. & S. A. LIEBHABER. 1994. Erythroid-cell specific determinants of α-globin mRNA stability. Mol. Cell. Biol. **14**: 8123–8132.
10. WEISS, I. M. & S. A. LIEBHABER. 1995. Erythroid-cell specific mRNA stability elements in the α2-globin 3' untranslated region. Mol. Cell. Biol. **15**: 2457–2465.
11. WANG, X., M. KILEDJIAN, I. M. WEISS & S. A. LIEBHABER. 1995. Detection and characterization of a 3' untranslated region ribonucleoprotein complex associated with human α-globin mRNA stability. Mol. Cell. Biol. **15**: 1769–1777.
12. KILEDJIAN, M., W. WANG & S. A. LIEBHABER. 1995. Identification of two KH domain proteins in the α-globin mRNP stability complex. EMBO J. **14**: 4357–4364.
13. WANG, X. & S. A. LIEBHABER. 1996. Complementary change in cis determinants and trans factors in the evolution of an mRNP stability complex. EMBO J. **15**: 5040–5051.
14. HOLCIK, M. & S. A. LIEBHABER. 1997. RNP complexes sharing cis and trans components assemble at the 3'UTR of four highly stable mRNAs. Proc. Natl. Acad. Sci. **94**: 2410–2414.
15. ALBITAR, M., M. KATSUMATA & S. A. LIEBHABER. 1991. Human α-globin genes demonstrate autonomous developmental regulation in transgenic mice. Mol. Cell Biol. **11**: 3786–3794.
16. LIEBHABER, S. A., Z. WANG, F. E. CASH, B. MONKS & J. E. RUSSELL. 1996. Developmental silencing of the embryonic ζ-globin gene: concerted action of promoter and 3' flanking region combined with stage-specific silencing by the transcribed segment. Mol. Cell. Biol. **16**: 2637–2646.
17. SABATH, D. E., E. A. SPANGLER, E. M. RUBIN & G. STAMATOYANNOPOULOS. 1993. Analysis of the human ζ-globin gene promoter in transgenic mice. Blood **82**: 2899–2905.

18. SHARPE, J. A., D. J. WELLS, E. WHITELAW, P. VYAS, D. R. HIGGS & W. G. WOOD. 1993. Analysis of the human α-globin gene cluster in transgenic mice. Proc. Natl Acad. Sci. **90**: 11262–11266.
19. SPANGLER, E. A., K. A. ANDREWS & E. M. RUBIN. 1991. Developmental regulation of the human zeta-globin gene in transgenic mice. Nucl. Acids Res. **18**: 7093–7097.
20. RUSSELL, J. E., J. MORALES, A. MAKEYEV & S. A. LIEBHABER. 1998. Sequence divergence in the 3′ untranslated regions of human ζ- and α-globin mRNAs mediates a difference in their stabilities and contributes to efficient α-to-ζ-gene developmental switching. Mol. Cell. Biol. **18**: 2173–2183.
21. JACOBSON, A. & S. W. PELTZ. 1996. Interrelationships of the pathways of mRNA decay and translation in eukaryotic cells. Annu. Rev. Biochem. **65**: 693–739.
22. MORALES, J., J. E. RUSSELL & S. A. LIEBHABER. 1997. Destabilization of human α-globin mRNA by anti-termination is controlled during erythroid differentiation and is paralleled by phased shortening of the poly(A) tail. J. Biol. Chem. **272**: 6607–6613.
23. BEELMAN, C. A & R. PARKER. 1995. Degradation of mRNA in eukaryotes. Cell **81**: 179–183.
24. MATUNIS, M. J., W. M. MICHAEL & G. DREYFUSS. 1992. Characterization and primary structure of the poly(C)-binding heterogeneous nuclear ribonucleoprotein complex K protein. Mol. Cell. Biol. **12**: 164–171.
25. SIOMI, H., M. J. MATUNIS, W. M. MICHAEL & G. DREYFUSS. 1993. The pre-mRNA binding K protein contains a novel evolutionarily conserved motif. Nucl. Acids Res. **21**: 1193–1198.

Transcriptional Factors for Specific Globin Genes[a]

J. J. BIEKER,[b] L. OUYANG, AND X. CHEN

Mount Sinai School of Medicine, Brookdale Center for Molecular Biology, One Gustave L. Levy Place, New York, New York 10029, USA

ABSTRACT: Correct temporal control of the ß-like globin cluster is generated in part by the binding of tissue-restricted transcriptional regulators to their cognate sites. Erythroid Krüppel-like Factor (EKLF) is one of these red cell-specific activators that is particularly important for switching on adult β-globin gene expression. However, its simple presence is not sufficient to activate the β-globin promoter, as primitive erythroid cells and a number of erythroid cell lines express EKLF yet do not express adult ß-globin. One explanation that may account for these observations is that post-translational modification of EKLF differs within these cell populations. To address this issue, we are investigating whether phosphorylation plays a role in modulating EKLF activity. *In vitro* and *in vivo* approaches have been used to demonstrate that EKLF is a phosphoprotein whose ability to bind DNA and transcriptionally activate an adjacent promoter is critically dependent on its phosphorylation status. Of particular interest is a casein kinase II site within the EKLF minimal transactivation domain.

The correct regulation of gene expression relies on the combinatorial interplay between cell-restricted and generally-expressed transcription factors.[1,2] Such protein-protein interactions can be modified by secondary changes in any individual component.[3] In addition, these events occur within the context of chromatin, where structural constraints, and their attendant modulators, add yet another layer of potential cellular control points for regulation.[4,5]

All of these issues come into play when studying the transcriptional control of the ß-like globin cluster, as the globins combine tissue-specificity with developmentally regulated switching in expression.[6,7] At a primary level, the identification of tissue-specific DNA binding proteins that direct globin transcription have begun to illuminate the molecular mechanisms that establish and maintain this process.[8]

One of these tissue-specific regulators is Erythroid Krüppel-like Factor (EKLF). EKLF is a zinc finger DNA binding protein that interacts with the CACCC element in the adult β-globin promoter and, through its proline-rich transactivation domain, directs high-level expression of β-globin expression.[9,10] Its interaction with the adult ß-globin CACCC element is quite specific,[11] as EKLF does not interact well with the closely-related bh1/γ CACCC element and is thereby implicated as a potential globin switching factor.[12] Consistent with this idea, genetic ablation of EKLF leads to profound β-thalassemia and embryonic lethality yet leaves expression of yolk sac β-like globins unaffected.[13,14] In addition, EKLF expression is critical for consolidating the switch from fetal to adult globin and for generating an open chromatin structure around the adult β-globin transcription unit.[15,16]

However, a paradox that has emerged from these and other EKLF studies is that it is expressed within erythropotential tissues and cell lines that do not produce adult β-globin. For example, murine EKLF is first expressed during development within the blood islands of the day 7.5 embryo, which produce primitive erythroid cells that only express the

---

[a]This work was supported by a fellowship from the Cooley's Anemia Foundation to XC, and by PHS Grant DK46865 to JJB, who is a Scholar of the Leukemia Society of America.
[b]Corresponding author: Tel: 212-241-4143; Fax: 212-860-9279 E-mail: jbieker@smtplink.mssm.edu

embryonic globins.[17] EKLF is then expressed later in the fetal liver, where it helps generate optimal adult β-globin expression within the definitive erythroid cell compartment. Translational regulation cannot account for this difference in effect, as EKLF protein is present in both primitive and definitive erythroid populations.[17] To address whether post-translational modification may be playing a role in differential EKLF activity, we investigated whether changes in EKLF phosphorylation alters its DNA binding or transactivational properties *in vitro* and *in vivo*.

RESULTS

Our previous studies had demonstrated that the EKLF transactivation region contains subdomains that are important for both inter- and intra-molecular interactions.[10,18] We had postulated that phosphorylation might play a role in either/both of these processes (FIG. 1). Because there are a number of potential phosphorylation sites in both the minimal activation and the inhibitory subdomains,[19] we were interested in determining if this is indeed the case. As a result, we directed our attention towards the proline-rich transactivation region of EKLF, rather than towards its zinc finger domain.

To begin our analyses, we addressed whether the phosphorylation status of EKLF affects its DNA binding function. We transiently transfected COS cells with pSG5/EKLF,[9] which expresses the full-length EKLF product, or with pSG5/Δpro,[10] which synthesizes only the zinc finger domain. Upon comparison with extracts from pSG5-transfected COS cells, gel shift assays with the β-globin CACCC element probe reveals a new, fast-migrating shift uniquely present in the extracts from EKLF-expressing cells. A portion of each of these extracts was treated with calf intestine phosphatase prior to the gel shift assay. The results show that the zinc finger domain is unaffected by this treatment; however, the full-length product is adversely affected by phosphatase treatment. We conclude that the phosphorylation status of EKLF has a direct affect on its ability to bind DNA, and that this effect is localized to the proline-rich transcriptional activation domain.

We next wished to assess which amino acid might be the primary EKLF target(s) for the putative MEL kinase. Extracts were prepared from uninduced MEL cells and from cells at 24, 48, and 72 hours post-HMBA induction. In addition, extracts were prepared from CV1 cells that had been transfected with pSG5 or with pSG5/EKLF. Proteins were

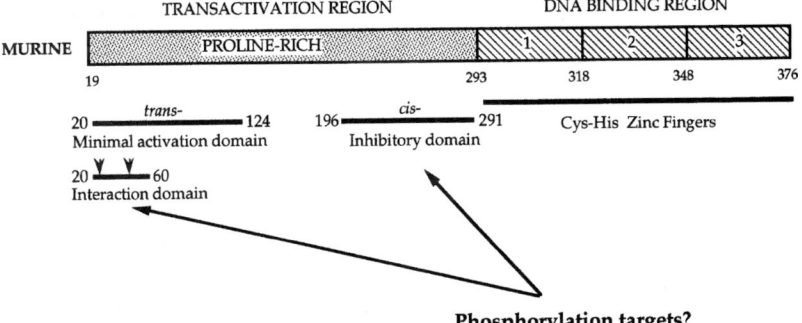

FIGURE 1. Domain map of murine EKLF. This schematic summarizes the locations along the linear EKLF amino acid sequence of DNA binding, activation, and inhibitory domains that were mapped by *in vivo* and *in vitro* functional studies.[9,10,18] Locations of potential phosphorylation target sites are also indicated. Arrows within the interaction domain show the positions of the two site-directed mutants discussed in the text.

resolved by SDS-PAGE and probed with an anti-phosphotyrosine antibody. Although there are a number of reactive proteins in these extracts, none of them comigrate with EKLF. As an additional test, the extracts were immunoprecipitated with the anti-phosphotyrosine antibody and the precipitated proteins were resolved by electrophoresis and probed with the anti-EKLF antibody. Again, no EKLF-reactive band was seen. These results suggest that tyrosine may not be the amino acid that is the primary target for the MEL kinase.

The alternate target would be serine and/or threonine. If modification of these residues is prevented, one prediction would be that globin expression would be directly affected, since de-phosphorylated EKLF has a much lowered affinity for its site, and since EKLF is a necessary component for inducing high levels of β-globin.[13,14] To address this issue, MEL cells were treated at a non-toxic concentration with H7, which is a serine/threonine kinase inhibitor.[20] These cells were then induced with HMBA, and hemoglobin synthesis was monitored at 24, 48, 72, and 96 hours post-induction. The results show that hemoglobin synthesis is extensively delayed, such that at 48 hours, these cells still present no evidence of hemoglobin synthesis, whereas the untreated controls are 36% hemoglobin positive. This data implicates serine/threonine kinases as important players in terminal differentiation of MEL cells, consistent with the prediction above. However, these experiments do not directly implicate EKLF in this type of control.

To obtain more direct evidence for involvement of serine/threonine kinase(s) in EKLF function, we compared the murine and human EKLF amino acid sequences,[21] particularly within the minimal transactivation domain, in search of conserved kinase target sequences. This uncovered a threonine within one consensus casein kinase II (CKII) site (TQE/DD) located 23 residues from the amino terminus (FIG. 2). The importance of this sequence was tested in two ways. Both tests relied on construction of a mutated derivative at this site within the mouse gene, converting $TQED_{44}$ to $TQAG_{44}$ by site-directed mutagenesis (numbering of the mouse gene is based on the initiator methionine as aa 19). One test, already published,[18] utilized an *in vivo* competition assay which demonstrated that increasing amounts of wild-type EKLF could compete with a positive-acting factor for transcription of a reporter in the 32DEpo1 erythropotential cell line. This competitive effect was localized to the amino terminal 40 amino acids of EKLF, a region containing the putative CKII site. Importantly, the competitive ability of this fragment was lost when the site-directed mutant described above ($TQAG_{44}$) was used for these experiments. However, other site directed mutants (*e.g.*, $SAET_{24}$ to $SAAG_{24}$) still retained their competitive ability.

The second functional test was performed by cotransfection of the GAL/EKLF chimeric activator with the pG5BCAT reporter into 32DEpo1 cells. This reporter is extensively activated by GAL/EKLF, and only slightly affected by a derivative that contains the

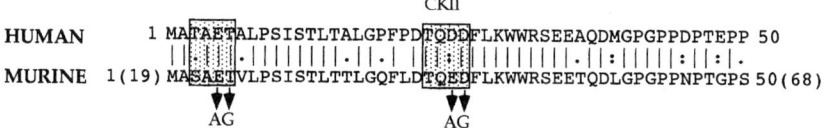

FIGURE 2. Comparison of human and murine EKLF amino acid sequences within the minimal activation domain. The homology within the first 50 amino acids is shown,[9,21] as is the putative CKII site and the site-directed mutations used for the analyses described in the text.

$SAAG_{24}$ mutation. However, the $TQAG_{44}$ mutation completely abolishes its transcriptional activity. We conclude from these two tests that the putative CKII site located 23 residues from the amino terminus is critically important both for protein-protein interactions and for efficient transcriptional activation. These data also more directly implicate an important role for serine/threonine kinase(s) in EKLF function, particularly within its minimal transcriptional activation domain.

We next utilized a number of approaches to determine if CKII might be responsible for modulating EKLF activity. Our substrate for the *in vitro* experiments was HIS-tagged EKLF that was affinity purified to homogeneity. The ability of MEL extracts to phosphorylate this substrate was tested in two ways. First, in solution we found that the MEL extract contains a kinase activity that phosphorylated EKLF. Second, we used an in-gel kinase assay as a means to direct our attention to potential kinase activities. In the in-gel kinase assay,[22] the polyacrylamide gel is made in the presence of EKLF. MEL extracts were then electrophoresed through this gel, and kinase activities *in situ* were determined by incubation with labeled ATP after renaturation. The data demonstrate that there are a number of discrete activities of various molecular weights that are able to phosphorylate EKLF. Of particular interest was the one at ~40,000 MW, a size that corresponds to the catalytic α subunit of CKII.[23] Appearance of this band is selectively inhibited by heparin, a known inhibitor of CKII.[24] In addition, the band comigrates with purified CKIIα. From this data we felt that MEL extracts contain CKII, and that this is one of the kinases that is able to modify EKLF.

Further characterization of this activity was performed in solution using purified EKLF and CKII. By optimizing the reaction conditions, we found that a 5′ incubation with 25 units was sufficient for efficient phosphorylation of EKLF. To further demonstrate a potential interaction between these two molecules in MEL cells, a "pull-down" experiment, using the HIS-tag of HIS/EKLF, was performed by incubating purified HIS/EKLF with MEL extract. We found that CKII from the extract could coprecipitate with HIS-EKLF. These and the previous results demonstrate that EKLF is a substrate for MEL-derived CKII.

Finally, to garner evidence that CKII has a functional effect on EKLF, we cotransfected 32DEpo1 cells with pG5BCAT reporter, GAL/EKLF(20-124) which contains the minimal transcriptional activation subdomain (aa 20-124)[18], and varying amounts of a CKIIα-expressing plasmid (25). We found that reporter levels, which are already active in these cells in the presence of GAL/EKLF(20-124), were additionally increased up to four-fold depending on the amount of cotransfected CKII. From these data we conclude that the primary effect of CKII on EKLF is to increase its transcriptional activity, likely through its interaction with the minimal transactivation domain which contains the putative CKII site described earlier.

DISCUSSION

EKLF is a transcriptional activator whose function is crucial for generating optimal levels of β-globin transcription in the erythroid cell.[9] Part of the specificity of this effect resides within its zinc fingers, which readily discriminate amongst various closely-related CACCC elements.[11,26] However, the transactivation domain is another potential target for EKLF functional control. Our previous deletion and mutagenic analyses revealed that this 270 amino acid region contains stimulatory and inhibitory subdomains.[18] The possibility that these opposite effects can be modulated post-transcriptionally arises when one considers that potential phosphorylation target sites reside within both of these subdomains. Our present study suggests that the phosphorylation status of EKLF effects its DNA binding and transactivational activity. EKLF is thus one of a large number of transcription factors that are regulated by phosphorylation.[3]

The effects of modification status on EKLF DNA binding, however, are not typical of most transcription factors, as dephosphorylated EKLF does not bind well to its target site. In this sense, it behaves more like p53, whose conformation and activity is modified by phosphorylation.[27] Whether phosphorylation of the EKLF inhibitory domain is involved in augmenting its DNA binding, and whether conformational changes lead to such effects have not been addressed by the present studies.

However, what the present studies have uncovered is the potential importance of a putative casein kinase II site within the minimal activation domain. CKII is a ubiquitously expressed and highly conserved heterotetrameric enzyme that has been shown to modify the transcriptional activity of a number of transcription factors, including p53,[27] ATF,[28] and c-Jun.[29] Although our present studies have focused on CKII/EKLF interactions, there are numerous examples of transcriptional activation domains being modulated by interactions with other kinases, such as CREB,[30] c-Jun,[31,32] Elk-1,[33] and ATF-2.[34]

These analyses raise intriguing possibilities concerning the control of EKLF activity during a variety of differentiative processes. For example, even though EKLF protein levels remain unchanged after induction of MEL cells, changes in its phosphorylation status may be part of the cellular response to HMBA and other inducers of MEL terminal differentiation. In addition, the modification status of EKLF may be different in cells which contain EKLF yet do not express β-globin when compared to committed, definitive erythroid cells, such as is the case in primitive erythroblasts,[17] HEL cells,[21] and FDCP-mix cells.[35] Resolution of these issues will likely illuminate whether events that control the status of EKLF modification play any role in the control of β-globin gene switching during erythroid ontogeny.

REFERENCES

1. STRUHL, K. 1991. Mechanisms for diversity in gene expression patterns. Neuron **7:** 177–181.
2. TJIAN, R. & T. MANIATIS. 1994. Transcriptional activation: A complex puzzle with few easy pieces. Cell **77:** 5–8.
3. HUNTER, T. & M. KARIN. 1992. The regulation of transcription by phosphorylation. Cell **70:** 375–387.
4. WOLFFE, A. P. & D. PRUSS. 1996. Targeting chromatin disruption: Transcription regulators that acetylate histones. Cell **84:** 817–819.
5. FELSENFELD, G. 1996. Chromatin unfolds. Cell **86:** 13–19.
6. ORKIN, S. H. 1990. Globin gene regulation and switching: Circa 1990. Cell **63:** 665–672.
7. MARTIN, D. I. K., S. FIERING & M. GROUDINE. 1996. Regulation of ß-globin gene expression: Straightening out the locus. Curr. Opin. Gen. & Devel. **6:** 488–495.
8. ORKIN, S. H. 1995. Transcription factors and hematopoietic development. J. Biol. Chem. **270:** 4955–4958.
9. MILLER, I. J. & J. J. BIEKER. 1993. A novel, erythroid cell-specific murine transcription factor that binds to the CACCC element and is related to the *Krüppel* family of nuclear proteins. Mol. Cell Biol. **13:** 2776–2786.
10. BIEKER, J. J. & C. M. SOUTHWOOD. 1995. The Erythroid Krüppel-like Factor (EKLF) transactivation domain is a critical component for cell-specific inducibility of a β-globin promoter. Mol. Cell. Biol. **15:** 852–860.
11. FENG, W. C., C. M. SOUTHWOOD & J. J. BIEKER. 1994. Analyses of β-thalassemia mutant DNA interactions with erythroid Krüppel-like factor (EKLF), an erythroid cell-specific transcription factor. J. Biol. Chem. **269:** 1493–1500.
12. DONZE, D., T. M. TOWNES & J. J. BIEKER. 1995. Role of Erythroid Krüppel-like Factor (EKLF) in human γ- to β-globin switching. J. Biol. Chem. **270:** 1955–1959.
13. NUEZ, B., D. MICHALOVICH, A. BYGRAVE, R. PLOEMACHER & F. GROSVELD. 1995. Defective haematopoiesis in fetal liver resulting from inactivation of the EKLF gene. Nature (London) **375:** 316–318.

14. PERKINS, A. C., A. H. SHARPE & S. H. ORKIN. 1995. Lethal ß-thalassemia in mice lacking the erythroid CACCC-transcription factor EKLF. Nature (London) **375**: 318–322.
15. WIJGERDE, M., J. GRIBNAU, T. TRIMBORN, B. NUEZ, S. PHILIPSEN, F. GROSVELD & P. FRASER. 1996. The role of EKLF in human ß-globin gene competition. Genes & Devel. **10**: 2894–2902.
16. PERKINS, A. C., K. M. L. GAENSLER & S. H. ORKIN. 1996. Silencing of human fetal globin expression is impaired in the absence of the adult ß-globin gene activator protein EKLF. Proc. Natl. Acad. Sci., USA **93**: 12267–12271.
17. SOUTHWOOD, C. M., K. M. DOWNS & J. J. BIEKER. 1996. Erythroid Kruppel-like Factor (EKLF) exhibits an early and sequentially localized pattern of expression during mammalian erythroid ontogeny. Devel. Dyn. **206**: 248–259.
18. CHEN, X. & J. J. BIEKER. 1996. Erythroid Krüppel-like Factor (EKLF) contains a multifunctional transcriptional activation domain important for inter- and intramolecular interactions. EMBO J. **15**: 5888–5896.
19. KENNELLY, P. J. & E. G. KREBS. 1991. Consensus sequences as substrate specificity determinants for protein kinases and protein phosphatases. J. Biol. Chem. **266**: 15555–15558.
20. HIDAKA, H., M. WATANABE & R. KOBAYASHI. 1991. Properties and use of H-series compounds as protein kinase inhibitors. Meth. Enzymol. **201**: 328–339.
21. BIEKER, J. J. 1996. Isolation, genomic structure, and expression of human Erythroid Krüppel-like Factor (EKLF). DNA and Cell Biol. **15**: 347–352.
22. CAVIGELLI, M., F. DOLFI, F. X. CLARET & M. KARIN. 1995. Induction of c-fos expression through JNK-mediated TCF/Elk-1 phosphorylation. EMBO J. **14**: 5957–5964.
23. MEISNER, H. & M. P. CZECH. 1991. Phosphorylation of transcriptional factors and cell cycle dependent proteins by casein kinase II. Curr. Opin. Cell Biol. **3**: 474–483.
24. HATHAWAY, G. H., M. J. ZOLLER & J. A. TRAUGH. 1981. Identification of the catalytic subunit of casein kinase II by affinity labelling with 5'-p-fluorosulfonylbenzoyl adenosine. J. Biol. Chem. **256**: 11442–11446.
25. CZECH, M. P. 1991. Enhanced casein kinase II activity in COS-1 cells upon overexpression of either its catalytic or non-catalytic subunit. J. Biol. Chem. **266**: 14435–14439.
26. BIEKER, J. J. 1994. Role of Erythroid Krüppel-like Factor (EKLF) in erythroid-specific transcription. *In* Molecular Biology of Hemoglobin Switching. G. Stamatoyannopoulos, Ed. **1**: 231–241. Intercept, Ltd. Andover, MA.
27. HUPP, T. R. & D. P. LANE. 1994. Allosteric activation of latent p53 tetramers. Current Biol. **4**: 865–875.
28. WADA, T., T. TAKAGI, Y. YAMAGUCHI, H. KAWASE, M. HIRAMOTO, A. FERDOUS, M. TAKAYAMA, K. A. W. LEE, J. C. HURST & H. HANDA. 1996. Copurification of casein kinase II with transcription factor ATF/E4TF3. Nucl. Acids. Res. **24**: 876–884.
29. LIN, A., J. FROST, T. DENG, T. SMEAL, N. AL-ALAWI, U. KIKKAWA, T. HUNTER, D. BRENNER & M. KARIN. 1992. Casein Kinase II is a negative regulator of c-Jun DNA binding and AP-1 activity. Cell **70**: 777–789.
30. GONZALEZ, G. A. & M. R. MONTMINY. 1989. Cyclic AMP stimulates somatostatin gene transcription by phosphorylation of CREB at serine 133. Cell **59**: 675–680.
31. PULVERER, B. J., J. M. KYRIAKIS, J. AVRUCH, E. NIKOLAKAKI & J. R. WOODGETT. 1991. Phosphorylation of c-jun mediated by MAP kinases. Nature (London) **353**: 670–674.
32. BINETRUY, B., T. SMEAL & M. KARIN. 1991. Ha-Ras augments c-Jun activity and stimulates phosphorylation of its activation domain. Nature (London) **351**: 122–127.
33. MARAIS, R., J. WYNNE & R. TREISMAN. 1993. The SRF accessory protein Elk-1 contains a growth factor-regulated transcriptional activation domain. Cell **73**: 381–393.
34. LIVINGSTONE, C., G. PATEL & N. JONES. 1995. ATF-2 contains a phosphorylation-dependent transcriptional activation domain. EMBO J. **14**: 1785–1797.
35. HU, M., D. KRAUSE, M. GREAVES, S. SHARKIS, M. DEXTER, C. HEYWORTH & T. ENVER. 1997. Multilineage gene expression precedes commitment in the hemopoietic system. Genes & Devel. **11**: 774–785.

Silencing and Activation of Embryonic Globin Gene Expression

GORDON D. GINDER,[a-e] RAKESH SINGAL,[a,b] JANE A. LITTLE,[a,b,d] NANCY DEMPSEY,[a,b] RICHARD FERRIS,[a,b] AND SHOU ZHEN WANG[a,b,d]

[a]*Division of Oncology,* [b]*Department of Medicine,* [c]*Institute of Human Genetics, and* [d]*Cancer Center, University of Minnesota, Minneapolis, Minnesota, USA*

ABSTRACT: An understanding of the mechanisms that control developmental stage-specific transcription of globin genes offers the promise of successful therapeutic activation of fetal or embryonic β-type genes in β-thalassemia syndromes. A large body of evidence supports the notion of conservation of such mechanisms across vertebrate species and validates the use of pre-clinical studies of silencing and activation of fetal or embryonic globin genes in animals. Using globin gene transfections into primary avian erythroid cells and cultured murine erythroleukemia cells, we have studied mechanisms involved in stage-specific embryonic β-type globin gene silencing and activation. These studies show that 1) methylation of the exact CpG nucleotides that are methylated in normal adult erythroid cells *in vivo is* capable of blocking transcription of a transfected embryonic globin gene promoter via binding of a methyl DNA binding protein in primary erythroid cells. 2) Activation of embryonic β-type globin gene transcription in adult erythroid cells by short chain fatty acids is mediated through specific DNA sequences both in the promoter and downstream of the promoter.

The differential regulation of globin gene transcription in embryonic, fetal, and adult erythroid cells has provided an illuminating model of the mechanisms of developmental control of vertebrate gene expression and has direct relevance to potential molecular therapy of β-thalassemia syndromes.

Among the current models proposed to account for developmental β-type globin gene switching the two most accepted are one that emphasizes competition between embryonic/fetal and adult globin gene promoters for the activating effects of the locus control region (LCR) and one that emphasizes autonomous silencing of the embryonic β-type globin genes in adult erythroid cells. Much of the focus of the latter model has been on identifying specific *cis*-acting sequences required for autonomous silencing and the *trans*-acting nuclear factors that mediate these effects. However, both epigenetic modifications of DNA, specifically site-specific DNA methylation, and alterations in chromatin structure have long been implicated as having a role in the silencing and activation of embryonic globin genes. We report here results that support an important role for both

[e]Address correspondence to: Gordon D. Ginder, M.D., Professor of Internal Medicine and Human Genetics, Director, Massey Cancer Center, Virginia Commonwealth University, 401 College Street, P. O. Box 980037, Richmond, VA 23298-0037; Tel: (804) 828-0450; Fax: (804) 828-8853; E-mail: gginder@mcc1.mcc.vcu.edu

DNA methylation and chromatin protein acetylation in silencing transcription of embryonic β-type globin genes in two vertebrate animal model systems.

RESULTS

DNA Methylation within the Avian Embryonic ρ Gene Promoter Silences Transcription in Primary Erythroid Cells

An inverse correlation between site-specific DNA methylation and structural gene transcription was first described in the vertebrate globin genes.[1-3] Subsequently, animal model studies[4] and eventually clinical intervention trials were aimed at increasing fetal γ-globin gene expression and Hb-F levels in patients with β-thalassemia and sickle cell anemia by treatment with the DNA cytosine methyl transferase inhibitor and cytotoxic nucleoside analog, 5 azacytidine.[5,29] The evidence for a role for DNA methylation in silencing globin gene transcription *in vivo* has, perhaps, been most straight-forward in the case of embryonic β-type globin genes, including the avian ρ-globin gene.[6,7] We have examined the role and mechanism of physiologically correct DNA methylation in the silencing of the avian ρ globin gene in primary erythroid cells. The details of the methods used in these studies are published elsewhere.[8]

Analysis of CpG Methylation of the ρ-Globin Gene Promoter in Primitive (Embryonic) and Definitive (Adult) Erythroid Cells

The ρ-globin gene is highly expressed in 5-day embryonic red blood cells (RBC) but is completely silenced in adult RBC.[9] Using the bisulfite genomic sequencing method, the pattern of methylation of the 235 bp DNA fragment containing the ρ-gene promoter was determined in genomic DNA from both five-day embryonic and adult avian erythroid cells.

As shown in FIGURE 1, all CpG's in the minimal 235 bp promoter were unmethylated in five-day embryonic erythroid cells in which the gene is expressed and fully methylated in adult RBC's in which it is silenced.

Physiologically Correct Methylation of the ρ Gene Minimal Promoter Silences Transcription in Primary Erythroid Cells.

As described by Minie *et al.*[10] the major activity of the ρ-globin gene promoter resides in a minimal sequence of 246 bp immediately upstream from the transcription start site. This promoter is capable of conferring high-level, stage-specific transcription in primary avian erythroid cells, and all of the *trans*-acting factor binding sites identified in the ρ promoter are located in the first 230 bp from the transcription start site.

In order to test the ability of CpG methylation in the minimal ρ promoter to silence transcription, a 235 bp promoter DNA fragment was isolated and methylated at every CpG *in vitro*, using the bacterial Sss I DNA methyl transferase. This methylated fragment was then ligated into a chloramphenicol acetyl transferase (CAT) reporter gene construct containing a potent erythroid-specific enhancer consisting of 5′ hypersensitive sites (HSS) 2 and 3 from the avian β-type globin gene cluster. These HSS have been shown to be critical to high-level expression of the ρ gene in transgenic mice and in cell transfection assays.[11,12] Control experiments included construction of an identical expression vector with a mock methylated 235 bp ρ promoter and another construct with only the ρUC vector methylated at every CpG. As shown in FIGURE 2, methylation of the ρ promoter at the

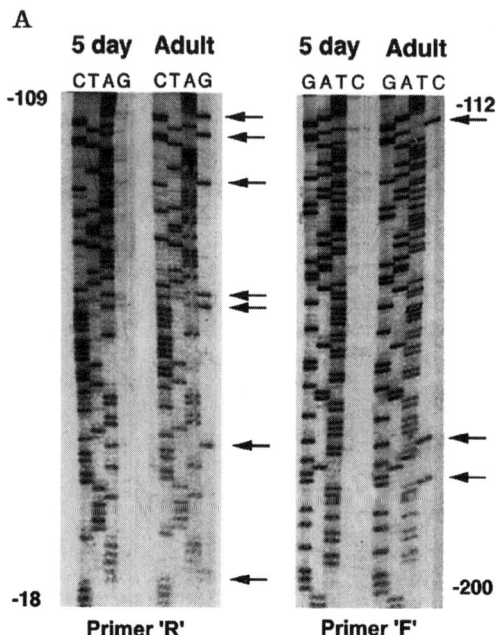

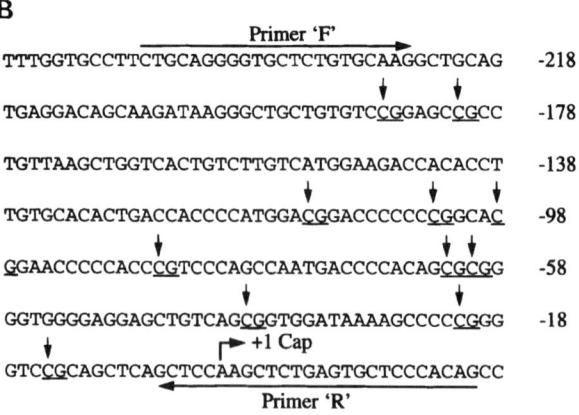

FIGURE 1. *In vivo* methylation of CpG dinucleotides of the ρ promoter in 5-day and adult chicken erythroid cells using the 'bisulfite conversion technique. Arrows indicate methylated cytosines. Positions indicated are relative to the transcription start site (**A**). Cytosines which are not associated with CpG dinucleotides (sequence shown in **B**) have all been converted to thymidines in both 5-day and adult erythroid cells. FIGURE 1B shows the ρ-globin gene promoter sequence. Arrows indicate methylated cytosines that are clearly seen in FIGURE 1A (data not shown for CpG dinucleotide at position -15). Primer 'R' and 'F' indicate the sequence of ρ globin gene promoter used for designing internal primers and for sequencing.

same sites that are methylated *in vivo* caused an ~20-fold decrease in expression in primary avian erythroid cells, while methylation of 157 CpGs in the vector alone had no effect. These data strongly support the notion that methylation of the ρ-gene promoter can cause a marked silencing of transcription even in the presence of a strong enhancer/LCR element in primary erythroid cells which contain all of the transacting factors needed to support very high levels of globin gene transcription.

The Methylated ρ-Gene Promoter Preferentially Binds to a Methyl DNA Binding Protein

Several mechanisms have been proposed to account for the repressive effect of DNA methylation upon transcription. One proposed mechanism is through direct interference with transcription factor binding by the methylated cytosine bases.[13] Examination of the ρ-gene promoter and detailed footprinting of the factors from primary erythroid cell nuclei that bind to them revealed only one putative binding site that contains a methylatable CpG dinucleotide within its recognition sequence.[10] This is a canonical SP-1 site, and SP-1 is one nuclear factor that has been shown to bind equally well to methylated or unmethylated cognate DNA recognition sequences.[14] This suggests that methylation of the ρ-gene promoter does not directly interfere with nuclear protein factor binding to the ρ-promoter DNA binding proteins and led us to investigate a possible indirect effect mediated by methylated DNA-specific binding proteins, such as those described by Bird and co-workers.[15–17] Of interest, the ρ minimal 235 bp promoter fits the criteria for CpG islands, which are CpG-rich DNA sequences generally found within or near the promoters of housekeeping-type genes. The methyl DNA binding protein, MeCP-1, has been shown to bind to methylated CpG islands containing at least 12 symmetrically methylated CpG's. MeCP-1 has been shown to block transcription of the human α globin gene promoter in cultured non-erythroid cells and in cell-free *in vitro* transcription assays.[16,17]

In order to test for the presence of MeCP-1 in primary avian erythroid cells, gel mobility shift assays were carried out using the proto-typical MeCP-1 binding target CG-11[15] as probe with methylated or unmethylated CG-11 DNA as the specific competitor. As

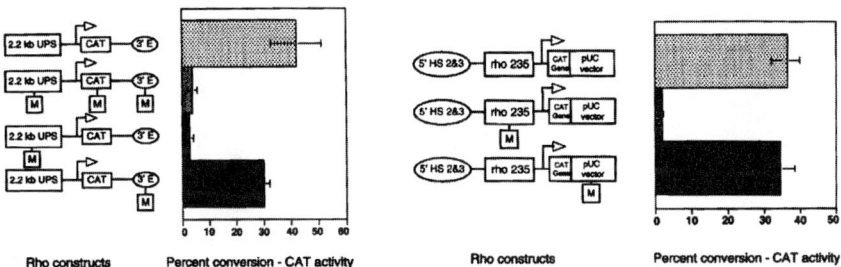

FIGURE 2. Levels of ρ-globin gene promoter activity in primary chicken erythroid cells transiently transfected with the methylated or mock methylated ρ-globin gene constructs depicted. Complete methylation of all CpGs in a particular region of a given construct is represented by attached 'M.' Each experiment was carried out in triplicate and levels of CAT conversion percentages presented represent the mean values and standard deviations. Methylation of an extended 2.2 kb upstream promoter resulted in significant reduction in promoter activity in the presence of the strong erythroid 3′ β/ε enhancer (*left panel*). Methylation of a 235 bp ρ-globin gene promoter also resulted in significant reduction in promoter activity even in the presence of the strong 5′ enhancer, which includes erythroid-specific hypersensitive sites 2 and 3, while methylation of the pUC vector alone had no effect (*right panel*).

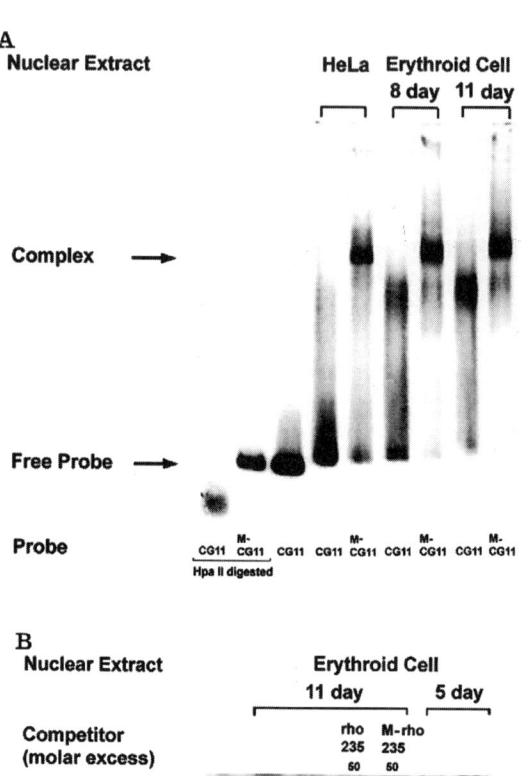

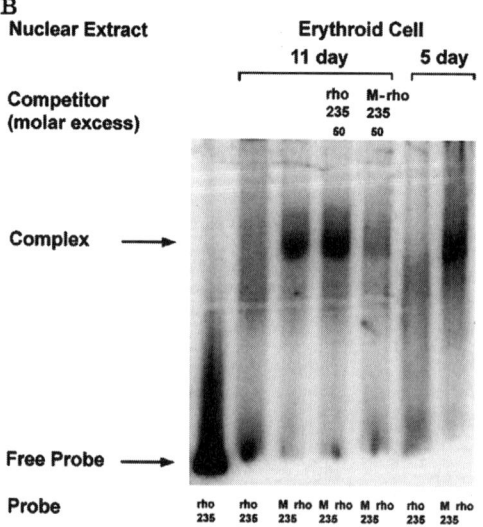

FIGURE 3. Mobility shift assay for the presence of MeCPC in chicken erythroid cell or control HeLa cell nuclear extracts. End-labeled, methylated CG11 probe (M-CG11) but not mock-methylated CG11 (CG11) forms a complex with erythroid cell nuclear extract that has similar mobility as the MeCP-1 complex seen with HeLa cell nuclear extract (**A**). Similar results were seen with 5-day chicken erythroid cell nuclear extract (data not shown). Panel **B** demonstrates binding of MeCPC in chicken erythroid cell nuclear extract to methylated ρ 235 (M-ρ 235) probe. End-labeled M-ρ 235 but not mock methylated ρ 235 forms a complex with erythroid cell nuclear extract. This complex was competed effectively by an excess of unlabeled methylated but not mock methylated ρ 235.

shown in FIGURE 3A, both 5-day and 11-day embryonic erythroid cells are capable of forming an MeCP-1-like complex with an identical mobility as the complex formed in HeLa cell extracts.[15]

To test for an analog of this methylated cytosine-specific DNA binding protein activity in the same primary erythroid cells used to demonstrate the silencing effect that CpG methylation exerted upon the ρ promoter, a similar binding assay was carried in which methylated or unmethylated ρ 235 bp promoter DNA was used as probe and as specific competitor. As shown in FIGURE 3B, only methylated ρ235 DNA bound a specific complex when incubated with nuclear extracts from primary primitive (5 day) and definitive (11 day) erythroid cells. Cold competitor experiments showed that methylated but not unmethylated ρ 235 DNA could compete for this binding complex, thus confirming the specificity of this binding activity for methylated ρ-gene promoter sequences and providing the first direct demonstration of such a methylated DNA-specific complex binding to an actual gene promoter sequence. We term this binding activity MeCPC for *M*ethyl *C*ytosine binding *P*rotein *C*omplex, since both its exact composition and its relationship to MeCP-1 has not been determined.

A Short-Chain Fatty Acid (SCFA) Response Element within the Murine Epsilon Y Minimal Promoter Mediates Increased Expression in Adult Phenotype Murine Erythroid Cells

The short-chain fatty acid, butyrate, was originally shown to be capable of inducing erythroid differentiation and increased adult globin gene mRNA in murine erythroleukemia (MEL) cells. Subsequently, butyrate was shown to be capable of inducing expression of normally silent embryonic β-type globin genes in adult erythroid cells in an avian animal model[6] and in murine cell culture.[19] In the case of the avian ρ globin gene, the effect of butyrate was shown to be sequence-specific and separable from the earlier reported effect on differentiation in MEL cells.[20] Short-chain fatty acids have also been shown to be capable of increasing expression of fetal β-type globin genes in animal models[21,22] and in patients with β-thalassemia.[23,24] Previously, we have reported that propionic acid is a potent inducer of murine embryonic epsilon Y gene expression in adult phenotype MEL cells.[19] In an attempt to define the promoter sequences involved in this activation of embryonic epsilon-Y gene in adult erythroid cells, deletion mutant constructs consisting of various lengths of epsilon-Y promoter driving a *neo*-gene were stably transfected into MEL cells. These cells were subsequently treated with either dimethyl sulfoxide (DMSO), which induces differentiation and increased endogenous adult β-globin expression but not endogenous embryonic epsilon-Y gene expression, or propionic acid, which induces both differentiation and expression of endogenous epsilon-Y.[19] As shown in FIGURE 4, DMSO did cause increased expression from the epsilon-Y promoter in reporter constructs containing between 900 bp and 210 bp of promoter sequence, in contrast to the lack of effect on the endogenous epsilon-Y gene.[19] This suggests that some of the sequences required for complete suppression of epsilon-Y transcription may be lacking in the epsilon-Y *neo*-constructs. However, propionic acid treatment resulted in a further two-to-threefold induction of epsilon-Y expression relative to expression of the endogenous constituitive triose phosphate isomerase (TPI) gene in all constructs that contained at least 210 bp of the epsilon-Y promoter. Those constructs containing only 145 bp of promoter were not inducible in this assay and had minimal detectable basal activity, although some small amount of basal expression can be inferred from the fact that these stable transfectants were viable under G-418 drug selection. These data are evidence for a 65 bp sequence element located between 210 bp and 145 bp from the epsilon-Y gene origin of

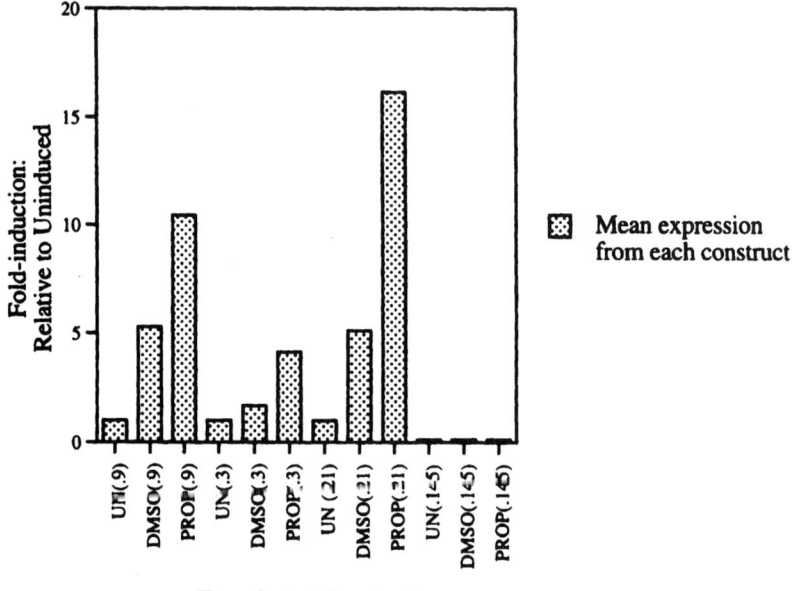

FIGURE 4. A 65 bp fragment of the embryonic epsilon γ globin gene promoter mediates preferential response to propionate. Recombinant constructs consisting of either 0.9 kb, 0.3 kb, 0.21 kb, or 0.145 kb of ε^Y promoter ligated into a *neo*-gene plasmid were stably transfected into MEL cells. After selection in G418 antibiotic, resistant cell pools were treated with either saline control (UN), 2% dimethyl sulfoxide (DMSO), or 5 mM propionic acid (Prop.). Cytoplasmic RNA was harvested and assayed for ε^Y RNase protection assay followed by quantitation on a Molecular Dynamics phosphorimager. For each assay ε^Y RNA levels were calculated relative to the level of expression of constitutively expressed triose phosphate isomerase RNA.

transcription that is able to mediate a preferential increase in embryonic epsilon-Y gene expression in adult phenotype MEL cells.

Examination of the potential nuclear protein binding sites within this 65 bp element responsible for the preferential induction of the embryonic epsilon-Y gene by propionate reveals cognate sites for the erythroid Krüppel-like factor EKLF[25] and the stage selector element (SSE).[26] DNA footprinting analysis of these sequences in the presence of nuclear extracts from control cells versus extracts from propionate-treated cells demonstrated DNA protein contacts at the adjacent EKLF and SSE binding sites that were induced by propionate (data not shown).

DISCUSSION

The mechanisms that control the developmental switching of globin gene transcription in vertebrates are both multiple and complex. The studies reported here have focused on mechanisms involving epigenetic and chromatin-mediated processes. In the case of the avian embryonic ρ globin gene it seems clear that DNA methylation is capable of exerting a dominant silencing effect on transcription even in the presence of potent erythroid

LCR/enhancer elements and in an optimum nuclear environment of erythroid-specific transcription factors. This could explain the observation that in both an avian animal model[6,7] and in yeast artificial chromosome mediated transgenic mouse models of human gamma globin gene regulation in the context of the entire β-globin locus,[27] the DNA methyl transferase inhibitor, 5 azacytidine, is required to obtain measurable transcription of embryonic β-type globin genes. However, neither chickens nor mice have fetal-specific erythroid development. The role of DNA methylation in silencing fetal γ-globin gene transcription is not likely as dominant and certainly not as complete given the fact that the γ-globin gene is normally expressed at up to 1-2% of the level of the β-globin gene in adults. This conclusion is also supported by the results of studies in which human γ globin gene constructs which were methylated and transfected into non-erythroid cells were incompletely silenced in the presence of a strong enhancer[16] although a fully methylated γ-globin gene was more completely silenced in non-erythroid cells in the absence of an enhancer.[28] The reason for the lesser effect of DNA methylation on γ-globin expression may be the lower density of CpG sites in the human γ-globin gene promoter.[17] As such, MeCP-1 or the analogous factor, MeCPC, which we detect in primary avian erythroid cells and which is likely responsible for the strong suppression of transcription of the methylated ρ-gene promoter, may not be able to bind effectively to the γ-globin gene promoter.[17] Nonetheless, DNA methylation has been implicated in negative regulation of primate fetal globin gene expression through studies demonstrating activation of these genes by 5-azacytidine.[4] Despite the uncertainty of the relative contribution of DNA methylation versus other mechanisms related to the cell cycle-specific actions of cytotoxic agents on hematopoietic progenitors, 5-azacytidine has been shown to cause therapeutic increases in γ-globin gene expression and, consequently, therapeutically elevated fetal hemoglobin levels in patients with β-thalassemia and sickle cell anemia.[5,29,30] A more important role for DNA methylation in the silencing of embryonic globin genes is likely based upon studies in animal models, such as those reported here and on those in transgenic mouse models of human embryonic and fetal β-type globin gene expression in adult erythroid cells.[27]

The precise mechanism(s) by which short-chain fatty acids (SCFA), such as butyrate and propionate, mediate increased expression of embryonic and fetal β-type globin gene transcription in adult erythroid cells remains to be determined. However, the demonstrated effect of these compounds in a range of animal models and humans suggests that highly evolutionarily conserved mechanisms exist. Studies in the avian globin gene system have shown that the effect is not due to bulk changes in histone acetylation or overall chromatin structure as determined by intermediate DNAase I sensitivity,[7,20,31,32] but rather that the effect is relatively sequence specific within the β-globin locus.[7,20] Similarly, studies of the human fetal γ-type globin genes in a transgenic animal model have revealed sequence-specific SCFA response elements.[33] Interestingly, there is yet to be identified a single consensus SCFA response sequence, and in the case of the γ-globin gene more than one response region has been identified in the same promoter and 5′ flanking sequences.[33]

The most well-documented effect of SCFA's, especially the prototype butyric acid, on cells is their ability to inhibit histone deacetylase activity.[34,35] Recent studies of the transcription factor complexes that bind to promoter activator and silencer sequences of a wide variety of promoters have revealed the presence of histone deacetylases (HDAC) in these complexes.[36-38] It appears that one or more histone deacetylases can associate with sequence-specific DNA binding protein(s) and mediate repressive effects on transcription by deacetylating the core histones that are in contact with transcription factor binding sequences, thus preventing the formation of a stable transcription initiation complex by rendering the histone-DNA contacts of nucleosomes tighter. Alternatively, the HDAC may deacetylate some other protein, acetylation of which is necessary for establishment of a transcription initiation complex. In either case association of HDAC with sequence-specific binding proteins is a plausible mechanism for the observed sequence specificity of the effect of SCFA's on globin gene transcription. Since HDAC have been found to bind to more than one type of sequence-specific DNA-binding protein complex, there is reason to expect the observed findings of more than one cis-sequence capable of mediating a stimulating effect of SCFA's on embryonic/fetal globin gene transcription, and transcription of other genes as well. A full elucidation of the factors involved in the stimulation of embryonic/fetal β-type globin gene expression by SCFA's could provide multiple molecular targets for therapeutic manipulation of globin gene expression in the thalassemia syndromes.

REFERENCES

1. MCGHEE, J. D. & G. D. GINDER. 1979. Specific DNA methylation sites in the vicinity of the chicken β-globin genes. Nature **280:** 418–420.
2. SHEN, C.-K. J. & T. MANIATIS. 1980. Tissue-specific DNA methylation in a cluster of rabbit (β-like globin genes. Proc. Natl. Acad. Sci.USA **77:** 6634–6638.
3. VAN DER PLOEG, L. H. & R. A. FLAVELL. 1980. DNA methylation in the human γ-δ-β-globin locus in erythroid and nonerythroid tissues. Cell **19:** 947–958.
4. DESIMONE, J., P. HELLER, L. HALL & D. ZWIERS. 1982. 5-Azacytidine stimulates fetal hemoglobin synthesis in anemic baboons. Proc. Natl. Acad. Sci. USA **79:** 4428–4431.
5. LEY, T., J. DESIMONE, N. P. ANAGNOU, G. H. KELLER, R. K. HUMPHRIES, P. H. TURNER, N. S. YOUNG, P. KELLER & A. W. NIENHUIS. 1982. 5-Azacytidine selectively increases γ-globin synthesis in a patient with β+ thalassemia. N. Engl. J. Med. **307:** 1469–1475.
6. GINDER, G. D., M. J. WHITTERS & J. K. POHLMAN. 1984. Activation of a chicken embryonic globin gene in adult erythroid cells by 5-azacytidine and sodium butyrate. Proc. Natl. Acad. Sci. USA **81:** 3954–3958.
7. BURNS, L. J., J. G. GLAUBER & G. D. GINDER. 1988. Butyrate induces selective transcriptional activation of a hypomethylated embryonic globin gene in adult erythroid cells. Blood **72:** 1536–1542.
8. SINGAL, R., R. FERRIS, J. A. LITTLE, S. Z. WANG & G. D. GINDER. 1997. Methylation of the minimal promoter of an embryonic globin gene silences transcription in primary erythroid cells. Proc. Natl. Acad. Sci. USA **94:** 13724–13729.
9. BROWN, J. L. & V. M. INGRAM. 1974. Structural studies on chick embryonic hemoglobins. J. Biol. Chem. **249:** 3960–3972.
10. MINIE, M. E., T. KIMURA & G. FELSENFELD. 1992. The developmental switch in embryonic ρ-globin expression is correlated with erythroid lineage-specific differences in transcription factor levels. Development **115:** 1149–1164.
11. MASON, M. M., E. LEE, H. WESTPHAL & M. REITMAN. 1995. Expression of the chicken β-globin gene cluster in mice: Correct developmental expression and distributed control. Mol. Cell. Biol. **15:** 407–414.
12. WANDERSEE, N. J., R. C. FERRIS & G. D. GINDER. 1996. Intronic and flanking sequences are required to silence enhancement of an embryonic β-type globin gene. Mol. Cell. Biol. **16:** 236–246.
13. BIRD, A. 1992. The essentials of DNA methylation. Cell **70:** 5–8.
14. JANE, S. M., D. L. GUMUCIO, P. A. NEY, J. M. CUNNINGHAM & A. W. NIENHUIS. 1992. The effect of DNA methylation on protein binding to the stage selector element of the γ-globin gene promoter. Blood **80:** 958
15. MEEHAN, R. R., J. D. LEWIS, S. MCKAY, E. L. KLEINER & A. P. BIRD. 1989. Identification of a mammalian protein that binds specifically to DNA containing methylated CpGs. Cell **58:** 499–507.
16. BOYES, J. & A. BIRD. 1991. DNA methylation inhibits transcription indirectly via a methyl-CpG binding protein. Cell **64:** 1123–1134.
17. BOYES, J. & A. BIRD. 1992. Repression of genes by DNA methylation depends on CpG density and promoter strength: Evidence for involvement of a methyl-CpG binding protein. EMBO J. **11:** 327–333.
18. LEDER, A. & P. LEDER. 1975. Butyric acid, a potent inducer of erythroid differentiation in cultured erythroleukemic cells. Cell **5:** 319–322.
19. LITTLE, J. A., N. J. DEMPSEY, M. TUCHMAN & G. D. GINDER. 1995. Metabolic persistence of fetal hemoglobin. Blood **85:** 1712–1718.

20. GLAUBER, J. G., N. J. WANDERSEE, J. A. LITTLE & G. D. GINDER. 1991. 5'-flanking sequences mediate butyrate stimulation of embryonic globin gene expression in adult erythroid cells. Mol. Cell. Biol. **11:** 4690–4697.
21. PERRINE, S. P., A. RUDOLPH, D. V. FALLER, C. ROMAN, R. A. COHEN, S. J. CHEN & Y. W. KAN. 1988. Butyrate infusions in the ovine fetus delay the biologic clock for globin gene switching. Proc. Natl. Acad. Sci. USA **85:** 8540–8542.
22. CONSTANTOULAKIS, P., T. PAPAYANNOPOULOU & G. STAMATOYANNOPOULOS. 1988. α-Amino-N-butyric acid stimulates fetal hemoglobin in the adult. Blood **72:** 1961–1967.
23. PERRINE, S. P., G. D. GINDER, D. V. FALLER, G. H. DOVER, T. IKUTA, H. E. WITKOWSKA, S. P. CAI, E. P. VICHINSKY & N. F. OLIVIERI. 1993. A short-term trial of butyrate to stimulate fetal-globin-gene expression in the β-globin disorders. N. Engl. J. Med. **328:** 81–86.
24. PERRINE, S. P., N. F. OLIVIERI, D. V. FALLER, E. P. VICHINSKY, G. J. DOVER & G. D. GINDER. 1994. Butyrate derivatives: New agents for stimulating fetal globin production in the β-globin disorders. Am. J. Pediatr. Hematol. Oncol. **16:** 67–71.
25. MILLER, I. J. & J. J. BIEKER. 1993. A novel, erythroid cell-specific murine transcription factor that binds to the CACCC element and is related to the Krüppel family of nuclear proteins. Mol. Cell Biol. **13:** 2776–2786.
26. JANE, S. M., P. A. NEY, E. F. VANIN, D. L. GUMUCIO & A. W. NIENHUIS. 1992. Identification of a stage selector element in the human γ-globin gene promoter that fosters preferential interaction with the 5' HS2 enhancer when in competition with the β-promoter. EMBO J. **11:** 2961–2969.
27. PACE, B., Q. LI, K. PETERSON & G. STAMATOYANNOPOULOS. 1994. α-Amino butyric acid cannot reactivate the silenced γ gene of the β locus YAC transgenic mouse. Blood **84:** 4344–4353.
28. BUSSLINGER, M., J. HURST & R. A. FLAVELL. 1983. DNA methylation and the regulation of globin gene expression. Cell **34:** 197–206.
29. CHARACHE, S., G. DOVER, K. SMITH, C. C. TALBOT, M. MOYER & S. BOYER. 1983. Treatment of sickle cell anemia with 5-azacytidine results in increased fetal hemoglobin production and is associated with nonrandom hypomethylation of DNA around the γ-δ-β-globin gene complex. Proc. Natl. Acad. Sci. **80:** 4842–4846.
30. LOWREY, C. H. & A. W. NIENHUIS. 1993. Brief report: Treatment with azacitidine of patients with endstage β-thalassemia. N. Engl. J. Med. **329:** 845–848.
31. BROTHERTON, T. W., J. RENEKER & G. D. GINDER. 1990. Binding of HMG 17 to mononucleosomes in the avian β-globin gene cluster in erythroid and non-erythroid cells. Nucleic Acids Res. **18:** 2011–2016.
32. CRANE-ROBINSON, C., T. R. HEBBES, A. L. CLAYTON & A. W. THORNE. 1997. Chromosomal mapping of core histone acetylation by immunoselection. Methods: A Companion to Methods in Enzymology **12:** 48–56.
33. PACE, B. S., Q. LI & G. STAMATOYANNOPOULOS. 1996. *In vivo* search for butyrate responsive sequences using transgenic mice carrying A γ gene promoter mutants. Blood **88:** 1079–1083.
34. RIGGS, M. G., R. G. WHITTAKER, J. R. NEUMAN & V. M. INGRAM. 1977. n-Butyrate causes histone modification in HeLa and Friend erythroleukaemia cells. Nature **268:** 462–464.
35. KRUH, J. 1982. Effects of sodium butyrate, a new pharmacological agent on cells in culture. Mol. Cell. Biochem. **42:** 65–82.
36. ALLAND, L., R. MUHLE, HOU H. JR., POTES J., CHIN L., N. SCHREIBER-AGUS, AND R. A. DEPINHO. 1997. Role for N-CoR and histone deacetylast in Sin3-mediated transcriptional repression. Nature **387:** 49–55.
37. LAHERTY, C. D., W. M. YANG, J. M. SUN, J. R. DAVIE, E. SETO & R. N. EISENMAN. 1997. Histone deacetylases associated with the mSin3 corepressor mediate mad transcriptional repression. Cell **89:** 349–356.
38. HEINZEL, THORSTEN, R. M. LAVINSKY, T. M. MULLEN, M. SÖDERSTRÖM, C. D. LAHERTY, J. TORCHIA, W. M. YANG, G. BRARD, S. D. NGO, JAMES R. DAVIE, E. SETO, R. N. EISENMAN, D. W. ROSE, C. K. GLASS & M. G. ROSENFELD. 1997. A complex containing N-CoR, mSin3 and histone deacetylase mediates transcriptional repression. Nature **387:** 43–48.

Hemoglobin Switching Protocols in Thalassemia

Experience with Sodium Phenylbutyrate and Hydroxyurea[a]

GEORGE J. DOVER[b]

Department of Pediatrics, Johns Hopkins University School of Medicine, 600 N. Wolfe Street, CMSC 2-116, Baltimore, Maryland 21287, USA

ABSTRACT: Homozygous β thalassemia affects thousands of people around the world. Current management of this condition includes regular transfusion of red cells, which leads to transfusional iron overload requiring chelation therapy: increasing hemoglobin levels while decreasing or eliminating iron overload is therefore a major therapeutic goal in the treatment of thalassemia. Bone marrow transplantation may achieve this goal, but it is not an option for most patients. This study reports on efforts to increase γ-globin transcription and HbF production using sodium phenylbutyrate (SPB) and hydroxyurea (HU). It was found that 36% (4/11) of all patients or 50% (4/8) of non-transfused patients responded to SPB (increase in Hb levels of 1g/dL). A positive correlation between baseline serum erythropoietin level and likelihood of response to SPB was observed. Since HU may also increase HbF production, evaluation of combination therapy with these drugs is underway and preliminary results are reported.

Homozygous β thalassemia, a disease in which there is inadequate production of β globin leading to severe anemia, affects thousands of individuals worldwide. Current management of this condition includes the use of regular red cell transfusions and iron chelation therapy. The development of an effective therapy to increase hemoglobin levels in homozygous β thalassemia without the use of red cell transfusions could allow normal growth and development while decreasing or eliminating transfusional iron overload, which remains the major cause of death, reduced life expectancy and morbidity in individuals with this disease.[1] While bone marrow transplantation can achieve these aims,[2] it is not a therapeutic option for the majority of patients.

For some years, there has been interest in increasing γ-globin transcription and fetal hemoglobin (HbF) production in patients with beta hemoglobinopathies.[3,4] For patients with homozygous β thalassemia, increased γ-globin production and a reduction in the ratio of α to non-α globin could reasonably be expected to ameliorate the severity of the anemia. To this end, trials of chemotherapeutic agents including 5-azacytidine[3,5–7] and hydroxyurea[3,8,9] have been conducted; but myelotoxicity, fears of long-term carcinogenesis and only modest responses to treatment have limited the clinical usefulness of these agents. Erythropoietin has also been used, but responses to this therapy have been variable.[10,11]

---

[a]This study was supported by funding of the Cooley's Anemia Foundation and National Institutes of Health Grant RO1-H28028. This report has been previously published in The Thalassemia Intermedia; The Genetic Resource: Special Issue, 1997, Vol. 11 (2), U.S. Department of Health and Human Services Public Health Service.

[b]Tel: (410)955-5976; Fax: (410)955-9850; E-mail: gdover@welchlink.welch.jhu.edu

There is considerable evidence that butyrate analogues induce erythroid differentiation[12-14] and stimulate hemoglobin F production in human erythroid progenitors *in vitro*.[15-17] In vivo, these agents have also been shown to reactivate embryonic globin production in an avian model,[19] delay the switch from fetal to adult globin in ovine fetuses,[18] and to increase HbF production in adult primates.[17,20-22]

In humans, several fatty acids including α-amino-butyric acid,[23] arginine butyrate,[24,25] isobutyramide,[26,27] sodium phenylbutyrate,[28,29] propionic acid[30] and 2-propylpentanoic (dipropylacetic) acid (unpublished data) have now been demonstrated to stimulate fetal hemoglobin production, suggesting that they may play a role in the treatment of the β-globin disorders. Previous clinical trials of these agents in β thalassemia however, have been limited to relatively short-term trials of the intravenous agent, arginine butyrate[24,25,31] and oral isobutyramide.[26,27]

Sodium phenylbutyrate (SPB) is an orally administered agent originally developed to promote waste nitrogen excretion in the treatment of urea cycle disorders[32] and currently used for this purpose in an FDA approved Phase III trial. Over 100 patient years experience with this drug has now accumulated with no untoward effects being found. The finding of increased hemoglobin F levels in these patients[28] stimulated clinical trials of sodium phenylbutyrate in patients with β hemoglobinopathies.

We have begun a preliminary trial of oral SPB in patients with homozygous β thalassemia. This represents the largest clinical trial of any hemoglobin switching agent used in thalassemic patients to date.

Our preliminary data demonstrate that sodium phenylbutyrate can safely be administered to patients with homozygous β thalassemia and is well tolerated by the majority. The need to take 40 tablets daily, epigastric discomfort, and the body odor created in some patients are problematic. Poor compliance with this regimen, based on previous experience with this drug was expected to be a frequent problem,[29] but surprisingly was not, possibly related to the fact that many of these patients had had prior experience with other cumbersome medical interventions including transfusion schedules and iron chelation therapy. The oral route of administration, however, has clear advantages over the intravenous route needed for arginine butyrate, particularly as all the evidence available suggests that in the management of the β hemoglobinopathies, these therapies, if effective, will be needed long term.

We found that 36% (4/11) of all patients or 50% (4/8) of non-transfused patients responded to sodium phenylbutyrate when a response was defined as a sustained increase in hemoglobin of more than 1g/dL over pre-treatment values. Clearly, sodium phenylbutyrate can increase hemoglobin in some patients with homozygous β thalassemia, but is not effective in all of them. While it seems evident that β-globin mutation alone does not predict response, the fact that two siblings treated in this study both responded to sodium phenylbutyrate therapy raises the possibility that some other genetic factor is involved. Other genetic factors linked and unlinked to the β-globin locus have been shown to effect hemoglobin F levels in normal individuals and patients with β hemoglobinopathies.[39,40]

The failure of hemoglobin to increase in patients showing a decrease in levels of lactate dehydrogenase and indirect bilirubin is disappointing and raises interesting questions as to the cause of these changes if not related to decreased hemolysis. Similarly we have observed increased production in F reticulocytes in all patients treated with this agent to date and the persistence of levels of F reticulocytes higher than baseline in some patients up to a month or more after the cessation of therapy with an agent known to be rapidly metabolized and excreted. Similar observations have been reported following the use of arginine butyrate.[24,27] This uniformity of F reticulocyte response, persistence of response in some patients long after the cessation of therapy and lack of correlation between changes in F reticulocytes and increased total hemoglobin or increased absolute hemoglobin F production may indicate suboptimal increases in hemoglobin F insufficient to decrease ineffective erythropoiesis.

We observed an inconsistent response to therapy, a decrease in traditional indicators of hemolysis in all non-transfused patients which were not predictive of an increase in hemoglobin and increases in hemoglobin not entirely explained by increased hemoglobin F in those patients who did respond to therapy. This suggests that "classic" hemoglobin switching, increase in gamma globin production with resultant decrease in globin chain imbalance, could not explain the increases in hemoglobin seen. Three possible explanations exist: that sodium phenylbutyrate 1) caused non-specific induction of all globin production, α, β and γ, and not just γ alone; 2) caused non-specific expansion of red cell mass by the release of thalassemic red cells previously sequestered in the marrow or due to an increase in production of thalassemic red cells; 3) caused a prolongation of red cell survival without a change in red cell production. There is evidence to support the first of these (personal communication, G. Stamatoyannopoulos) and the latter two lead to testable hypotheses in further patients.

A positive correlation between baseline serum erythropoietin level and the likelihood of responding to SPB therapy was observed. This observation, together with the fact that erythropoietin levels in homozygous beta thalassemia are generally elevated, but inappropriately so for the degree of anemia, suggests that clinical trials of combination therapy using erythropoietin with sodium phenylbutyrate may be of value. It must be remembered however, that in these patients erythropoietin levels are related to other factors, such as baseline HbF%[11] and as such erythropoietin may only be a marker of some other factor affecting response.

Both oral Hydroxyurea and subcutaneous/intravenous erythropoietin have been shown to increase hemoglobin levels in some thalassemia patients.[8-10] Combinations of both of these drugs have been shown by Rachmilewitz to also increase hemoglobin levels but it is not clear whether together these drugs are additive. Fibach has shown that SPB and HU in human erythroid cultures have a synergistic effect on increasing HbF.[16] Since not all subjects with thalassemia respond to SPB, we believe initial trials of combination therapy (Hu and SPB, Epo and SPB) are warranted.

Predictors of Increased Hemoglobin in Response to SPB Therapy

Response to sodium phenylbutyrate therapy, as defined by a sustained increase in total hemoglobin of > 1g/dL above baseline, did not appear to be predicted by β globin mutation; baseline % HbF, absolute HbF or F reticulocyte levels; baseline hemoglobin or baseline α to non-α globin ratios. Similarly, significant falls in lactate dehydrogenase and indirect bilirubin, traditional measures of hemolysis, could be demonstrated in all those non-transfused patients with no differences being observed between responders and non-responders. Interestingly, those patients with baseline erythropoietin levels greater than 120 mU/mL were significantly ($p < 0.05$) more likely to experience an increase in hemoglobin (4/6) than those whose baseline erythropoietin level was below 120 mU/mL (0/6). A similar trend existed between baseline HbF% in those patients not receiving regular red cell transfusions and response to sodium phenylbutyrate therapy, although this did not reach statistical significance. Of the 4 patients with baseline HbF% <40, none responded to therapy. In contrast, 4 of the 5 patients with baseline HbF% >40 did respond ($p = 0.075$).

Compliance with SPB Therapy

Sodium phenylbutyrate tablets were provided to the patients 25 days supply at a time with a further supply being provided only when the patient specifically requested more tablets. In this way compliance was calculated for each patient by comparing the number of tablets dispensed to that prescribed. Compliance with therapy was a problem in only one patient, #3, who abruptly discontinued therapy after 100 days, having been 95% compliant up until that time. For the patients as a group, compliance with medication was 97 ± 3%.

Adverse Events Occurring on SPB Therapy.

The daily dose of 20g of sodium phenylbutyrate contributes 2460 mg (107 mmol) of sodium to the diet, a significant proportion of the recommended daily intake. One of the twelve patients (#6), developed ankle edema while in hospital associated with a 3.5% increase in body weight which resolved spontaneously with dietary modification. Following discharge from hospital, one patient (# 1) required intermittent treatment with a thiazide diuretic and one (#8) required an increase in her previous diuretic dose to control peripheral edema. No patient developed hypertension. Epigastric discomfort following the ingestion of the tablets was the most common adverse effect, being reported by seven of the twelve patients. Two patients, both splenectomized and not on regular penicillin prophylaxis, had non-fatal episodes of bacterial septicemia: patient #4 developed streptococcus pneumonia at day 71 and plesiomonas shigelloides at day 200 and patient #6 staphylococcus epidermidis septicemia related to a indwelling central venous catheter at day 24. Patient 8 suffered a hemorrhage from a gastric ulcer at day 220 soon after the commencement of aspirin therapy for longstanding pulmonary hypertension. Patient l, who had spun hemoglobin levels between 5.1 and 7.5 g/dL associated with marked erythroblastosis, developed spinal cord compression requiring irradiation at day 323 and ceased sodium phenylbutyrate therapy. Patient 10 developed a deep venous thrombosis at day 28 with a hemoglobin 5.9 g/dL. Three patients experienced bad body odor while on therapy, which in one, # 12, caused her to be unable to tolerate the medication long term even at half the usual dose. These complaints are probably related to the *in vivo* β-oxidation of phenylbutyrate to phenylacetate, a compound with an offensive odor secreted as a defense mechanism by the stinkpot turtle.[38]

Arginine Butyrate then SPB

We have treated one patient in collabortion with Dr. Olivieri (Hospital for Sick Children, Toronto) with SPB after she was taken off intravenous arginine butyrate. The patient was treated for 30 days, maintained her hemoglobin level, but was removed from therapy when she had a reoccurrence of neurologic toxicity secondary to expansion of her marrow which required irradiation. Dr. Olivieri does not attribute this side-effect to SPB, but further patients will have to be treated to determine whether SPB can safely maintain the hemoglobin levels of patients already treated with arginine butyrate.

Hydroxyurea and SPB

We have treated two transfusion-dependent thalassemia patients with combinations of HU and SPB. Both patients were maintained on their usual transfusion schedule and response was monitored by their pretransfusion Hb levels. The first patient showed no response after 60 days and was discontinued. The second patient, treated longer has shown a steady increase in his pretransfusion hemoglobin level and a decrease in his transfusion requirements.

Update of SPB/HU

To date between patients treated through Baltimore/Yale/Penn (4) and Toronto (10) we have enrolled 14 patients on SPB/HU protocols. All four from Baltimore/Yale/Penn are off study (3 completed SPB/HU trials for >200 days and one stopped therapy without reaching toxicity with HU). The two thalassemia intermedia patients showed no synergistic effect on SPB/HU and the transfusion-dependent patient showed only a questionable effect according to Dr. A. Cohen.

We originally proposed over three years to treat 10 patients with SPB/HU for >200 days and have completed evaluation of five (three Baltimore/Yale/Penn patients and #9, #10–120 days) and have started two more.

We have treated the Toronto patients for a total of 61 patient months on SPB (18 patient months on SPB/HU) on this protocol, and have seen no significant increase in hemoglobin levels. The two Baltimore/Yale patients were treated for 11 months each on SPB/HU (total of 22 patient months).

Only two out of the present 14 non-transfusion–dependent thalassemic patients treated with SPB have shown any increase in hemoglobin levels with SPB alone. An additional patient not in the study has had an increase in hemoglobin for over two years of SPB, but she does not wish to add HU or EPO.

REFERENCES

1. ZURLO M. C., P. DE STEFANO, C. BORGNA-PIGNATTI, A. DI PALMA, A. PIGA, C. MELEVENDI, F. DI GREGORIO, M. G. BURATINI & S. TERZOLI. 1989. Survival and causes of death in thalassemia major. Lancet **2:** 27.
2. LUCARELLI, G., M. GALIMBERTI, P. POLCHI, E. ANGELUCCI, D. BARONCIANI, C. GIARDINI, M. ANDREANI, F. AGOSTINELLI, F. ALBERTINI & R. A. CLIFT. 1993. Marrow transplantation in patients with thalassemia responsive to iron chelation therapy. New Engl. J. Med. **329:** 840.
3. NIENHUIS, A. W., T. J. LEY, R. K. HUMPHRIES, N. S. YOUNG & G. DOVER. 1985. Pharmacological manipulation of fetal hemoglobin synthesis in patients with severe β-thalassemia. Ann. N.Y. Acad. Sci. **445:** 198.
4. STAMATOYANNOPOULOS, J. A. & A. W. NIENHUIS. 1992. Therapeutic approaches to hemoglobin switching in treatment of hemoglobinopathies. Annu. Rev. Med. **43:** 497.
5. LEY, T. J., J. DESIMONE, N. P. ANAGNOU, G. H. KELLER, R. K. HUMPHRIES, P. HELLER & A. W. NIENHUIS. 1982. 5-Azacytidine selectively increases γ-globin synthesis in a patient with β+ thalassemia. N. Engl. J. Med. **307:** 1469.
6. DUNBAR, C., W. TRAVIS, Y. W. KAN & A. NIENHUIS. 1989. 5-Azacytidine treatment in a β⁰-thalassemic patient unable to be transfused due to multiple alloantibodies. Br. J. Hematol. **74:** 467.
7. LOWREY, C. H. & A. W. NIENHUIS. 1993. Treatment with azacytidine of patients with end-stage β-thalassemia. N. Engl. J. Med. **329:** 845.
8. MCDONAGH, K. T., E. P. ORRINGER, G. J. DOVER & A. W. NIENHUIS. 1990. Hydroxyurea improves erythropoiesis in a patient with homozygous beta thalassemia. Clin. Res. **38:** 346A, Abstract.
9. FUCHAROEN, S., N. SIRITANARATKUL, P. WINICHAGOON, W. SIRIBOON, J. CHOWATHAWORN, W. MUANGSUP, S. CHAICHAROEN, N. POOLSUP, B. CHINDAVIJAK, P. POOTRAKUL, A. PIANKIJAGUM, A. N. SCHECHTER & G. P. RODGERS. 1993. Hydroxyurea increases HbF levels and improves the effectiveness of erythropoiesis in β-thalassemia/HbE disease. Blood **82:** 357a, Abstract.
10. RACHMILEWITZ, E. A., A. GOLDFARB & G. DOVER. 1991. Administration of erythropoietin to patients with β thalassemia intermedia: A preliminary trial. Blood **78:** 1145, Letter.
11. OLIVIERI, N. F., B. SHERIDAN, M. FREEDMAN, G. DOVER, S. PERRINE & R. S. NAGEL. 1992. Trial of recombinant human erythropoietin in thalassemia intermedia. Blood **80:** 3258, Letter.
12. ORKIN, S. H., D. SWAN & P. LEDER. 1975. Differential expression of α- and β-globin genes during differentiation of cultured erythroleukemic cells. J. Biol. Chem. **250:** 8753.
13. ANDERSON, L. C., M. JOKINEN & C. G. GAHMBERG. 1979. Induction of erythroid differentiation in the human leukemia cell line K562. Nature **278:** 364.

14. SAMID, D., S. SHACK & L. T. SHERMAN. 1992. Phenylacetate: A novel nontoxic inducer of tumor cell differentiation. Cancer Res. **52:** 1988.
15. PERRINE, S. P., B. A. MILLER, D. V. FALLER, R. A. COHEN, E. P. VICHINSKY, D. HURST, B. H. LUBIN & TH. PAPAYANNOPOULOU. 1989. Sodium butyrate enhances fetal globin expression in erythroid progenitors of patients with HbSS and β-thalassemia. Blood **74:** 454.
16. FIBACH, E., P. PRASANNA, G. P. RODGERS & D. SAMID. 1993. Enhanced fetal hemoglobin production by phenylacetate and 4-phenylbutyrate in erythroid precursors derived from normal blood donors and patients with sickle cell anemia and β-thalassemia. Blood **82:** 2203.
17. STAMATOYANNOPOULOS, G., B. NAKAMOTO, B. JOSEPHSON, Q. LI, A. BLAU, E. LIAKAPOULOU, TH. PAPAYANNOPOULOU, S. BRUSILOW & G. DOVER. 1993. Acetate, a product of butyrate catabolism, stimulates γ-globin expression in adult cells in vivo and in culture. Blood **82:** 313a, Abstract.
18. PERRINE, S. P., A. RUDOLPH, D. V. FALLER, C. ROMAN, R. A. COHEN, S-J. CHEN & Y. W. KAN. 1988. Butyrate infusions in the ovine fetus delay the biologic clock for globin gene switching. Proc. Natl. Acad. Sci. USA **85:** 8540.
19. GINDER, G. D., M. J. WHITTERS & J. K. POHLMAN. 1984. Activation of a chicken embryonic globin gene in adult erythroid cells by 5-azacytidine and sodium butyrate. Proc. Natl. Acad. Sci. USA **81:** 3954.
20. CONSTANTOULAKIS, P., TH. PAPAYANNOPOULOU & G. STAMATOYANNOPOULOS. 1988. Alpha-amino-N-butyric acid stimulates fetal hemoglobin in the adult. Blood **72:** 1961.
21. CONSTANTOULAKIS, P., G. KNITTER & G. STAMATOYANNOPOULOS. 1989. On the induction of fetal hemoglobin by butyrates: In vivo and in vitro studies with sodium butyrate and comparison of combination treatment with 5-azaC and Ara C. Blood **74:** 1963.
22. BLAU, C. A., P. CONSTANTOULAKIS, C. M. SHAW & G. STAMATOYANNOPOULOS. 1993. Fetal hemoglobin induction with butyric acid: Efficacy and toxicity. Blood **81:** 529.
23. PERRINE, S. P., M. F. GREENE & D. V. FALLER. 1985. Delay in the fetal globin switch in infants of diabetic mothers. New Engl. J. Med. **312:** 334.
24. PERRINE, S. P., G. D. GINDER, D. V. FALLER, G. J. DOVER, T. IKUTA, H. E. WITKOWSKA, S-P. CAI, E. P. VICHINSKY & N. F. OLIVIERI. 1993. A short term trial of butyrate to stimulate fetal-globin-gene expression in the β- globin disorders. New Engl. J. Med. **328:** 81.
25. SHER, G. D., B. ENTSUAH, G. GINDER, G. DOVER, J. LITTLE, J. DONSKY, M. BERKOVITCH, N. LEWIS, L. CHANG, S. PERRINE & N. F. OLIVIERI. 1993. Intravenous infusion of arginine butyrate increases γ-globin mRNA expression and F-reticulocytes in patients with homozygous β-thalassemia and sickle cell disease. Blood **82:** 312a, Abstract.
26. COSTIN, D., G. DOVER, N. OLIVERI, E. BEUTLER, C. T. WALSH, S. TORKELSON, C. PANTAZIS, M. BRAUER, D. V. FALLER & S. P. PERRINE. 1993. Clinical use of the butyrate derivative isobutyramide in the β-globin disorders. Blood **82:** 357a.
27. PERRINE, S. P., N. F. OLIVIERI, D. V. FALLER, E. P. VICHINSKY, G. J. DOVER & G. D. GINDER. 1994. Butyrate derivatives: New agents for stimulating fetal globin production in the β-globin disorders. Am. J. Ped. Hem.-Onc. **16:** 67.
28. DOVER, G. J., S. W. BRUSILOW & D. SAMID. 1992. Increased fetal hemoglobin in patients receiving sodium 4-Phenylbutyrate. New Engl. J. Med. **327:** 569. Letter.
29. DOVER, G. J., S. W. BRUSILOW & S. CHARACHE. 1994. Induction of HbF production in subjects with sickle cell anemia by oral sodium phenylbutyrate. Blood **84:** 339.
30. LITTLE, J., M. TUCHMAN & G. D. GINDER. 1994. Elevated fetal hemoglobin levels in propionic acidemia. Clin. Res. **42:** 238A. Abstract.
31. PERRINE, S., G. DOVER, D. COSTIN, C. PANTAZIS, S. EMBURY, G. LAZZARI, E. VICHINSKY, P. DAFTARI, A. XIN & N. OLIVIERI. 1993. Correction of globin chain imbalance in thalassemia major by arginine butyrate therapy. Blood **82:** 312a, Abstract.
32. BRUSILOW, S. W. 1991a. Treatment of urea cycle disorders. *In* Treatment of Genetic Disease. R. J. Desnick, Ed.: 79. Churchill-Livingstone.
33. Coulter Electronics. 1985. How to handle abnormal blood results for Coulter Counter instruments. Coulter Education Center, Miami FL 33014. September.
34. TICHELLI, A., A. GRATHWOHL, A. DRIESSEN, S. MATHYS, E. PFEFFERKORN, A. REGENASS, P. SCHUMACHER, C. STEBLER, M. WERNLI, C. NISSEN & B. SPECK. 1990. Evaluation of the Sysmex R-1000: An automated reticulocyte analyzer. J. Clin. Path. **93:** 70.
35. DOVER, G. J., S. H. BOYER & W. R. BELL. 1978. Microscopic method for assaying F-cell production: Illustrative changes during infancy and aplastic anemia. Blood **52:** 664.

36. HUISMAN, T. H. J. & J. H. P. JONXIS. 1977. The hemoglobinopathies: Techniques of identification. In Clinical and biochemical analysis, Vol 6: 192. M. K. Schwartz, Ed. N. Y., New York. Marcel Dekker Inc.
37. BRUSILOW, S. W. 1991b. Phenylacetylglutamine may replace urea as a vehicle for waste nitrogen excretion. Pediatr. Res. **29:** 147.
38. EISNER, T., W. E. CONNER, K. HICKS, K. R. DODGE, K. R. ROSENBERG, T. H. JONES, M. COHEN & J. MEINWALD. 1977. Stink of stinkpot turtle identified: Phenylalkanoic acids. Science **196:** 1347.
39. DOVER G. J., K. D. SMITH, Y. C. CHANG, S. PURVIS, A. MAYS, D. A. MEYERS, C. SHEILS & G. SERJEANT. 1992. Fetal hemoglobin levels in sickle cell disease and normal individuals are partially controlled by an X-linked gene located at Xp22.2. Blood **80:** 816.
40. THEIN, S. L., M. SAMPIETRO, K. ROHDE, J. ROCHETTE, D. J. WEATHERALL, G. M. LATHROP & F. DEMENAIS. 1994. Detection of a major gene for heterocellular hereditary persistence of fetal hemoglobin after accounting for genetic modifiers. Am. J. Hum. Genet. **54:** 214.
41. GALANELLO, R., S. BARELLA, M. P. TURCO, N. GIAGU, A. CAO, F. DORE, N. L. LIBERATO, R. GUARNONE & G. BAROSI. 1994. Serum erythropoietin and erythropoiesis in high- and low-fetal hemoglobin β-thalassemia intermedia patients. Blood **83:** 561.

Cellular and Molecular Effects of a Pulse Butyrate Regimen and New Inducers of Globin Gene Expression and Hematopoiesis

TOHRU IKUTA, GEORGE ATWEH, VASSILIKI BOOSALIS, GARY L. WHITE, SILVANA DA FONSECA, MICHAEL BOOSALIS, DOUGLAS V. FALLER, AND SUSAN P. PERRINE[a]

Hemoglobinopathy-Thalassemia Research Unit, Departments of Medicine, Pediatrics, Pharmacology and Experimental Therapeutics, Boston University School of Medicine, Boston, Massachusetts, USA

Department of Medicine, Mt. Sinai School of Medicine, New York, New York, USA

Department of Animal Resources, University of Oklahoma Health Sciences Center, Oklahoma City, Oklahoma, USA

ABSTRACT: Cooley's anemia is characterized by a deficiency of β-globin chains, a relative excess of α-globin chains, and consequent accelerated programmed death of developing erythroid cells in the bone marrow. Increasing expression of the γ-globin genes to adequately balance excess α-globin chains can ameliorate this disorder. Butyrates induce γ-globin experimentally, but can also cause cell growth arrest with prolonged exposure or high concentrations, which in turn can accelerate apoptosis. To determine if these potentially opposing effects can be balanced to enhance therapeutic efficacy, an intermittent "pulsed" regimen of butyrate was evaluated. Following induction of γ-globin mRNA and protein synthesis, total hemoglobin increased in β-thalassemia patients by more than 2 g/dl above baseline, and Hb F increased above 20% in 5/8 sickle cell patients from baseline levels of 2% Hb F. Specific regulatory regions were identified in the γ- and β-globin gene promoters to which new binding of transcription factors, including αCP2 (an activator of γ globin) occur during therapy solely in the butyrate-responsive patients. Other compounds which induce γ globin, derivatives of acetic, phenoxyacetic, propionic, and cinnamic acids, and dimethylbutyrate, are under investigation. Some of these newer γ-globin inducers (designated hemokines) provide better potential as therapeutics by also acting to increase hematopoietic cell viability and proliferation. Pharmacologic induction of expression of the endogenous γ-globin genes is a realistic approach to therapy of the β-globin disorders for many patients, with some effective agents available now and new therapeutics, with enhanced activities, under development.

[a]Address correspondence to: Susan P. Perrine M.D., Hemoglobinopathy-Thalassemia Research Unit, Boston University School of Medicine, 80 East Concord St, L-911, Boston, MA 02118; Tel: 617 638-5639; Fax: 617 638-4176; E-mail: sperrine@med-med1.bu.edu

Cooley's anemia becomes clinically apparent only after the fetal (γ) globin genes are developmentally suppressed and the mutant adult (β) globin genes become active, resulting in diminished non-α : α globin chains in red blood cells.[1-4] The toxicity of unmatched α-globin chains results in early programmed cell death with intramedullary hemolysis of thalassemic erythroid progenitors.[5] Analyses of different globin gene mutations and clinical studies have demonstrated that increased expression of fetal globin can ameliorate the β-thalassemias, as γ-globin chains can balance the excess α globin and improve red blood cell survival.[1-4,6,7] However, a narrow window exists in which any γ-globin stimulant must act before cell death occurs in thalassemia, making it difficult to reverse the cell destruction. A class of naturally occurring compounds, short-chain fatty acids such as butyrates, phenylbutyrate, and propionates, have been found in several experimental systems to stimulate expression of γ globin selectively from a transfected $\gamma\delta\beta$ globin gene complex, in globin promoter-reporter gene assays, in animal models, in cells cultured from patients, and in short-term clinical trials.[8-19] However, these simple fatty acids have two limitations as therapeutics: they are rapidly metabolized as energy sources, and they inhibit cell growth when used at high concentrations for prolonged periods.[9,20,21-26] Phenylbutyrate, a short-acting butyrate derivative, has been demonstrated to significantly increase Hb F in sickle cell patients and total hemoglobin in 36% of Cooley's anemia patients by a mean of 2.1 g/dl, a higher increase than the level (1.0 g/dl), which was the end point in clinical trials which resulted in approval of recombinant erythropoietin.[27-28] Higher plasma levels of erythropoietin were observed in the phenylbutyrate-responsive patients, suggesting that higher basal rates of erythropoiesis or enhanced erythroid cell viability induced by erythropoietin may contribute to the efficacy of Hb F stimulants.[28]

Arginine butyrate is a potent stimulant of γ-globin expression through transcriptional activation of the γ-globin promoter, despite having a short plasma half-life *in vivo* and inducing growth arrest in cancer cells.[8,9,13,15,22-25] To determine if adequate γ-globin induction could be elicited with butyrate while avoiding its suppressive effects on erythroid cell growth, an intermittent "pulsed" regimen of intravenous arginine butyrate was studied in 13 patients with β-hemoglobinopathies. The hypothesis for this method of use was that drug-exposed erythroblasts might be able to proliferate and survive better if the drug was given briefly to induce γ-globin expression and was then withdrawn. When this pulsed regimen was used following an initial period of frequent therapy as a "priming" period in thalassemia patients, an increase in γ-globin gene expression and an increase in total hemoglobin up to 4 g/dl above baseline was observed. The results of this regimen were in contrast to a previous study by Scher *et al.*, who gave high-dose, continuous 24-hour/day therapy, for six or seven days/week, a regimen which would be expected to inhibit cell proliferation and inhibit the synthesis of proteins such as globin.[26]

Potential molecular mechanisms of this agent have been examined in some of the established globin gene regulatory regions. *In vivo* footprinting and electrophoretic mobility shift assays with nuclear extracts from patients' erythroblasts before and during butyrate therapy have been employed to identify the sites of butyrate's molecular action on the globin genes. The new binding of transcription factors in globin gene promoter regions with effective butyrate therapy has identified two butyrate-responsive promoter regions (Ikuta *et al.*, submitted). Other potential genetic regulatory regions, particularly the LCR, remain to be analyzed. Finally, a search for additional γ-globin–inducing agents which do not share the limitation of butyrates in inhibiting cell growth has identified several compounds which stimulate both γ-globin gene expression and proliferation of hematopoietic cells.[25] These dual activities make such compounds likely to be more effective agents for the treatment of the β-hemoglobinopathies.

MATERIALS AND METHODS

Treatment Regimens and Biochemical Analyses

Nineteen different patients with beta globin disorders have been studied for either biochemical effects alone, (if transfusions were continued) or for hematologic effects of an intermittent butyrate regimen in 13 patients. Patients ranged in age from 3 to 55 years, with equivalent proportions of both genders represented. Studies were performed with approval of the Institutional Review Boards of the Boston Medical Center, the University of California at San Francisco, and the Mt. Sinai Medical Center. A regimen of weekly therapy, usually administered over 8-10 hours at night for 4 or 5 nights per week, was evaluated initially, with intra-patient dose escalations from 250 mg/kg/dose up to a maximum of 1800 mg/kg/dose administered. An intermittent pulse regimen, which provided at least 10 days between treatment courses, was subsequently evaluated in 13 patients.[20] In sickle cell patients, effective doses for inducing Hb F were between 250 and 500 mg/kg; in thalassemia patients, effective doses for induction of γ-globin mRNA and protein were usually 500–1500 mg/kg/dose, while optimal doses for increasing red blood cell counts were lower, usually 800 mg/kg/dose for thalassemia patients. Once Hb F or total hemoglobin initially increased, treatment regimens were reduced in frequency to three or four day intervals, once or twice per month, with at least 10 days between treatment courses. The time required for maintenance of therapeutic effects was usually 4-6 nights per month. The total doses used for maintenance therapy in this pulse regimen were 2–4.5 g/kg/month. This is less than 10% of the total monthly doses (48–56 g/kg/month) which had been used by Scher *et al.* in a less successful continuous 24 hour/day regimen.[26] Iron and folic acid supplements were provided, as additional iron has been demonstrated to be required for hematologic responses to other Hb F-inducing agents.[30,31] This was a second difference from the treatment regimen used by Scher *et al.*, which did not provide iron supplements.

Biochemical analyses were performed at different dose levels. Globin chain synthetic analyses, F-reticulocyte quantitation, and analyses of α, β and γ-globin mRNA by primer extension were performed as previously described.[20,29,32] Five micrograms of mRNA were analyzed for each condition and γ-globin levels were compared to the patient's β or α globin in the same mRNA sample by PhosphoImager.[32–34] Optimal responses were usually detected at 24–72 hours following a treatment course, but were often suppressed during the treatment course.

In Vivo *Footprinting and Electrophoretic Mobility Shift Assays*

In vivo footprinting was performed as previously described[33–35] on erythroblasts obtained before and with butyrate therapy and demonstrated four regions of new protein binding (Ikuta *et al.,* submitted). Nuclear extracts were prepared from circulating nucleated erythroblasts obtained from patients before, during, or immediately following butyrate therapy as previously described.[30–31,35–36] Purification was performed in samples in which there were fewer than 75% nucleated erythroblasts by using negative selection with CD45 antibody-coated flasks (Applied Immune Sciences, Santa Clara, CA) to which all cells adhered except for erythroid cells.[5] Electrophoretic mobility shift assays were carried out using double-stranded oligonucleotides containing a proximal γ-globin gene promoter sequence which had been identified in *in vivo* footprinting analyses to which new protein binding was induced during butyrate therapy, and which had been found to be functional sites of butyrate activity previously in reporter gene assays.[15,17] The new protein-DNA binding patterns observed were compared to sites of HPFH point mutations and to other established functional sites for γ-globin expression.[17,37–39] The BRE-G1 proximal region contained a region to which the Stage Selector Protein complex, an activator of γ-globin expression, binds.[40–41] Oligonucleotides corresponding to the –530 region upstream of β-globin were also used as a probe in gel shift assays, as this sequence has been shown to bind the silencer protein BP-1 more intensively in sickle cell patients with the Indian-Arabian haplotype, in whom β-globin expression is suppressed.[42–44]

Cell Proliferation Studies Using a Multi-lineage Hematopoietic Cell Line

An IL-3-dependent cell line (32Dcl3), which also differentiates along erythroid or myeloid lineages with the addition of EPO or G-CSF respectively when IL-3 concentrations are reduced by 50-fold, was used to evaluate the growth-promoting effects of some newly developed compounds, which had already been identified as inducing both γ-globin expression and erythroid progenitor growth in previous studies.[25,45] 32Dc13 cells were cultured in RPMI media with 10% fetal bovine serum, glutamine, and antibiotics and with 0, 0.5, or 25 U/ml of IL-3. Cells were incubated in a humidified atmosphere at 37°C and in 5% CO_2. Hb F-stimulating compounds to be tested were added at final concentrations of 1 mM. Viable cells were enumerated after trypan blue staining at days 1, 5, and 10 and compared between controls and treated cells. Proportions of cells in different parts of the cell cycle and in which apoptosis had occurred were also examined by FACScan analysis after incubation with propidium iodide using established methods.[45]

In Vivo Studies

Animal studies were performed with the approval of the Committee on Animal Studies at the University of Oklahoma as previously described.[15] Five prototype compounds which had been shown to stimulate γ-globin and cell proliferation *in vitro* were evaluated in anemic baboons. Baboons were maintained with sterile indwelling vascular catheters for blood sampling. Oral doses of several prototype compounds were administered via nasogastric tube and blood was sampled for determination of plasma levels of the compounds from 30 minutes to 48 hours after administration as previously described.[15] Sampling was also performed and plasma levels analyzed after intravenous administration of the compounds to determine bio-availability.[46]

RESULTS

An example of representative globin mRNA isolated from circulating erythroid cells of patients before and during butyrate therapy and analyzed by primer extension is shown in FIGURE 1. Five β-thalassemia patients and one sickle cell patient studied here responded to butyrate administration with an increase in γ-globin mRNA, compared to pre-treatment levels, with inductions ranging from 3.0- to 6.1-fold (mean = 4.1-fold increase). γ : α globin ratios were compared in each sample as an internal control. The inductions in γ-globin mRNA reverted to the patients' baseline (untreated) levels a few days after butyrate therapy was completed, but were present for at least three days (*e.g.*, patient 4, the sample designated -* demonstrated persistent γ-globin induction 2 days after therapy, although less than the peak effect observed one day after therapy).

The peak increase in γ-globin mRNA usually occurred 24 to 48 hours after a course of butyrate, and was followed 24 hours later by a peak increase in γ-globin protein synthesis, usually one to three days after the maximal γ-globin mRNA level was detected. An example of improvement in globin chain balance following a 2-day treatment course of 750

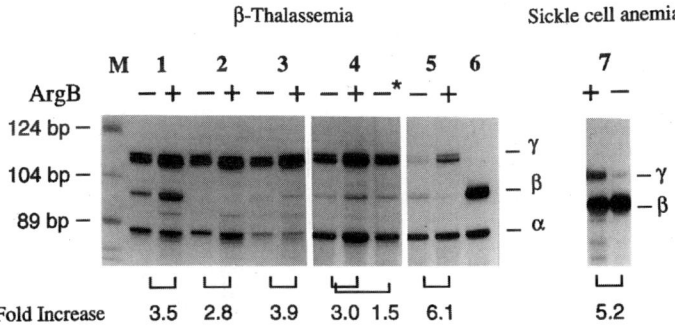

FIGURE 1. Induction of γ-globin mRNA with butyrate therapy in β-thalassemia patients. Analysis of globin mRNAs by primer extension in 5 patients with β-thalassemia (*Lanes 1–5*) and a normal adult subject (*Lane 6*). Samples obtained prior to therapy and during therapy are designated with − and + above the lane, respectively. Patient 4 was analyzed before (-), 24 hours after therapy was completed (+), and 44 hours after therapy ended (-*). Fold increases above baseline ratios of γ globin compared to α globin in the same sample by PhosphoImager are shown at the bottom of the lanes. M designates molecular weight markers. The positions of migration of the α, β and γ products are indicated.

mg/kg/dose in a patient with transfusion-dependent thalassemia major is shown in FIGURE 2. Beta-globin synthesis was initially suppressed within one day of therapy, followed by a peak increase in γ-globin three days after therapy. Increases in total hemoglobin in patients with β-thalassemia were observed from 2.4–4.3 g/dl above well-established baseline levels with corresponding increases in hematocrit and red blood cell counts. In five sickle cell patients, Hb F increased to above 20%, a level which is generally associated with a marked reduction in clinical symptoms. Two patients, who had baseline levels of less than 1% Hb F, did not respond. This pulsed regimen has proven to be safe, well-tolerated, and efficacious in small studies, and should undergo pivotal testing in larger trials.

Butyrate-responsive regions in the human γ-globin promoter have been identified in two ways, with *in vivo* footprinting and with gel shift assays, performed with nuclear extracts derived from patients' purified erythroblast samples. A schematic illustration of new protein-DNA binding detected in the proximal γ-globin promoter with butyrate therapy is shown in FIGURE 3A, designated by the circles. This region has been termed Butyrate Response Element - Gamma 1 or BRE-G1, extending from −50 to −70 nt relative to the transcription start site. Four Butyrate-responsive elements (BRE-Gs) have been identified in the γ-globin gene promoter (Ikuta *et al.*, submitted). Several of these regions of new protein binding were close to, or at, positions of point mutations that occur with hereditary persistence of fetal hemoglobin (HPFH) syndromes which result in changes in transcription factor binding.[37] BRE-G1 has been demonstrated to be a major site of butyrate activity and has been functionally related to activity of isobutyramide and other carboxylic acids in reporter gene studies (refs. 15, 17, and Ikuta *et al.*, submitted).

Butyrate-induced alterations in the binding of nuclear proteins to BRE-G1 were detected by electrophoretic mobility shift assay using nuclear extracts prepared from patients before or during butyrate treatment (FIG. 3B). A new set of protein-DNA complexes (a, b and c) appeared when extracts from butyrate-treated patients were used (*Lanes 2 and 4*), with some bands migrating in positions similar to those seen when extracts from the fetal-like cell line K562 (*Lane 3*) were used. The binding pattern shown in *Lane 4* used nuclear extract from a thalassemic patient with mutations at −87 nt and at codon 39. Nuclear extracts prepared from bone marrow erythroblasts of a normal subject (*Lane 5*), or from the same thalassemic patient prior to treatment (*Lane 1*) do not demonstrate the

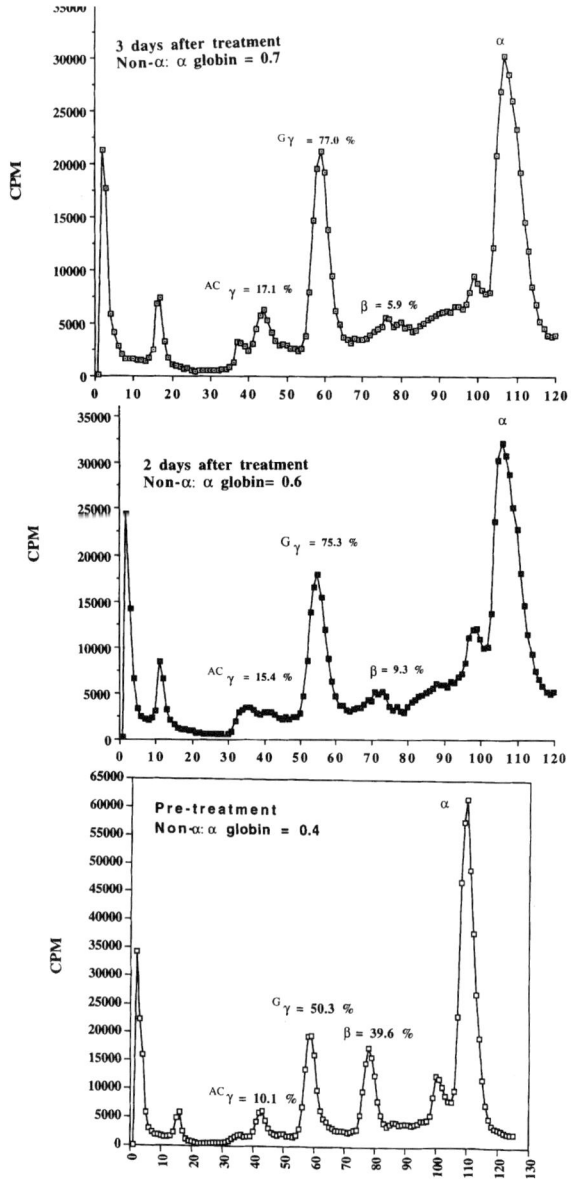

FIGURE 2. Improvement in non-α : α globin synthetic ratios in a transfusion-dependent β⁺-thalassemia patient following treatment with arginine butyrate. Baseline profiles for the patient is shown in the *bottom panel*. An initial *decrease* in β globin was observed two days after treatment with two doses of 750 mg/kg butyrate. A maximal increase in γ globin and optimal improvement in globin chain ratios was observed three days *after* treatment (*top panel*). The peak protein synthetic response followed the peak mRNA response by approximately one day.

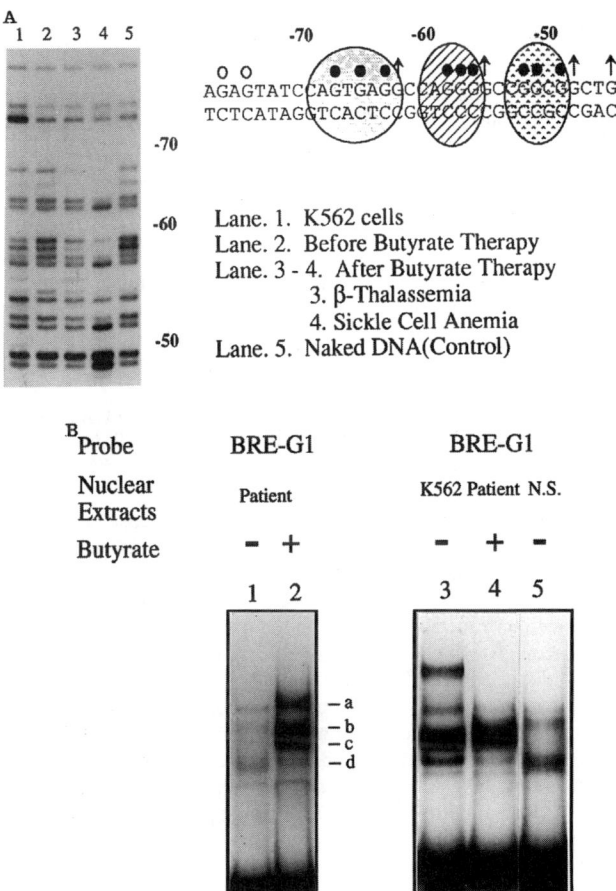

FIGURE 3. Butyrate-responsive regions in the γ-globin gene promoter, identified by electrophoretic mobility shift assays and *in vivo* footprinting. **A.** *In vivo* footprints of BRE-G1 in the γ-globin gene promoter. *In vivo* footprinting analysis of the proximal region of the γ-globin gene promoter. *Lane 1,* Hemin-induced K562; *Lane 2,* DNA from a sickle cell anemia patient before therapy; *Lane 3,* from a β-thalassemia patient during therapy; *Lane 4,* from a sickle cell anemia patient during therapy; *Lane 5,* naked DNA. Positions relative to the transcription start site are shown on the top of figure. The summary of *in vivo* footprints is also shown. *Closed* and *open circles* indicate footprinted and unfootprinted G residues, respectively. *Upward arrows* indicate G residues that showed hyperreactivity to dimethyl sulfate. This region from −48 to −70 has been designated as BRE-G1 and contains the region to which the Stage Selector Protein complex binds. **B.** Analysis of transcription factors binding to BRE-G1 by electrophoretic mobility shift assay. Origins of probe and nuclear extracts are shown on the top of figure. Nuclear extracts prepared before butyrate treatment are depicted by the -, and those with butyrate treatment by the +. The patient shown in *Lane 4* is a thalassemic patient with mutations at −87 and codon 39. K562 designates nuclear extracts made from this fetal-like erythroleukemic cell line. N.S. indicates nuclear extracts prepared from purified erythroblasts of a normal subject. Protein-DNA complexes which change with butyrate treatment are designated a, b, c, and d. Competition assays have identified the slowest migrating (top) band (a) as αCP2, a component of the Stage Selector Protein complex.

three prominent shifted protein complexes. The fast-migrating complex, which is intense in the normal subject, may represent a repressor protein, and is diminished in the extracts prepared from the thalassemic patient during butyrate therapy. One of the proteins binding to this region in response to butyrate was found to be entirely competed away by cold oligonucleotide corresponding to αCP2, which has been considered a "bridging" component of the Stage-Selector Protein complex identified by Cunningham and Jane et al.[39–41] It is likely that new binding of transcription factors may also occur in other regulatory regions in response to butyrate, particularly in the Locus Control Region and in the β-globin promoter (Ikuta et al., submitted), as β-globin gene expression often diminishes before γ-globin synthesis increases. We have recently also found that BP-1 (a silencer of β-globin gene expression) binding to the β-globin gene promoter region occurs during therapy solely in butyrate-responsive patients (Ikuta et al., submitted), and is not observed in patients who do not respond to butyrate therapy.

Studies in the murine cell line 32Dcl3 demonstrated that several new chemical inducers of γ globin also stimulated proliferation of a hematopoietic cell line which has multi-lineage potential, at rates which were similar to growth rates induced by erythropoietin or G-CSF. As shown in FIGURE 4, depletion of IL-3 resulted in apoptotic cell death of 32Dcl3 within 3 days, while a 50-fold decrease in IL-3 resulted in cessation of proliferation, with minimal cell survival. Addition of several of the new compounds, which we have designated hemokines, increased proliferation of these cells to rates similar to those induced by erythropoietin or G-CSF. This result indicates that these new compounds maintain hematopoietic cell viability and stimulate proliferation, perhaps through a mechanism similar to activities of the growth factors IL-3, erythropoietin or G-CSF, through induction of growth-related genes, or by stimulation of metabolic pathways, as well as inducing γ globin.

This erythropoietic growth effect was also observed *in vivo*. Significant increases were observed in hemoglobin and red blood cell counts with administration of the prototype hemokines methylhydrocinnamic acid and phenoxyacetic acid to baboons for three to five days, as shown in FIGURE 5. Oral administration of several different hemokine compounds, including methylhydrocinnamic acid, phenoxyacetic acid, and dimethylbutyrate, have produced millimolar plasma levels in baboons. The shortest half-lives were 7.4 hours after a small 20 mg/kg dose of dimethylbutyrate, and prolonged millimolar plasma levels were achieved for more than 24 hours, depending on the doses given (data not shown). Thus, both oral bio-availability and biologic activity have been demonstrated with other simple γ-globin inducers.

DISCUSSION

Clinical studies of the first generation butyrate-derived drugs (arginine butyrate, phenylbutyrate, isobutyramide) in β-hemoglobinopathy patients with diverse molecular mutations in the globin locus have demonstrated that different doses are required for optimal efficacy in different subjects. In general, more intense therapy was required for β-thalassemia patients than was required to elicit optimal responses in sickle cell patients. A period of weekly therapy, "induction," analogous to a priming period for initial gene reactivation, was required for β-thalassemia patients, but was not necessary for sickle cell subjects. Induction could then be followed by intermittent (pulsed) therapy to produce and maintain optimal increases in red blood counts in both types of disorders. As previously demonstrated by Fibach in *in vitro* studies using phenylbutyrate and phenylacetate, suppression of erythropoiesis in a given patient appeared to occur with the same concentrations that maximally increased γ-globin protein synthesis and mRNA. Decreasing the doses of butyrate and giving the drugs intermittently, with at least 10 days between treatment cycles, appeared to induce better overall erythropoietic responses, despite providing

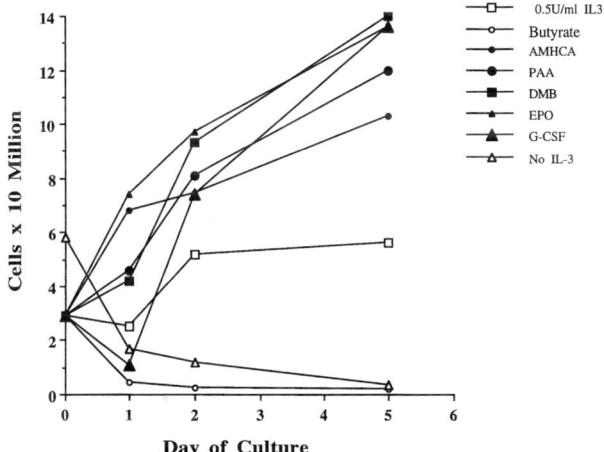

FIGURE 4. Cellular effects of new γ globin inducing agents (hemokines) *in vitro*. The IL-3–dependent cell line 32Dcl3 demonstrates loss of cell proliferation when IL-3 is depleted by 50-fold (to 0.5 U/ml) or entirely (*open symbols*), and when butyrate (*open circles*) was added in addition to the low concentration of IL-3 (0.5 U/ml). Addition of hemokine compounds (*closed symbols*) phenoxyacetic acid (PAA), dimethylbutyrate (DMB), or methylhydrocinnamic acid (AMHCA) at the same concentrations prevented the decrease in viability and stimulated proliferation of the cells. This degree of proliferation induced by these compounds was similar to the growth rates induced by addition of erythropoietin or G-CSF (*closed triangles*) in the same IL-3 deprived cells.

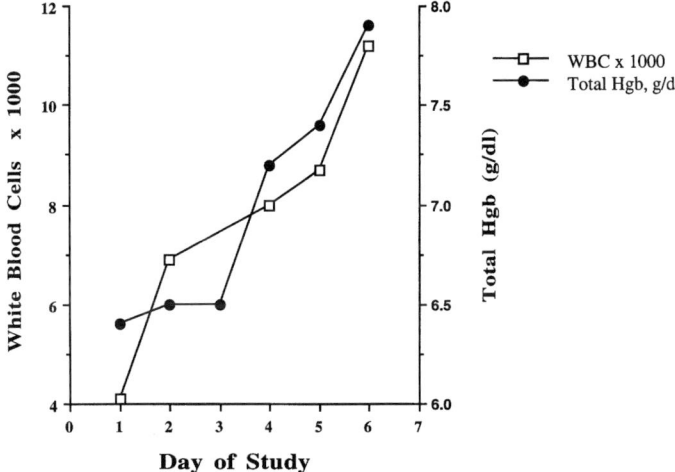

FIGURE 5. Example of hematopoietic stimulation by a new γ-globin gene inducer, a hemokine compound. An increase in multiple blood cell lineages resulted when a prototype hemokine compound (α methylhydrocinnamic acid) was administered for 5 days to an anemic baboon, which was being phlebotomized 5% of its blood volume daily. An increase in both white blood cells and total hemoglobin was observed.

less correction of globin-chain imbalance. The results strongly suggest that despite the narrow therapeutic window, the two potentially antagonistic effects of butyrate (induction of γ globin and inhibition of erythroid cell growth) can be balanced for substantial therapeutic effect in thalassemia. Despite the complexities of the requirement for intravenous administration and the need to identify an optimal dose for each patient, treatment with arginine butyrate has become a preferable alternative to transfusions and iron chelation for some patients who initially entered the study for a limited time-frame, but have since remained on treatment indefinitely, on a compassionate basis. This patient acceptance and preference may be related in large part to the substantially lower cumulative amount of time required for medical intervention with butyrate (six nights per month, compared to 20 nights/month for Desferol chelation and transfusions). More importantly, this pulsed method of administering butyrate has eliminated requirements for regular transfusions in some patients, and provides an alternative method of therapy for patients with alloantibodies who cannot receive the transfusions they would otherwise require. Thus, even at this relatively early stage of clinical development, butyrate therapy represents a therapeutic advance, as transfusion-related complications, such as infections as well as iron loading, are the major causes of mortality in Cooley's anemia patients. The long-term efficacy, as well as long-term side effects, of this therapy must be evaluated in larger studies. However, it is encouraging that tolerance has not been observed in patients treated with the intermittent regimen for over two years, as a decline in response was evident in patients previously treated with weekly therapy within several months.

The molecular mechanisms through which these promising therapeutics act are beginning to be elucidated. Two sites of butyrate activity in the β-globin complex, identified by butyrate-dependent binding of two transcription factors to these regions, were identified in butyrate-responsive patients. No such binding activity was detected in a non-responding patient. αCP2, a protein component of the Stage Selector complex,[40-41] binds to the proximal γ promoter in response to butyrate. Second, BP-1, a silencer of β globin,[42-44] also binds more tightly during therapy (Ikuta *et al.*, submitted). This latter effect, if apparent at the level of β-globin chain synthesis, might suggest that close monitoring be necessary in patients with β+ thalassemia early in therapy, as butyrate might make the over-all globin chain ratios transiently worse if the β-suppression effect were excessive. Suppression of β-globin synthesis would not be detrimental in sickle cell disease, however, where dilution of $β^s$ chains combined with stimulation of γ chains, could synergistically inhibit the tendency towards sickling. These transcriptional effects on the individual β and γ genes can be potentially individually targeted with new generations of globin-gene–inducing agents.

The studies above demonstrating stimulation of both γ globin and of erythroid cell growth are encouraging developments in the quest for better therapeutics, including orally active agents. Because there is already marked ineffective erythropoiesis in β thalassemia, an increase in red cell proliferation without an improvement in globin chain balance would not be expected to be beneficial. Application of agents with actions which induce both γ globin and cell viability would likely also require a careful balance of effects, in a fashion opposite to the balance required for effective application of butyrate compounds. Pulsed administration would also be expected be necessary to avoid excessive proliferation of erythroid cells with globin chain imbalance which are susceptible to rapid programmed cell death. However, the increase in survival and proliferation of a multi-lineage cell line which otherwise underwent apoptotic cell death in the absence of IL-3 indicates that these compounds may increase cell survival and may provide a broader therapeutic window than naturally exists. Demonstration of both Hb F stimulating and erythropoietic actions of these new compounds in a primate animal model after oral administration indicates that they are indeed orally bioavailable. Extensive safety testing and dose-range studies are required before any of these compounds can be considered for evaluation in patients, but administration in primates has not demonstrated adverse effects so far.

As all patients who survive to birth have some functional γ-globin genes, these genes are available for reactivation with no donor or stem cell manipulation required to provide an endogenous source of alternative globin protein for deficient β globin in β thalassemia. For the past fourteen years, the primary therapeutic agents under study to induce the γ-globin genes in Cooley's anemia have been myelosuppressive chemotherapeutic agents. Now, in small clinical trials, other compounds which act through transcriptional control appear safe and efficacious in some of the patients studied. New generations of γ-globin–inducing compounds, which overcome many of the limitations of the first agents, and even stimulate hematopoiesis, are in late stages of preclinical development. Larger clinical trials are necessary to confirm the results of initial studies of the currently available therapies and to investigate new generations.

REFERENCES

1. STAMATOYANOPOULOS, J. A. *et al.* 1992. Therapeutic approaches to hemoglobin switching in the treatment of hemoglobinopathies. Ann. Rev. Med. **43**: 497–522.
2. GALLO, E. *et al.* 1979. The importance of the genetic picture and globin synthesis in determining the clinical and hematological features of thalassemia intermedia. Brit. J. Haematol. **41**: 211–221.
3. KARLSSON, S. & A.W. NIENHUIS. 1985. Development regulation of human globin genes. Ann. Rev. Biochem. **54**: 1071–1108.
4. WOOD, W. G. & D. J. WEATHERALL. 1983. Development genetics of the human haemoglobins. Biochem. J. **215**: 1–10.
5. YUAN, J. *et al.* 1993. Accelerated programmed cell death (apoptosis) in erythroid precursors of patients with severe β-thalassemia (Cooley's Anemia). Blood **82**: 374–377.
6. LEY, T. J. *et al.* 1982. 5-Azacytidine selectively increases γ-globin synthesis in a patient with β^+ thalassemia. N. Engl. J. Med. **307**: 1469–1475.
7. LOWREY, C. H. & A. W. NIENHUIS. 1993. Treatment with azacytidine of patients with end stage β-thalassemia. N. Engl. J. Med. **329**: 845–849.
8. PARTINGTON, G. A., N. J. YARWOOD & T. R. RUTHERFORD. 1984. Human globin gene transcription in Xenopus oocytes: Enhancement by sodium butyrate. EMBO J. **3**: 2787–92.
9. FALLER, D. V. & S. P. PERRINE. 1995. Butyrate in the treatment of sickle cell disease and β-thalassemia. Curr. Opin. in Hematol. **2**: 109–117.
10. PERRINE, S. P., M. F. GREENE & D. V. FALLER. 1985. Delay in the fetal globin switch in infants of diabetic mothers. N. Engl. J. Med. **312**: 334–338.
11. GLAUBER, J. G. *et al.* 1991. 5′-Flanking sequences mediate butyrate stimulation of embryonic globin gene expression in adult erythroid cells. Mol. Cell. Biol. **11**: 4690–4697.
12. PERRINE, S. P. *et al.* 1988. Butyrate infusions in the ovine fetus delay the biologic clock for globin gene switching. Proc. Natl. Acad. Sci. USA **85**: 8540–8542.
13. CONSTANTOULAKIS, P., T. PAPAYANOPOULOU & G. STAMATOYANNOPOULOS. 1988. Alpha-amino-n-butyric acid stimulates fetal hemoglobin in the adult. Blood **72**: 1961–67.
14. LIAKOPOULOU, E. *et al.* 1995. Stimulation of fetal hemoglobin production by short chain fatty acids. Blood **86**: 3227–3235.
15. PERRINE, S. P. *et al.*. 1994. Isobutyramide, an orally bioavailable butyrate analogue, stimulates fetal globin gene expression *in vitro* and *in vivo*. Brit. J. Haematol. **88**: 555–561.
16. PACE, B. S. *et al.* 1996. *In vivo* search for butyrate responsive sequences using transgenic mice carrying $^A\gamma$ gene promoter mutants. Blood **88**: 1079–1083.
17. SAFAYA, S., A. IBRAHIM & R. F. RIEDER. 1994. Augmentation of γ-globin gene promoter activity by carboxylic acids and components of the human β-globin locus control region. Blood **72**: 3929–3935.
18. PERRINE, S. P. *et al.* 1989. Sodium butyrate enhances fetal globin gene expression in erythroid progenitors of patients with HbSS and β thalassemia. Blood **74**: 454–459.
19. PERRINE, S. P. *et al.* 1993. N: A short-term trial of butyrate to stimulate fetal-globin gene expression in the β-globin disorders. N. Engl. J. Med. **328**: 81–86.
20. ATWEH, G. *et al.* 1996. Sustained hematologic response to pulse butyrate therapy in beta globin disorders. Blood **88**: 652a.

21. FIBACH, E. *et al.* 1993.Enhanced fetal hemoglobin production by phenylacetate and 4-phenylbutyrate in erythroid precursors derived from normal donors and patients with sickle cell anemia and β-thalassemia. Blood **82**: 2203–2209.
22. TOSCANI A., D. R. SOPRANO & K. J. SOPRANO. 1988. Molecular analysis of sodium butyrate-induced growth arrest. Oncogene Res. **3**: 223–238.
23. WINTERSBERGER E., I. MURDRAK & U. WINTERBERGER. 1983. Butyrate inhibits mouse fibroblasts at a control point in the G_1 phase. J. Cell. Biochem. **21**: 239–247.
24. CHAROLLAIS R. H., C. BUGUET & J. MESTER. 1990. Butyrate blocks the accumulation of mRNA in the late G^1 phase but inhibits both the early and late G^1 progression in chemically transformed mouse fibroblasts BP-A31. J. Cell. Phys. **145**: 46–52.
25. TORKELSON, S. *et al.* 1996. Erythroid progenitor proliferation is stimulated by phenoxyaceticand phenylalkyl acids. Blood Cells, Mol. Dis. **20**: 150–158.
26. SHER, G. D. *et al.* 1995. Extended therapy with intravenous arginine butyrate in patients with β-hemoglobinopathies. N. Engl. J. Med. **332**: 1606–1610.
27. DOVER, G. J., S. BRUSILOW & D. SAMID. 1992. Increased fetal hemoglobin in patients receiving sodium 4-phenylbutyrate. N. Engl. J. Med. **327**:569–570.
28. COLLINS, A. F., *et al.* 1995. Oral sodium phenylbutyrate therapy in homozygous beta thalassemia: A clinical trial. Blood **85**: 43–49.
29. CLEGG, J. B., *et al.* 1996. Abnormal human haemoglobins: Separation and characterization of the α and β chains by chromatography, and the determination of two new variants, Hb Chesapeake and Hb J (Bangkok). J. Mol. Biol. **19**: 91–108.
30. NAGEL, R. L., *et al.* 1993.F-reticulocyte response in sickle cell anemia treated with recombinant human erythropoietin: A double-blind study. Blood **1**: 9–14.
31. RODGERS, G. P. *et al.* 1993. Augmentation by erythropoietin of the fetal-hemoglobin response to hydroxyurea in sickle cell disease. N.Engl J.Med. **328**: 73–80.
32. CHOMCZYNSKI, P. & N. SACCHI. 1987. Single-step method of RNA isolation by acid guanidinium thiocyanate-phenol-chloroform extraction. Anal. Biochem. **162**: 156–159.
33. IKUTA, T. *et al.* 1996. Globin gene switching: *In vivo* protein-DNA interactions of the human β-globin locus in erythroid cells expressing the fetal or the adult globin gene program. J. Biol. Chem. **271**: 14082–14091.
34. IKUTA, T. & Y. W. KAN. 1991. *In vivo* protein-DNA interactions at the β-globin gene locus. Proc. Natl. Acad. Sci. USA **88**: 10188–10192.
35. MULLER, P. R. & B. WOLD. 1989. *In vivo* footprinting of a muscle specific enhancer by ligation mediated PCR. Science **246**: 780–78.
36. KIM, C. G. *et al.* 1988. Purification of multiple erythroid cell proteins that bind the promoter of the α-globin gene. Mol. Cell. Biol. **10**: 4270–4281.
37. LIN, H. J., C. Y. HAN & A. W. NIENHUIS. 1992. Functional profile of the human fetal γ-globin gene upstream promoter region. Am. J. Hum. Genet. **51**: 363–370.
38. GUMUCIO, D. L. *et al.* 1988. Nuclear proteins that bind the human γ-globin gene promoter: Alterations in binding produced by point mutations associated with hereditary persistence of fetal hemoglobin. Mol. Cell. Biol. **8**: 5310–5322.
39. MCDONAGH, K. T. *et al.* 1991. The upstream region of the human γ-globin gene promoter: Identification and functional analysis of nuclear protein binding site. J. Biol. Chem. **266**: 11965–11974.
40. JANE, S. M., *et al.* 1992. Identification of a Stage Selector Element in the human γ-globin gene promoter that fosters preferential interaction with the 5'HS2 enhancer when in competition with the β-promoter. EMBO J. **11**: 2961–2969.
41. JANE, S. M., A. W. NIENHUIS & J. M. CUNNINGHAM. 1995. Hemoglobin switching in man and chicken is mediated by a heteromeric complex between the ubiquitous transcription factor CP2 and a developmentally specific protein. EMBO J. **14**: 97–105.
42. BERG, P. E., *et al.* 1989. A common protein binds to two silencers 5' to the human β globin gene. Nuc. Acids Res. **17**: 8833–8852.
43. BERG, P. E., *et al.* 1996. Cloning of BP-1, a repressor of the human beta globin gene. Blood **88**: 472a.
44. ELION, J. *et al.* 1992. DNA sequence variation in a negative control region 5' to the beta globin gene correlates with phenotypic expression of the $β^s$ mutation. Blood **79**: 787–92.

45. PATEL G., et al. 1996. Transcriptional activation potential of normal and tumor-associated myb isoforms does not correlate with their ability to block G-CSF-induced terminal differentiation of murine myeloid precursor cells. Oncogene **13**: 1197–1208.
46. TSUCHIYA, N. et al. 1982. High performance liquid chromatography of carboxylic acids using 4 bromomethyl-7acetoxy-coumarin as fluorescent reagent. J. Chromatog. **234**: 121–130.

Elimination of Transfusions Through Induction of Fetal Hemoglobin Synthesis in Cooley's Anemia[a]

NANCY F. OLIVIERI,[b] DAVID C. REES,[f] GORDON D. GINDER,[d] SWEE LAY THEIN,[f] JOHN S. WAYE,[c] LEBE CHANG,[b] GARY M. BRITTENHAM,[e] AND DAVID J. WEATHERALL[f]

[b]*The Hospital for Sick Children, Toronto, Canada*

[c]*DNA Diagnostic Laboratory, McMaster University Medical Centre, Hamilton, Canada*

[d]*The University of Minnesota School of Medicine, Minneapolis, Minnesota, USA*

[e]*MetroHealth Medical Center, Case Western Reserve University, Cleveland, Ohio, USA*

[f]*MRC Molecular Hematology Unit, Institute of Molecular Medicine, John Radcliffe Hospital, Oxford, United Kingdom*

ABSTRACT: Pharmacological stimulation of fetal hemoglobin production is of considerable interest as an alternative approach to therapy for Cooley's anemia. While intravenous compounds have been effective in inducing short-term increases in fetal hemoglobin in a few patients, long-term elimination of transfusion requirement has not been reported. In patients with Cooley's anemia, treatment with oral sodium phenylbutyrate alone, sodium phenylbytyrate combined with hydroxyurea, and hydroxyurea alone, has augmented fetal hemoglobin production and increased total hemoglobin concentration as much as 5 g/dl over baseline eliminating transfusion requirement in two patients. Parallel declines in circulating nucleated red cell count, and concentrations of serum transform receptor and erythropoietin. are consistent with more effective erythropoiesis. Over extended periods of treatment, no induction of other fetal proteins and no adverse effects were observed. Particular disease mutations and other genetic factors may be of prime importanec in determining the response to agents that induce production of fetal hemoglobin.

For many years, the search for treatment aimed at reduction of globin chain imbalance in patients with Cooley's anemia has focused on the pharmacologic manipulation of fetal hemoglobin ($\alpha 2\gamma 2$; HbF). If the γ globin genes could be reactivated in these patients,

---

[a]Research reported here was supported by The Connaught Transformative Research Grant Program, University of Toronto, Canada; The Medical Research Council of Canada; The Ontario Heart and Stroke Foundation; The Cooley's Anaemia Foundation; National Institutes of Health Grant DDK 29902; and The Medical Research Council, United Kingdom. Dr. Olivieri is a Scientist of the Medical Research Council of Canada.

[g]Address reprint requests and other correspondence to Dr. N.F. Olivieri, Director, Hemoglobinopathy Program, The Hospital for Sick Children, Room 9413, 555 University Avenue, Toronto, Ontario, Canada M5G 1X8.

functional hemoglobin synthesis could be maintained during adulthood, ameliorating the severity of the disease.[1] Clinical trials aimed at augmentation of fetal hemoglobin synthesis in Cooley's anemia and thalassemia intermedia have included those of of 5-azacytidine, hydroxyurea, recombinant human erythropoietin, butyric acid compounds, and combinations of these agents.[2] Stimulation of fetal hemoglobin synthesis by *hydroxyurea* in experimental animals[3] first prompted study of this agent in sickle cell disease. In a multicenter, double-blinded, placebo-controlled clinical trial of 299 adults with sickle cell disease, hydroxyurea therapy was associated with reduction of clinical complications.[4] By contrast, hydroxyurea has been administered to relatively few patients with Cooley's anemia; in initial studies, no significant effect on red cell production, fetal hemoglobin or γ globin mRNA synthesis was observed.[5] Trials of hydroxyurea in patients with non-transfusion–dependent thalassemia have demonstrated increases in fetal hemoglobin over four to five months of therapy, but no parallel change in total hemoglobin concentration.[6] Increases in hemoglobin concentration during hydroxyurea treatment have been described in a non-transfusion-dependent patient[7] and more recently in a transfusion–dependent patient[8] with homozygous β thalassemia, and in a series of patients with hemoglobin E/β thalassemia.[9]

The *butyrate* compounds, derivatives of natural short-chain fatty acids, have offered potential therapy for Cooley's anemia following the observation that elevated plasma concentrations of α amino-*n*-butyric acid in infants of diabetic mothers delayed the normal switch from γ to β globin.[10,11] The observation that *sodium phenylbutyrate*, used for years as treatment for children with inherited urea-cycle disorders,[12] resulted in increased fetal hemoglobin production in K562 cells[13] led to early trials of this compound in patients with sickle cell disease[14] and Cooley's anemia.[15] Extended therapy with phenylbutyrate in 11 adults with homozygous β thalassemia induced modest increases in hemoglobin (1.2 to 2.8 gdl over baseline) in four non-transfusion–dependent patients, but neither percentage nor absolute fetal hemoglobin increased significantly during therapy.[15] None of the patients with Cooley's anemia showed hematologic responses during phenylbutyrate therapy. In a Phase I trial in which six patients with sickle cell disease and severe β thalassemia were treated with intravenous *arginine butyrate*, two or three weeks of therapy induced 2- to 6-fold increases in the levels of γ-globin mRNA; increases were observed in all three patients with Cooley's anemia.[16] The percentage of γ-globin synthesis over that of γ/γ+ β-globin synthesis reportedly increased from 6 to 45 percent above pre-treatment levels in all patients, while proportions of F-reticulocytes increased 1.5 to 3-fold over those determined at baseline. Despite these changes, no increases in hemoglobin concentration were observed during short-term arginine butyrate therapy.

The first patient with Cooley's anemia to be treated with extended butyrate therapy was a 21-year-old woman with the genotype of homozygous hemoglobin Lepore.[16] During administration of 2000 milligrams of arginine butyrate per kilogram as a 24-hour intravenous infusion six days per week for seven weeks, an increase in total hemoglobin concentration from 4.7 to 10.2 gdl was observed. In parallel, continuous arginine butyrate therapy reportedly eliminated globin chain imbalance. Reduction from 24 to 9 hours of infusion per day was reportedly associated with a subsequent worsening of globin chain imbalance.[16] No evidence of marrow suppression during administration of these high doses of arginine butyrate was observed. These findings do not appear to support subsequent concerns that continuous high-dose butyrate may be cytotoxic to red cell precursors.[17,18] Less encouraging results were reported during extended therapy with intravenous arginine butyrate in a subsequent trial of 10 patients,[19] 5 with different point mutations responsible for severe thalassemia syndromes (TABLE 1). Arginine butyrate was rapidly escalated to 2000 mg/kg and administered 24 hours a day, 5 to 6 days a week for approximately 10 weeks. Although modest increases in F-reticulocytes and fetal hemoglobin concentration were observed, no changes in globin chain imbalance or total hemoglobin concentration were demonstrated. No evidence for butyrate-induced marrow suppression was noted. Again, these findings do not appear to support concerns of cytotoxicity during continuous high-dose arginine butyrate.[17,18] Because these observations in patients with common mutations of the β-globin genes differed from those of the first study in which identical treatment of a patient with homozygous hemoglobin Lepore induced a striking hematologic response, the potential influence of this genotype on the hematologic response to switching agents is being investigated. The results of long-term treatment of the first two patients homozygous for hemoglobin Lepore are reported here.

TABLE 1. α- and β-Globin Genotypes, and Status of the Xmn I Polymorphism, in Patients with Thalassemia Treated with 10 Weeks of Continuous Intravenous Arginine Butyrate[19]

β Globin Mutations	α Cluster	Xmn I[30]
codon 41/42 (CTTT)/codon 17	$-\alpha^{3.7}/\alpha\alpha$	Xmn I -/-
-619 bp deletion/-619 bp deletion	$-\alpha^{3.7}/\alpha\alpha$	Xmn I -/-
IVS-1#6/IVS-1#110	αα/αα	Xmn I -/-
IVS-1#6/IVS-1#110	αα/αα	Xmn I -/-
codon 41/42 (CTTT)/Hb E	αα/αα	Xmn I +/-

PATIENTS AND METHODS

Patient 1

The first patient was a 23-year-old female, diagnosed at the age of two years to have Cooley's anemia due to homozygosity for the δβ fusion hemoglobin variant, hemoglobin Lepore Boston-Washington. Monthly red cell transfusions were commenced at the age of four years and splenectomy was performed at age six years to reduce red cell requirements. Transfusions were discontinued after three years because of red cell allo-immunization, after which the hemoglobin concentrations varied between 4 and 6 g/dl. This severe anemia led to poor exercise tolerance, growth failure, delayed sexual maturation and extensive bone marrow hyperplasia, resulting in gross, progressive skeletal deformities. At the age of 21 years, a short-term increase in hemoglobin concentration was observed during a seven-week course of intravenous arginine butyrate, reported previously.[16] Subsequently, arginine butyrate was administered intermittently, but had to be discontinued owing to difficulties with parenteral drug administration. Oral sodium phenylbutyrate, 10 g/m²/day, was therefore commenced in 1993; hydroxyurea 10 mg/g/day, increased over six months to 15 mg/g/day, was added to the treatment regimen after approximately four months of therapy with sodium phenylbutyrate alone.

Patient 2

The patient's 12-year-old brother (FIG.) was found to have Cooley's anemia due to homozygosity for hemoglobin Lepore at the age of six months. He began red cell transfusions at age 15 months when his hemoglobin concentration was 5.5 g/dl. Every four weeks he received 15 ml packed red cells/kg to maintain pre-transfusion hemoglobin concentrations of 9.5 g/dl. In 1991 his transfusion requirements increased, necessitating splenectomy. In 1995, therapy with sodium phenylbutyrate, 10 g/m²/day, was introduced; red cell transfusions, administered monthly for the next three months, maintained baseline hemo-

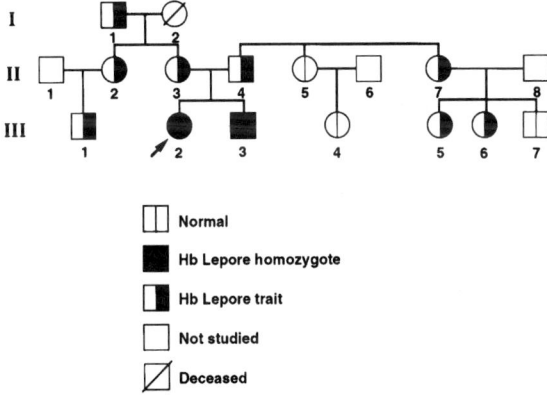

FIGURE. Pedigree of family. Arrow indicates the propositus (III-2); the brother (patient 2) is III-3.

globin concentrations of 9.5 g/dl. After the third transfusion during therapy with sodium phenylbutyrate, transfusions were withheld. Hydroxyurea, 6 mg/g/day, was added after phenylbutyrate had been administered for approximately six months and after transfusions had been withheld for approximately three months; the dose of hydroxyurea was increased over six months, to 13.5 mg/g/day.

Drug Regimen

Throughout the study the patients were maintained on 5 mg of oral folic acid per day. Sodium phenylbutyrate was administered in 500 mg tablets in three divided doses. The first patient received sodium phenylbutyrate supplied by Triple Crown America (parent company Fyrklo Venn, Scandanavia, AB) under a United States Investigational New Drug application IND #38405 to Dr. Nancy F. Olivieri and with permission of the Health Protection Branch, Health Canada, Ottawa, Canada. The second patient received sodium phenylbutyrate supplied by Pharmaceutics International Inc., Hunt Valley, Maryland 21031 USA under a United States Investigational New Drug application #17123 to Drs. George Dover and Saul Brusilow, under a research protocol supported in part by the United States' Cooley's Anemia Foundation. Administration of sodium phenylbutyrate and hydroxyurea was approved by The Research Ethics Board of The Hospital for Sick Children, Toronto, Canada.

Hematological Analysis

Hematological studies, hemoglobin electrophoresis on cellulose acetate and starch gel, estimation of fetal hemoglobin, and the relative rates of α, β and γ globin chain synthesis followed standard methods.[20] The relative numbers of F cells were determined by immunofluorescence-staining of fixed blood smears and by fluorescence-activated cell sorting, using a mouse monoclonal anti-γ chain antibody.[21] Serum transferrin receptor levels were determined using previously described methods.[22] Estimations of serum erythropoietin were determined by ELISA (R and D Systems, Minneapolis, MN).

Markers of Fetal Erythropoiesis

The $^G\gamma/^A\gamma$ content of fetal hemoglobin was determined by mass spectroscopy.[23] Alpha-feto-protein levels were measured by radioimmunoassay designed to give maximal sensitivity in the range 0–14 IU/ml. Carcinoembryonic antigen levels were measured by radioimmunoassay using standard methods.

DNA Analysis

Genomic DNA, isolated from peripheral blood lymphocytes, was analyzed by Southern hybridization.[24] The deletion breakpoint fragment for hemoglobin Lepore was amplified by PCR[25] using appropriate primers.[26] Polymorphisms in the β-globin gene cluster were analyzed after PCR amplification,[27] which was also used to amplify the region immediately upstream from the $^A\gamma$-globin gene from positions -653 to +50 relative to the CAP site; this region was sequenced in DNA from the first patient and her mother. In the PCR the upstream primer was 5′-biotinylated to facilitate preparation of a single stranded (SS) template by using magnetic beads. The SS DNA was directly sequenced using the dideoxy chain termination method.[28]

RESULTS

Hematological Responses

During therapy with sodium phenylbutyrate in the first patient, hemoglobin concentrations were maintained between 8.5 and 9.5 g/dl, approximately 4 g/dl over baseline. Following addition of hydroxyurea, hemoglobin concentrations increased further to 11 to 11.8 g/dl. The fetal hemoglobin concentration increased from approximately 3.9 g/dl at baseline to approximately 10.5 g/dl during combined therapy with sodium phenylbutyrate and hydroxyurea. In the second patient, during the period on regular transfusions in parallel with the administration of sodium phenylbutyrate, no change in pre-transfusion hemoglobin concentrations was observed. Over the three months after stopping transfusions, the hemoglobin concentration gradually declined to 5.8 g/dl, in parallel with an increase in nucleated red blood cells and of fetal hemoglobin to approximately 5 g/dl, the latter reflecting endogenous erythropoiesis that had been previously suppressed by transfusions. Following the addition of hydroxyurea, the hemoglobin concentration gradually increased to 10 g/dl, in parallel with an increase of approximately 5 g/dl of fetal hemoglobin and a decline in nucleated red blood cell count. The patient has maintained this hemoglobin level for 18 months, during which no transfusions have been required. Hydroxyurea induced a modest reduction in absolute neutrophil count in both patients (data not shown).

Hematological Findings

Hemoglobin analysis showed that both patients are homozygotes for the δβ fusion variant, hemoglobin Lepore Washington Boston.[20,26] Globin-chain synthesis studies demonstrated a progressive decline in the synthesis ratio of α/γ + δβ Lepore globin chains, reflecting an increase in γ chain synthesis during treatment. Declines in nucleated red cell counts, in parallel with a reduction in serum transferrin receptor and erythropoietin concentrations (TABLE 2), indicated a reduction in erythroid expansion[22] during therapy.

TABLE 2. Consecutive Data on II.2 and II.3

Pedigree Designation	Date	Hb (g/dl)	Hb F (%) (normal 0.3-1.1)	F Cells (%) (normal 0-4.4)	Gγ/Aγ Chain Ratio (normal adults, 0.5-0.8)	α/non-α Chain Ratio (normal 1.0)	Starch Gel Electrophoresis (normal adults (CA 1+2)	α-FP (IU/ml) (normal 0-9)	CEA (μg/ml) (normal <10)	sTfR (μg/ml) (normal 0.85-3.05)	EPO (IU/ml) (normal 3.9-14.9)
III.2	7/1/92	4.5				4.0				47.6	955
	2/4/92	4.5									955
	16/8/93	7.9									
	11/24/94	8.5									
	30/1/96	11.0	89	100	0.68		CA 1+2	<2		19.5	34.4
	4/3/96	11.5	91	100	0.71			<2		19.2	28.8
	29/3/96	11.2		100				<2		20.9	79.0
	26/4/96	11.8		100						16.4	36.1
	24/5/96	11.6				2.9	CA 1+2			18.3	31.8
	1/4/97	11.9					CA 1+2		9	10.6	
III.3	30/1/96	9.1	36	56.7	0.57	4.0	CA 1+2	<2		24.9	75.7[a]
	4/3/96	5.8	71	85.7	0.57			<2		37.7	825
	29/3/96	6.5		100				<2		33.1	874
	3/5/96	7.8	91	100			CA 1+2			30.7	203
	24/5/96	9.5		100	0.55	2.6	CA 1+2		10	19.8	46.7
	3/9/96	10.3	90								
	9/12/96	9.7									
	1/4/97	10.3								14.0	

NM = Gγ/Aγ not measurable when % Hb F <1%; sTfR = soluble transferrin receptor; α-FP =α-fetoprotein; CEA = carcinoembryonic antigen; CA = carbonic anhydrase; EPO = serum erythropoietin concentration.
[a]While on transfusions.

TABLE 3. Hematologic Data on Family

Pedigree Designation	Hb Analysis	HbA$_2$ (%)	Hb F (%)	F Cells (%)	Gγ/Aγ Ratio	Starch Gel	sTfR (μg/ml)	α-FP (IU/ml)
I.1	A+Lepore	2.4	0.8		NM[b]	CA 1+2	3.3	<2
II.2	A+Lepore	2.8	2.5	16.2	<1	CA 1+2	2.7	<2
II.3	A+F+Lepore	2.3	3.4	23.2	0.3	CA 1+2	2.3	<2
II.4	A+Lepore	3.1	1.2	4.4	<1	CA 1+2	3.1	4.7
II.5	A	2.5	0.3	2.0	NM	CA 1+2	2.8	<2
II.7	A+Lepore	2.5	0.9	16.0	NM	CA 1+2	2.4	4.2
III.1	A+Lepore	2.1	1.2	10.7	<1	CA 1+2	2.1	<2
III.2	F+Lepore[a]	0	89	100	0.68	CA 1+2	47.6	<2
III.3	F+Lepore[a]	0	91	100	0.55	CA 1+2	37.7	<2
III.4	A	2.2	0.3	2.5	NM	CA 1+2	1.5	2.0
III.5	A+Lepore	3.7	2.4	16.0	<1	CA 1+2	2.4	<2
III.6	A+Lepore	2.9	1.2	13.0	<1	CA 1+2	2.4	<2
III.7	A	2.8	0.4	2.1	NM	CA 1+2	1.8	2.6
Normal range		2.2 - 3.3	0.3 - 1.1	0-4.4			0.85 - 3.05	0-9

NM = Gγ/Aγ not measurable when % Hb F <1%.
sTfR = soluble transferrin receptor, α-FP = alpha feto-protein.
[a]Consecutive data given in TABLE 2.

Markers of Fetal Erythropoiesis

Estimations of the $^G\gamma/^A\gamma$ globin chains demonstrated that the output of both γ globin loci was increased, with a preponderance of $^A\gamma$ chain synthesis (TABLE 3). Analysis of red cell carbonic anhydrase by starch electrophoresis showed that isozymes 1 and 2, virtually absent from cord blood cells,[20] were present at normal adult levels in several samples obtained from the patients after they had synthesized high concentrations of fetal hemoglobin. Serum concentrations of alpha feto-protein and carcinoembryonic antigen were also within adult range. Together with an adult pattern of synthesis of $^A\gamma$ globin chains, these findings provide no evidence for reversion to a fetal form of erythropoiesis or reactivation of other genes expressed in fetal life.

DNA Analysis and Family Studies

Heterozygosity for hemoglobin Lepore, with values of fetal hemoglobin and F cells within those reported in the literature,[20,29] was observed in both parents and several members of the family (TABLE 3). Southern hybridization with β and γ gene probes revealed the deletion responsible for hemoglobin Lepore Washington-Boston.[26] Both patients were homozygous for absence of the Xmn I polymorphic site (-/-) at position -158 of the $^G\gamma$ globin gene. The region immediately upstream from the $^A\gamma$ globin gene, positions -653 to +50 relative to the CAP site, in the first patient and her mother, showed no abnormalities. No unaffected relatives had increased levels of fetal hemoglobin or F cells.

DISCUSSION

The magnitude and duration of augmentation of fetal hemoglobin seen in these patients, associated with doubling of hemoglobin concentration and independence from transfusion, have not been observed previously in Cooley's anemia. The sustained response of the first patient represents the longest reported period of therapy aimed at stimulating fetal hemoglobin in a patient with thalassemia. The marked decrease in nucleated red blood cell count and serum transferrin receptor concentration, as well as the reduction in globin chain imbalance, indicate a genuine augmentation of fetal hemoglobin synthesis, and not cell selection or increased proliferation of erythroid marrow. These long-term responses, in the absence of adverse effects, provide the first evidence for the effectiveness and safety of the combination of sodium phenylbutyrate and hydroxyurea in the reactivation and long-term maintenance of high levels of fetal hemoglobin. Supporting the safety of prolonged administration of these agents is the observation that, while the switch from fetal to adult hemoglobin is part of a coordinated series of changes in the enzyme and antigen constitution of the red cell,[20] there was no evidence for reversion to fetal erythropoiesis or for augmented synthesis of other fetal proteins. This suggests that, even in the face of this profound switch to fetal hemoglobin synthesis, neither agent reactivates other genes normally switched off after fetal life, a finding consistent with an avian model in which butyrate-induced selective activation of an embryonic globin gene was unassociated with a change to primitive erythropoiesis.[31]

Previous attempts to reactivate fetal hemoglobin synthesis in Cooley's anemia *in vivo* have proved disappointing. The laboratory responses to short-term arginine butyrate in a pilot study[16] were not observed in a larger trial,[19] while administration of sodium phenylbutyrate alone has been ineffective in Cooley's anemia.[15] Although increases in fetal hemoglobin, and modest changes in total hemoglobin, have been reported during administration of hydroxyurea to patients with thalassemia,[5-9] neither this agent nor recombinant erythropoietin[32,33] induce consistent hematological improvement in patients with Cooley's anemia.[2] Only 5-azacytidine, when administered intravenously, has induced increases in hemoglobin concentration in patients with Cooley's anemia.[34,35] Why, therefore, have these patients shown such a dramatic response in fetal hemoglobin production to these agents? It has been suggested that butyrate-associated induction of fetal hemoglobin in mice may require the presence of pre-activated γ–globin genes.[36] Nonetheless, sodium phenylbutyrate and hydroxyurea have, so far, failed to induce a similar response in small series of patients with thalassemia intermedia in whom sustained synthesis of fetal hemoglobin has been observed (Dover, G. J., unpublished observations). Is the response observed the result of another gene segregating in this family, or a reflection of the unusual thalassemia mutation?

There is no evidence for an associated genetic basis for increased fetal hemoglobin synthesis,[37] hereditary persistence of fetal hemoglobin (HPFH),[20] in the patients or their relatives. The absence of a deletion of the β-globin gene cluster apart from that responsible for hemoglobin Lepore, and the normal DNA sequence in the promoter regions of the $^A\gamma$ genes predominant in fetal hemoglobin production in these patients, argue against a determinant for deletion or non-deletion HPFH in either patient. The slight elevations in fetal hemoglobin levels in the parents and other heterozygotes for hemoglobin Lepore do not exceed those reported previously.[20,29] No normal family member has elevated levels of fetal hemoglobin or F cells, offering no evidence for heterocellular HPFH.[37] Finally, both the proband and her brother lack the polymorphism, identified by the restriction enzyme *Xmn* I 158 nucleotides 5′ to the $^G\gamma$ globin genes which, in homozygotes, is associated with augmented fetal hemoglobin production in response to anemic stress.[30,37]

The deletion underlying the fusion gene that codes for hemoglobin Lepore could be responsible for this unusual response. It might alter the relationship between regulatory sequences and structural loci in the $\delta\beta$ globin gene cluster, making persistent γ chain production more likely; heterozygotes for hemoglobin Lepore usually have slightly higher levels of fetal hemoglobin than those for thalassemia.[20,29] Furthermore, the mutation responsible for hemoglobin Lepore deletes a region of the globin gene cluster with features of an origin of replication, the only sequence of this type in this cluster.[38,39] DNA replication may be linked to a number of transcriptional functions, notably to the form of repression known as silencing.[40] The hemoglobin Lepore rearrangement could thereby interfere with the post-natal repression of the γ globin genes, increasing responsiveness to agents that augment fetal hemoglobin synthesis. This hypothesis is supported by a recent single case report of a patient with double heterozygosity for β thalassemia and hemoglobin Lepore.[41] These questions may be clarified by further studies of the fetal hemoglobin response to these agents in patients with hemoglobin Lepore or forms of β thalassemia created by similar deletions of the β-globin gene cluster.

Considering the remarkable (previously unreported) clinical improvement that can be achieved with this treatment, it is now extremely important to determine why the outcome is so variable and, in particular, whether this reflects the nature of the thalassemia mutation or other genetic factors. Furthermore, although the sustained fetal hemoglobin response in the patients described here was not associated with side effects or augmented synthesis of other fetal proteins, the recent report of the reactivation of the latter in patients with renal failure treated with erythropoietin[42] indicates that the overall effects of these agents on the expression of fetal genes requires further study. These problems are of particular importance now that the possibility of reactivating other fetal genes for the management of genetic disease is being explored.[43]

REFERENCES

1. WOOD, W. G. & D. J. WEATHERALL. 1983. Developmental genetics of the human hemoglobins. Biochem. J. **215:** 1–10.
2. OLIVIERI, N. F. 1996. Reactivation of fetal hemoglobin in patients with thalassemia. Sem. Hematol. **33:** 24–42.
3. PLATT, O. S., S. H. ORKIN, G. DOVER, et al. 1984. Hydroxyurea enhances fetal hemoglobin production in sickle cell anemia. J. Clin. Invest. **74:** 652–656.
4. CHARACHE, S., M. L. TERRIN, R. D. MOORE, et al. 1995. Effect of hydroxyurea on the frequency of painful crises in sickle cell anemia. N. Engl. J. Med. **332:** 1317–1322.
5. NIENHUIS, A. W., T. J. LEY, R. K. HUMPHRIES, et al. 1985. Pharmacological manipulation of fetal hemoglobin synthesis in patients with severe beta thalassemia. Ann. N. Y. Acad. Sci. **445:** 198–211.
6. LOUKOPOULOS, D., E. VOSKARIDOU, A. STAMOULAKATOU, et al. 1995. Clinical trials with hydroxyurea and recombinant human erythropoietin. In Molecullar Biology of Hemoglobin Switching. G. Stamatoyannopoulos, Ed.: Volume 1: 365–372. Intercept Ltd.
7. MCDONAGH, K. T., E. P. ORRINGER, G. J. DOVER, et al. 1990. Hydroxyurea improves erythropoiesis in a patient with homozygous beta thalassemia. Clin. Res. **38:** 346A, Abstract.
8. ARRUDA, V. R., C. S. P. LIMA, S. T. O. SAAD, et al. 1997. Successful use of hydroxyurea in β-thalassemia major. N. Engl. J. Med. **336:** 964, Letter.
9. FUCHAROEN, S., N. SIRITANARATKUL, P. WINICHAGOON, et al. 1997. Hydroxyurea increases hemoglobin F levels and improves the effectiveness of erythropoiesis in β-thalassemia/hemoglobin E disease. Blood **87:** 887–892.
10. BARD, H. & J. PROSMANNE. 1985. Relative rates of fetal hemoglobin and adult hemoglobin synthesis in cord blood of infants of insulin–dependent diabetic mothers. Pediatr. **75:** 1143–1147.
11. PERRINE, S. P., M. F. GREENE, D. V. FALLER. 1985. Delay in the fetal globin switch in infants of diabetic mothers. N. Engl. J. Med. **312:** 334–338.
12. FINKELSTEIN, J. E., E. R. HAUSER, C. O. LEONARD, et al. 1990. Late onset ornithine transcarbamylase deficiency in male patients. J. Pediatr. **117:** 897–902.
13. SAMID, D., A. YEH & P. PRASANNA. 1992. Induction of erythroid differentiation and fetal hemoglobin production in human leukemic cells treated with phenylacetate. Blood **80:** 1576–1581.
14. DOVER, G. J., S. BRUSILOW, S. CHARACHE. 1994. Induction of fetal hemoglobin production in subjects with sickle cell anemia by oral sodium phenylbutyrate. Blood **84:** 339–343.
15. COLLINS, A. F., H. A. PEARSON, P. GIARDINA, et al. 1995. Oral sodium phenylbutyrate therapy in homozygous beta thalassemia. Blood **85:** 43–49.
16. PERRINE, S. P., G. D. GINDER, D. V. FALLER, et al. 1993. A short–term trial of butyrate to stimulate fetal–globin–gene expression in the beta–globin disorders. N. Engl. J. Med. **328:** 81–86.
17. FALLER, D. V. & S. P. PERRINE. 1995. Butyrate in the treatment of sickle cell disease and β-thalassemia. Curr. Opin. Hematol. **2:** 109–117.

18. ATWEH, G. F., G. J. DOVER, D. V. FALLER, et al. 1996. Sustained hematologic response to pulse butyrate therapy in beta globin disorders. Blood **88:** 652A, Abstract.
19. SHER, G. D., G. GINDER, J. A. LITTLE, et al. 1995. Extended therapy with arginine butyrate in patients with thalassemia and sickle cell disease. N. Engl. J. Med. **332:** 106–110.
20. WEATHERALL, D. J. & J. B. CLEGG. 1981. The Thalassaemia Syndromes. Blackwell Scientific Publications. Oxford.
21. THORPE, S. J., S. L. THEIN, M. SAMPIETRO, et al. 1994. Immunochemical estimation of hemoglobin types in red blood cells by FACS analysis. Br. J. Haematol. **87:** 125–132.
22. HUEBERS, H. A., Y. BEGUIN, P. POOTRAKUL, et al. 1990. Intact transferrin receptors in human plasma and their relation to erythropoiesis. Blood **75:** 102–107.
23. SHACKLETON, C. H. L. & H. E. WITKOWSKA. 1991. Mass spectrometry in the characterization of variant hemoglobins. *In* Mass spectrometry: Clinical and biomedical applications. D. M. Desiderio, Ed.: 135. Plenum. New York.
24. SOUTHERN, E. M. 1975. Detection of specific sequences among DNA fragments separated by gel electrophoresis. J. Mol. Biol. **98:** 503–507.
25. SAIKI, R. A., D. H. GELFAND, S. STOFFEL, et al. 1988. Primer-directed enzymatic amplification of DNA with thermostable DNA polymerase. Science **239:** 487–491.
26. BAIRD, M., H. SCHREINER, C. DRISCOLL, et al. 1981. Localization of the site of recombination of the Hb Lepore Boston globin gene. J. Clin. Invest. **58:** 560–564.
27. SUTTON, M., E. BOUHASSIRA & R. NAGEL. 1989. Polymerase chain reaction amplification applied to the determination of β-like globin cluster haplotypes. Am. J. Hematol. **32:** 66–69.
28. CRAIG, J. E., S. M. SHEERIN, R. BARNETSON, et al. 1993. The molecular basis of HPFH in a British family identified by heteroduplex formation. Br. J. Haematol. **84:** 106–110.
29. EFREMOV, G. D. 1978. Hemoglobins Lepore and anti-Lepore. Hemoglobin **2:** 197–233.
30. MILLER, B. A., N. F. OLIVIERI, M. SALAMEH, et al. 1987. Molecular analysis of the high F phenotype in Saudi Arabian sickle cell anemia. N. Engl. J. Med. **316:** 244–250.
31. BURNS, L. J., J. G. GLAUBER & G. D. GINDER. 1988. Butyrate induces selective transcriptional activation of a hypomethylated embryonic globin gene in adult erythroid cells. Blood **72:** 1536–1542.
32. OLIVIERI, N. F., M. FREEDMAN, S. PERRINE, et al. 1992. Trial of recombinant human erythropoietin in thalassemia intermedia. Blood **80:** 3258–3260.
33. RACHMILEWITZ, E. A., M. AKER, D. PERRY, et al. 1995. Sustained increase in hemoglobin and RBC following long-term administration of recombinant human erythropoietin to patients with homozygous beta thalassemia. Br. J. Haematol. **90:** 341–345.
34. LOWREY, C. H. & A. W. NIENHUIS. 1993. Brief report: treatment with azacytidine of patients with end-stage—thalassemia. N. Engl. J. Med. **329:** 845–849.
35. LEY, T. J., J. DESIMONE, N. P. ANAGNOU, et al. 1982. 5-Azacytidine selectively increases gamma-globin synthesis in a patient with $β^+$ thalassemia. N. Engl. J. Med. **307:** 1469–1475.
36. PACE, B, Q. LI, K. PETERSON, et al. 1994. α-amino butyric acid cannot reactivate the silenced γ gene of the β locus *YAC* transgenic mouse. Blood **84:** 4344–4453.
37. WOOD, W. G. 1993. Increased HbF in adult life. Clin. Haematol. **6:** 177–213.
38. KITSBERG, D., S. SELIG, I. KESHET, et al. 1993. Replication structure of the human β-globin gene domain. Nature **366:** 588–590.
39. ALADJEM, M. I., M. GROUDINE, L. L. BRODY, et al. 1995. Participation of the human beta-globin locus control region in initiation of DNA replication. Science **270:** 815–819.
40. KELLY, T. J., P. V. JALLEPALLI & R. K. CLYNE. 1994. Silence of the ORCs. Curr. Biol. **4:** 238–241.
41. RIGANO, P., L. MANFRÉ, R. LA GALLA, et al. 1997. Clinical and hematological response to hydroxyurea in a patient with Hb lepore/β-thalassemia. Hemoglobin **21:** 219–226.
42. BALLIZZI, V., L. DE NICOLA, P. AMES, et al. 1997. Fetal proteins and chronic treatment with low-dose erythropoietin. J. Lab. Clin. Med. **129:** 193–199.
43. TINSLEY, J. M., A. C. POTTER, S. T. PHELPS, et al. 1996. Amelioration of the dystrophic phenotype of mdx mice using a truncated utrophin transgene. Nature **384:** 349–353.

Butyrate Trials[a]

MARIA DOMENICA CAPPELLINI,[b,d] GIOVANNA GRAZIADEI,[b]
LAURA CICERI,[b] ALESSIA COMINO,[b] PAOLO BIANCHI,[b]
MAURO POMATI,[c] AND GEMINO FIORELLI[b]

[b]*Centro Anemie Congenite, Ospedale Maggiore Policlinico IRCCS,
Università di Milano, Milano, Italy*

[c]*Servizio di Ematologia - Ospedale Maggiore Policlinico IRCCS,
Milano, Italy*

ABSTRACT: The aims of this study were to ascertain tolerability, safety and efficacy of oral isobutyramide (150 mg/kg bw/day) in stimulating fetal hemoglobin production in twelve thalassemia intermedia patients. Patients were treated for 28 days and followed for a further 28 days. Efficacy was monitored by non-α/α globin chain ratio and percentage of HbF. Five patients experienced increases of non-α/α ratio ranging between 5.3 and 100% at the end of treatment. Five patients show an increase of HbF ranging between 4.4 and 26%. Their HbF% continues to increase during follow-up period. The analysis of variance for HbF showed a time effect close to significance both in treatment period ($p = 0.06$) and in follow-up period ($p = 0.08$). Moreover, to evaluate a possible erythropoietic modification, serum Erythropoietin (sEpo) and serum Transferrin Receptor (sTfR) were evaluated. Serum Epo and sTfR levels were significantly increased during treatment ($p < 0.05$ vs baseline).

Clinical and experimental data indicate that increased levels of fetal hemoglobin (HbF) are of benefit in ameliorating the clinical severity of the β-globin disorders.[1] The presence of HbF through life, as shown by patients with Hereditary Persistence of Fetal Hemoglobin, is compatible with a normal life.[2] Small increments in fetal globin synthesis can ameliorate β-thalassemia by decreasing the imbalance of excess unmatched α-globin chains in the red blood cell. The unmatched α-globin chains damage the red cell and cause rapid red blood cell destruction and life-threatening anemia.[3]

Different chemiotherapic agents, including 5-azacytidine, cytosine arabinoside and hydroxyurea, have been shown to stimulate γ-globin synthesis and HbF.[4–7] However, cytotoxicity from these drugs has been suggested to have some risk and has generated renewed urgency for identifying safe and effective agents for stimulating HbF.[8]

Increased plasma levels of α amino-*n*-butyric acid have been identified in fetuses developing in the presence of maternal diabetes. These fetuses do not suppress fetal globin before birth as a normal fetus does and experimental evidence indicates that α amino-*n*-butyric acid and some analogues induce the expression of HbF.[9]

---

[a]This study was partly supported by Fondazione Italiana "Leonardo Giambrone" per la guarigione della Thalassemia and by MURST 60% and was presented in part at the 38th Annual Meeting of the American Society of Hematology, Orlando, FL.

[d]Corresponding author: Maria Domenica Cappellini, M.D., Centro Anemie Congenite, Istituto di Medicina Interna e Fisiopatologia Medica, Università di Milano, Ospedale Maggiore Policlinico IRCCS, Via Francesco Sforza 35, 20122 Milano, Italy; Tel: 39-2-55033752; Fax: 39-2-55180241; E-mail: Maria.Cappellini@unimi.it

In fetal sheep the infusion of butyric acid in utero during the time of the normal gene switch stimulates the γ globin gene.[10] In erythroid cells cultured from normal fetuses and patients with β-thalassemia or sickle cell anemia butyrate enhances fetal globin gene expression.[11,12]

The mechanism by which butyrates stimulate γ-globin production is not fully understood, but they have been shown to modify histone acetylation[13] and more recently to interact with silencer sequences in the γ-gene promoter.[14]

Two phase I/II studies of intravenous arginine butyrate administration in a limited number of patients with sickle-cell disease and β-thalassemia, heterogenous with respect to genotype and transfusion requirement, have been reported.[15,16] Although the protocol was almost identical, the results of the second study were disappointing compared to those reported in the earlier pilot study.

Apparently arginine butyrate has few short-term side effects; however in baboons, prolonged infusion of high doses (8 to 10 g/kg/day) were complicated with neurotoxicity.[17] However butyric acid is rapidly metabolized as an energy source. In animals and in humans, it is cleared rapidly within 5 to 15 minutes when given intravenously requiring continuous infusion.[18]

Isobutyramide is a branched chain amide derivative of the fatty acid butyric acid with oral bioavailability. *In vitro* isobutyramide at a concentration of 0.3 mM is able to stimulate the γ-globin synthesis. Isobutyramide has a long plasma half life (7.5-10 h) and no demonstrable toxicity, even in the fetal sheep in whom drug levels of 18 mM were achieved. Treatment of fetal sheep with Isobutyramide results in profound inhibition of globin gene switching, with 80 to 90% fetal globin actively synthesized at the time of birth.[19] Oral administration of isobutyramide to adult non-human primates has resulted in prompt elevations of fetal globin chain synthesis. Single oral doses of 115, 150 and 300 mg/kg body weight have been administered to two normal adults: the lower dose has been shown to be able to maintain isobutyramide plasma levels above 0.3 mM concentration that is required *in vitro* to stimulate fetal hemoglobin production.[19]

We performed a pilot phase II open study on 12 transfusion-independent adult patients with thalassemia intermedia given oral isobutyramide (150mg/kg body weight/day) in order to ascertain the tolerability, safety and efficacy of the compound in stimulating fetal hemoglobin production. Moreover, to evaluate a possible erythropoietic modification during isobutyramide treatment, serum Erythropoietin (sEpo) and serum Transferrin Receptor (sTfR) were evaluated. The results support the notion that isobutyramide is capable of increasing HbF in a subset of thalassemia intermedia patients, possibly through a cellular and/or molecular mechanism.

MATERIALS AND METHODS

This was a pilot phase II, open study of the safety and efficacy of oral isobutyramide approved by the Italian National Health Committee for Drug Investigation and by the Ethic Committee on Clinical Investigation of the University of Milan.

The study was designed including a screening phase, a treatment phase of 28 days (evaluation of safety and efficacy on days 0, 4, 8, 14, 21 and 28), and a post-treatment follow-up period of 28 days (evaluation on days 35, 42 and 56). The drug was administered orally over 28 days at a dose of 150 mg per kg body weight once a day. An orange or mint flavored isobutyramide powder was provided as a solid formulation in sachets for instant reconstitution in water or fruit juice.

Patients

Twelve Caucasian patients with thalassemia intermedia (7 men, 5 women, mean ± SE age 31 ± 2 years, range 20-43) were enrolled in this study, according to the inclusion (age > 18 years, Hb ≥ 10g/dL, negative HIV antibodies, informed consent) and exclusion criteria (pregnancy, clinical evidence of primary renal, cardiovascular, respiratory, other hematologic, neurologic and endocrine diseases, treatment with any other investigational drug, uncooperative attitude). Patients participated in the study as outpatients. They all started to take folic acid (5-methyltetrahydrofolic acid 15 mg/day per os) 2 weeks before starting the study and continued throughout the study period. Ten of the 12 patients had been occasionally transfused during their life but none of them underwent blood transfusion the year before entering the study. Nine were splenectomized. The diagnosis of thalassemia intermedia was based on hematological and clinical features. The α and β genotypes were determined as previously described.[20] The C——T nucleotide substitution at position -158 from the 5' end of the $^G\gamma$-globin gene was determined by restriction enzyme XmnI. The presence of this substitution is noted as XmnI+ and its absence as XmnI-(TABLE I).

Methods

Safety was evaluated by physical examination, vital signs, clinical laboratory evaluations (blood biochemistry, urinalysis) ECG, chest X ray and adverse events. Changes in laboratory indexes or development/deterioration of symptoms were evaluated according to the WHO recommendations for assessment of toxicity.[21] Efficacy was monitored by determining the non-α/α globin chain ratio and HbF%. Globin chain synthesis was evaluated by HPLC separation on a Variant machine adapted for a globin chain program (HPLC, Bio-Rad Laboratories, USA). The analysis was performed in triplicate and the results reported as the mean of 3 evaluations. Hemoglobin F was quantified by HPLC (Bio-Rad Variant Hemoglobin Testing System).

Serum Epo and sTfR were assayed using a commercially available enzyme immuno assay (Predicta Epo Kit, Genzyme and TfR Quantikine R&D Systems, Minneapolis USA), according to the manufacturer's directions. All samples were analyzed in duplicate after appropriate dilution (1:6 for sEpo, 1:600 for sTfR). Absorbance was readed at 450 nm, with dual wavelength correction at 630 nm, using Vmax EASIA Reader and Medgenix

TABLE 1. Characteristics of Thalassemia Intermedia Patients Treated with Oral Isobutyramide

Patient No	Age (yrs)	Sex	Total Hb (g/dl)	HbF %	Non-α/α Ratio	Genotype	Xmn I Site	Blood Transfusion	Splenectomy
1	38	M	8.7	35.1	0.41	IVS1-110/IVS1-6	-/-	Occasionally	Yes
2	36	M	7.0	64.6	0.41	Cod 39/IVS1-6	-/-	Occasionally	No
3	24	M	9.8	97.5	0.45	Cod 39/IVS1-110	+/-	One	No
4	19	F	9.2	39.4	0.38	-87/IVS1-6	-/-	Occasionally	Yes
5	32	F	6.9	95.8	0.46	δb/Cod 39	+/-	One	Yes
6	33	M	6.5	50.1	0.44	Cod 39/IVS1-6	+/-	Occasionally	Yes
7	26	M	8.4	27.7	0.59	-87/IVS1-6	-/-	Occasionally	Yes
8	43	F	7.6	51.8	0.43	IVS2-1/IVS1-6	+/-	Occasionally	Yes
9	41	M	8.0	3.8	0.50	IVS1-6/IVS1-6	-/-	Occasionally	Yes
10	27	M	9.6	87.3	0.34	IVS1-110/δβ	-/-	Occasionally	Yes
11	30	F	9.0	97.8	0.51	Cod 39/Cod 39	+/+	Never	Yes
12	24	F	8.6	11.2	0.52	Cod 39/β+ mild	-/-	Occasionally	No

ELISA-AID Software. Absorbance of the test wells was compared with the Standard Curve (four parameter logistic fit), converted to a numerical value, and expressed as mU/ml for sEpo and µg/ml for sTfR.

Statistical Evaluation

The analysis, as planned in the protocol, focused on the change over time of the two main efficacy parameters. We calculated the percentage change in each variable between day 0 and the other 5 assessments under treatment (days 4, 8, 14, 21 and 28) and the percentage change between day 28 and the 3 drug-free assessments (days 35, 42 and 56). Two separate analyses were performed for each phase using a 2-way analysis of variance with the time of assessment as within-subject factor. The two hypotheses tested with this analysis concern the constant effect (to test for an overall change from baseline) and the time effect (to test for variations along time of the percent differences). Patients were considered treatment responders when they showed an improvement of the efficacy parameters (non-α/α ratio and/or HbF%) either on day 28 or on day 56 versus baseline. A percent increase versus baseline less than 2% was considered as negligible.

Serum Epo and sTfR values were analyzed using a commercially available computer program (Labstat 4.0 bio-Rad Laboratories, Srl). Student's t-test was used for comparison between means. Correlation coefficients were calculated with Pearson's test and linear regression analysis, to assess correlation between variables. Considering that subjects with iron deficiency anemia represent the predicted physiological sEpo and sTfR response to anemia, the Observed/Predicted log sEpo and log sTfR ratio (O/P ratio) was calculated for each patient, using reference regression line obtained from literature.[22,23] The 95% confidence limits were calculated to define a range of reference for O/P values. These limits were: 0.76–1.16 for sEpo and 0.91–1.09 for O/P sTfR.

RESULTS

Twelve patients were enrolled in this study according to the protocol. Their genotypes and clinical profile are shown in TABLE 1. All the patients completed the treatment (28 days) and the follow-up (28 days). Patients compliance to treatment was 100% and no treatment schedule had to be changed. No drug-related adverse events were recorded. The non α/α ratio and HbF% were evaluated as the two major efficacy parameters. The two efficacy parameters were determined at baseline and on days 4, 8, 14, 21, 28, 35, 42 and 56. FIGURE 1 shows the plot of the mean values over time of the non α/α ratio of all the patients. Patient by patient analysis revealed that 5 patients (4,7,8,9 and 10) presented a percent increase of this ratio ranging between 5.3 and 100% at the end of treatment. In patients 4 and 7 the ratio returned to the pretreatment levels by the end of the follow-up period. The value reached by patients 8, 9 and 10 at the end of the treatment was either maintained or increased. Surprisingly, an increase of the non α/α ratio was observed also in 3 other patients (1, 5, and 6) at the end of the follow-up (range 4.5–56.5%) (TABLE 2). FIGURE 2 shows the plot of the mean values over time of the HbF% of all the patients. For HbF we found a slight but constant increase during the follow-up period. Analysis of variance showed a time effect very close to significance in both the treatment period (p = 0.06) and follow-up (p = 0.08). The 95% CIs (lower limit close to 0) for HbF% on days 28 and 56 versus baseline was consistent with a near significant increase. Six patients (4,6,7,8,9, and 12) showed an increase ranging between 4.4 and 26%. In these patients, except in one (12), HbF% continued to rise during the follow-up period. Two of the remaining 6 patients (1 and 2) showed no relevant improvement and in 4 patients

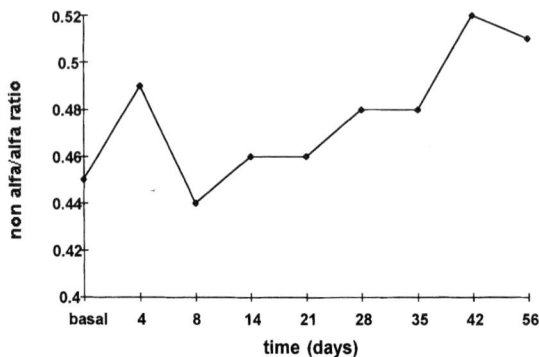

FIGURE 1. Plot of the mean values over time of the non α/α ratio in 12 thalassemia intermedia patients treated with oral isobutyramide.

(3,5,10, and 11) HbF% was already ≥ 90% at baseline making impossible to evaluate any significant increase (TABLE 3). Significant decreases in total Hb, although slow and moderate, were observed over time (FIG. 3).

Serum Epo values at baseline were spread from 20.99-253.33 mU/ml (mean 145.07 ± 22). At baseline, 4 patients had inadequate endogenous sEpo production for their degree of anemia (three with high and one with low O/P sEpo level). sEpo levels increased significantly during treatment as shown in FIGURE 4. sTfR values at baseline were ranging from 5.05 to 16 µg/ml (mean 10.77 ± 0.93 µg/ml) significantly higher ($p < 0.05$) than normal values in non-anemic subjects (normal range 0.85–3.05 µg/ml). At day 4 during treatment and at day 35 during follow-up a significant increase of the mean sTfR values versus baseline ($p < 0.05$) was observed (FIG. 5).

DISCUSSION

Induction of HbF with butyrate-based compounds has been demonstrated *in vitro*[11-14] and *in vivo*.[9,15,16] Their potential therapeutic use in thalassemia and hemoglobinopathies

TABLE 2. Individual Patient Results for non-α/α Ratio at Day 28 and Day 56

Patient No	Genotype	Raw Data			$\Delta\%^a$	$\Delta\%^a$
		Baseline	Day 28	Day 56	Day 28	Day 56
1	IVS1-110/IVS1-6	0.415	0.40	0.62	−3.61	49.40
2	β°39/IVS1-6	0.41	0.33	0.37	−19.51	−9.76
3	β°39/IVS2-1	0.45	0.40	0.45	−11.11	0.00
4	IVS1-6/-87	0.38	0.40	0.36	5.26	−5.26
5	δβ°/ β°39	0.46	0.40	0.72	−13.04	56.52
6	β°39/IVS1-6	0.44	0.42	0.46	−4.55	4.55
7	IVS1-6/-87	0.59	0.65	0.51	10.17	−13.56
8	IVS2-1/IVS1-6	0.44	0.51	0.56	15.91	27.27
9	IVS1-6/IVS1-6	0.34	0.68	0.41	100.00	20.59
10	IVS1-110/δβ°	0.50	0.62	0.74	24.00	48.00
11	β°39/ β°39	0.51	0.42	0.44	−17.65	−13.73
12	β°39/ β +mild	0.52	0.53	0.50	1.92	−3.85

$^a\Delta\%$: percent variation vs baseline.

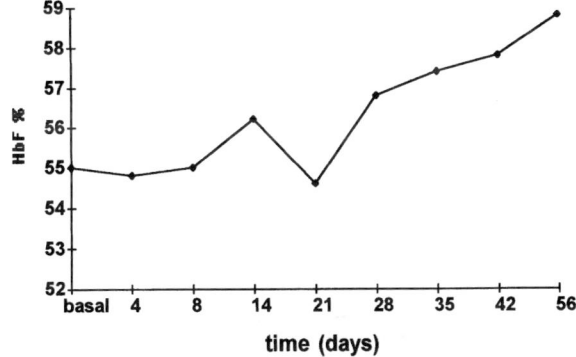

FIGURE 2. Plot of the mean values over time of the HbF% in 12 thalassemia intermedia patients treated with oral isobutyramide. $p < 0.01$ "time effect": mean values of the raw data have been analyzed over time (day 0,4,8,14,21,28,42 and 56) by two-way ANOVA analysis.

remains an exciting prospect. Unfortunately, the most effective compounds so far used in patients, such as arginine butyrate and phenylbutyrate, have disadvantages caused by the mode of administration.[8] The results presented here show that HbF stimulation can be achieved in thalassemia intermedia patients with a branched-chain derivative of butyric acid, isobutyramide. This agent has two enormous advantages: it can be administered orally and it reaches high plasma levels with a single dose.[19] Previous trials with arginine butyrate[15,16] and other compounds[24] in a limited number of patients with sickle cell disease or β thalassemia have been difficult to interpret because of differences in the treatment schedule, the extent of drug supplementation (iron or folic acid), and the threshold used to evaluate the hematologic response. Moreover, the patients treated were heterogeneous with respect to their transfusion regimen. In this pilot phase II open study, we administered 150 mg/kg body weight of isobutyramide once a day to thalassemia intermedia patients in order to evaluate the safety and efficacy of the drug in stimulating HbF production. The dosage was chosen to maintain plasma levels above 0.3 mM, which was reported to be required to stimulate fetal globin production *in vitro*[19] and *in vivo*.[25] Thalassemia in

TABLE 3. Individual Patient Results for HbF % at Day 28 and Day 56

Patient No	Genotype	Raw Data			$\Delta\%^a$	$\Delta\%^a$
		Baseline	Day 28	Day 56	Day 28	Day 56
1	IVS1-110/IVS1-6	35.1	31.3	32.3	−10.83	−7.98
2	β°39/IVS1-6	64.4	63.3	65.1	−2.01	0.77
3	β°39/IVS2-1	97.5	98	98.2	0.51	0.72
4	IVS1-6/-87	39.4	46.6	49.5	18.27	25.63
5	δβ°/b°39	95.8	95.5	96.3	−0.31	0.52
6	β°39/IVS1-6	50.1	52.3	57.5	4.39	14.77
7	IVS1-6/-87	27.7	34.9	36.8	25.99	32.85
8	IVS2-1/IVS1-6	51.8	58.3	63.2	12.55	22.01
9	IVS1-6/IVS1-6	3.8	4.5	6.2	18.42	63.16
10	IVS1-110/δβ°	87.3	85.2	86.1	−2.41	−1.37
11	β°39/ β°39	97.8	98.8	98.3	1.02	0.51
12	β°39/ β+mild	11.25	11.9	11.8	5.78	4.89

$^a\Delta\%$: percent variation vs baseline

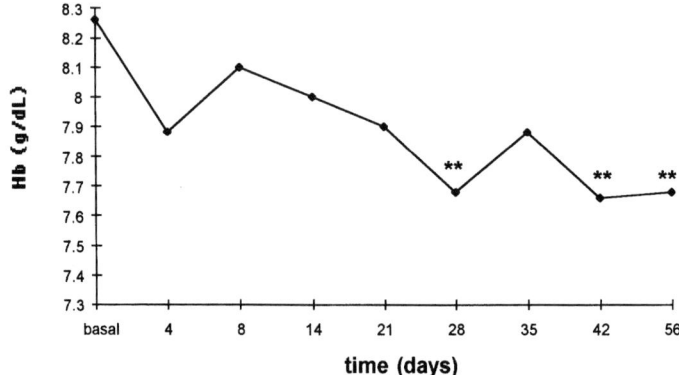

FIGURE 3. Plot of the mean values over time of the total Hb in 12 thalassemia intermedia patients treated with oral isobutyramide. $p < 0.01$ "time effect": mean values of the raw data have been analyzed over time (day 0,4,8,14,21,28,42 and 56) by two way ANOVA analysis. $**p < 0.01$ vs baseline.

termedia patients were deemed good candidates for this study as they are transfusion-independent, adults, and cooperative. Compliance was excellent and no patient experienced gastric discomfort or any other side effects related to oral ingestion of the drug. The criteria for effective therapy have still to be defined, with no drug having been shown to enhance HbF synthesis in thalassemia. The aim of this study was to investigate if isobutyramide is able to increase HbF levels. We were also interested in investigating its clinical effect. For this reason we arbitrarily defined as responders patients showing an increase of the globin chain synthesis ratio and/or HbF of over 2% compared to baseline values at the end of the treatment and or at the end of follow-up. Because of the possible variability of the methods used and the likelihood of some individual variations in hematological values over time in patients of this kind, analyses were performed in triplicate at each timepoint (the reported values are the mean of 3 determinations). Two years of observation of 7 patients before the study (8 assessments) had shown that natural oscillations over time were within 5% for the non-α/α ratio and less than 2% for HbF (data not shown). Taking these observations into account and according to our definition of responders, our findings

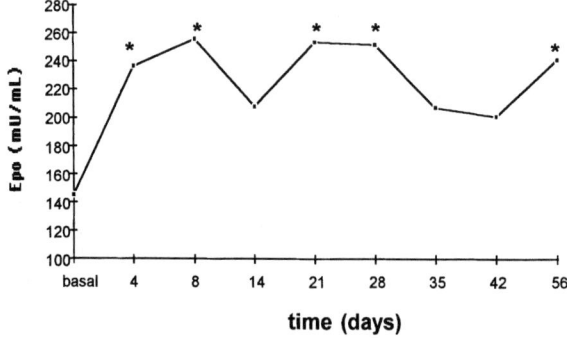

FIGURE 4. Plot of the mean values over time of the Epo in 12 thalassemia intermedia patients treated with oral isobutyramide. $*p < 0.05$ vs baseline.

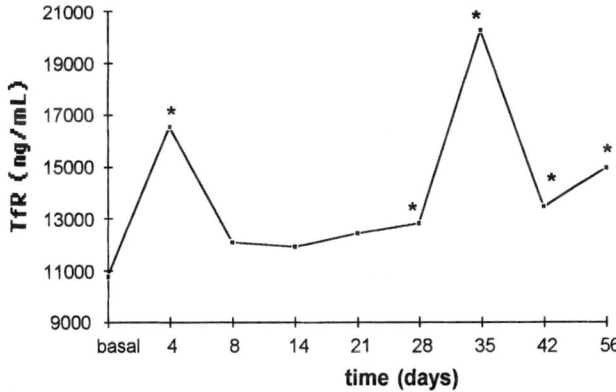

FIGURE 5. Plot of the mean values over time of the TfR in 12 thalassemia intermedia patients treated with oral isobutyramide. $*p < 0.05$ vs baseline.

that 58% of the patients responded to one or both of the efficacy parameters at the end of treatment (7/12) and 75% (9/12) at the end of follow-up appears reliable. The most impressive result was the continuous progressive increase of HbF in 5 patients up to 1 month after the cessation of therapy. Persistent F reticulocyte levels higher than baseline have also been reported in some patients up to a month or more after the withdrawal of sodium phenylbutyrate and arginine butyrate treatment.[15,24] The lack of a rise in total Hb concentration is disappointing and raises several questions about the mechanisms through which isobutyramide enhances HbF production. In order to evaluate possible modification of erythropoiesis induced by isobutyramide treatment we measured the sEpo and sTfR. The soluble form of transferrin receptor is a truncated form of the entire cell membrane transferrin receptor molecule and derived from bone marrow erythroid precursors. Circulating levels have been demonstrated to be related to the erythropoietic activity in normal subjects as well as in different types of anemia. Erythrokinetic studies have confirmed also that sTfR provides a simple and reliable quantitative method to evaluate the total erythropoiesis *in vivo*.[26] The significant increase of sTfR few days after drug introduction and few days after withdrawal, supports the hypothesis that the erythroid cell population is at least partly changed. We also observed a significant increase in the common indirect indexes of hemolysis such as serum LDH, indirect bilirubin and reticulocytes. Moreover, circulating erythroblasts rose significantly and returned to baseline 3 weeks after completing the study treatment (data not shown). Thalassemia intermedia is a very complex disorder in which a severe defective erythropoiesis results in a heterogeneous cell population. It is well known that F cells and RBCs with high amounts of HbF have a preferential survival.[27] Since we observed an inconsistent response to total hemoglobin, a consistent increase in HbF in at least 5 patients, and increases of hemolysis and peripheral nucleated red cells, it may be hypothesized that isobutyramide causes a) an erythropoietic stress due to a direct hemolytic effect on peripheral cells or b) a nonspecific expansion of RBC mass in the bone marrow, increasing both the large part of ineffective erythropoiesis and the small part of effective erythropoiesis. This suggests that more than one mechanism may be involved at either a cellular or molecular level. The key issue in the treatment of thalassemia would be to obtain steady and unequivocal rises in hemoglobin concentration and absolute level of HbF concentration in peripheral blood. On the basis of our results and on those reported by others with different compounds, we suggest that further studies of longer periods treatment are warranted.

ACKNOWLEDGMENTS

The authors are indebted to Dr. Cristina Le Grazie and Dr. Anna Giudici for their assistance in planning the trial, BASF and Vertex Phamaceuticals for providing the drug and to Dr. Gabrielle Boissard for statistical analysis.

REFERENCES

1. THEIN, S. L. 1993. β-thalassemia. In The Haemoglobinopathies: Bailliere's Clinical Haematology, Vol 6. D.R. Higgs & D.J. Weatherall, Eds: 151–175. London.
2. CAPPELLINI, M. D., G. FIORELLI, C. F. BERNINI. 1981. Interaction between homozygous β^0 thalassemia and the Swiss type of hereditary persistence of fetal hemoglobin. Br. J. Haematol. **48**: 561–572.
3. WEATHERALL D. J., J. B. CLEGG, D. R. HIGGS & W. G.WOOD. 1995. The hemoglobinopathies. In The Metabolic and Molecular Bases of Inherited Disease. C. R. Scriver, A. L. Beaudet, W. S. Sly, & D. Valle, Eds,; 3417–3484. McGraw Hill. New York
4. LEY, T. Y., J. DE SIMONE, C. T. NOGUCHI, et al. 1983. 5-azacytidine increases gamma globin synthesis and reduce the proportion of dense cells in patients with sickle cell anemia. Blood **62**: 370–380.
5. RODGERS, G. P., G. J. DOVER & N. UYESAKA. 1993. Augmentation by erythropoietin of the fetal-hemoglobin response to hydroxyurea in sickle cell disease. New Engl. J. Med. **328**: 74–86.
6. ZENG, Y. T., S. Z. HUANG, Z. R. REN, et al. 1995. Hydroxyurea therapy in beta-thalassemia intermedia: inprovment in hematological parameters due to enhanced beta-globin synthesis. Brit. J. Haematol. **90**: 557–563.
7. CHARACHE, S., M. L. TERRIN, R. D. MOORE, et al. 1995. Effect of hydroxyurea on the frequency of painful crises in sickle cell anemia. New Engl. J. Med. **322**:1317–1322.
8. RODGERS, G. P. & E. A. RACHMILEWITZ. 1995. Novel treatment options in the severe β-globin disorders. Br. J. Haematol. **91**: 263–268.
9. PERRINE, S. P., M. F. GREENE & D. V. FALLE. 1985. Delay in fetal globin switch in infants of diabetic mothers. New Engl. J. Med. **312**: 334–338.
10. PERRINE, S. P., A. RUDOLPH, D. V. FALLER, et al. 1988. Butyrate infusions in the ovine fetus delay the biologic clock for globin gene switching." Proc. Natl. Acad. Sci. USA **85**: 8540–8542.
11. PERRINE, S. P., B. A. MILLER & D. V. FALLER. 1989. Sodium butyrate enhances fetal globin expression in erythroid progenitors of patients with HbSS and thalassemia. Blood **74**: 454–459.
12. FIBACH, E., P. PRASANNA, G. P. RODGERS & D. SAMID. 1993. Enhanced fetal hemoglobin production by phenylacetate and 4-phenylbutyrate in erythroid precursor derived from normal donors and patients with sickle cell disease. Blood **82**: 2203–2206.
13. GLAUBER, J. G., N. J. WANDERSEE, J. A. LITTLE & G. D. GINDER. 1991. 5'-flanking sequences mediate butyrate stimulation of embryonic globin gene expression in adult erythroid cells. Mol. Cell.Biol. **11**: 4690–4697.
14. PACE, B., Q. LI, K. PETERSON & G. STAMATOYANNOPOULOS. 1994. α-Amino butyric acid fails to reactive the totally silenced γ gene of the β locus YAC. Blood **84**: 4344–4353.
15. PERRINE, S. P., G. GINDER, D. V. FALLER, et al. 1993. A short- term trial of butyrate to stimulate fetal globin gene expression in the β globin gene disorder. New Engl. J. Med. **328**: 81–86.
16. SHER G. D., G. D. GINDER, J. LITTLE, et al. 1995. Extended therapy with intravenous original butyrate in patients with beta-hemoglobinopathies. New Engl. J. Med. **24**: 1606–1610.
17. BLAU, C. A., P. CONSTANTOULAKIS, C. M. SHAW & G.STAMATOYANNOPOULOS. 1993. Fetal hemoglobin induction with butyric acid: Efficacy and toxicity. Blood **81**: 529–537.
18. PERRINE, S. & D. V. FALLER. 1993. Butyrate-induced reactivation of fetal globin genes: A molecular treatment for the β-hemoglobinopathies. Experientia **49**: 133–137.

19. PERRINE S. P., G. H. DOVER, P. DAFTARI, et al. 1994. Isobutyramide, an orally bioavailable butyrate analogue, stimulates fetal globine gene expression in vitro and in vivo. Br. J. Haematol. **88**: 555–561.
20. CAMASCHELLA, C., U. MAZZA, A. ROETTO, et al. 1995. Genetic interactions in thalassemia intermedia: analysis of β-mutations, α-genotype, γ-promoters and β-LCR hypersensitive sites 2 and 4 in Italian patients. Am. J. Hematol. **48**: 82–87.
21. MILLER A. B., B. HOOGSTRATEN, M. STAQUET, et al. 1981. Reporting results of cancer treatment. Cancer **47**: 207–214.
22. BAROSI, G. 1994. Inadequate erythropoietin response to anemia: definition and clinical relevance. Ann. Hematol. **68**: 215–223.
23. CAMASCHELLA C., C. CONELLA, C. CALABRESE, et al. 1996. Serum erythropoietin and circulating transferrin receptor in thalassemia intermedia patients with heterogeneous genotypes. Haematologica **81**: 397-403.
24. COLLINS A. F., H. A. PEARSON, P. GIARDINA, et al. 1995. Oral sodium phenylbutyrate therapy in homozygous β thalassemia: A clinical trial. Blood **85**: 43-49.
25. BRETTMAN, L. R., P. R. CHATURVEDI. 1996. Pharmacokinetics and safety of single oral doses of VX-366 (Isobutyramide) in healthy volunteers. J. Clin. Pharmacol. **36**: 617–622.
26. BEGUIN, Y., G. K. CLEMOINS, P. POOTRAKUL, et al. 1993. Quantitative assessment of erythropoiesis and functional classification of anemia based on measurements of serum transferrin receptor and erythropoietin. Blood **81**: 1067–1076.
27. STAMATOYANNOPOULOS, G. & A. W. NIENHUIS. 1994. Hemoglobin switching. *In* Molecular Bases of Blood Diseases. G. Stamatoyannopoulos, A. W. Nihenuis, P. Majerus, H. Varmus, Eds.: 107–127. W. B. Saunders. Philadelphia.

Hydroxyurea Therapy in Thalassemia[a]

DIMITRIS LOUKOPOULOS,[b,g] ERSI VOSKARIDOU,[c]
ALEXANDRA STAMOULAKATOU,[d] YANNIS PAPASSOTIRIOU,[d]
VASILIKI KALOTYCHOU,[b] APHRODITE LOUTRADI,[c] GABRIEL
COZMA,[e] HELENI TSIARTA,[f] AND NIKOS PAVLIDES[f]

[b]*First Department of Medicine, University of Athens*

[c]*Thalassemia Center, Laikon Hospital, Athens*

[d]*Hematology Laboratory, Aghia Sophia Children's Hospital, Athens*

[e]*Research Division, CILAG Company, Zug, Switzerland*

[f]*Thalassemia Center, Nikosia Hospital, Cyprus*

ABSTRACT: The clinical effectiveness of Hydroxyurea in thalassemia is still controversial. The present paper puts together the authors' experience in two groups of patients with thalassemia intermedia and sickle cell/β-thalassemia treated with varying dosages of hydroxyurea over several months. A third group received hydroxyurea along with recombinant human erythropoietin. Our observations are summarized in that treatment with hydroxyrea results in a significant increase of fetal hemoglobin with no change of the total hemoglobin levels. The drug causes also a considerable increase of the erythrocyte volume and hemoglobin content while the MCHC values remain unchanged. As a rule, and without objective criteria so far, patients state feeling better and having more energy. The authors postulate that this feeling may reflect the significant decrease of ineffective erythropoiesis resulting by the replacement of the poorly hemoglobinized, prematurely dying erythroid progenitor and red cell population by another population of cells with higher hemoglobin content and longer survival, the regeneration of which requires less energy and consumption. As expected, patients with sickle cell/β-thalassemia have also fewer crises and painful episodes. The above findings are in keeping with the few available reports in the literature.

Hydroxyurea (HU), a potent ribonucleotide reductase inhibitor, is a well known chemotherapeutic agent which has been used largely for the treatment of various myeloproliferative conditions over the past 20 years. HU is easy to use because its main toxicity, *i.e.*, leukopenia and thrombocytopenia, is usually fully reversible a few days after its discontinuation. The potential of HU to induce hemoglobin F (HbF) synthesis both in anemic monkeys[1] and in patients with sickle cell disease[2–4] was reported from several Centers simultaneously in 1984. These results were in keeping with previous studies where a similar effect was reported for 5′-azacytidine.[5,6]

---

[a]These studies were supported by grants 91 ED 97 (Secretariat of R and D) to D.L. and Y3A/3440 (Ministry of Health) to E.V.

[g]Corresponding author: Dimitris Loukopoulos, MD, Professor of Medicine, First Department of Medicine, University of Athens, Laikon Hospital, 115 27 Athens, Greece; Tel: 30-1-777 11 61; Tel. 30-1-363 33 79 (home); Fax: 301-360 7089; E-mail: dloukop@atlas.uoa.gr

Re-activation of γ-chain synthesis is of utmost importance in the sickle cell syndromes because the dispersion of a varying number of HbF molecules among those of HbS and the formation of $\alpha 2\beta^S\gamma$ hybrids markedly decrease the process of polymerization and sickling, with obvious potential clinical benefits. Moreover, in β-thalassemia, the addition of a varying number of γ-chains in the poorly hemoglobinized red cells not only complements their low MCH, but it mainly neutralizes the noxious excess of α-chains and allows a better survival of the erythroid precursors in the marrow and of the red cells in the peripheral blood.

The potential of HU to preferentially promote proliferation and differentiation of erythroid precursors with HbF synthetic capacity but without any major toxicity has soon led to the systematic evaluation of a large number of patients with sickle cell disease all over the US and has conclusively shown that the frequency of pain crises and other complications significantly decreased while on the drug.[7] A study from our Center in 14 Greek (Caucasian) compound β^S/β-thalassemia heterozygotes using an empirically developed scale of pain produced similar results not only with regards to major crises, but also with regards to other details such as ability to work or study and strength of the necessary analgesic medications.[8] Today, the beneficial efficacy of HU in sickle cell disease is being evaluated in several European Centers taking care of such patients.

The efficacy of HU in thalassemia is still controversial; the drug has been used in thalassemia major in an attempt to rapidly reduce the total volume of bone marrow, when this causes severe bone pain, or the size of extramedullary erythropoietic masses, when these compress vital organs or tissues. Unfortunately, these reports do not contain any information on HbF.[9] In other instances, HU has been given to patients with thalassemia intermedia in the hope that it may induce HbF synthesis and improve the overall condition. These experiments remain still mostly anecdotal. The goal of this paper is to report our own experience in this field and compare it with other published or personally communicated information.

PATIENTS AND METHODS

Our report summarizes our results in three groups of patients with a thalassemic component:

a) patients with thalassemia intermedia treated with HU alone,

b) patients with thalassemia intermedia treated with HU in combination with recombinant human erythropoietin (r-huEPO), and

c) compound heterozygotes for β-thalassemia and the β^S gene who received hydroxyurea alone.

In group a) the interacting β-thalassemia genes were mostly of the mild type, *i.e.*, IVS1-nt 6, -87 and, rarely IVS1-nt 110. Groups b) and c) included patients with various β^0 or β^+-thalassemia defects, common in the East Mediterranean; one patient in group b) was a $\beta^0/\delta\beta$ compound with 98% HbF.[10] All patients were adults, had no medical problems apart those associated with their condition, and were considered as fully reliable since we had followed them up closely over the last several years. The studies were approved by the Ethical Committee of the Hospital.

HU (Myers-Squibb, USA) was administered in dosages ranging from 15 up to 35 mg/kg-day over 4 to 7 days/week. Further details will given separately. The patients were closely followed up during the first months of therapy; monitoring was loosened when both patients and physicians felt safe with regards to potential side effects. Laboratory parameters were determined using conventional techniques.

RESULTS AND COMMENTS

Thalassemia Intermedia Treated with HU Alone (Group a)

The drug has been administered at the standard dose of 1.5 g daily (20 mg/kg rounded up to the next 500 mg) over 7 days/week and, as a rule, it was well tolerated. To our surprise, most patients repeatedly reported "feeling better" from the onset of the trial; this statement should not be disregarded *a priori*, although it cannot be expressed objectively. The pattern of response was similar in all patients. Red cells became larger and their MCH (but not their MCHC) increased (FIG. 1). Hemoglobin and hematocrit levels did not change. Reticulocyte counts were not consistent; however, the number of nucleated red cells in the peripheral blood gradually decreased in most cases. Hemoglobin F started augmenting soon after initiation of the trial and reached a plateau of 2-4 times the base line after approximately three months of therapy. Increasing the dose of HU to toxicity (up to

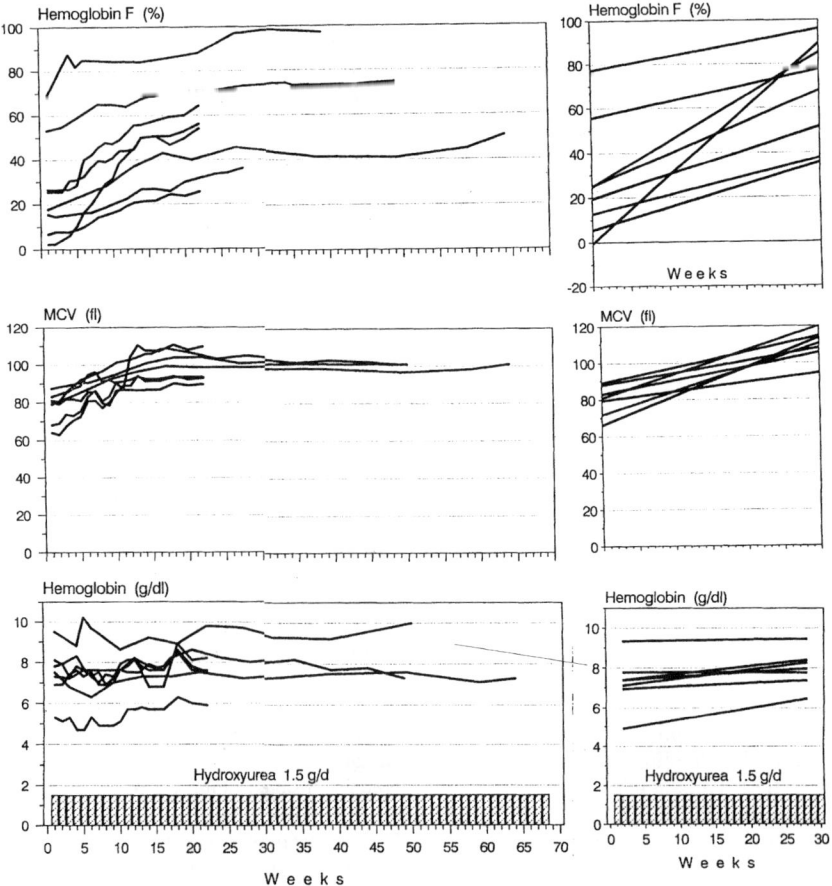

FIGURE 1. Response of 8 patients with thalassemia intermedia (group a) to a standard dose (1.5 g/d) of hydroxyurea administered over 30 weeks. Results are expressed as actual values and as trends.

2.5 g daily 4 days/week) did not appear to push the reponse any further, implying either that HU was becoming toxic or that the potential of the bone marrow to preferentially expand the HbF synthesizing erythroid population is not unlimited (FIG. 2). As the value of these results is not clear yet, continuation of the trial is recommended.

Patients with Thalassemia Intermedia Treated with Hydroxyurea in Combination with r-huEPO (Group b)

This trial was carried out following the reports by Rachmilewitz et al.[11] and by Olivieri et al.[12] that administration of r-huEPO in thalassemia intermedia may increase the red cell

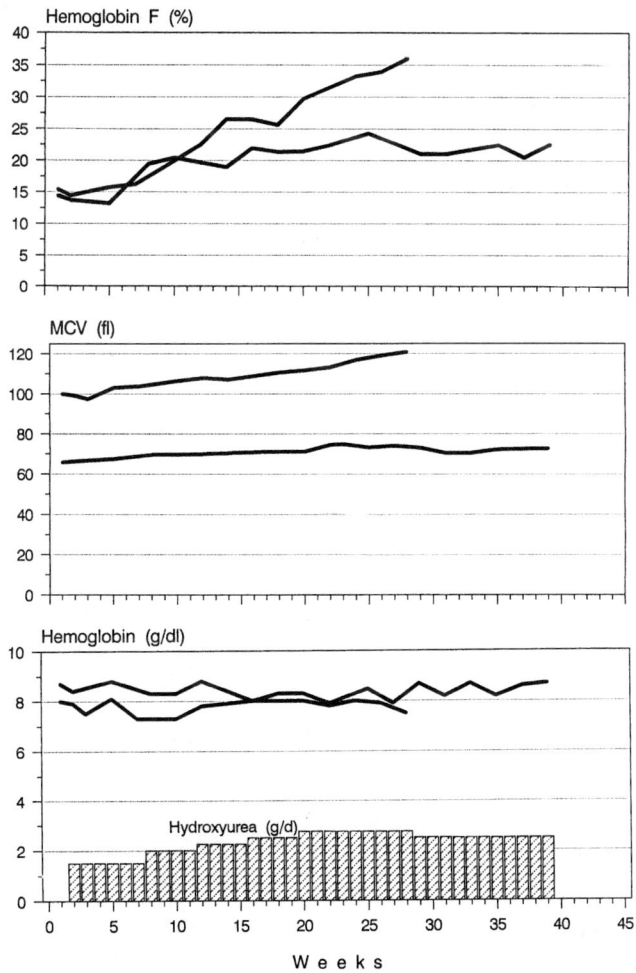

FIGURE 2. Response of 2 patients with thalassemia intermedia to an escalating dose of hydroxyurea (1.0 up to 2.75 g/d) administered over several weeks. The increase of dose does not result in a proportional intcrease of HbF.

mass, and the report of Rodgers et al.[13] that addition of r-huEPO to patients already responding to HU resulted in a further increase of HbF. The trial involved 10 patients, 3 males and 7 females, age 21 to 48 years. All of them received 1.0 g of HU daily over 4 consecutive days/week along with 50,000 U of r-huEPO (CILAG, Switzerland) administered im 3 times/week over 12 weeks; they were also given folic acid (5 mg/day) and iron sulfate (300 mg/day), in keeping with the idea that expansion of erythropoiesis may be facilitated by the presence of promptly available iron. Following this period, the 8 responders were randomly assigned to one group who continued with 50,000 U of r-huEPO once a week for an additional 12 weeks (2 with and 2 without HU) and another group who received 10,000 U of r-huEPO once a week (2 with and 2 without HU) over 12 weeks. FIGURE 3 depicts the results. Hemoglobin values increased in 8 out of 10 patients; the increase was significant and, in most instances it was made up mainly by HbF. The increase lasted only as long the the dose of r-huEPO was very high; administration of the hormone in lesser dosages failed to sustain the initial dramatic result (FIG. 3). Splenectomy did not appear to influence the reponse. The patients stated feeling much better and having increased appetite and strength. These effects do not appear to relate to the amount of additional oxygen which can be delivered to the tissues as a result of the increased red cell mass. When the latter was calculated taking into consideration the high oxygen affinity of HbF, the gain in oxygen delivery almost vanished.

Patients with Sickle Cell/β-Thalassemia Treated with HU (Group C)

That HU can increase HbF bringing about a clear clinical benefit in patients with homozygous sickle cell disease has been repeatedly confirmed.[7,8] The question which is addressed in this review is whether the thalassemic component of the compound β^S/β-thalassemia heterozygotes of our studies may have any additional or different role. Up to now, this study includes 29 evaluable β^S/β^o-thalassemia and 15 β^S/β^+-thalassemia compound heterozygotes. Some of them have now completed more than five years on HU. With a few exceptions only, all patients have responded with a spectacular increase of their usually very low HbF, which has reached percentages as high as 30 or even 40% in some instances. In parallel, their red cells became larger and heavier and reveal a strikingly normalized morphology on microscopy. Total hemoglobin and MCHC values did not change appreciably. In several instances the reticulocyte number decreased. The increase of HbF was higher in the females in both the β^S/β^+-thalassemia and the β^S/β^o-thalassemia subgroups. Moreover, after several months on HU, the increase of HbF in the β^S/β^+-thalassemia patients was clearly lower than that of the β^S/β^o-thalassemia compounds (24% vs 36%), with the β^S/β^S homozygotes falling in the middle (30%). As most of the patients are Xmn negative, the effect of this factor cannot be correctly evaluated. As expected, the number and severity of crises rapidly came down to none, while most patients stated, here again, feeling much better since the first weeks of treatment and prior to any evidence of HbF increase. The antisickling effects of HU will not be discussed any further in this review; however, to explain the sense of "feeling better," especially in the patients of groups a) and b), our hypothesis is that this effect reflects a significant reduction of ineffective erythropoiesis, which clearly diminishes the erythropoietic "effort" of the patients along with their fatigue and decreased activity. The frequent observation that the usually abundant circulating erythroblasts markedly decrease following cytoreductive treatment along with the fact that total hemoglobin levels remain unchanged throughout the trials clearly supports the idea of an extensive replacement of the poorly hemoglobinized, promptly sickling red cells by a population of cells which have a hemoglobin content more than the usual one, a considerably lesser excess of deleterious α-chains and a high proportion of HbF, a pigment

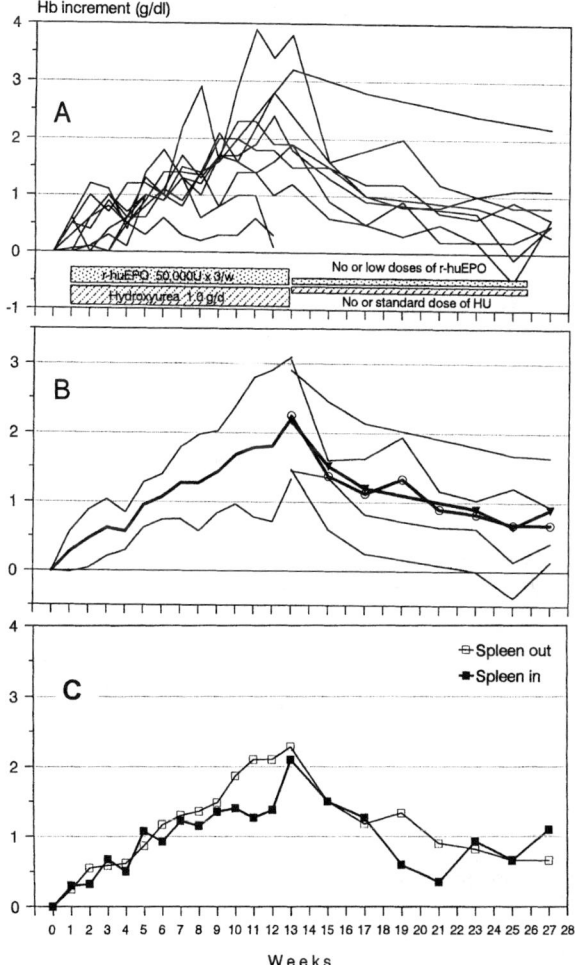

FIGURE 3. Response of 10 patients with thalassemia intermedia (group b) to a standard dose of hydroxyurea (1.0 g/d over 4 days/week) administered along with 50,000 U of recombinant human erythropoietin (plus folic acid and iron sulfate) over 12 weeks; continuation of therapy with lower doses of r-huEPO (with or without HU) did not sustain the result.

with high oxygen affinity which definitely inhibits HbS polymerization and prevents sickling crises.

Our studies in thalassemia intermedia have their laboratory counterpart. Using a two-phase erythroid cell culture system, Fibach et al. have shown that the addition of HU results in a pronounced increase of HbF, and they proposed that this may recapitulate the enhanced proliferation of HbF-containing erythroid cells which is thought to occur in vivo.[14] However, in an abstract presented at this meeting, Kollia et al. show that the increase of HbF also reflects increased transcription and more efficient processing of the respective γ-mRNA.[15]

TABLE 1. Main Features of the Patients of This Study

Underlying Molecular Defects
Group a: IVS1-nt6, -87, IVS1-nt1570, and IVS1-nt110
Groups b and c: β° : IVS1-nt1, IVS2-nt1, β° 39
β^+ : -87, IVS1-110, IVS2-nt745

	Group a			Group b			Group c		
	A[a]	B	C	A	B	C	A	B	C
Hemoglobin (g/dl)									
Mean	7.5	7.7	0.2	7.7	9.4	1.7	8.9	9.3	0.4
Standard deviation	1.3	1.2	1.3	1.0	1.3	1.4			
Hemoglobin F (%)									
Mean	32.9	59.2	16.3	55.0	63.2	8.2	6.7	23.1	16.3
Standard deviation	27.1	22.3		23.9	23.2		4.7	9.2	
Hemoglobin F (g/dl)									
Mean	2.5	4.6	2.1	4.24	6.35	2.11	0.6	2.2	1.8
Standard deviation	0.4	0.3		0.3	0.2		0.61	0.13	
MCV (fl)									
Mean	77.5	98.2		80.0	84.0	4.0	75.7	98.1	22.1
Standard deviation	8.4	7.0		11.6	12.2		11.3	15.5	
MCHC (%)									
Mean	28.9	29.4	0.5	28.9	29.2		30.9	32.1	1.3
Standard deviation	2.2	1.0		2.1	1.5		1.4	1.2	

[a]A: Base line values; B: Values after 6 months of treatment; C: Increments.
Group a, thalassemia intermedia treated with hydroxyrea alone (10 patients, ages 21–38). Group b, thalassemia intermedia treated with hydroxyurea and recombinant human erythropoietin (10 patients, ages 21–48). Group c, patients with sickle cell/β-thalassemia (44 patients, ages 18–50).

At the clinical level, other instances where administration of HU in thalassemia intermedia resulted in a significant increase of HbF, are the two adults reported by Hiajjar and Pearson in 1994[16] and the HbE/β-thalassemia compound heterozygotes in Thailand recently reported by Fucharoen et al.[17] Interestingly, the latter group displayed also a considerable increase of total hemoglobin levels as well as a clearcut improvement of the clinical status of the patients, most probably as a result of cutting down the ineffective erythropoiesis and severe hemolysis associated with HbE disease. In contrast, the study of Zeng et al., where administration of HU to two Chinese patients with thalassemia intermedia resulted in a net increase of the β over α-chain biosynthetic ratio with no effects on HbF, has no interpretation so far and needs further exploration.[18]

Assuming that HU may have a clinical benefit in thalassemia intermedia, the question now comes to assessing its long-term safety, especially with regards to potential leukemogenicity, which has been noticed in various myeloproliferative conditions.[19] Our group have approached this problem by caryotype (sister chromatid exchange and other chromosomal abnormalities) and molecular studies (ras and p53 mutations) in several patients who have received HU over many years. Up to now, results are negative, but the study is not yet complete.

In conclusion, HU has a clear effect in all β-thalassemic syndromes in the sense of replacing the poorly hemoglobinized, readily sickling and short-lived erythroid cell population with a new cohort of precursors with an active HbF synthesis program which end up in a better-functioning and longer-living red cell population. In some instances the event is associated with considerable clinical improvement; in others, the clinical relevance is still controversial. The question of administering HU in thalassemia should not be considered as closed; instead, it requires further systematic exploration and trials of HU in combination with other HbF-inducing agents.

REFERENCES

1. LETVIN N. L., D. C. LINCH, P. BEARDSLEY, K. W. MCINTYRE & D. G. NATHAN. 1984. Augmentation of fetal hemoglobin production in anemic monkeys by hydroxyurea. N. Engl. J. Med. **310**: 317–323.
2. CHARACHE S., G. J. DOVER, R. D. MOORE, S. ECKERT, S. K. BALLAS, M. KOSHY, P. F. A. MILNER, B. P. ORRINGER, G. J. PHILLIPS, O. S. PLATT & G. H. THOMAS. 1992. Hydroxyurea: Effects on hemoglobin F production in patients with sickle cell anemia. Blood **79**: 2555–2565.
3. PLATT, O. S., S. H. ORKIN, G. J. DOVER, G. P. BEARDSLEY, B. MILLER & D. G. NATHAN. 1984. Hydroxyurea enhances fetal hemoglobin production in sickle cell anemia. J. Clin. Invest. **74**: 652–656.
4. VEITH, R., R. GALANELLO, TH. PAPAYANNOPOULOU & G. STAMATOYANNOPOULOS. 1995. Stimulation of F-cell production in patients with sickle-cell anemia treated with cytarabine or hydroxyurea. N. Engl. J. Med. **313**: 1571–1575.
5. DESIMONE, J., P. HELLER, L. HALL & D. ZWIERS. 1982. 5′-Azacytidine stimulates fetal hemoglobin synthesis (HbF) in anemic baboons. Proc. Natl. Acad. Sci. USA **79**: 4428–4431.
6. LEY T. J., J. DE SIMONE, N. P. ANAGNOU & A. W. NIENHUIS. 1982. 5′-Azacytidine selectively increases γ-globin synthesis in a patient with β$^+$-thalassemia. N. Engl. J. Med. **307**: 1469–1475.
7. CHARACHE S., M. L. TERRIN, R. D. MOORE, G. J. DOVER, F. B. BARTON, S. V. ECKERT, R. P. MAC MAHON, D. R. BONDS & THE INVESTIGATORS OF THE MULTICENTER STUDY OF HYDROXYUREA IN SICKLE CELL DISEASE. 1995. Effect of hydroxyurea on the frequency of painful crises in sickle cell anemia. N. Engl. J. Med. **332**: 1317–1322.
8. VOSKARIDOU E., V. KALOTYCHOU & D. LOUKOPOULOS. 1995. Clinical and laboratory effects of long term administration of hydroxyurea to patients with sickle cell/α-thalassemia. Brit. J. Haematol. **89**: 479–484.
9. KONSTANTOPOULOS, K., G. VAGIOPOULOS, R. KANTOUNI, S. LYMBERI, PATRIARCHEAS, D. GEORGAKOPOULOS & P. FESSAS. 1992. A case of spinal cord compression by extramedullary haemopoiesis in a thalassaemic patient: A putative role for hydroxyurea. Haematologica **77**: 352–354.
10. KOLLIA, P., P. KARABABA, K. SINOPOULOU, E. VOSKARIDOU, M. BOUSSIOU, M. PAPADAKIS & D. LOUKOPOULOS. 1992. β-thalassemia mutations and the underlying β gene cluster haplotypes in the Greek population. Gene Geography **6**: 59–70.
11. RACHMILEWITZ, E. A., A. GOLDFARB & G. J. DOVER. 1991. Administration of erythropoietin to patients with beta-thalassemia intermedia. Blood **78**: 1145–1147.
12. OLIVIERI, N. F., M. H. FRIEDMAN, S. P. PERRINE, G. J. DOVER & B. SHERIDAN. 1992. Trial of recombinant human erythropoietin: Three patients with thalassemia intermedia. Blood **80**: 3258–3260.
13. RODGERS, G. P., G. J. DOVER, N. UYESAKA, C. T. NOGUCHI, A. N. SCHECHTER & A. W. NIENHUIS. 1993. Augmentation by erythropoietin of the fetal hemoglobin response to hydroxyurea in sickle cell disease. N. Engl. J. Med. **328**: 73–80.
14. FIBACH, E., L. P. BURKE, A. N. SCHECHTER, C. T. NOGUCHI & G. P. RODGERS. 1993. Hydroxyurea increases fetal hemoglobin in cutured erythroid cells derived from normal individuals and patients with sickle cell anemia or β-thalassemia. Blood **81**: 1630–1635.
15. KOLLIA, P., M. POLITOU & D. LOUKOPOULOS. 1998. Hydroxyurea and hemin affect both the transcriptional and post-transcriptional mechanisms of some globin genes in human adult erythroid cells. Ann. N.Y. Acad. Sci. **850**. This volume.
16. HAJJAR, F. M. & H. A. PEARSON. 1994. Pharmacologic treatment of thalassemia intermedia with hydroxyurea. J. Pediatrics **125**: 490–492.
17. FUCHAROEN, S., N. SIRITINARATKUL, P. WINICHAGOON, J. CHAWTHAWORN, SIRIBOON, W. MUANSUP, S. CHAICHAROEN, N. POOOLSUP, B. CHINDAVIJAK, P. POOTRAKUL, A. PIANKIJAGUM, A. N. SCHECHTER & G. P. RODGERS. 1996. Hydroxyurea increases hemoglobin F levels and improves the effectiveness of erythropoiesis in β-thalassemia/hemoglobin E disease. Blood **87**: 887–892.

18. ZENG, Y-T., S-Z. HUANG, A-R. REN, Z-H. LU, F-Y. ZENG, A. N. SCHECHTER & G. P. RODGERS. 1995. Hydroxyurea therapy in β-thalassaemia intermedia: Improvement in haematological parametes due to enhanced β-globin synthesis. Brit. J. Haematol. **90**: 557–563.
19. WEINFELD, A, B. SWOLIN & J. WESTIN. 1994. Acute leukemia after hydroxyurea therapy in polycythemia vera and allied disorders: Prospective study of efficacy and leukaemogenicity with therapeutic implications. Eur. J. Haematol. **52**: 134–139.

The Role of Recombinant Human Erythropoietin in the Treatment of Thalassemia

ELIEZER A. RACHMILEWITZ[a,c] AND MEMET AKER[b]

[a]*Department of Hematology,* [b]*Department of Pediatrics, Hadassah University Hospital, Jerusalem, Israel*

ABSTRACT: The rationale for treatment with recombinant human erythropoietin (rHuEPO) in thalassemia came from studies in baboons, thalassemic mice and in erythroid cultures. The results demonstrated an increase in γ globin synthesis and consequently in fetal Hb (Hb F) resulting in improvement in erythropoietic parameters. In addition, endogenous serum Epo levels in various forms of thalassemia were inconsistent and not related to the severity of the anemia. Therefore, several preliminary studies with rHuEPO were performed, mainly on patients with β thalassemia intermedia. The results indicate: a) a significant, dose-related (500 u/kg to 1000 u/kg × 3/week) increase in thalassemia erythropoiesis without changes in % of Hb F, MCV and MCH, mainly in splenectomized patients; b) the minimum effective dose is 500 u/kg × 3/week; c) there were no major side effects during the continuous treatment period of 9 months. In order to improve both quantitative and qualitative thalassemia erythropoiesis, several trials were undertaken combining rHuEPO with hydroxyurea (HU), which is known to increase % Hb F, MCV and MCH without a major effect on Hb levels. The designed trial included 3 to 6 months of HU alone (20 mg/kg × 4/week), or with rHuEPO alone (500 u/kg × 3/week or 375 u/kg × 2/week) or a combination of the two drugs. The results show an additive effect of the two drugs, in some of the patients. It is not known whether the addition of oral iron to rHuEPO is warranted for maximal erythropoietic response. The major limiting factor in designing large scale clinical trials is the relatively high cost of the drug. Nevertheless rHuEPO alone or in combination with other Hb F modulating drugs may have a positive effect in thalassemia with resulting improvement in the quality of life.

Erythropoiesis is tightly regulated by the hormone erythropoietin, a glycoprotein hormone which induces the formation of red blood cells by stimulating proliferation, differentiation and maturation of erythroid progenitor cells.[1] Recombinant human erythropoietin (rHuEPO) became available for clinical use in a variety of primary and secondary anemias after cloning of the gene more then ten years ago.[2] Among the different types of anemia, a major component consists of congenital hemolytic anemia caused by mutations in the hemoglobin molecule, particularly sickle cell anemia and the thalassemia syndrome. The initial rationale of rHuEPO administration in hemoglobinopathies came following observations in anemic and non-anemic baboons[3] in thal. mice[4] and in thalassemia erythroid cultures,[5] where a significant increase in the percentage of fetal hemoglobin (HbF) concomitant with improvement in all erythroid parameters was observed. HbF was expected to ameliorate the severity and incidence of sickle cell crisis,[6] and to

---

[c]Corresponding author: E. A. Rachmilewitz, MD, Head, Department of Hematology; Hadassah University Hospital, Ein Kerem; P.O. Box 12,000, Jerusalem, 91120 Israel; Tel: 972 2 677-6744; Fax 972-2-642-3067; E-mail erach@hadassah.org.il

decrease the degree of hemolysis in thalassemia.[7] In the following review, we would like to summarize the available information on the role of rHuEPO in various forms of the thalassemia syndrome.

ENDOGENOUS SERUM EPO LEVELS IN THALASSEMIA

To date, there are no consistent results regarding endogenous EPO levels in thalassemia. The studies of Hammond et al.,[8] Manor et al.,[9] Beumi et al.,[10] and Nisli et al.,[11] failed to demonstrate a direct inverse relationship between severity of the anemia in transfused or non-transfused patients with β thalassemia intermedia (TI) and major (TM). In patients with sickle cell anemia, Sherwood et al.[12] showed that serum EPO levels were lower than expected for the degree of their anemia. These findings are in contrast to the reports of Alessi et al.[13] and Dore et al.[14] who showed a significant increase in serum EPO levels in patients with TI and TM. The reasons for the variable results in the different studies are multifold. Among them are 1) different methodology of serum EPO determination, 2) the presence or absence of blood transfusions and the time of the assay *vis à vis* the most recent transfusion, 3) the age of the patients, since very high serum EPO levels were found in young patients with TM and TI, comparable to the levels found in patients with aplastic anemia,[9] which were different from the levels found in older thalassemia patients with the same degree of anemia, 4) the presence or absence of the spleen[11] and 5) last but not least, the circadian rhythm of EPO levels may also play a role.[15] Consequently, the decision whether to treat a patient with TI or TM with rHuEPO cannot be made on the basis of endogenous serum EPO levels as in other anemic disorders such as MDS or cancer-induced anemia.

THE EFFECT OF rHuEPO ON HbF SYNTHESIS IN EXPERIMENTAL SYSTEMS

The preliminary results of rHuEPO in experimental animals such as baboons[3] and thalassemia mice[4] were very encouraging and suggested that γ-globin chain synthesis is markedly increased following administration of rHuEPO at a dose at least 5- to 10-fold higher than that used to correct the anemia of patients with chronic renal failure.[16] Encouraging results were also obtained in synchronous erythroid cultures from TI and TM patients where alteration of rHuEPO concentrations resulted in a marked increase in HbF synthesis. On the basis of these results as well as the preliminary trials in patients with sickle cell anemia,[17] the foundation has been laid for preliminary trials of rHuEPO therapy in thalassesmia.

THE EFFECT OF rHuEPO ON PATIENTS WITH THALASSEMIA AND CHRONIC RENAL FAILURE

One of the first successful indications for treatment with rHuEPO was to correct the anemia of patients with chronic renal failure either before or after instituting dialysis.[16] The effective dose is in a range of 25 to 100 u/kg given subcutaneously twice a week. By coincidence, a certain percentage of the patients with anemia of chronic renal failure who were treated with rHuEPO, had α- or β-thalassemia trait. One study[18] included 3 patients with β-thalassemia trait and one with α-thalassemia trait. The dose requirements of rHuEPO in order to achieve a target Hb level of > 10g/dl and the ongoing maintenance dose were higher when compared to matched dialysis patients without thalassemia trait (FIG.1). One

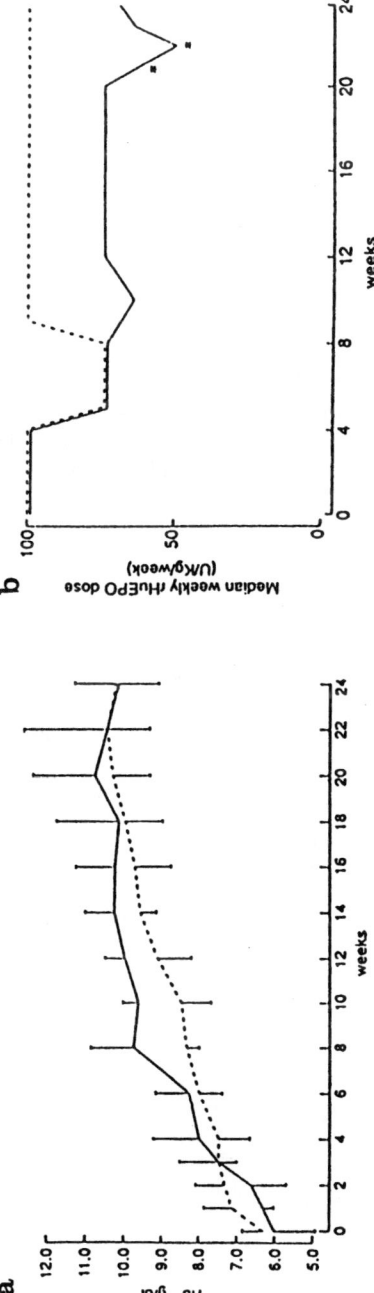

FIGURE 1A AND B. 1a: Hb levels in dialysis patients with (- - -) and without (——) thalassemia trait; Figure 1b: Median weekly rHuEPO dose in dialysis patients with (- - -) and without (——) thalassemia trait p < 0.05 between the two patient groups. (From Cheng et al.[18])

patient with HbH disease did not respond to 250 u/kg/week, unlike the patient with HbH disease reported by Winearls *et al.* who did respond to a dose of 600 u/kg/week.[19]

In another study, 4 patients with β thalassemia minor required higher doses of rHuEPO (75 u/kg × 3/week) compared with non-thalassemic controls.[20] Lai *et al.*[21] also observed a smaller and delayed increase in Hb levels in three patients with α-thalassemia trait and one with β-thalassemia trait using a higher rHuEPO dose of 175 u/kg/w compared to non-thalassemia dialysis patients who received an average of 120 u/kg/w. In two patients with end-stage renal failure and β-thalassemia trait, who were transfusion dependent, administration of rHuEPO resulted in stable Hb levels obviating the need for further transfusions.[22] A very intriguing observation has been recently reported in a group of 12 anemic hemodialyzed patients, in whom the level of HbF increased from <3% to a peak value of 48% after one month of treatment with rHuEPO (45 u/kg m × 3/week). A correlation was found between % HbF and the reticulocyte count, indicating the influence of the changes of erythroid activity on HbF levels.[23] These astonishing results will have to be verified by additional studies. If indeed rHuEPO administration in thalassemia will increase the amount of HbF production, one could expect that patients with thalassemia and chronic renal failure would respond better to rHuEPO when compared to controls without thalassemia. However, as mentioned above, the available reports to date do not demonstrate the advantage expected from the results of the study by Bellizi *et al.*[23]

The conclusion from the present studies indicate that the presence of α- or β-thalassemia trait does not prevent correction of the anemia by rHuEPO in patients with chronic renal failure undergoing dialysis. But in order to reach a satisfactory therapeutic target of Hb level in such patients, one needs more time and higher doses of rHuEPO when compared to patients with end-stage renal failure without thalassemia

THE ROLE OF rHuEPO FOR PATIENTS WITH β THALASSEMIA INTERMEDIA

The theoretical rationale for treatment of patients with thalassemia with rHuEPO was based on several observations: 1) the preliminary observations in experimental animals and in erythroid cultures that resulted in increase in the synthesis of HbF,[24] 2) the discrepancy between endogenous serum EPO levels and the severity of the anemia in patients with thalassemia minor and intermedia, 3) a significant improvement in the quality of life in patients with β-thalassemia intermedia who underwent splenectomy, which resulted in a temporary increase in Hb levels of 1–3g/dl.[25] In the first trial, a relatively large dose of rHuEPO (1000 u/kg/week) was given twice a week to three patients with β-thalassemia intermedia.[26] The selected dose of rHuEPO was based on the doses used in baboons. The results showed an increase in total Hb levels by 2g/dl without any changes in % of HbF and in RBC indices. In a second preliminary trial,[27] 2 out of 3 patients responded to a dose of subcutaneous injections of rHuEPO, (200–1000 u/kg × 3/week), by a 2–3 g/dl increase in Hb without changes in other erythroid parameters. An additional six patients treated for 10 weeks with similar amounts of rHuEPO failed to respond.[7]

The longest trial of rHuEPO in β-thalassemia intermedia was carried out in ten patients for 5–12 months. The results showed an increase in total Hb concentrations of 2–3 g/dl which was dependent on the dose of rHuEPO from 500 to 950 u/kg × 3/week (FIG.2). Seven splenectomized patients responded much better than three non-splenectomized patients. As in the preliminary reports, there were no changes in the percent of HbF, in globin-chain synthetic ratios, and in RBC indices throughout the period of study. Additional studies on the effects of rHuEPO in thalassemia were carried out by Nizli *et al.* in Turkey following administration of 500–1000 u/kg × 3/week for three months to ten patients with TI. In three patients, total Hb increased by at least 2 g/dl, which lasted as long as rHuEPO was given.[29] In a second study, a sustained increase in Hb levels in 3 out of 16 patients with transfusion-dependent TM was observed, negating the need for further transfusions. Two patients did not require transfusions for more than 2 years. The positive response was confined to splenectomized patients, but apparently splenectomy was not the only factor that characterized the patients who responded to rHuEPO.[29] As in the previous studies, there were no changes in any other erythroid parameters as well as in the levels of HbF. In one patient with thalassemia and severe iron overload, where iron chelation was not adequate, administration of rHuEPO was able to maintain higher Hb levels that permitted chronic phlebotomy and reduced the requirement for iron chelation therapy.[7] A similar therapeutic approach has been successfully applied in patients with chronic renal failure.[30]

THE IMPORTANCE OF ORAL IRON SUPPLEMENTATION WITH rHuEPO

In patients with anemia and chronic renal failure, several studies of iron metabolism and kinetics have indicated that oral or even intravenous (I.V.) iron supplementation is required in order to obtain an optimal hemopoietic response to rHuEPO.[30] The basic difference between patients with anemia of chronic renal failure and patients with thalassemia is the fact that the latter have excess iron stored as ferritin or hemosiderin in many organs. In addition, their RBC also contain considerable amounts of iron that is not in the form of hemoglobin. The key question is whether upon administration of rHuEPO, the iron in their stores can be mobilized to meet the requirements created by the increased erythropoietic drive. From the present available data, the answer to the former question is not clear. Hypochromic microcytic RBC were formed following administration of rHuEPO

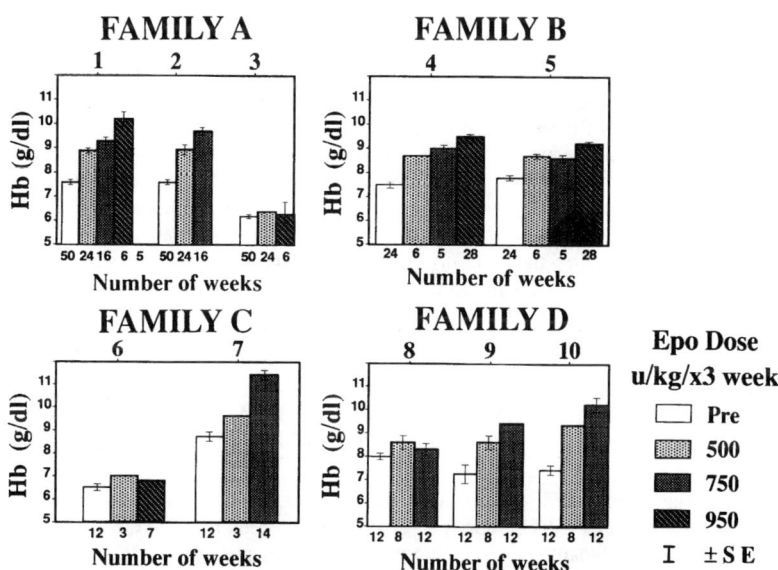

FIGURE 2: Changes in mean Hb levels in 10 patients with β-thalassemia intermedia from four different families following treatment with rHuEPO (500–900 u/kg × 3/week). Each bar represents a mean of ± 0.1 of serial determinations performed every two weeks (SE < 0.1 is not illustrated). The numbers below each bar indicate the number of weeks of treatment with a different dose of rHuEPO. Patients 3, 5, 6 and 8 were splenectomized. (From Rachmilewitz et al.[28])

without oral iron supplementation to five patients with sickle cell anemia, associated with a decrease in serum ferritin in three of them. This finding indicates that under erythropoietic stress, iron deficient erythropoiesis can occur in iron repleted subjects.[31] The availability of iron is rate limiting in response to rHuEPO in normal individuals.[32,33] On the other hand, iron supplementation together with rHuEPO may increase the existing iron overload.[34] The available data on oral iron in thalassemia patients who received rHuEPO is not sufficient to draw any conclusions. In most of the reported cases, oral iron supplementation was given in order to make sure of its availability for rHuEPO-mediated erythropoiesis,[26,27] although in some patients the positive response to rHuEPO occurred without the addition of oral iron.[7] The only way to answer this question is by designing a well-controlled study of iron kinetics associated with an evaluation of the possible erythropoietic response in thalassemia patients who receive rHuEPO with or without oral iron supplementation.

Another approach is to try the effect of the oral iron chelator L1, which, unlike desferrioxamine (DF), is capable of removing free iron from iron-loaded thalassemic RBC.[35] Since it is a weaker binder to iron than DF, it might release the chelated iron to meet the increased demands following administration of rHuEPO. A preliminary result of the positive role of L1 in promoting erythropoiesis in patients with rheumatoid arthritis and anemia has been previously reported.[36]

As pointed out by Olivieri,[7] rHuEPO in thalassemia patients may increase the risk of bone marrow expansion with the potential outcome of cortical destruction. Indeed, in one patient, mild bone pain was observed following a marked increase in Hb levels after receiving rHuEPO.[37] However, in all the other reported cases, there were no major side effects that could be attributed to rHuEPO other than some intermittent skeletal discomfort which was controlled by bed rest and mild analgesics. An accelerated linear growth was found in the seven out of ten responding patients as expressed by changes in height standard deviation score for chronological age.[28]

The conclusions that can be drawn from the available data suggest that rHuEPO is capable of inducing erythropoietic response in patients with TI who are not regularly transfused. The magnitude of the response is dose related and was not uniform in all patients. Splenectomized patients seem to do better. It was rather disappointing that the erythropoietic drive resulted mainly in the production of thalassemic RBC since there were no changes in γ-chain synthesis, increased levels of HbF, and improvement of RBC indices.

One of the major drawbacks of this treatment is the need for relatively high doses of rHuEPO in order to obtain a meaningful response. Since rHuEPO is an expensive drug, at this point its cost effectiveness will not allow it to be used worldwide, particularly in less developed countries where the number of thalassemia patients is relatively high and regular blood transfusion programs are still unavailable.

COMBINED ADMINISTRATION OF rHuEPO WITH MODULATORS OF HbF SYNTHESIS

As previously mentioned, the effect of rHuEPO was confined to an increase in the quantity of newly formed RBC. Therefore an attempt has been made to combine rHuEPO with drugs which are capable of improving the quality of thalassemic RBC by stimulating HbF synthesis. Most of the data has been obtained with hydroxyurea (HU), an antitumor agent that was initially tried in experimental animals.[38] The use of HU was found to significantly decrease painful crises and the frequency of transfusions in patients with sickle cell anemia.[6,17] On the other hand, the preliminary data on the use of HU in thalassemia suggests that although an increase in the percentage of HbF or in β-globin chain synthesis,[39] together with a consequent improvement in RBC indices has been found, it was not sufficient to increase significantly the level of total Hb and to modify the clinical course of the disease.[7] Therefore, the idea of combining an agent like rHuEPO which is capable of inducing a quantitative erythropoietic drive, together with an agent like HU, which is capable of inducing qualitative changes in the newly formed RBC, is most appealing.[40] One can also assume that HU might spare non-cycling erythroid precursors which may undergo accelerated differentiation and maturation by adding rHuEPO.[41] This approach was first tried in sickle cell anemia and the results were not uniform. While Goldberg et al.[17] did not find any synergistic effect using the two drugs in 5 patients, Rodgers et al.[6] did find a synergistic effect of the two drugs in 4 patients with sickle cell anemia. The differences could be related to the dose of HU and rHuEPO, and to iron supplementation.

In thalassemia patients another theoretical advantage for the use of the two drugs in combination is that although rHuEPO may cause further bone marrow expansion, it may be neutralized to some extent by the effect of HU. In the first trial, rHuEPO was given alone s.c. for 12 weeks (500 u/kg × 3/w) together with oral iron and folic acid. In a subsequent period of 12 weeks HU was given (20 mg/kg) for 4 days every week while rHuEPO was given in the remaining 3 days of the week and was followed by an additional 12 weeks where HU (20 mg/kg × 4/w) was given alone. When each drug was given by itself, there was an increase in total Hb compared with pre-treatment levels. When the two drugs were given together, an additive positive effect on total Hb levels was found only in 2 out of 7 patients (FIG. 3). In all patients, the percent of Hb F and RBC indices improved when HU was given with or without rHuEPO. There were no significant HU-induced changes in other laboratory parameters or any major side effects which could be related to either drug throughout the trial period. In another short trial, rHuEPO (400 u/kg × 3/w and 800 u/kg × 2/w) was given together with HU (1500 mg/day × 4 days/week) for 12 weeks. In 8 out of 10 patients, total Hb increased with an average increment of 1.5g/dl. In some patients the percent HbF increased from 5% to 20% above baseline values in addition to improvement in RBC indices.[43]

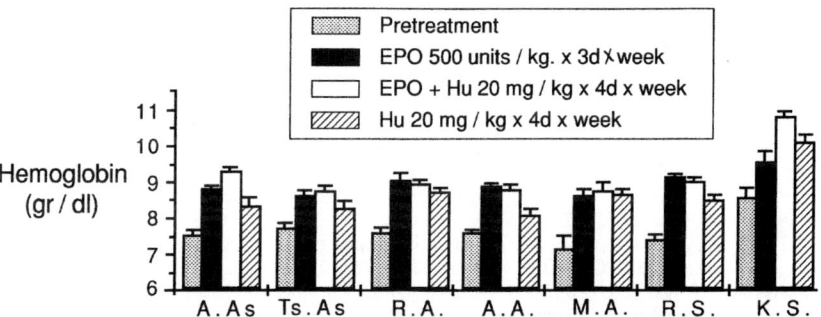

FIGURE 3: Changes in mean Hb levels (mean ± SD) in 7 patients with β-thalassemia intermedia, following administration of rHuEPO (500 u/kg × 3 d/week) for 12 weeks, rHuEPO (500 u/kg × 3d/week) and Hydroxyurea (HU) (20 mg/kg × 4d/week) for 12 weeks and HU (20 mg/kg × 4d/week) alone for 12 weeks. All patients received oral iron (ferrous citrate 246 mg/day) and folic acid (5 mg/day) throughout the trial period.

SUMMARY AND CONCLUSIONS

From all the available data to date, one can conclude that treatment with rHuEPO increases the erythropoiesis of thalassemia RBC in patients with TI, in a dose-related pattern with an average increase of 1–3 g/dl over baseline levels. The minimum effective dose is at least 5 to 10 times higher than the dose used to correct the anemia in patients with chronic renal failure, starting in a range of 400 to 500 u/kg × 3/week and higher. It is not known why the response is not uniform in all patients. It seems that splenectomized patients respond better, most likely since in the absence of the spleen, the newly formed thalassemic RBC survive longer than in patients with an intact enlarged spleen. The response to rHuEPO does not correlate with the levels of endogenous serum EPO levels. At this point it is not known whether the addition of oral iron is mandatory for optimal response to rHuEPO. In order to improve the quality of the newly formed RBC, by increasing the synthesis of HbF and consequently the RBC indices, several agents have been tried. Among them are HU, short chain fatty acids[44] and hemin.[45] The preliminary data on combinations of rHuEPO with HU showed positive effects in several erythroid parameters but an additive effect on hemoglobin levels was not obtained in all treated patients. It is imperative to design well controlled clinical trials in order to ascertain what patient characteristics are predictive of a positive response to rHuEPO, the minimal effective dose, the time schedule and whether the addition of agents capable of inducing γ-globin chain synthesis besides HU will produce a synergistic effect that will improve both the quality and the quantity of erythropoiesis in patients with various forms of the thalassemia syndrome.

REFERENCES

1. SPIVAK, J. L. 1986; The mechanisms of action of erythropoietin. Int. J. Cell Cloning. **4:** 139–143.
2. LIN, F. K., S. SUGGS, et al. 1985. Cloning and expression of human erythropoietin gene. Proc. Natl. Acad. Sci. USA. **82:** 7580–7584.
3. AL-KHATTI, A., R. VEITH, et al. 1987. Stimulation of Hb F synthesis by erythropoietin in baboons. New Eng. J. Med. **317:** 415–420.
4. LEROY-VIARD, K., P. ROUGER-FESSARD, et al. 1991. Improvement of mouse beta-thalassemia. Blood **78:** 1596–1602.
5. FIBACH, E., A. N. SCHECHTER, et al. 1994. Reducing erythropoietin in cultures of human erythroid precusors elevates the proportion of fetal hemoglobin. Br. J. Haematol. **88:** 39–45.
6. RODGERS, G. P., G. J. DOVER, et al. 1993. Augmentation by erythropoietin of the fetal hemoglobin response to hydroxyurea in sickle cell disease. New Eng. J. Med. **328:** 71–80.
7. OLIVIERI, N. F. 1996. Reactivation of fetal hemoglobin in patients with thalassemia. Semin. Hematol. **33:** 24–42.
8. HAMMOND, G. D., A. ISHIKAWA, et al. 1962. Relationship between erythropoiesis and severity of anemia in hypoplastic and hemolytic states. In Erythropoiesis: 351. Grune and Stratton. Philadelphia, PA.
9. MANOR, D., E. FIBACH, et al. 1986. Erythropoietin activity in the serum of thalassemia patients. Scand. J. Haematol. **37:** 221–228.
10. BUEMI, M., A. SARDO, et al. 1987. Pattern of plasma erythropoietin in Cooley's Disease. In Thalassemia Today. G. Sirchia & A. Zanella, Eds.: 627–631. Centro Transfusionale, Milan.
11. NISLI, G., K. KAVAKLI, et al. 1997. Serum erythropoietin levels in patients with B thalassemia major and intermedia. Pediatr. Hematol. Oncol. **14:** 161–167.
12. SHERWOOD, J. B., E. GOLDWASSER, et al. 1986. Sickle cell anemia patients have low erythropoietin levels for their degree of anemia. Blood **67:** 46–49.
13. ALESSI, M., G. LONGO, et al. 1990. Erythropoietin serum levels in thalassemia. Ann. N.Y. Acad. Sci. **612:** 534–535.
14. DORE, F., S. BONGIGLI, et al. 1993. Serum erythropoietin levels in thalassemia intermedia. Ann. Hematol. **67:** 183–186.

15. ANDRE, M., P. BERGMAN, et al. 1991. Serum immunoreactive erythropoietin level: a new parameter for monitoring transfusion management in thalassemia. Nouv. Rev. Fr. Hematol. **33:** 299–302.
16. ESCHBACH, J. W. 1989. The anemia of chronic renal failure: Pathophysiology and the effect of recombinant erythropoietin. Kidney Int. **35:** 134–148.
17. GOLDBERG, M. A., C. BRUGNARA, et al. 1990. Treatment of sickle cell anemia with hydroxyurea and erythropoietin. N. Eng. J. Med. **323:** 366–372.
18. CHENG, I. K. P. & M. B. LU, et al. 1993. Influence of thalassemia on the response to recombinant human erythropoietin in dialysis patients. Am. J. Nephrol. **13:** 142–148.
19. WINEARLS, C. G. & R. T. HUGHES, et al. 1992. Erythropoietin dose requirement in a patient with Hb H disease and renal failure. Nephrol. Dial. Transplant. **7:** 1052–1054.
20. COZMA, G. & M. C. COZMA, et al. 1992. Beneficial effect of recombinant human erythropoietin in thalassemic patients on dialysis. Nephrol. Dial. Transplant. **7:** 82–83.
21. LAI, K. N., K. C. WONG, et al. 1992. Use of recombinant erythropoietin in thalassemic patients on dialysis. Am. J. Kid. Dis. **19:** 239–245.
22. KAGAN, A., L. SINAY-TREIMAN, et al. 1992. Recombinant human erythropoietin for anemia of end-stage renal failure in thalassemia trait. Nephron **62:** 229–230.
23. BELLIZZI, V., L. DE NICOLA, et al. 1997. Fetal proteins and chronic treatment with low dose erythropoietin. J. Lab. Clin. Med. **129:** 193–199.
24. STAMATOYANNOPOLOS, G., R. VEITH, et al. 1990. Induction of fetal hemoglobin by cell-cycle specific drugs and recombinant erythropoietin. Am. J. Ped. Hematol. Oncol. **12:** 21–26.
25. ENGELHARD, D., G. CIVIDALLI, et al. 1975. Splenectomy in homozygous beta thalassemia: A retrospective study of 30 patients. Brit. J. Haemal. **31:** 391–403.
26. RACHMILEWITZ, E. A., A. GOLDFARB, et al. 1991. Administration of erythropoietin to patients with beta thalassemia intermedia: A preliminary trial. Blood **78:** 1145–1147.
27. OLIVIERI, N. F., M. H. FREEDMAN, et al. 1992. Trial of recombinant erythropoietin to patients with beta-thalassemia intermedia. Blood **80:** 3258–3260.
28. RACHMILEWITZ, E. A., M. AKER, et al. 1995. Sustained increase in haemoglobin and RBC following long-term administration of recombinant human erythropoietin to patients with homozygous beta-thalassemia. Br. J. Haematol. **90:** 341–345.
29. NISLI, G., K. KAVAKLI, et al. 1996. Recombinant human erythropoietin trial in thalassemia intermedia. J. Trop. Pediatr. **42:** 330–334.
30. VAN WYCK, D. B. 1989. Iron management during recombinant human erythropoietin therapy. Am. J. Kidney Dis. **14:** 9–13.
31. NAGEL, R. L., E. VICHINSKKY, et al. 1993. F reticulocyte response in sickle cell anemia treated with recombinant human erythropoietin: a double-blind study. Blood **81:** 9–14.
32. BRUGNARA, C., L. A. CHAMBERS, et al. 1993. Red cell regeneration induced by subcutaneous recombinant erythropoietin in iron-replete subjects. Blood **81:** 956–964.
33. BRUGNARA, C., G. M. COLELLA, et al. 1994. Effects of subcutaneous human erythropoietin in normal subjects: Development of decreased reticulocyte hemoglobin content and iron-deficient erythropoiesis. J. Lab. Clin. Med. **123:** 660–667.
34. KOOISTRA, M. P., A. VAN ES, et al. 1991. Iron metabolism in patients with anemia of end stage renal disease. Br. J. Haem. **79:** 634–639.
35. SHALEV, O., T. REPKA, et al. 1995. Deferriprone (L-1) chelates pathologic iron deposits from membranes of intact thalassemic and sickle RBC both in vitro and in vivo. Blood **86:** 2008–2013.
36. VREUGDENHIL, G., G. J. KONTOGHIORGHES, et al. 1991. Impaired erythropoietin responsiveness to the anaemia in rheumatoid arthritis. A possible inverse relationship with iron stores and effects of the oral iron chelator 1,2-dimethyl-3hydroxypyrid-4-one. Clin. Exp. Rheumatol. **9:** 35–40.
37. OLIVIERI, N. R., G. D. SHER, et al. 1995. Long-term treatment with recombinant human erythropoietin in patients with thalassemia: Reduction in requirement for transfusion and chelation therapy. *In* Sickle Cell Disease and Thalassemias: New Trends in Therapy. Colloque INSERM: 234–305. John Libbey Euro-text Ltd. Montrouge, France.
38. SAUVAGE, C., P. ROUGER-FESSARD, et al. 1993. Improvement of mouse thalassemia by hydroxyurea. Br. J. Haematol. **84:** 492–498.

39. ZENG, Y. T., S. Z. HUANG, *et al.* 1996. Hydroxyurea therapy in thalassemia intermedia: Improvement in hematological parameters due to enhanced β-globin synthesis. Br. J. Haematol. **90:** 557–563.
40. DEFRANCESCHI, L. & P. ROUYEV-FESSARD, *et al.* 1996. Combination chemotherapy of erythropoietin, hydroxyurea, and clotrimaxzole in a thalassemic mouse: A model for human therapy. Blood **87:** 1188–1195.
41. ALTER, B. P. & C. K. WAGNER, *et al.* 1989. Modulation of mouse hemoglobin expression by hydroxyurea and erythropoietin in vivo. Prog. Clin. Biol. Res. **316B:** 317–335.
42. AKER, M. & G. DOVER, *et al.* 1995. Combination of erythropoietin and hydroxyurea results in improved quality and quantity of RBC in 7 patients with thalassemia intermedia. *In* Sickle Cell Disease and Thalassemia: New Trends in Therapy. Colloque INSERM. John Libbey Eurotext Ltd. **234:** 197–199.
43. LOUKOPOULOS, D., E. VASKARDOU, *et al.* 1993. Effective stimulation of erythropoiesis in thalassemia intermedia with recombinant Human Erythropoietin and Hydroxyurea [abstract]. Blood **82:** 357.
44. PERRINE, S. P. & N. F. OLIVIERY, *et al.* 1994. Butyrate derivatives: New agents for stimulating fetal globin production in the beta-globin disorders. Am. J. Ped. Hematol. Oncol. **16:** 67–71.
45. FIBACH, E. & P. KOLLIA, *et al.* 1995. Hemin induced acceleration of hemoglobin production in immature cultured erythroid cells: Preferential enhancement of fetal hemoglobin. Blood **85:** 2967–2974.

Improved Amphotropic Retrovirus-Mediated Gene Transfer into Hematopoietic Stem Cells

DAVID M. BODINE,[a,c] CYNTHIA E. DUNBAR,[b] LAURIE J. GIRARD,[a] NANCY E. SEIDEL,[a] AMANDA P. CLINE,[a] ROBERT E. DONAHUE,[b] AND DONALD ORLIC[a]

[a]*Hematopoiesis Section, Laboratory of Gene Transfer, National Center for Human Genome Research, NIH, Bethesda, Maryland 20892-4442*

[b]*Hematology Branch, National Heart Lung and Blood Institute, NIH, Bethesda, Maryland*

ABSTRACT: The efficiency of amphotropic retrovirus-mediated gene transfer into human Hematopoietic Stem Cells (HSC) is less than 1%. This has impeded gene therapy for hematopoietic diseases.[1-3] In this study we demonstrate that populations of mouse and human HSC contain low to undetectable levels of the amphotropic virus receptor mRNA (ampho R mRNA), and are resistant to transduction with amphotropic retroviral vectors. In a subpopulation of mouse HSC expressing 7-fold higher levels of ampho R mRNA, transduction with amphotropic retrovirus vectors was 30-fold higher. We conclude that retrovirus transduction of HSC correlates with ampho R mRNA levels. Our results predict that alternative sources of HSC or retroviruses will be required for human gene therapy of hematopoietic diseases. One alternative source of stem cells is from individuals treated with cytokines. We have previously shown that mice treated with G-CSF and SCF have an immediate increase in peripheral blood HSC immediately after treatment, followed by a 10-fold increase in bone marrow HSC 14 days after treatment.[4] In this report we show that when rhesus monkey bone marrow cells collected 14 days after G-CSF and SCF treatment were transduced with amphotropic retroviruses, gene transfer levels were approximately 10%, which was easily detected by Southern blot analysis. We conclude that the increased gene transfer may be the result of increased expression of the amphotropic retrovirus receptor, increased numbers of cycling HSC or both.

Hematopoietic Stem Cells (HSC) are among the most attractive targets for retrovirus-mediated gene transfer.[5-6] Since HSC can completely and permanently repopulate the hematopoietic system following bone marrow transplantation,[7] integration of proviral DNA into the genome[8] of HSC would result in continuous production of hematopoietic cells with the transferred gene. The concept has been demonstrated in murine models using mouse-specific ecotropic retrovirus vectors.[9-14] As examples, retrovirus mediated gene transfer of the β-glucuronidase gene has cured murine β-glucuronidase deficiency,[15] and retrovirus mediated gene transfer of the Multiple Drug Resistance gene has protected the hematopoietic system from taxol treatment.[16] In these studies, gene transfer was observed into 20% or more of hematopoietic cells for over 1 year.[9-16]

[c]Corresponding author: David M. Bodine, PhD, National Center for Genome Research, Nitt, Hematopoiesis Section/LGT, 49 Covent Drive, MSC 4442, Bldg. 49/Rm. 3A14, Bethesda, MD 20892-4442.

Amphotropic murine retroviruses have been used as gene transfer vectors for human gene therapy.[5,6] Studies using different transduction protocols have reported gene transfer efficiencies of less than 0.1% to 1.0% using amphotropic retroviral vectors. A fundamental obstacle to gene therapy of human hematopoietic diseases has been the low level of gene transfer observed in human[1-3] or primate[17,18] studies using amphotropic retroviral vectors.

Ecotropic and amphotropic retroviruses differ in the gp70 proteins in the retrovirus envelope.[8] The gp70 protein of ecotropic viruses uses an amino acid transport protein on the surface of target cells as its receptor.[19,20] The gp70 binding site on this protein is not conserved among mammals. This restricts ecotropic retrovirus transduction to mouse cells.[20] The gp70 protein of amphotropic virus uses as its receptor a phosphate channel protein in which the gp70 binding site is conserved, allowing amphotropic viruses to transduce most mammalian cells.[21-23] We hypothesized that the relatively poor transduction of HSC with amphotropic viruses may be due to low levels of the amphotropic retrovirus receptor.

Recent studies have shown that murine HSC can be enriched over 1000-fold so that as few as 10–50 cells can repopulate irradiated or W/W^v mice. A variety of HSC enrichment strategies have been developed,[24] including removal of cells expressing lineage markers (Lin-), and positive selection for cells expressing Sca-1, c-kit, or other markers.[25-27] We have previously shown that a population of murine Lin- cells expressing high levels of c-kit (c-kit^{HI}) was highly enriched for HSC,[21] and we have used these cells to study mRNA expression in HSC.[28,29] Studies with human bone marrow have shown that the most primitive hematopoietic cells express the CD34 antigen, but not the CD38 antigen, while less primitive hematopoietic progenitor cells expressed both the CD34 and CD38 antigens.[30,31]

In all of these studies, only 3% or less of the enriched HSC have been demonstrated to be progressing through the cell cycle.[24,25] The number of cycling HSC may be higher in other populations of HSC other than bone marrow. Cytokine treatment of both mice and patients can mobilize HSC into the peripheral blood,[32] with an accompanying decrease in the repopulating ability of the bone marrow.[33,34] We have previously shown that the number of HSC in the bone marrow recovers to 10-fold greater than normal levels after treatment with G-CSF and SCF.[4] Because retroviruses preferentially integrate into cycling cells,[8] we hypothesized that conditions which would cause the stem cell number to increase would improve gene transfer efficiency.

In this study, we assayed amphotropic retrovirus receptor mRNA (ampho R mRNA) expression in both mouse and human HSC. The level of ampho R mRNA was nearly undetectable in enriched populations of HSC. In contrast, ecotropic retrovirus receptor mRNA (eco R mRNA) was easily detected in the same cells. We isolated a subpopulation of murine HSC comprising approximately 15% of the total number which express higher levels of ampho R mRNA. In most HSC populations, transduction with ecotropic retrovirus vectors was more than 10-fold more efficient than with amphotropic retrovirus vectors. The exception was the subpopulation expressing higher levels of ampho R mRNA where transduction with amphotropic retrovirus vectors was comparable to ecotropic retrovirus vectors. We also examined gene transfer into mouse and rhesus monkey peripheral blood and bone marrow cells collected after treatment with G-CSF and SCF. Amphotropic retrovirus mediated gene transfer into G-CSF and SCF primed Rhesus monkey was estimated at up to 10%, a level 10-fold higher than previous attempts, and detectable by Southern Blot analysis. We conclude that the low levels of expression of ampho R mRNA in HSC is be responsible for the inefficient gene transfer observed in human and primate gene transfer experiments. We propose that the increased gene transfer we observed in cytokine pretreated rhesus monkeys may be the result of increased expression of the amphotropic retrovirus receptor, increased numbers of cycling HSC or both.

METHODS

Mice and Cells

All mice were purchased from the Jackson laboratory, Bar Harbor ME. Young adult C57BL/6J female mice, 3 to 5 weeks old, were used for hematopoietic stem cell enrichment. WBB6F$_1$-W/W^v mice were used as recipients of transduced hematopoietic stem cells. The ψ-CRE MFG-lacZ and ψ-CRIP MFG-NLSlacZ cell lines were maintained in Dulbecco's Modified Eagle's Medium (DMEM) supplemented with 10% Newborn Calf serum (NCS; both from GIBCO, Gaithersburg, MD). The LNL6 and G1Na retroviral vectors carry an identical bacterial phosphotransferase gene.[35,36] Supernatants from all 4 cell lines were harvested from producer cell lines grown to confluence in Dulbecco's modified Eagle's medium (DMEM) supplemented with 10% fetal calf serum (Gibco/BRL, Gaithersburg, MD).

Enrichment of HSC

Mouse bone marrow HSC were isolated as previously described.[27] Briefly, cells were fractionated by counterflow centrifugal elutriation and collected at flow rates of 25 ml/min, 30 ml/min (discarded), and 35 ml/min (FR25, FR35). FR25 or FR35 cells were incubated in a cocktail of rat anti-mouse monoclonal antibodies directed against lineage and cells expressing lineage markers were removed using antibody coated immunomagnetic beads. Lin-cells were incubated with biotinylated anti-c-kit antibody (ACK-4; a gift of Dr. S. I. Nishikawa), and high levels of c-kit (c-kit^{HI}) were collected. We have previously shown that all hematopoietic stem cells (HSC) reside in the c-kit^{HI} population.[27]

Human bone marrow cells were obtained with informed consent from volunteer donors. Mononuclear cells were enriched population for CD34 positive cells and stained with antibodies to FITC-labeled human lineage markers, APC labeled CD34, and PE labeled CD38. Lin-CD34+ CD38- cells (90% pure) were collected by cell sorting.

Isolation and Analysis of RNA

Total cellular RNA was isolated according to the manufacturer's instructions using RNAzol B. First strand cDNA synthesis was performed on an aliquot of RNA according to the manufacturer's instructions (Perkin Elmer Cetus, Norwalk, CT). An estimate of the amount of cDNA in each sample was obtained by limiting dilution RT-PCR (Perkin Elmer Cetus, Norwalk, CT), using the b-2 microglobulin (b-2 M) (primers and conditions shown below), with 0.1 μl of α^{32}PdCTP added per reaction. Phosphorimager analysis was used to identify the linear range of the β-2 M amplification curve. These values were used to determine equivalent quantities of cDNA for amplification with primers specific for the retrovirus receptor mRNAs shown in TABLE 1.[28]

Rhesus Stem and Progenitor Cell Harvesting

Young adult (age 3–5 years) rhesus macaques (*Macaca mulatta*) were housed and handled in accordance with the guidelines set by the Committee on Care and Use of Laboratory Animals of the Institute of Laboratory Animal Resources, National Research Council (DHHS Publication No. NIH 85–23). Recombinant human stem cell factor (200

Table 1. Primers and PCR conditions.

Gene		Primer Sequence	Conditions
Mouse	Ecotropic R	sense: 5'CTG CCT CAA CAC CTA TGA CC3'	94°C-1 min.
		anti-sense: 5'TGC TGA CGT GAG AAC TCT CC3'	58°C-1 min.
		Fragment size: 308 bp	72°C-2 min.
Mouse	Amphotropic R	sense: 5'CGG GCG GAA GAC GAG AAG GA3'	94°C-1 min.
		anti-sense: 5'GAA GCC ACT GGA CGG TGT GA3'	65°C-1 min.
		Fragment size: 309 bp	72°C-2 min.
Mouse	β-2 Microglobulin	sense: 5'TGC TAT CCA GAA AAC CCC TC3'	94°C-1 min.
		anti-sense: 5'GTC ATG CTT AAC TCT GCA GG3'	55°C-1 min.
		Fragment size: 258 bp	72°C-2 min.
Human	Ecotropic R	sense: 5'CTG CCT GAA CAC TTT TGA TCT GGT GGC3'	94°C-1 min.
		anti-sense: 5'GAG GTC ATG TGT GTC CGT GAG AAC TCC3'	58°C-1 min.
		Fragment size: 371 bp	72°C-2 min.
Human	Amphotropic R	sense: 5'CGG AAC ATC TTC GTG GCC TG3'	94°C-1 min.
		anti-sense :5'GCT GGT CAT GAG AGA GCC GTG3'	62°C-1 min.
		Fragment size: 220 bp	72°C-2 min.
Human	β-2 Microglobulin	sense: 5'CTC GCG CTA CTC TCT CTT TC3'	94°C-1 min.
		anti-sense: 5'CAT GTC TCG ATC CCA CTT AAC3'	55°C-1 min.
		Fragment size: 330 bp	72°C-2 min.
Lac Z		sense: 5'GCC GAC ACC AGA CTA AGA AC3'	94°C 1 min.
		anti-sense: 5'CCT CTT CGC TAT TAC GCC AG3'	58°C 1 min.
		Fragment size: 289 or 310 bp	72°C 2 min.
Neo		sense: 5'CGG ATC GCT CAC AAC CAG TC3'	94°C 1 min.
		antisense: 5' AGC CGA ATA GCC TCT CCA CC3'	60°C 1.5 min.
		Fragment size: 483 or 467	72°C 2 min.

Cycle number for all primer pairs = 35

µg/kg/day) and recombinant human granulocyte colony-stimulating factor 10 µg/kg/day) were given as subcutaneous injections for 5 days. Peripheral blood apheresis of 2.5 times the animal's blood volume was performed as described on day 5.[37] Bone marrow was harvested from the femurs, iliac crests, and ischial tuberosities under general anesthesia, either prior to G-CSF and SCF treatment, or 14 days after discontinuation of cytokine treatment.

Retrovirus Transduction

For transduction of mouse hematopoietic stem cells, 70% confluent plates of the producer cell lines were grown overnight in DMEM supplemented with 15% Hyclone FCS. The medium was aspirated from the plates, cytokines (f.c. mouse IL-3 10 ng/ml; rat SCF 100 ng/ml; human IL-6 100 ng/ml) and polybrene (f.c.: 6 µu/ml) were added, and the mixture was filtered (0.45 mm) and added to the target cells. The cells were cultured for 96 hours at 37°C (4 changes of medium) before being returned to recipient W/W^v mice. Proviral integration was analyzed by PCR of DNA extracted from peripheral blood cells using the following MFG-lacZ primers shown below. For rhesus monkey transduction CD34+ cells were transduced in undiluted LNL6 or G1Na supernatants supplemented with 4 µg/ml protamine sulfate, 20 ng/ml human IL-3, 100 ng/ml human SCF, 50 ng/ml human IL-6. Cells were cultured 96 hours at 37°C (4 changes of medium). After transduction the cells were cryopreserved. Seven to 10 days after BM harvesting the animals received 650 rads total body irradiation on each of two days. The next day, the transduced CD34-

enriched cells thawed and infused. Standard supportive care and transfusion support for rhesus transplantation recipients were given.

After reconstitution, peripheral blood and bone marrow cells were collected at 1–3 month intervals. PCR was performed using the neo primers shown. For Southern blotting, 10 μg of DNA were digested with either Sac I or Bgl II, electrophoresed on a 1% agarose gel, transferred to a nylon membrane and before hybridized with a Neo probe.

RESULTS

Analysis of Retrovirus Receptor mRNA Expression in Mouse Hematopoietic Stem Cells

We compared ampho R and eco R mRNA levels in unfractionated bone marrow RNA and RNA isolated from a variety of cell lines by both Northern blot and RT-PCR analysis. We demonstrated that our RT-PCR primers and conditions gave identical results to the Northern analysis (data not shown). Because of the scarcity of HSC in the bone marrow we compared ampho R and eco R mRNA levels by RT-PCR in two populations of enriched murine HSC. Lin- c-kit^{HI} cells elutriated at a flow rate of 25 ml/min. (FR25) represent approximately 25% of the HSC in C57BL/6 mice, and Lin- c-kit^{HI} cells elutriated at a flow rate of 35 ml/min. FR35 cells represent approximately 15% of the HSC in C57BL/6 mice.[27,38] Eco R mRNA was present in similar levels in 3T3 cells, four independent isolates of unfractionated bone marrow cells, and 7 independent isolates of FR35 Lin-c-kit^{HI} cells, and was approximately 50% of the 3T3 cell level in FR25 Lin-c-kit^{HI} cells (FIG. 1). The level of ampho R mRNA in unfractionated bone marrow cells was approximately 50% the level in 3T3 cells. Ampho R mRNA was present at low but detectable levels in FR35 Lin-c-kit^{HI} cells, but was nearly undetectable in FR25 Lin-c-kit^{HI} cells ($p = 0.035$; FIG. 1).

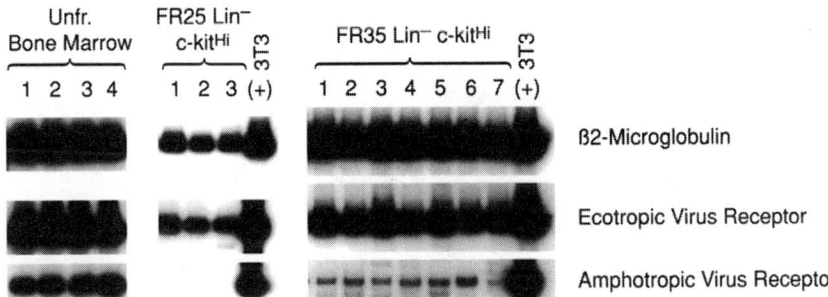

FIGURE 1. Retrovirus receptor mRNA expression in enriched populations of mouse hematopoietic stem cells. The level of expression of the mRNAs encoding the mouse ecotropic and amphotropic retrovirus receptors were compared by Reverse Transcriptase PCR analysis using primers specific for each mRNA. The level of mouse β-2 microglobulin mRNA was measured to quantify the amount of c-DNA analyzed in each reaction. RNA isolated from NIH 3T3 cells (which are efficiently transduced by both amphotropic and ecotropic retroviruses) served as a positive control. **Top Panel:** Mouse β-2 microglobulin mRNA expression in unfractionated bone marrow cells (4 independent RNA isolates; *left of panel*); FR25 Lin- c-kit^{HI} cells (3 independent RNA isolates; *center of panel*); and 3T3 cells (*right of panel*). **Center Panel:** Mouse ecotropic retrovirus receptor mRNA expression in the same RNA populations. **Bottom Panel:** Mouse amphotropic retrovirus receptor mRNA expression in the same RNA populations.

Analysis of Retrovirus Receptor mRNA Expression in Human Hematopoietic Stem Cells

Expression of retrovirus receptor mRNAs was analyzed in two populations of human primitive hematopoietic cells. Cells co-expressing the CD34 and CD38 antigens are enriched for progenitor cells, while CD34+/CD38- cells are enriched for more primitive cells.[30,31] Human ampho R mRNA was expressed in CD34+/CD38+ cells, but was nearly undetectable in CD34+/CD38- cells. These results were similar to the pattern of expression seen in mouse HSC. The human homologue of the ecotropic virus receptor does not serve as a retrovirus receptor on human cells owing to changes in the virus binding site. This mRNA was expressed in CD34+/CD38+ cells, and at lower levels in CD34+/CD38- cells (FIG. 2).

Transduction of Mouse HSC with Ecotropic and Amphotropic Retroviruses

To determine the relationship between eco R and ampho R mRNA expression and gene transfer efficiency, a co-transduction assay was developed. Two cell lines producing ecotropic and amphotropic lacZ retroviruses (ψ-Cre MFG-lacZ and ψ-Crip MFG-NLSlacZ, respectively) were selected. These retroviruses differ by a 21 base pair nuclear localization signal (NLS) and could be distinguished by either PCR or Southern blot analysis (FIG. 3). Equal volumes of supernatant from the two producer cell lines were combined and used to transduce 3T3 cells, FR25 Lin-c-kit[HI] cells, and FR35 Lin-c-kit[HI] cells. Southern blot analysis of DNA extracted from transduced 3T3 cells demonstrated that the producer cell lines produced equivalent titers of each retrovirus (FIG. 3). Ecotropic MFG-

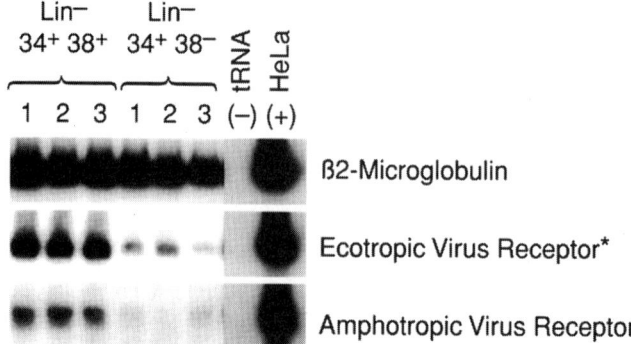

FIGURE 2. Retrovirus receptor mRNA expression in enriched populations of human primitive hematopoietic cells. The level of expression of the mRNAs encoding the human equivalent of the mouse ecotropic retrovirus receptor (this molecule does not function as a retrovirus receptor in human cells) and the human amphotropic retrovirus receptor were compared with Reverse Transcriptase PCR using primers specific for each mRNA. The level of β-2 microglobulin mRNA was measured to quantify the amount of c-DNA analyzed in each reaction. RNA isolated from HeLa cells (which are efficiently transduced by amphotropic retroviruses) served as a positive control. **Top Panel:** Human β-2 microglobulin mRNA expression in Lin- CD34+ CD38+ cells (3 independent RNA isolates; *left of panel*), Lin-CD34+CD38- cells (3 independent RNA isolates; *center of panel*), and negative control (tRNA) and positive control (HeLa cell) RNA samples. **Center Panel:** Human ecotropic retrovirus receptor equivalent mRNA expression in the same RNA populations. **Bottom Panel:** Human amphotropic retrovirus receptor mRNA expression in the same RNA populations.

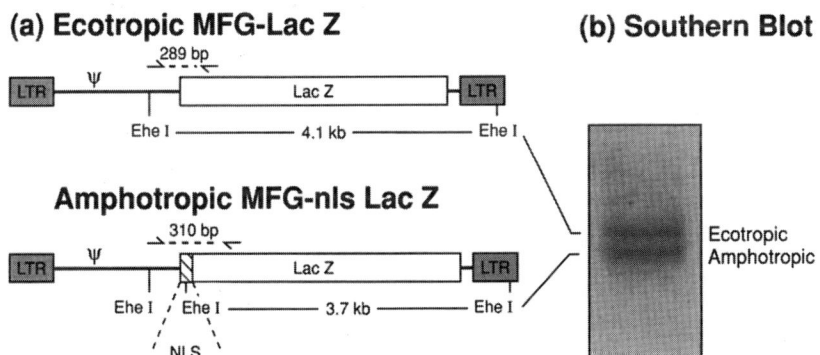

FIGURE 3. Co-transduction assay using the MFG-lacZ and MFG-NLS lacZ virus vectors. (**a**) The two proviruses, MFG-Lac Z (ecotropic) and MFG-nls Lac Z (amphotropic). The provirus from the amphotropic producer cell line can be distinguished from the provirus from the ecotropic producer cell line by either Southern blot analysis using Ehe I for digestion (**b**) or PCR analysis based on the presence of a 21 base pair Nuclear Localization Signal (nls) in the MFG-nls Lac Z provirus using the primers shown in (**a**).

lacZ proviral sequences were detected in DNA extracted from peripheral blood cells of 10 of 13 recipients of transduced FR25 Lin-c-kit^{HI} cells. No proviral sequences were detected in 3 recipients. Consistent with the low level of expression of amphotropic retrovirus receptor mRNA detected in FR25 Lin- c-kit^{HI} cells, amphotropic MFG-NLSlacZ proviral sequences were detected in only one animal, at a low level. The ratio of amphotropic to ecotropic retrovirus transduction of FR25 Lin- c-kit^{HI} cells was 0.022±0.07 (FIG. 4). Ecotropic MFG-lacZ proviral sequences were detected in DNA extracted from peripheral blood cells of all 11 recipients of transduced FR35 Lin- c-kit^{HI} cells. Consistent with the higher level of expression of amphotropic retrovirus receptor mRNA detected in FR35 Lin- c-kit^{HI} cells, amphotropic MFG-NLSlacZ proviral sequences were detected in 6 of the 11 animals. In three mice, the level of amphotropic proviral sequences was greater than or equal to the ecotropic proviral sequences in the same animal. The ratio of amphotropic to ecotropic retrovirus transduction into FR35 Lin- c-kit^{HI} cells was 0.625±0.7 (p =0.018; FIG. 4). To exclude the possibility that transduction of progenitors among the FR35 Lin- c-kit^{HI} cells was responsible for the positive signals, animals were analyzed 16 weeks post transplantation, and complete repopulation with donor cells was demonstrated using polymorphisms in the mouse β-globin gene.[10,16]

Retroviral Transduction Efficiency of G-CSF/SCF–Primed BM and PB in the Rhesus Autologous Transplantation Model

We have previously shown that following a 5 day course of treatment with G-CSF and SCF, mice have an immediate increase in the number of peripheral blood HSC, followed by a 10-fold increase in bone marrow HSC activity the peaks at 14 days after cytokine treatment.[4] We hypothesized that the increase in HSC activity might be accompanied by an increase in cycling HSC which would facilitate retrovirus mediated gene transfer. To test this hypothesis, we compared amphotropic retrovirus transduction into rhesus monkey peripheral blood and bone marrow collected after G-CSF/SCF treatment. Two animals were treated with SCF and G-CSF for five days and peripheral blood cells were collected via apheresis on the fifth day. Previous studies in rhesus monkeys and baboons by ourselves and others have shown maximal CFU-GM mobilization on days 4–6 after initiation of SCF and G-CSF.[39] CD34-enriched peripheral blood stem and progenitor cells were transduced for 96 hours in suspension culture with either LNL6 or G1Na neo vectors (titer: 1-5×10^5) using a protocol similar to that used in human clinical trials.[2] Fourteen days after discontinuation of the G-CSF/SCF treatment, bone marrow was harvested, enriched for cells expressing CD34, and transduced under identical conditions as the peripheral blood, using whichever vector was NOT used to transduce the peripheral blood cells.

All animals received over 10 million CD34-enriched and cultured cells per kilogram. Both peripheral blood and bone marrow cells were reinfused after total body irradiation. The two animals recovered granulocyte counts to greater than 500/µl on days 10 and 14 respectively, faster than rhesus monkeys in our previous studies transplanted with CD34-enriched steady-state BM that engrafted on days 18–24.[17] The animals were followed for the presence and the origin of the Neo gene after engraftment. Similar to the strategy described in FIGURE 3, the LNL6 and G1Na vectors can be distinguished by the presence of additional polylinker sequences in G1Na. Both proviruses can be amplified in the same reaction with one set of primers and separated by denaturing gel electrophoresis.

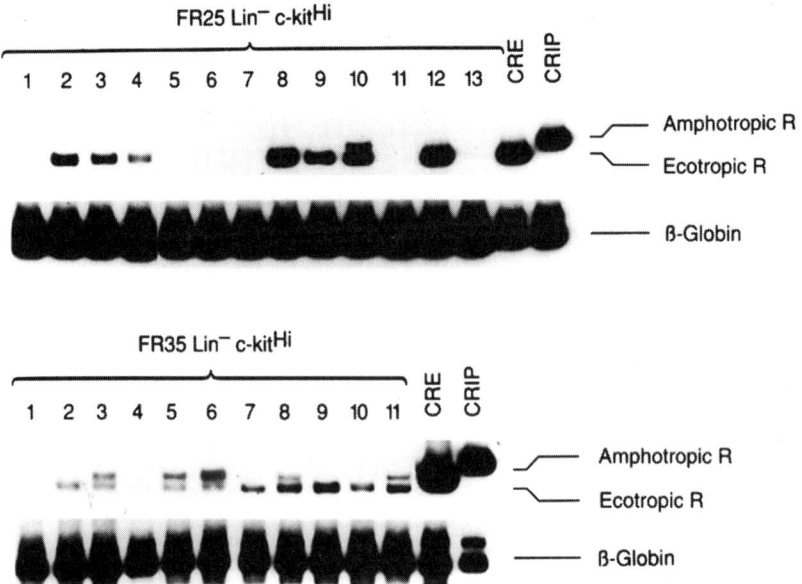

FIGURE 4. Co-transduction of mouse FR25 Lin- c-kit^{HI} and FR35 Lin- c-kit^{HI} stem cells. Equal volumes of supernatant from the MFG-lacZ and MFG-NLS lacZ producer cell lines were mixed and used to transduce enriched stem cell populations (96 hours; 4 changes). **Top panel:** Analysis of DNA extracted from the peripheral blood of *W/W^v* mice 16 weeks after transplantation with transduced FR25 lin- c-kit^{HI} cells. DNA was amplified using the PCR primers shown in FIGURE 3. The sizes of the fragments corresponding to the amphotropic and ecotropic retroviruses are 311 and 290 bp respectively. These mice represent two independent experiments. The mouse adult β-globin genes (4 genes per cell) was co-amplified as an internal control (*bottom*). **Lower panel:** Analysis of DNA extracted from the peripheral blood of *W/W^v* mice 16 weeks after transplantation with transduced FR35 Lin- c-kit^{HI} cells. These mice represent two independent experiments. The mouse β-globin gene was co-amplified as an internal control (*bottom*).

Semiquantitative PCR analysis demonstrated high levels of the vectors exposed to the post cytokine treatment marrow and lower levels of the vector exposed to the peripheral blood cells. Mononuclear cells, granulocytes and BM cells had Neo gene signals corresponding to a copy number of .05/cell (5%). FACS-sorted populations of T cells in both animals, and B cells in one animal were also positive for the marker gene, at levels of 3–5%.

The relatively high level of vector-containing blood cells we observed using semi-quantitative PCR was confirmed by Southern blot analysis. A band hybridizing to a Neo probe could be detected after digestion of DNA from animal J370 (FIG. 5). The intensity was estimated to be between 5–10%. The band size indicates origin from the G1Na vector, which was used to mark the primed BM. When the samples were cut with a restriction enzyme cutting once within the provirus in order to study the number of insertion sites, no bands were detectable, suggesting that more than one clone was contributing to the marking (data not shown).

DISCUSSION

Retrovirus binding to target cells and cell cycle status are two factors recognized to be important for retrovirus transduction.[6] Our results indicate that amphotropic retroviruses transduce mouse HSC at lower frequencies than ecotropic retroviruses, and at ratios consistent with the level of ampho R mRNA. In a previous study, Osborne et al.[40] showed that amphotropic retrovirus-mediated gene transfer into mouse HSC was inefficient, requiring preselection for transduced bone marrow cells to achieve detectable levels of transduction. This study did not compare the efficiency of transduction of ecotropic and amphotropic retroviral vectors. In another study, Richardson et al.[41] were unable to detect amphotropic retrovirus-mediated gene transfer to unfractionated fetal liver cells, while transduction

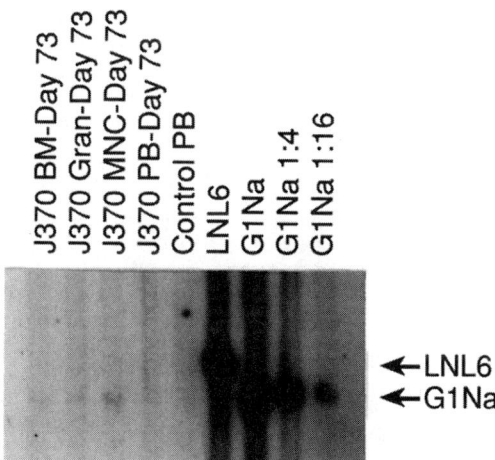

FIGURE 5. Southern blotting for the presence of the Neo gene in samples from monkey J370 at the indicated times post-transplantation. DNA samples from nucleated bone marrow cells (BM), purified granulocytes (GRAN) and mononuclear cells (MNC), and unfractionated peripheral blood nucleated cells (PB) from J370, negative control PB from a non-transplanted monkey, and positive control standards of dilutions of (single copy) producer cell line DNA into normal BM DNA were cut with Sac1, an enzyme which flanks the Neo transgene in bothLNL6 and G1Na, and probed with a neo gene probe.

with ecotropic retroviruses was detected. Gene transfer into repopulating HSC from fetal liver was not analyzed.

Our results are consistent with the hypothesis that the low level of retrovirus-mediated gene transfer into murine and primate HSC is a consequence of a low level of expression of ampho R mRNA. Higher levels of amphoR mRNA were present in human hematopoietic progenitor cells (CD34+ CD38+), which are efficiently transduced by amphotropic retroviruses. The similarity of gene transfer efficiencies into mouse and primate HSC using amphotropic vectors[17,18] indicates that the mouse may be a suitable model system to develop improved amphotropic retrovirus-mediated gene transfer protocols.

There are potential solutions to the problems presented by the low level of expression of ampho R mRNA. We have shown that we can isolate a subpopulation of mouse HSC expressing higher levels of ampho R mRNA, which are more efficiently transduced by amphotropic retrovirus vectors. We predict that if a population of HSC expressing higher levels of ampho R receptor mRNA can be isolated, gene transfer efficiency can be improved. Our results in rhesus monkeys indicate that amphotropic retrovirus-mediated gene transfer efficiency is greater in G-CSF and SCF primed bone marrow and peripheral blood. We hypothesize that this may be due to an increase in the number of HSC expressing higher levels of the mRNA encoding the amphotropic retrovirus receptor mRNA. Additional cell populations to examine would include cord blood stem cells, which have been identified as excellent targets for gene transfer using amphotropic retroviral vectors based on a greater efficiency of gene transfer into progenitor cells.[42–43]

In both murine and human experiments the percentage of cells with the HSC phenotype (Lin- Sca-1+ Thy-1.1-; Lin- c-kitHI; Lin- CD34+ CD38-) which are in the G2 or M stage of the cell cycle is less than 3%.[24] This low level of cycling among HSC remains a problem for retrovirus-mediated gene transfer into HSC since retroviral integration requires cell division.[8] We have shown that treatment of normal mice with G-CSF and SCF causes a transient increase in HSC number first in the peripheral blood and later in the bone marrow.[4] Cytokine priming may cause the treated HSC to engraft more efficiently or causes an increase in the absolute number of HSC. A critical experiment will be to determine the cell cycle status and the level of ampho R mRNA in these cells. The results of these experiments should help to determine whether the increase in amphotropic retrovirus-mediated gene transfer is due to increased levels of ampho R mRNA, increased HSC cycling, or a combination of the two.

REFERENCES

1. BRENNER, M. K. *et al.* 1993. Gene marking to determine whether autologous marrow infusion restores long-term haemopoiesis in cancer patients. Lancet **342:** 1134–1137.
2. DUNBAR, C. E. *et al.* 1995. Retrovirally marked CD34-enriched peripheral blood and bone marrow cells contribute to long-term engraftment after autologous transplantation. Blood **85:** 3048–3057.
3. KOHN, D. B. *et al.* 1995. Engraftment of gene-modified umbilical cord blood cells in neonates with adenosine deaminase deficiency. Nature Med. **1:** 1017–1023.
4. BODINE, D. M., N. E. SEIDEL & D. ORLIC. 1996. Bone marrow collected 14 days after in vivo administration of Granulocyte Colony-Stimulating Factor and Stem Cell Factor to mice has 10-fold more repopulating ability than untreated bone marrow. Blood **88:** 89–97.
5. ANDERSON, W. F. 1984. Prospects for human gene therapy. Science **226:** 401–409.
6. MULLIGAN, R. C. 1993. The basic science of gene therapy. Science **260:** 926–932.
7. THOMAS, E. D. *et al.* 1975. Bone marrow transplantation. (two parts) N. Eng. J. Med. **292:** 832–902.
8. VARMUS, H. 1988. Retroviruses Sci. **240:** 1427–1435.
9. DZIERZAK, E. A., TH. PAPAYANNOPOULOU & R. C. MULLIGAN. 1988. Lineage specific expression of a human β-globin gene in murine bone marrow transplant recipients reconstituted with retrovirus-transduced stem cells. Nature **331:** 35–41.

10. BODINE, D. M., S. KARLSSON & A. W. NIENHUIS. 1989. Combination of interleukins 3 and 6 preserves stem cell function in culture and enhances retrovirus-mediated gene transfer into hematopoietic stem cells. Proc. Nat. Acad. Sci. USA **86**: 8897–8901.
11. LIM, B., J. F. APPERLY, S. H. ORKIN & D. A. WILLIAMS. 1989. Long-term expression of human adenosine deaminase in mice transplanted with retrovirus infected hematopoietic stem cells. Proc. Nat. Acad. Sci. USA **86**: 8892–8896.
12. BELMONT, J. W. et al. 1988. Expression of adenosine deaminase in murine hematopoietic cells. Mol. Cell. Biol. **8**: 5116–5125.
13. WILSON, J. M., O. DANOS, M. GROSSMAN, D. H. RAULET & R. C. MULLIGAN. 1990. Expression of human adenosine deaminase in mice reconstituted with retrovirus-transduced hematopoietic stem cells. Proc. Nat. Acad. Sci. USA **87**: 439–443.
14. JORDAN, C. T. & I. R. LEMISCHKA. 1990. Clonal and systemic analysis of long-term hematopoiesis in the mouse. Genes & Dev. **4**: 220–232.
15. WOLF, J. H. et al. 1993. Reversal of pathology in murine mucoploysaccharidosis type VII by somatic gene transfer. Nature **360**: 749–753.
16. SORRENTINO, B. P. et al. 1992. Selection of drug-resistant bone marrow cells in vivo after retroviral transfer of human MDR1. Science **257**: 99–103.
17. BODINE, D. M. et al. 1993. Long-term in vivo expression of a murine adenosine deaminase gene in Rhesus monkey hematopoietic cells of multiple lineages after retroviral mediated gene transfer into CD34+ bone marrow cells. Blood **82**: 1975–1980.
18. VAN BEUSECHEM V. W., A. KAKLER, P. J. MEIDT & D. VALERIO. 1992. Long-term expression of human adenosine deaminase in Rhesus monkeys transplanted with retrovirus infected bone marrow cells. Proc. Nat. Acad. Sci. USA **89**: 7640–7644.
19. ALBRITTON, L. M., L. TSENG, D. SCADDEN & J. M. CUNNINGHAM. 1989. A putative murine ecotropic retrovirus receptor encodes a multiple membrane-spanning protein and confers susceptibility to virus infection. Cell **57**: 659–666.
20. ALBRITTON, L. M., J. W. KIM, L. TSENG & J. M. CUNNINGHAM. 1993. Envelope-binding domain in the cationic amino acid transporter determines the host range of ecotropic murine viruses. J. Virol. **67**: 2091–2096.
21. MILLER, D. G., R. H. EDWARDS & A. D. MILLER. 1994. Cloning of the cellular receptor for amphotropic murine retroviruses reveals homology to that for gibbon ape leukemia virus. Proc. Nat. Acad. Sci. USA **91**: 78–82.
22. VAN ZEIJL, M., S. V. JOHANN, E. CLOSS, J. CUNNINGHAM, R. EDDY, T. B. SHOWS & B. O'HARA. 1994. A human amphotropic retrovirus receptor is a second member of the gibbon ape leukemia virus receptor family. Proc. Nat. Acad. Sci. USA **91**: 1168–1172.
23. KAVANAUGH, M. P., D. G. MILLER, W. ZHANG, W. LAW, S. L. KOZAK, D. KABAT & A. D. MILLER. 1994. Cell-surface receptors for gibbon ape leukemia virus and amphotropic murine retrovirus are inducible sodium-dependent phosphate symporters. Proc. Nat. Acad. Sci. USA **91**: 7071–7075.
24. SPANGRUDE, G. J., L. SMITH, N. UCHIDA, K. IKUDA, S. HIEMFELD, J. FRIEDMAN & I. L. WEISSMAN. 1991. Mouse hematopoietic stem cells. Blood **78**: 7835–7840.
25. SPANGRUDE, G. J., S. HEIMFELD & I. L. WEISSMAN. 1988. Purification and characterization of mouse hematopoietic stem cells. Science **241**: 58–62.
26. VISSER, J. W. M., J. G. J. BAUMAN, A. H. MULDER, J. F. ELIASON & A. M. DE LEEUW. 1984. Isolation of murine pluripotent hematopoietic stem cells. J. Exp. Med. **59**: 1576–1590.
27. ORLIC, D., R. FISCHER, S. I. NISHIKAWA, A. W. NEINHUIS & D. M. BODINE. 1993. Purification and characterization of heterogeneous pluripotent hematopoietic stem cell populations expressing high levels of c-kit receptor. Blood **82**: 762–770.
28. ORLIC, D., S. ANDERSON, L. G. BIESECKER, B. P. SORRENTINO & D. M. BODINE. 1995. Pluripotent hematopoietic stem cells contain high levels of mRNA for c-kit, GATA-2, p45 NF-E2, and c-myb and low mRNA for c-fms and the receptors for granulocyte colony-stimulating factor and interleukins 5 and 7. Proc. Nat. Acad. Sci. USA **92**: 4601–4605.
29. SORRENTINO, B. P., K. T. MCDONAGH, D. WOODS & D. ORLIC. 1995. Expression of retroviral vectors containing the human multidrug resistance 1 cDNA in hematopoietic cells of transplanted mice. Blood **86**: 491–501.

30. TERSTAPPEN L. W. M. M., S. HUANG, M. SAFFORD & M. R. LANSDORP LOKEN. 1991. Sequential generations of hematopoietic colonies derived from single nonlineage-committed CD34+CD38- progenitor cells. Blood **77:** 1218–1225.
31. BAUM, C. M., I. L. WEISSMAN, A. S. TSUKAMOTO, A. M. BUCKLE & B. PEAULT. 1992. Isolation of a candidate human hematopoietic stem-cell population. Proc. Nat. Acad. Sci. USA **89:** 2804–2808.
32. EAVES, C. J. 1993. Peripheral blood stem cells reach new heights. Blood **82:** 1957–1958.
33. BODINE, D. M., N. E. SEIDEL, K. M. ZSEBO & D. ORLIC. 1993. In vivo administration of stem cell factor to mice increases the absolute number of pluripotent hematopoietic stem cells. Blood **82:** 445–455.
34. BODINE, D. M., N. E. SEIDEL, M. S. GALE, A. W. NIENHUIS & D. ORLIC. 1994. Efficient retrovirus transduction of mouse pluripotent hematopoietic stem cells mobilized into the peripheral blood by treatment with granulocyte colony-stimulation factor and stem cell factor. Blood **84:** 1482–1491.
35. CASSEL, A., M. COTTLER-FOX, S. DOREN & C. E. DUNBAR. 1993. Retroviral-mediated gene transfer into CD-34 enriched human peripheral blood stem cells. Exp. Hematol. **21:** 585–591.
36. MILLER, A. D. & C. BUTTIMORE. 1986. Redesign of retrovirus packaging cell lines to avoid recombination leading to helper virus production. Mol. Cell. Biol. **6:** 2895–2902.
37. DONAHUE, R. E., M. R. KIRBY, M. E. METZGER, B. A. AGRICOLA, S. E. SELLERS & H. M. CULLIS. 1996. Peripheral blood CD34+ cells differ from bone marrow CD34+ cells in Thy-1 expression and cell cycle status in nonhuman primates mobilized or not mobilized with Granulocyte Colony-Stimulating Factor and/or Stem Cell Factor. Blood **87:** 1644–1653.
38. ORLIC, D. & D. M. BODINE. 1992. Pluripotent hematopoietic stem cells of low and high density can repopulate W/W^v mice. Exp. Hematol. **20:** 1291–1295.
39. ANDREWS, R. G., R. A. BRIDDELL, G. H. KNITTER, T. OPIE, M. BRONSDEN, D. MYERSON, F. R. APPELBAUM & I. K. MCNIECE. 1994. In vivo synergy between recombinant human Stem Cell Factor and recombinant human Granulocyte Colony-Stimulating Factor in baboons: Enhanced circulation of progenitor cells. Blood **84:** 800–810.
40. OSBORNE, W. R. A., R. A. HOCK, M. KALEKO & A. D. MILLER. 1990. Long-term expression of human adenosine deaminase in mice after transplantation of bone marrow infected with amphotropic retroviral vectors. Hum. Gene Ther. **1:** 31–41.
41. RICHARDSON, C., M. WARD, S. PODDA & A. BANK. 1994. Mouse fetal liver cells lack amphotropic retroviral receptors. Blood 433–439.
42. LU, L., M. XIAO, D. W. CLAPP, Z. H. LI & H. E. BROXMEYER. 1993. High efficiency retroviral mediated gene transduction into single isolated immature and replatable (CD34+++) hematopoietic stem/progenitor cells from human umbilical cord blood. J Exp. Med. **178:** 2089–2096.
43. HANLEY, M. E., J. A. NOLTA, R. PARKMAN & D. B. KOHN. 1994. Umbilical cord blood cell transduction by retroviral vectors: Pre-clinical studies to optimize gene transfer. Blood Cells **20:** 539–546.

Retroviral Vectors Aimed at the Gene Therapy of Human β-Globin Gene Disorders[a]

ROBERT PAWLIUK,[b] THOMAS BACHELOT,[b] HARRY RAFTOPOULOS,[c] CHRISTIAN KALBERER,[d] R. KEITH HUMPHRIES,[d] ARTHUR BANK[c] AND PHILIPPE LEBOULCH[b,e,f]

[b]*Harvard-MIT Division of Health Sciences and Technology, Massachusetts Institute of Technology, Cambridge, Massachusetts 02139*

[c]*College of Physicians & Surgeons, Columbia University, New York, New York 10032*

[d]*Terry Fox Laboratory, British Columbia Cancer Agency, Vancouver, BC V5Z1L3, Canada*

[e]*Harvard Medical School and Brigham & Women's Hospital, Hematology-Oncology Division, Boston, Massachusetts 02115.*

ABSTRACT: We are focusing on the development of complex retroviral vectors containing human β-globin gene and β-LCR for the gene therapy of sickle cell disease and β-thalassemias. First generation vectors containing mutated splice-sites to insure stability of proviral transfer enabled long-term reconstitution in 10/12 transplanted mice for a least 8 months with high expression levels in 2 out of 3 mice analyzed (5% and 20% murine β). Transfer and expression were also achieved in secondary recipients (range: 3–11% murine β). Position independent expression was not observed. In an effort to increase the efficiency of gene transfer and obtain complete reconstitution of recipient mice with exclusively transduced cells while enriching for proviral integration into active chromatin regions, we have incorporated a cassette expressing CD24 or the green fluorescent protein (GFP). Stable transfer to murine bone marrow cells allowed efficient FACS-sorting of pure populations of transduced cells. A family of vectors based on these principles and containing segments of γ- or δ-globin genes were also designed for systematic analysis of their anti-sickling properties.

Most current strategies for the gene therapy of β-globin gene disorders aim at obtaining stable integration of a normal human β-globin gene or an anti-sickling gene construct in the genome of hematopoietic stem cells (HSCs). Efficient and stable gene transfer into HSCs is a prerequisite for permanent correction of genetic defects, because transient gene transfer or transduction of more differentiated bone marrow cells would provide only temporary symptomatic relief. Appropriate *cis*-acting regulatory elements must be linked to the globin gene construct to achieve erythroid-specific expression of the transferred gene at therapeutic levels. Because bone marrow reconstitution in transplanted recipients

[a]This work was supported by grants from NIH HL48374 and HL55435.
[f]Corresponding Author: Dr. Philippe Leboulch, MIT E25-545, 77 Massachusetts Avenue, Cambridge, MA 02139; Tel: (617) 253-5818; Fax: (617) 253-3459; E-mail: paulvw@mit.edu

is often mono- or oligo-clonal,[1,2] it is also important to 1) maximize the efficiency of HSC transduction, 2) eliminate most non-transduced HSCs from the graft and the recipient, and 3) obtain expression of the transduced gene in erythroid cells relatively independently of chromosomal integration sites (position-independence of expression).

Hence, the ideal gene transfer vector, from the combined standpoints of targeting HSCs and expressing gene constructs suitable for the gene therapy of β-globin gene disorders, should meet the following requirements: 1) fidelity of gene transfer (no rearrangement), 2) high efficiency of stable chromosomal integration in HSCs, 3) control of the number of integrated genetic structures, 4) elimination of non-transduced cells, 5) safety, and 6) compatibility with high, erythroid-specific and position-independent expression of a normal β-globin gene or a potent anti-sickling gene construct, for β-thalassemias or Sickle-Cell disease (SCD), respectively. Based upon their capacity for highly efficient infection and non-toxic and stable integration into the genome of a wide range of cell types, recombinant retroviruses presently represent the most attractive vehicle for exogenous gene transfer into HSCs.[3,4]

Early studies have described the use of retroviral vectors to introduce a human β-globin gene along with its proximal cis-acting elements into murine bone marrow cells.[5-8] In these studies, stable proviral transmission was obtained, and erythroid-specific expression of the transduced β-globin gene was observed in transplanted mice. However, the expression of the human β-globin transgene was low and integration site-dependent (< 1 to 5% of human β-globin/murine $β_{maj}$-globin mRNA ratio).[5-8] In addition, only a few transplanted mice showed sustained production of hematopoietic cells transduced with the human β-globin gene, indicating that infection of long-term repopulating cells had been rarely obtained.[5-8] The discovery of the β-LCR has given new hope to achieving successful gene therapy of human globin disorders by providing a means to obtain high, position-independent expression of the transduced β-globin gene.[9-11] Since the activity of each DNase I hypersensitive (HS) site of the β-LCR has been localized to small DNA fragments,[12-21] it has become possible to construct retroviral vectors transducing β-LCR derivatives linked to the human β-globin gene and its proximal cis-acting elements. Unfortunately, the first attempts by many groups to produce such vectors resulted in low viral titers and very unstable proviral transmission with a high frequency of gross rearrangements.[22-25]

Our studies have first focused on this question of genetic instability of [β-globin/LCR] retroviral vectors by defining determinants of proviral transmission and identifying means to improve stability and viral titer.[26] These optimized vectors have enabled us to analyze the expression properties of various retrovirally transduced β-LCR derivatives in erythroid cells *in vitro*[26] and following bone marrow transplantation in mice.[27] With regard to SCD, we have also designed anti-sickling vectors by introducing, in our [β-globin/LCR] retroviruses, the codons of the δ-globin or the γ-globin gene that encode anti-sickling residues [ref. 28 and unpublished results]. In order to improve gene transfer efficiencies of [β-globin/LCR] retroviral vectors to HSC, we are exploring the use of a small gene cassette encoding the green fluorescence protein (GFP), as a dominant marker for efficient *ex vivo* selection/isolation of transduced HSCs.

PROVIRAL TRANSMISSION AND VIRAL TITERS OF [β-GLOBIN/LCR] RETROVIRAL VECTORS

The general design of our [β-globin/LCR] retroviral vectors, derived from the MoMLV/MoMSV retroviral vector LXSN [29], is represented in FIGURE 2. Details of the construction can be found in Leboulch *et al.*[26] We were constrained to use the β-globin gene instead of its cDNA, since it is well established that introns of the β-globin gene are

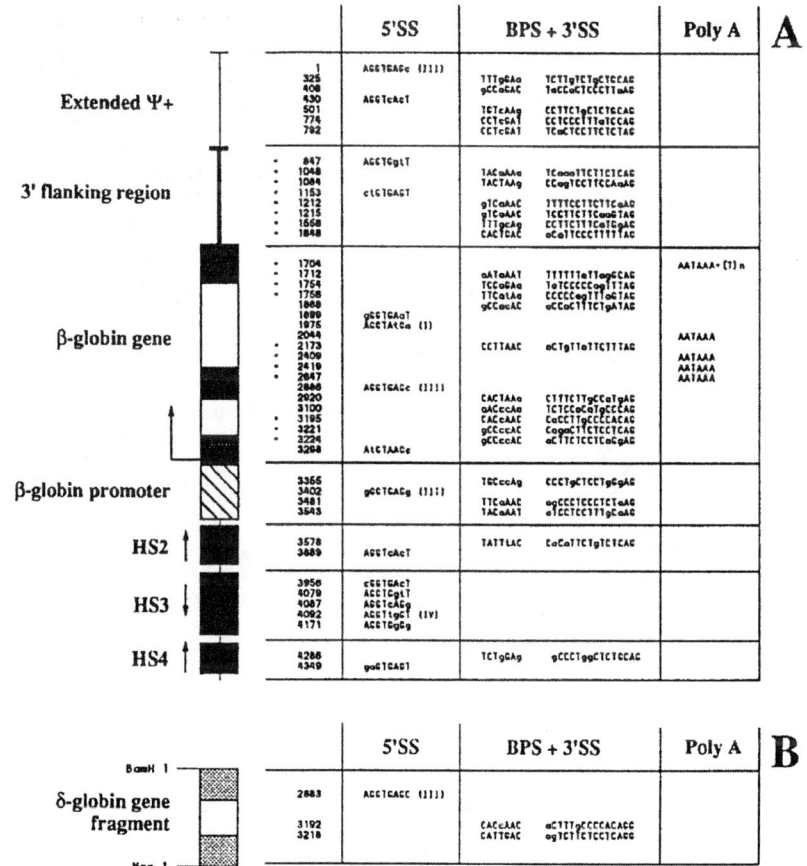

FIGURE 1. DNA sequence analysis in search for structures potentially responsible for instability of proviral transmission. Base 1 starts at the natural 5'SS of MoMSV. Matches or mismatches with 5'SS, 3'SS, BPS and polyA consensus sequences are indicated by capital letters or lowercases, respectively. 5'SS matching one of the five classes are indicated with roman numbers. Regions that we mutated for restoring stability of proviral transmission are indicated by asterisks. (**A**) (β-globin/LCR) retroviral vector (see Leboulch et al. [26]). (**B**) (Nco1-BamH1) DNA fragment from the δ-globin gene present in (β/δ-globin/HS2) retroviral vector, p#147 (see Takekoshi et al. [28]).

indispensable for high-level expression of this gene. The β-globin gene was inserted in reverse orientation with respect to the direction of transcription of the provirus to prevent splicing of the β-globin introns on the viral genomic RNA prior to packaging. Various β-LCR derivatives were inserted immediately upstream of the β-globin promoter. In our initial study, a self-inactivating vector was created by deletion of the viral enhancer in the right LTR, and an internal NeoR cassette was placed under the transcriptional control of several heterologous enhancers/promoters. Packaging cells Ψcre and Ψcrip were used to generate viral producers, as described in Leboulch et al [26]

To examine proviral transmission and to measure viral titers, NIH 3T3 and murine erythroleukemia (MEL) cells were infected by exposure to supernatants of producer cells and were subsequently selected with G418.[26] Proviral transmission was analyzed by Southern blot using NeoR and β-globin specific probes after appropriate restriction digestions of genomic DNA.[26] As observed by others with similar [β-globin/LCR] retroviral vectors, most of our initial vectors appeared very unstable for proviral transmission [26]. In an effort to surmount this major hurdle, we performed a DNA sequence analysis for the presence of structures potentially deleterious (FIG. 1).[26] Genetic instability of retroviruses often occurs by 1) inappropriate splicing or cleavage/polyadenylation of the viral genomic RNA and/or 2) rearrangements during the reverse transcription process (ref. 26; for review, see 30). Inappropriate splicing and polyadenylation of viral genomic RNA are observed relatively rarely when a cDNA is transduced, since intra-exonic polyA or SS are rarely functional. In contrast, non-transcribed genomic structures or inserts placed in complementary/reverse (C/R) orientation may reveal unwanted polyadenylation signals (polyA) or splice-sites (SS). This applies to [β-globin/LCR] retroviral constructs, in which the human β-globin gene is placed in C/R orientation to allow transmission of the full genomic structure. With regard to rearrangements occurring during reverse transcription, they can be triggerred by the presence of repeated sequences or motifs that mimic various cis-acting elements important for the life-cycle of the virus (ref. 26; for review, see 30). Besides isolated sequence motifs, it is believed that arrangements in *cis* of such motifs and modifications of the overall or local three-dimensional structure of an RNA can have a wide range of effects in activating or inactivating these sequence motifs, as observed for splice-site selection (ref. 26; for review, see 30). By screening our constructs for the presence of these deleterious features, we identified an A/T-rich segment in the second intron of the human β-globin gene (βIVS2) and many C/R polyA and SS (FIG. 1).[26] Instead of attempting to change the arrangement of the transduced structures by modifying, for instance, the position of the β-LCR derivatives, we decided to eliminate many of the potentially deleterious sequences by extensive mutagenesis of the transduced β-globin gene.[26] This extensive mutagenesis resulted in stable proviral transmission in infected cell lines and murine bone marrow repopulating cells, with viral titers up to 5×10^5/ml (ecotropic, from Ψcre).[26]

As additional support to our splicing hypothesis, we have now obtained direct physical evidence that splicing of non mutated [β-globin/LCR] viral RNA does operate actively in packaging cells (unpublished results). We have also obtained evidence that low retroviral titers observed with certain inserts can be in part explained by splicing of the packaging signal (Ψ+) or by inefficient nucleo-cytoplasmic export of full-length viral RNA in producer cells (unpublished results). Accordingly, we are now investigating specific complementary strategies to increase viral titers further.

EXPRESSION PROPERTIES OF [β-GLOBIN/LCR] RETROVIRAL VECTORS

These optimized vectors have enabled us to analyze the expression properties of various [β-globin/LCR] retroviral constructs in MEL cells and in mice reconstituted with infected marrow cells (FIG. 2).[26,27] Using our modified β-globin construct under the control of an [HS2 + HS3 + HS4] β-LCR derivative in a mouse transplant model, we demonstrated, for the first time, stable transfer and long-term, high-level expression of a transferred β-globin gene *in vivo*. Three of five mice transplanted with bone marrow cells transduced with high-titer β-globin virus showed the presence of unrearranged β-globin provirus at 4-8 months posttransplant.[27] Moreover, long-term expression of the transferred gene was seen in 2 of these mice at levels of 5% and 20% that of endogenous murine β-globin at 6 and 8 months posttransplantation.[27] Further proof that true long term–repopulating hematopoietic stem cells were transduced with our vector was obtained by the successful transfer and high-

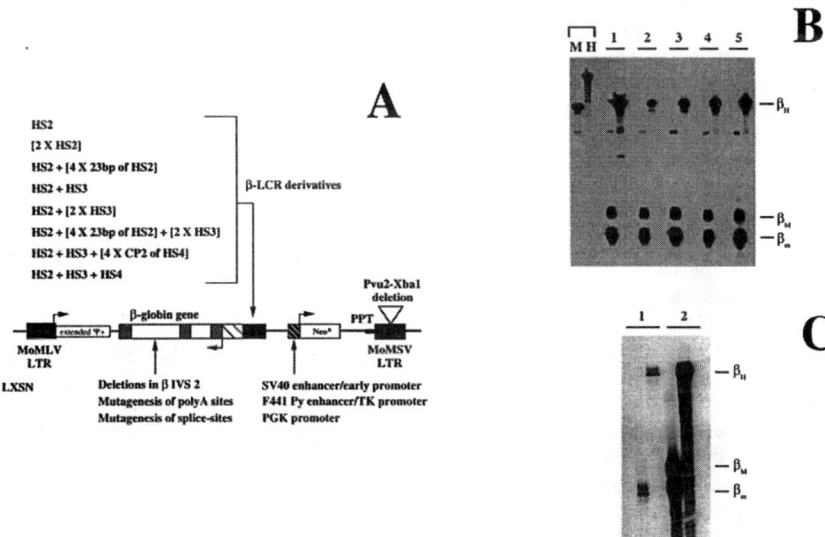

FIGURE 2. (**A**) General design of (β-globin/LCR) retroviral vectors. β-LCR derivatives transduced and internal enhancers/promoters driving NeoR are shown. Structures modified by extensive mutagenesis to obtain stable proviral transmission are also indicated. (**B**) and (**C**) RNA protection assays (see Leboulch et al. [26]). The left and right tracks of each lane contain a murine specific β-globin probe and a human specific β-globin probe, respectively. Positions of specific protected fragments are indicated: human β- ($β_H$), murine $β_{maj}$- ($β_M$), and murine $β_{min}$- ($β_m$). (**B**) Left side, positions of undigested murine (M) and human (H) probes. *Lane 1*, RNA extracted from pool (> 100) of electroporated (average of three copies per cell), G418 selected, and DMSO induced MEL cells, using a non-mutated (β-globin/HS2/PGK) construct. *Lanes 2–5*, RNA extracted from pool (> 100) of infected (one provirus per cell), G418 selected, and DMSO induced MEL cells, using stable, mutagenized (^{mut}) retroviral vectors: 2, (β-globin/HS2/SV40)^{mut}; 3, (β-globin/HS2/PGK)^{mut}; 4, (β-globin/(HS2+HS3+(4xCP2 HS4))/PGK)^{mut}; 5, (β-globin/(HS2+HS3+HS4)/PGK)^{mut}. Comparisons between *Lane 1* (~ 3 copies per cell) and *Lane 3* (one provirus per cell) indicate similar expression levels for the two samples on a per gene basis. *Lanes 2 to 5* show differential expression properties of LCR derivatives in retrovirally transduced and DMSO-induced MEL cells. (**C**) Inducibility of human β-globin mRNA expression upon DMSO induction, as shown in G418 selected MEL cells infected with (β-globin/HS2/F441 Py)^{mut}. *Lane 1*, no induction; *Lane 2*, DMSO-induction for 5 days.

level expression of the human β-globin gene into irradiated secondary recipient mice. Of four secondary recipients generated from the two human β-globin RNA positive primary mice, all were found to be contain the human β-globin gene and be expressing high-levels of human β-globin RNA (3%–12% of endogenous murine β-globin) at 6 weeks posttransplant.[27] The conclusions drawn from these studies can be summarized as follows: 1) the mutated [β-globin/LCR] retroviral vectors are stable, even in the presence of complex β-LCR derivatives, 2) viral titers high enough to achieve gene transfer into bone marrow repopulating cells consistently were obtained (1 x 10^5/ml; ecotropic, from E-86), 3) [HS2 + HS3 + HS4] is the most potent β-LCR derivative in the context of our vectors (80% ratios of human β-globin/murine $β^{maj}$-globin mRNA on a per gene basis in DMSO-induced MEL cells, significant enhancer effect in engrafted mice as described above), followed by HS2 alone (about 75% of the levels obtained with the three sites combined in MEL cells, no data in transplanted mice), 4) no other combination tested of β-LCR derivatives has higher activity than the aforementioned ones; and 5) retroviral LTRs and heterologous enhancers do not appear to interfere with β-globin expression *in vivo*.

To test whether expression of the transduced β-globin gene would be independent from chromosomal integration sites, we studied several independent MEL cell clones that had been infected with [β-LCR/HS2]^{mut}.[26] No G418 selection was applied in order to reduce the risk of selection bias for proviral integration into open chromatin regions, although retroviruses are believed to integrate preferentially into such sites. Complete position-independence was not observed, but the variation appears relatively modest.[26] However, This partial effect contrasts with the complete position-independence originally described[10] or the lack of position-independence reported in another study.[31] The reasons for these discrepancies are still poorly understood. In our *in vivo* studies, the presence of the β-globin LCR elements does not appear to confer site-independent chromosomal integration on the transferred human β-globin gene, as has been reported in transgenic mice.[10] Our results add to recent evidence that the β-LCR functions primarily as a strong erythroid-specific enhancer in retroviral constructs.[31] The properties of "copy number-dependence, position-independence," as originally assigned to LCR function,[10] are best observed in transgenic animal experiments with large genomic fragments integrated as tandem repeats. With single copies of the β-LCR, this position independence of expression is variable.[31] In addition, the μ-LCR components HS 2, 3, and 4 used in our experiments may not be optimal for conferring consistent high-level expression on a single copy retroviral integrant; the β-LCR elements may be more optimal.

We are currently seeking further increase in globin expression at the RNA and protein levels by several means, such as incorporating different LCR elements or the Insulator from the β-globin gene cluster.[32] We are also attempting to duplicate these elements by placing them in the U3 region of the right LTR. Additional optimization of these constructs for viral stability and titers are likely to be necessary.

SELECTION OF TRANSDUCED HEMATOPOIETIC STEM CELLS

A complementary strategy for overcoming current gene transfer limitations is to enrich for transduced cells by use of a dominant selectable marker. Genes that confer resistance to toxic compounds such as G418 or methotrexate have been disappointing, because of difficulties associated with metabolic co-operation, non-specific drug toxicity and/or the extended time in culture required for effective selection (unpublished results). As an alternative strategy, several investigators have developed cDNAs encoding a variety of cell surface antigens, such as the truncated nerve growth factor receptor,[33] CD24 (or the murine homologue HSA),[34-36] Thy-1,[37] CD8,[38] and MDR-1[39] as dominant selectable markers in retroviral vectors. These markers, in combination with fluorescence-activated cell sorting technologies (FACS), enable the identification and enrichment of retrovirally transduced cells containing a transferred gene of interest. This enrichment leads to a significant increase in the proportion of provirally marked cells following transplantation *in vivo*.[40] Unfortunately, the use of functional cell surface proteins as markers of retroviral transduction can cause alterations in the cell phenotype,[39] and may be associated with immunological rejection of transduced cells upon transplantation *in vivo*. More recently, an altered "humanized" version of the green fluorescence protein (GFP) has been developed which enables high-level expression in mammalian cells.[41] The green fluorescence protein represents an ideal marker owing to its neutrality, its intracellular location, and its ease and efficiency of detection. Initial studies in the murine system have documented that high levels of transduced GFP expression can be detected within 24 hours after infection.[42,43]

The small size of the GFP cDNA has made it possible to substitute it for the NeoR gene in our [β-globin/LCR] retroviral vectors (FIG. 3). We took advantage of this construction step to change the configuration of our vectors, by replacing the MoMLV/MoMSV LTRs and packaging signal by those of the Murine Stem Cell Virus (MSCV), which provides high expression levels of transduced cDNAs in HSCs (FIG. 3).[40] In these new vectors, the GFP cDNA is driven by the PGK promoter (FIG. 3). In preliminary experiments, bone marrow cells from day 4 5-FU treated mice infected with β-globin/HS2 virus containing supernatants on fibronectin coated petri dishes showed 30–65% GFP+ cells 48 hours post infection (FIG. 3). Irradiated recipient mice transplanted with non-FACS selected transduced bone marrow cells showed 30% GFP+ peripheral blood cells, determined out to 5 months post transplant (unpublished results). However, mice that received FACS selected GFP+ bone marrow showed nearly 100% repopulation with retrovirally transduced cells. The proportion of GFP+ mononuclear and red blood cells in the peripheral blood of recipient mice at 3 months post transplant was 80–95% and 85–95% respectively (FIG. 4). RT-PCR analysis revealed the presence of human β-globin mRNA in all animals analyzed at 5 months post transplant. Moreover, Southern analysis on bone marrow and spleen DNA showed the presence of full-length, unrearranged provirus demonstrating stable transfer of the human β-globin gene to HSCs (unpublished results).

[β/δ-GLOBIN AND β/γ-GLOBIN] RETROVIRAL VECTORS FOR THE GENE THERAPY OF SICKLE CELL DISEASE

Human γ-globin and δ-globin chains have been previously identified as strong inhibitors of the polymerization of hemoglobin S, as opposed to the β-globin chain which exerts a moderate anti-sickling effect (for review, see ref. 44). However, γ-globin and δ-globin are normally expressed a very low levels in adult erythroid cells, in contrast to β-globin (for review, see ref. 21). We have succeeded in assigning most of the *in vitro* anti-sickling properties of δ and γ chains to residues δ 22Ala and δ 87Gln (with a possible additional contribution of δ 12Asn) (FIG. 5) and γ80Asp and γ87Gln respectively.[45] The study of Lepore

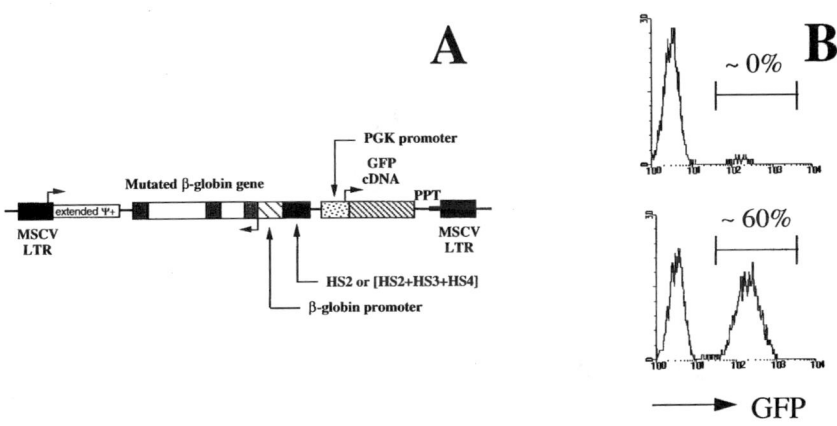

FIGURE 3. (A) Structure of the retroviral vector transducing/expressing GFP and (β-globin/HS2), as described in the text. Note that the neomycin resistance gene (FIG. 2) has been replaced by the GFP cDNA under the control of the PGK promoter. In addition, the LXSN LTRs and extended Ψ+ have been replaced by those of MSCV. (B) Flow cytometric analysis of GFP expression in murine day 4 5-FU bone marrow cells exposed to the [β-globin/HS2/GFP] recombinant retrovirus 48 hours post infection. *Top,* mock infected bone marrow; *Bottom,* p#703 infected bone marrow.

β/δ-hybrid globin genes has also provided insights into the differential expression properties of cis-acting elements proximal to the δ- and β-globin genes: the β-globin promoter and βIVS2 appear critical for high mRNA expression in adult erythroid cells (for review, see ref. 21). Interestingly, δ 22Ala and δ 87Gln are encoded by δ exons I and II.

Therefore, in an effort to obtain an efficient anti-sickling retroviral vector, we have designed two different vectors based upon our modified β-globin gene. The first vector is a chimeric β/δ globin gene, keeping in place the *cis*-acting sequences of the β-globin gene (β-globin promoter, βIVS-2) and β-LCR derivatives, while introducing the anti-sickling amino-acids of the δ-globin (δ22 and δ87) instead of the corresponding amino-acids of the β-globin (FIG. 5).[28] This vector, p#147, was constructed as follows: a 430 bp [Nco1-BamH1] fragment of the human δ-globin gene, which contains the first exon downstream of the initiator "ATG", the first intron and most of the second exon of the δ-globin gene, was used to replace the corresponding fragment of the human β-globin gene in the [β-globin/HS2/PGK]^{mut} retroviral vector (FIG. 5). This substitution introduces all the anti-sickling codons of the β-globin gene. Details of the construction process are described in Takekoshi *et al.*[28] Proviral transmission and expression properties were then tested *in vitro*. We found that our [β/δ-globin/HS2] retroviral vector was stable upon transmission of the proviral structure, gave viral titers up to 5 x 10^5/ml (ecotropic Ψcre), and expressed the anti-sickling β/δ hybrid globin mRNA in adult erythroid cells at levels equivalent to those obtained with the adult β-globin gene expressed from our [β-globin/HS2] retrovirus (FIG. 5).[28] The second vector, p#726, contains our modified β-globin gene in which the amino acid Threonine, normally present at position 87 of β-globin, was replaced with Glutamine, the amino acid responsible for at least part of the anti-sickling activity attributed to γ-globin, using a mutant oligo (unpublished results). This vector is now being tested for its expression and anti-sickling ability *in vivo*. Further evaluation of these vectors in transgenic animal models of SCD should assess their efficacy for the gene therapy of human patients.

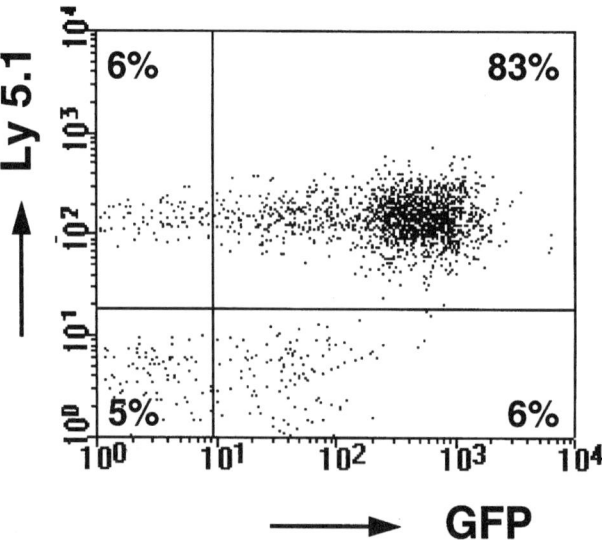

FIGURE 4. Flow cytometric analysis of peripheral blood mononuclear cells after Ficoll gradient, 2.5 months after transplantation of recipient mice with GFP$^+$ FACS selected bone marrow analyzed in FIGURE 3. Donor cell reconstitution was analyzed on the basis of Ly 5.1 expression. Ly 5.1 cells that are GFP$^+$ are probably red blood cells contaminating the lymphocyte preparation and not chimerism.

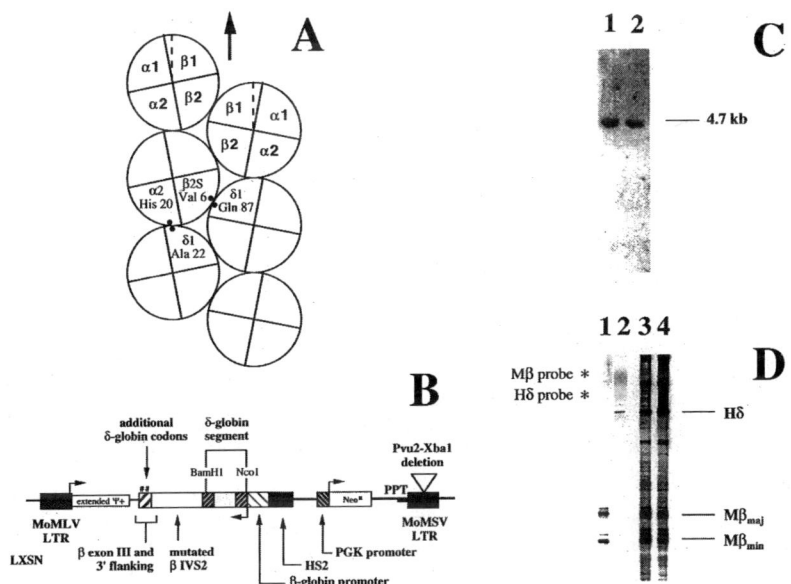

FIGURE 5. (**A**) Model of the structure of the Deoxy Hb S polymer (Wisher-Lowe double-strand) in which the subunits of the hemoglobin tetramer are symbolized by quadrants of a sphere. Putative locations of δ 87Gln and δ 22Ala, expected to impair lateral and axial contacts with $β_2^S$ 6Val and $α_2$ 20His, respectively, are indicated. (**B**) Structure of the (β/δ-globin/HS2) and [β/γ-globin/HS2] retroviral vectors as described in the text. (**C**) Southern blot analysis of proviral transmission of the (β/δ-globin/HS2) retroviral vector. Each lane contains Sac1-digested genomic DNA from a pool of MEL cells infected from a pool of Ψcrip producers. *Lane 1*, infection performed with the (β/δ-globin/HS2) retroviral vector; *Lane 2*, infection performed with the (β-globin/HS2/PGK)^{mut} virus, as size control for stable proviral transmission. (**D**) RNA protection assays. MEL cells were infected with amphotropic (β/δ-globin/HS2) virus obtained from a pool of Ψcrip producers, under conditions providing up to one provirus per cell. Infected MEL cells were subsequently selected with G418 and pooled. Total RNA was extracted from pools (> 100 independent clones) of infected and G418 selected MEL cells, either without induction or following induction with DMSO for 5 days (two independent experiments of DMSO-induction were performed). For each RNA sample from (β/δ-globin/HS2) infected cells, RNA protection assays were performed separately with the same amount of RNA, using a murine $β_{maj}$-globin specific probe or a human δ-globin specific probe. The digested samples were subsequently combined at 1:2 ratio ($β_{maj}$:δ) prior to loading onto a 6% polyacrylamide gel, so that *Lanes 2, 3* and *4* each contains protected bands obtained with both murine $β_{maj}$-globin and human δ-globin probes. Positions of undigested probes are indicated by asterisks. Positions of specific protected fragments are indicated, as follows: Hδ human δ; M$β_{maj}$ murine $β_{maj}$; M$β_{min}$, murine $β_{min}$. *Lanes: 1,* non-infected, DMSO-induced MEL cells, with the murine $β_{maj}$-globin probe alone; *2,* (β/δ-globin/HS2) virus infected, G418 selected, non-induced MEL cell pool; *2 and 3,* (β/δ-globin/HS2) virus infected, G418 selected, DMSO-induced MEL cell pools, corresponding to two independent DMSO inductions. (See Takekoshi *et al.*[28])

CONCLUSION

Human β-thalassemias and SCD are among the first genetic diseases to have been characterized at the molecular level. The β-globin gene cluster is among the first genes to have been cloned and studied, and our knowledge of the genetic regulation of very few genetic loci is as extended as that of the human β-globin gene. Nevertheless, gene therapy of human β-globin gene disorders remains an important challenge. The data presented here indicate that some of the major hurdles in regards to viral titers and stability, β-globin expression and gene transfer effiencies to HSCs can be surmounted. We are currently seeking further improvements in of the design of [β-globin/LCR] retroviral vectors to achieve our goal of high, position-independent expression of a normal β-globin gene or an efficient anti-sickling gene construct in erythroid cells and of obtaining complete and sustained reconstitution of bone marrow with the transduced HSCs in all transplanted recipients.

REFERENCES

1. LEMISCHKA, I. R., D. H. RAULET & R. C. MULLIGAN. 1986. Developmental potential and dynamic behavior of hematopoietic stem cells. Cell **45**: 917–927.
2. TURHAN, A. G., R. K. HUMPHRIES, G. L. PHILLIPS, A. C. EAVES & C. J. EAVES. 1989. Clonal hematopoiesis demonstrated by X-linked DNA polymorphisms after allogeneic bone marrow transplantation. New Engl. J. Med. **320**: 1655–1661.
3. HUGHES, P., J. D. THACKER, D. HOGGE, H. J. SUTHERLAND, T. E. THOMAS, P. M. LANSDORP, C. J. EAVES & R. K. HUMPHRIES. 1992. Retroviral gene transfer to primitive normal and leukemic hematopoietic cells using clinically applicable procedures. J. Clin. Invest. **89**: 1817.
4. SZILVASSY, S. J., C. C. FRASER, C. J. EAVES, P. M. LANSDORP, A. C. EAVES & R. K. HUMPHRIES. 1989. Retrovirus-mediated gene transfer to purified hemopoietic stem cells with long-term lympho-myelopoietic repopulating ability. Proc. Natl. Acad. Sci. USA **86**: 8798–8802.
5. BENDER, M. A., R. E. GELINAS & A. D. MILLER. 1989. A majority of mice show long-term expression of a human β-globin gene after retrovirus transfer into hematopoietic stem cells. Mol. Cell. Biol. **9**: 1426–1434.
6. DZIERZAK, E. A., T. PAPAYANNOPOULOU & R. C. MULLIGAN. 1988. Lineage-specific expression of a human β-globin gene in murine bone marrow transplant recipients reconstituted with retrovirus-transduced stem cells. Nature **331**: 35–41.
7. KARLSSON, S., T. PAPAYANNOPOULOU, S. G. SCHWEIGER, G. STAMATOYANNOPOULOS & A. W. NIENHUIS. 1987. Retroviral-mediated transfer of genomic globin genes leads to regulated production of RNA and protein. Proc. Natl. Acad. Sci. USA **84**: 2411–2415.
8. KARLSSON, S., D. M. BODINE, L. PERRY, T. PAPAYANNOPOULOU & A. W. NIENHUIS. 1988. Expression of the human β-globin gene following retroviral-mediated transfer into multipotential hematopoietic progenitors of mice. Proc. Natl. Acad. Sci. USA **85**: 6062–6066.
9. FORRESTER, W. C., S. TAKEGAWA, T. PAPAYANNOPOULOU, G. STAMATOYANNOPOULOS & M. GROUDINE. 1987. Evidence for a locus activation region: The formation of developmentally stable hypersensitive site in globin-expressing hybrids. Nuc. Acids Res. **15**: 10159–10177.
10. GROSVELD, F., G. B. VAN ASSENDELFT, D. R. GREAVES & G. KOLLIAS. 1987. Position-independent, high-level expression of the human β-globin gene in transgenic mice. Cell **51**: 975–985.
11. TUAN, D., W. SOLOMON, Q. LI & I. M. LONDON. 1985. The "β-like globin" gene domain in human erythroid cells. Proc. Natl. Acad. Sci. USA **82**: 6384–6388.
12. CATERINA, J. J., T. M. RYAN, K. M. PAWLIK, D. E. PALMITTER, R. L. BRINSTER, R. R. BEHRINGER & T. M. TOWNES. 1991. Human β-globin locus control region: Analysis of the 5′ DNase I hypersensitive site HS 2 in transgenic mice. Proc. Natl. Acad. Sci. USA **88**: 1626–1630.
13. COLLIS, P., M. ANTONIOU & F. GROSVELD. 1990. Detailed analysis of the site 2 region of the human β-globin dominant control region. EMBO J. **9**: 233–240.
14. CURTIN, P. T., D. LIU, W. LIU, J. C. CHANG & Y. W. KAN. 1989. Human β-globin gene expression in transgenic mice is enhanced by a distant DNase I hypersensitive site. Proc. Natl. Acad. Sci. USA **86**: 7082–7086.
15. FORRESTER, W. C., U. NOVAK, R. GELINAS & M. GROUDINE. 1989. Molecular analysis of the human β-globin locus activation region. Proc. Natl. Acad. Sci. USA **86**: 5439–5443.
16. PHILIPSEN, S., D. TALBOT, P. FRASER & F. GROSVELD. 1990. The β-globin dominant control region: Hypersensitive site 2. EMBO J. **9**: 2159–2167.
17. PRUZINA, S., O. HANSCOMBE, D. WHYATT, F. GROSVELD & S. PHILIPSEN. 1991. Hypersensitive site 4 of the human β globin locus control region. Nucleic Acids Res. **19**: 1413–1419.

18. RYAN, T. M., R. R. BEHRINGER, N. C. MARTIN, T. M. TOWNES, R. D. PALMITER & R. L. BRINSTER. 1989. A single erythroid-specific DNase I super-hypersensitive site activates high levels of human β-globin gene expression in transgenic mice. Genes & Develop. **3**: 314–323.
19. TALBOT, D., S. PHILIPSEN, P. FRASER & F. GROSVELD. 1990. Detailed analysis of the site 3 region of the human β-globin dominant control region. EMBO J. **9**: 2169–2178.
20. TUAN, D. Y. H., W. B. SOLOMON, I. M. LONDON & D. P. LEE. 1989. an erythroid-specific, developmental-stage-independent enhancer far upstream of the human "β-like globin" genes. Proc. Natl. Acad. Sci. USA **86**: 2554–2558.
21. STAMATOYANNOPOULOS, G. & A. W. NIENHUIS. 1994. Hemoglobin switching. *In* The Molecular Basis of Blood Diseases. G. Stamatoyannopoulos, A. W. Nienhuis, P. W. Majerus & H. Varmus, Eds. 107–155. W. B. Sanders Company. Philadelphia.
22. CHANG, J. C., D. LIU & Y. W. KAN. 1992. A 36-base-pair core sequence of locus control region enhances retrovirally transferred human β-globin expression. Proc. Natl. Acad. Sci. USA **89**: 3107–3110.
23. GELINAS, R., A. FRAZIER & E. HARRIS. 1992. A normal level of β-globin expression in erythroid cells after retroviral cells transfer. Bone Marrow Transpl. **9(Supp.1)**: 154–157.
24. NOVAK, U., E. A. S. HARRIS, W. FORRESTER, M. GROUDINE & R. GELINAS. 1990. High-level β-globin expression after retroviral transfer of locus activation region-containing human β-globin gene derivatives into murine erythroleukemia cells. Proc. Natl. Acad. Sci. USA **87**: 3386–3390.
25. PLAVEC, I., T. PAPAYANNOPOULOU, C. MAURY & F. MEYER. 1993. A human β-globin gene fused to the human β-globin locus control region is expressed at high levels in erythroid cells of mice engrafted with retrovirus-transduced hematopoietic stem cells. Blood **81**: 1384–1392.
26. LEBOULCH, P., G. M. S. HUANG, R. K. HUMPHRIES, Y. H. OH, C. J. EAVES, D. H. Y. TUAN & I. M. LONDON. 1994. Mutagenesis of retroviral vectors transducing human β-globin gene and β-globin locus control region derivatives results in stable transmission of an active transcriptional structure. EMBO J. **13**: 3065–3076.
27. RAFTOPOULOS, H., M. WARD, P. LEBOULCH & A. BANK. 1997. Long-term transfer and expression of the human β-globin gene in a mouse transplant model. Blood **90**: 3414–3422.
28. TAKEKOSHI, K. J., Y. H. OH, K. W. WESTERMAN, I. M. LONDON & P. LEBOULCH. 1995. Retroviral transfer of a human δ-globin / β-globin hybrid gene linked to β locus control region hypersensitive site 2 aimed at the gene therapy of Sickle Cell disease. Proc. Natl. Acad. Sci. USA **92**: 3014–3018.
29. MILLER, A. D. & G. J. ROSMAN. 1989. improved retroviral vectors for gene transfer and expression. BioTechniques **7**: 980–990.
30. COFFIN, J. M. 1991. Retroviridae and their replication. *In* Fundamental Virology. B. N. Fields & D. M. Knipe, Eds.: 645–708. Raven Press. New York.
31. SADELAIN M., C. H. WANG, M. ANTONIOU, F. GROSVELD & R. C. MULLIGAN. 1995. Generation of a high-titer retroviral vector capable of expressing high levels of the human beta-globin gene. Proc. Natl. Acad. Sci. USA **92**: 6728–1995.
32. CHUNG, J. H., M. WHITELEY & G. FELSENFELD. 1993. A 5' element of the chicken β-globin domain serves as an insulator in human erythroid cells and protects against position effect in Drosophila. Cell **74**: 505–514.
33. MAVILIO, F., G. FERRARI, S. ROSSINI, N. NOBILI, C. BONINI, G. CASORATI, C. TRAVERSARI & C. BORDIGNON. 1994 Peripheral blood lymphocytes as target cells of retroviral vector-mediated gene transfer. Blood **83**: 1988–1997.
34. CONNEALLY, E., P. BARDY, S. CHAPPEL, C. J. EAVES & R. K. HUMPHRIES. 1994. Expression of murine heat stable antigen (HSA) on human hematopoietic cells as a marker of retroviral infection. Blood **84**: 4140.
35. MIGITA, M., J. A MEDIN, R. PAWLIUK, S. JACOBSON, J. W. NAGLE, S. ANDERSON, M. AMIRI, R. K. HUMPHRIES & S. KARLSSON. 1995. Selection of transduced CD34+ progenitors ande enzymatic correction of cells from Gaucher patients, with bicistronic vectors. Proc. Natl. Acad. Sci. USA **92**: 12075–12079.
36. PAWLIUK, R., R. KAY, P. LANSDORP & R. K. HUMPHRIES. 1994. Selection of retrovirally transduced hematopoietic cells using CD24 as a marker of gene transfer. Blood **84**: 2868–2877.

37. PLANELLES, V., A. HAISLIP, E. S. WITHERS-WARD, S. A., STEWART, Y. XIE, N. P. SHAH & I. S. CHEN. 1991. A new reporter system for detection of retroviral infection. Gene Therapy **2:** 369–376.
38. HOLLANDER, G. A., B. D. LUSKEY, D. A. WILLIAMS & S. J. BURAKOFF. 1992. Functional expression of human CD8 in fully reconstituted mice after retroviral-mediated gene transfer of hemopoietic stem cells. J. Immunol. **149:** 438–444.
39. RICHARDSON, C. & A. BANK. 1995. Preselection of transduced murine hematopoietic stem cells populations leads to increased long-term stability and expression of the human multiple drug resistance gene. Blood **86:** 2579–2589.
40. PAWLIUK, R., C. J. EAVES & R. K. HUMPHRIES. 1997. Sustained high-level reconstitution of the hematopoietic system by preselected hematopoietic cells expressing a transduced cell-surface antigen. Hum. Gene Ther. **8:** 1595–1604.
41. ZOLOTUKHIN, S., M. POTTER, W. W. HAUSWIRTH, J. GUY & N. MUZYCZKA. 1996. A "humanized" green fluorescent protein cDNA adapted for high-level expression in mammalian cells. J. Virol. **70:** 4646–4654.
42. PERSONS, D. A., J. A. ALLAY, E. R. ALLAY, R. J. SMEYNE, R. A. ASHMUN, B. P. SORRENTINO & A. W. NIENHUIS. 1997. Retroviral-mediated transfer of the green fluorescent protein gene into murine hematopoietic cells facilitates scoring and selection of transduced progenitors in vitro and identification of genetically modified cells in vivo. Blood **90:** 1777–1786.
43. BIERHUIZEN, M. F. A., Y. WESTERMAN, T. P. VISSER, W. DIMJATI, A. W. WOGNUM & G. WAGEMAKER. 1997. Enhanced green fluorescent protein as selectable marker in retroviral mediated gene transfer in immature hematopoietic bone marrow cells. Blood **90:** 3304–3315.
44. BUNN, H. F. & B. G. FORGET. 1986. Hemoglobin: Molecular, Genetic and Clinical Aspects. W. B. Saunders Company. Philadelphia.
45. NAGEL, R. L., R. M. BOOKCHIN, J. FOHNSON, D. LABIE, H. WAJCMAN, W. A. ISAAC-SODEYRE, G. R. HONIG, G. SCHILIRO, J. H. CROOKSTON & K. MATSUTUMO. 1979. Structural bases of the inhibitory effects of hemoglobin F and hemoglobin A2 on the polymerization of hemoglobin S. Proc. Natl. Acad. Sci. USA **76:** 670.

Targeted Integration of a Recombinant Globin Gene Adeno-Associated Viral Vector into Human Chromosome 19[a]

JOAN BERTRAN, YANPING YANG, PHILLIP HARGROVE, ELIO F. VANIN, AND ARTHUR W. NIENHUIS[b]

Division of Experimental Hematology, Department of Hematology/Oncology, St. Jude Children's Research Hospital, Memphis, Tennessee 38105, USA

ABSTRACT: Transfer of a globin gene into stem cells along with the regulatory elements required to achieve high level expression in maturing erythroid cells would provide effective gene therapy for Cooley's Anemia. We have explored the use of recombinant adeno-associated viral (rAAV) vectors for this purpose. A vector designated rHS32$^A\gamma$3'RE that contains regulatory elements from the locus control and flanking regions, integrates as a stable head-to-tail concatamer in erythroleukemia cells at a high multiplicity of infection and exhibits high level, regulated γ globin gene expression. Inducible expression of the non-structural Rep proteins of wild-type AAV in HeLa cells transduced with rAAV vectors does not increase overall integration frequency, but targeted integration of rHS32$^A\gamma$3'RE into human chromosome 19 was documented.

Development of gene therapy for severe β-thalassemia will require methodology for inserting a globin gene into repopulating hematopoietic stem cells and achieving its expression in differentiating erythroid cells. Substantial efforts have been invested in the development of retroviral vectors based on murine leukemia virus for this purpose, but the relative inefficiency of gene transfer by such vectors into stem cells[1–4] and the instability of vector genomes containing regulatory elements from the locus control region[5–7] have prevented the successful application of this approach for human gene therapy of Cooley's Anemia. We have explored the use of an alternative vector system based on adeno-associated virus (AAV) for therapeutic globin gene transfer.[8–11]

AAV is a single stranded DNA virus with a genome of 4675 nucleotides that includes 145 nucleotide inverted terminal repeats (ITRs) and the coding sequences for non-structural (Rep) and structural (Cap) proteins.[12,13] During latent infection, many but not all genome integration events occur within a preferred site (AAVS1) on human chromosome 19.[14,15] Site-specific integration is mediated by DNA sequence specific interactions of the higher molecular weight Rep protein species, (p78 and p68) with sequences in the AAV ITRs and the host cell AAV integration site.[16–19]

---

[a]This work was supported in part by Cancer Center Support Grant P30CA 21765, NHBLI Program Project Grant P01HL 53749-02, the ASSISI Foundation of Memphis and by the American Lebanese Syrian Associated Charities (ALSAC).

[b]Corresponding Author: Arthur W. Nienhuis, MD, Director, St. Jude Children's Research Hospital, 332 N. Lauderdale, Memphis, Tennessee 38105; Tel: (901) 495-3301; Fax (901) 525-2720.

The ITRs are the only *cis*-active elements required for rAAV genome replication and encapsidation.[20,21] During production of rAAV, Rep and Cap genes are provided in trans, usually by a plasmid which includes the wild-type AAV genome that lacks ITRs.[13,20,22–24] Because site specific integration of the AAV genome depends on Rep functions, rAAV vectors without the Rep gene integrate randomly.[8,14]

AAV vectors have several potential advantages for gene therapy applications. Although 80% of humans have detectable serum antibodies, no disease has been associated with this virus.[12,13] AAV particles are relatively stable permitting their purification and concentration by physical techniques. Both the wild-type virus and rAAV vectors have a broad host range.[12,22,23] Indeed prolonged rAAV-mediated gene expression has been observed in brain and muscle following local injection and in the liver following intravenous administration of vector particles.[25–29]

Development of rAAV vectors for therapeutic applications has been limited by relatively inefficient, cumbersome methodology for vector preparation that includes infection of HeLa cells or human kidney cells with adenovirus and co-transfection with a vector plasmid containing one or more transcriptional units flanked by AAV ITRs and a helper genome consisting of the AAV Rep and Cap genes without AAV ITRs.[13,20,22–24] This limitation may be overcome by the recent development of strategies for deriving packaging cell lines and the identification and characterization of useful producer clones for rAAV.[30–32]

Our work has focused on the development of the rAAV vectors for transfer and expression of globin genes in erythroid cells.[8–11] Such vectors transfer, integrate and express globin genes in erythroleukemia cells when linked to a drug selection marker that facilitates recovery of clonal cell lines.[8,9] Furthermore, rAAV mediated expression of a globin gene has been documented in human progenitor derived, hematopoietic colonies although genome integration could not be evaluated.[10] More recent experiments have shown that an unselected rAAV genome containing a globin gene and linked regulatory elements will integrate and express a globin gene at high levels in erythroleukemia cells.[11] The vector studied, rHS32$^A\gamma^*$3'RE, contains hypersensitive sites (HS) 2 and 3 from the 5' locus control region, a regulatory element normally located just downstream from the $^A\gamma$ globin gene (3'RE) and a γ globin gene that had been mutationally marked ($^A\gamma^*$) to allow its transcript to be distinguished from those of the normal endogenous globin genes. The vector integrated as an intact, tandem head-to-tail concatamer with a median copy number of 6 and a globin gene expression level of 1–3 fold that of an endogenous globin gene. Consistent transduction and integration required a very high multiplicity of infection (MOI).

As detailed above, the non-structural Rep proteins of AAV mediate site specific integration into chromosome 19. We have designed experiments to determine whether Rep expression enhances integration frequency and whether its ability to facilitate site specific integration can be used to target a rAAV globin gene vector to chromosome 19.

MATERIALS AND METHODS

Cells and Plasmids

The following cell lines were used in these experiments: HtTA-22-a HeLa derived cell line which constitutively expresses the tet^R/VP16 transactivator (tTA),[33] Cos7 cells which constitutively express the SV40 T-antigen (American Tissue Culture Collection, Rockville, MD), and HAP7 cells—a rAAV packaging cell line which inducibly expresses the AAV Rep and capsid proteins upon infection with adenovirus.[32] These cell lines were maintained in Dulbecco's Modified Eagles Medium (DMEM) containing 10% fetal calf serum (FCS) and penicillin and streptomycin at standard concentrations.

The following plasmids were used in these studies: 1) *pAAV-EcoRec-DHFR:* This plasmid contains an expression cassette for the ecotropic retroviral receptor and a second expression cassette for a mutationally modified version of human dihydrofolate reductase (DHFR),[33] 2) *pAAV-Rep-NGFR*: This plasmid contains two expression cassettes, one having the Rep coding region from the AAV genome[20,24] under the control of a tetracycline modulated promoter[34] and a second expression cassette containing the coding sequences for the nerve growth factor receptor (NGFR) external and transmembrane domains.[35,36] The Rep fragment in this plasmid is a 2.1kb Alw26I-SacII fragment derived from pSUB201[20,24] and juxtaposed to the specified promoter and polyadenylation sites during a series of intermediate subcloning steps prior to insertion into a plasmid containing the AAV ITRs derived from pSUB201[20] using standard techniques.[37] The NGFR fragment was obtained by interrupting the coding sequences with PvuII digestion[35] and reconstruction of a termination codon flanked by convenient restriction sites using synthetic oligonucleotides. Again, this fragment was subcloned in a series of intermediate steps to juxtapose it to the SV40 promoter and polyadenylation sequences prior to insertion of the entire cassette into the pSUB201 derivative plasmid containing the Rep expression cassette, 3) *pHS32$^A\gamma$3'RE:* This plasmid contains the human $^A\gamma$ globin gene which has been mutationally marked to allow its transcript to be distinguished from that of the wild type gene, linked to the regulatory elements from the locus control region (HS2 and HS3) and a regulatory element (3'RE) located downstream of the chromosomal $^A\gamma$ globin gene,[11] and 4) *pSV40oriAAV:* This plasmid contains a SV40 origin of replication and a 4.5kb BalI fragment of the AAV genome containing the Rep and Cap genes without intact AAV inverted terminal repeats.[36]

Preparation of rAAV Particles

To produce rAAV, we used a previously published strategy[38] as modified in our laboratory which involves co-electroporating pSV40ori AAV and the relevant rAAV vector plasmid into Cos7 cells followed by infection with adenovirus (MOI = 10). The method for recovering rAAV particles was exactly as described[38] except that the trypsin digestion step was eliminated and two rather than three sequential isopycnic gradient centrifugations were performed.[33] In some cases, rAAV-EcoRec-DHFR was generated from a stable producer clone upon infection with adenovirus[32] and purified as described above. HS32$^A\gamma$3'RE, a rAAV containing a human globin gene and regulatory elements from the human β-globin gene cluster,[11] was prepared from a stable producer clone.[32] To prepare rAAV, helper adenovirus was used at a sufficient multiplicity of infection (MOI) to induce a marked cytopathic effect in all cells within 48 hours (approximate MOI of 5). All vector preparations were heat inactivated to destroy adenovirus by incubation at 56°C for 1 hour.

Titering of rAAV and Detection of Wild-type AAV

Each preparation was evaluated to estimate the concentration of physical particles (particle titer)[33] and infectious particles (infectious titer). The infectious titer of each rAAV preparation was determined as described[30] except that a rAAV packaging cell line (HAP7) developed in our laboratory[32] was utilized. Serial dilutions of rAAV were used to infect 1×10^5 HAP7 cells in a 1cm well (24 well plate) along with wild-type adenovirus (MOI 1-5). Sixty hours later, low molecular weight DNA was purified by the Hirt technique[39] and analyzed by Southern blot analysis[37] to detect the rAAV or wild-type AAV genome.

Adenovirus-5 was obtained from Advanced Biotechnologies, Inc. (Columbia, MD). The virus was amplified in 293 cells and purified by CsCl step and isopycnic gradient centrifugation according to standard protocols.[40] Viral titers were determined by plaque assay on 293 cells. The preparations of adenovirus used in these studies were screened for wild-type AAV contamination both by PCR analysis using primers specific for a segment of the capsid gene to amplify DNA prepared by standard techniques and by the infectious center assay as described above.

Transduction with rAAV

The protocol utilized was as previously described[33] except that periodic (every 15 minute) manual agitation was performed rather than mechanical rocking during the two hours of exposure of the target cells to rAAV in serum free medium. The MOIs specified in these experiments were based on particle titers.

DNA and Protein Analysis

Isolation of genomic[37] and low molecular weight DNA[39] was performed using standard protocols. The probes used in these analysis were as follows: a 476 base pair (bp) PstI-HpaI fragment for ecotropic receptor coding sequences[33] a 180bp PstI-BamHI fragment for detection of the AAVSI integration fragment,[15,17] a 900bp RsaII-HindIII fragment comprised of NGFR coding sequences derived from pAAV-Rep-NGFR and a 500bp HincII-SnaBI fragment containing AAV Cap coding sequences.[20] Probes were labeled by random priming with an oligo labelling kit (Pharmacia) following the manufacturer's instructions. Southern blot analysis was performed using standard methods. Protein extraction was performed by lysis of cells in a buffer containing SDS as described.[32] Western blot analysis was preformed using a monoclonal antibody (294.4) specific for the Rep proteins,[41] kindly provided by Jürgen Kleinschmidt.

FACS Analysis

Detection of expression of the ecotropic receptor (EcoRec) or nerve growth factor receptor (NGFR) utilized specific monoclonal antibodies and methodologies as previously described.[33,42]

Fluorescent in Situ *Hybridization (FISH)*

Colcemid-arrested HtTA22 cell clones containing an integrated vector genome were used as a source of metaphase chromosomes. Recombinant plasmid DNA (pAAV-EcoRec-DHFR or pHS32$^A\gamma$3′RE) was nick translated with digoxigenin-11-UTP and hybridized overnight at 37°C to fixed metaphase chromosomes with the inclusion of 0.5 mg/ml of Cot1 competitor DNA (Life Technologies, Gaithersburg, Maryland) according to previously described methods.[11,43] For the chromosome 19p specific probe, E2a cosmid DNA[43] was nick translated with biotin-16-dUTP. Signals were detected by incubating the slides with fluorescein-conjugated sheep antibodies to digoxigenin (Boehringer Mannheim) and Texas Red Avidin (Vector Laboratories, Burlington, CA). To counterstain, 4,6-diamidino-2-phenylindole (DAPI) was used. Individual fluorescein, Texas Red and DAPI labeled signals were collected with a Nikon epifluorescence microscope coupled to a CCD camera and merged using CytoVision software (Applied Imaging, Pittsburgh, Pennsylvania).

RESULTS

Transduction of Erythroleukemia Cells with rHS32$^A\gamma^*$3'RE

Transduction of the majority of erythroleukemia cells required a MOI of up to 10^8 (FIG. 1). Clones recovered after transduction at this MOI uniformly contained the $^A\gamma^*$ mRNA after 18 days of proliferation.[11] However, after continued passage for 6–8 weeks, only about 50% of the clones which expressed the $^A\gamma^*$ gene initially were found to have integrated the rHS32$^A\gamma^*$3'RE genome. Only at a MOI of 10^9 was integration consistently achieved (FIG. 1). In virtually all cases, the rHS32$^A\gamma^*$3'RE genome had integrated as a head-to-tail tandem concatamer.[11] These results prompted us to explore the ability of the AAV Rep protein to increase the frequency of rAAV genome integration and to target its integration to human chromosome 19.

Inducible Expression of the AAV Rep Proteins

rAAV-Rep-NGFR (FIG. 2) vector particles were used to transduce HtTA-22 cells at varying multiplicities of infection (MOI). These cells constitutively express the tet^R/VP16 chimeric transactivator. In the absence of tetracycline, Rep expression increased as a function of MOI. Tetracycline inhibited Rep expression in a concentration dependent manner (FIG. 2). These experiments established that the rAAV-Rep-NGFR vector could be used to obtain conditional expression of Rep in HtTA-22 cells.

rHS32$^A\gamma^*$ 3'RE

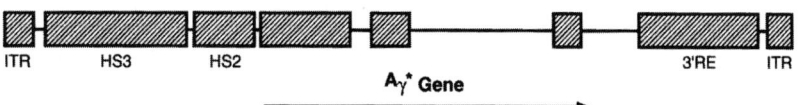

MOI	Expression mRNA-(RT-PCR) Day 18*	Integration - (Southern Blot)		
		Integrated*	Unrearranged*	Tandem Copies°°
4×10^8	10/10	8/18	8/8	6/8
4×10^9	10/10	23/24	23/23	22/23

FIGURE 1. Transduction of human erythroleukemia cells with rHS32$^A\gamma^*$3'RE. K562 erythroleukemia cells were transduced at the specified multiplicities of infection (MOI) as previously described.[11] After 24 hours cells were plated in semi-solid culture medium. Individual clones were plucked after 14 days and expanded for 3 days to provide cells for RNA extraction and for 2–4 weeks to provide cells for DNA analysis. (*) = ratio of positive clones to the total number analyzed. (oo) = proportion of clones in which the integrated, intact genome was in a tandem array of multiple head-to-tail copies. Abbreviations are as follows: HS = hypersensitive site, ITR = inverted terminal repeat and RE = regulatory element.

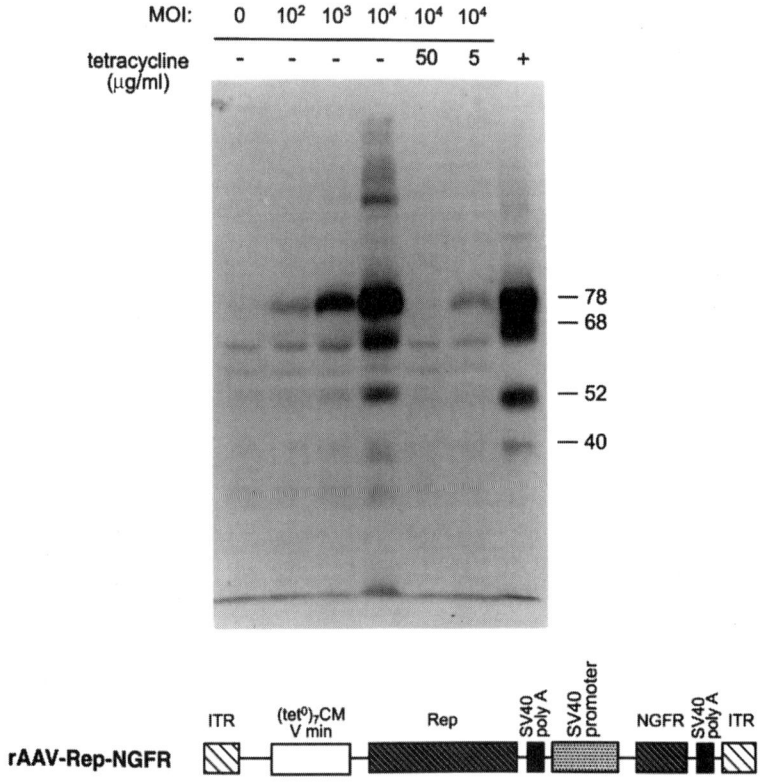

FIGURE 2. Inducible expression of the AAV Rep proteins. HtTA 22 cells were transduced with rAAV-Rep-NGFR at the specified multiplicities of infection (MOI) and cultured for 60 hours in the absence (−) or presence of tetracycline at the specified concentrations. Western blot analysis was performed on cellular extracts corresponding to 2×10^5 cells using the monoclonal anti-Rep antibody, 294.4.[40] For the positive control (+), HtTA-22 cells (10^7) were transfected with 20 μg of pAAV/Ad and infected with adenovirus (MOI = 5), an extract was prepared 48 hours later and an amount corresponding to 2×10^5 cells was loaded. The organization of the rAAV-Rep-NGFR genome is shown below. Abbreviations are as follows: ITR-inverted terminal repeats of the AAV genome; $(tet^O)_7CMV$-a minimal promoter element derived from the CMV genome flanked by a concatamer of seven binding sites for the prokaryotic tetracycline modulated repressor;[34] Rep-a fragment from the AAV genome containing the coding sequences for the replication proteins (p78, p68, p52 and p40); SV40 polyA-a fragment from Simian virus 40 genome containing polyadenylation sequences; SV40 promoter-a fragment from Simian virus 40 genome containing the early region promoter sequences; and NGFR- the coding sequences for the external and transmembrane domains of the nerve growth factor receptor.[36]

The Effect of Rep Expression on the Frequency of rAAV Integration

Our experimental design called for sequential transduction of a "reporter genome," in this case rAAV-EcoRec-DHFR, at a substantially higher MOI than the rAAV-Rep-NGFR vector in an effort to achieve preferential integration of the reporter vector genome (FIG. 3). rAAV mediated expression of the ecotropic retroviral receptor provides a surface displayed reporter gene product which is readily detected and quantified by

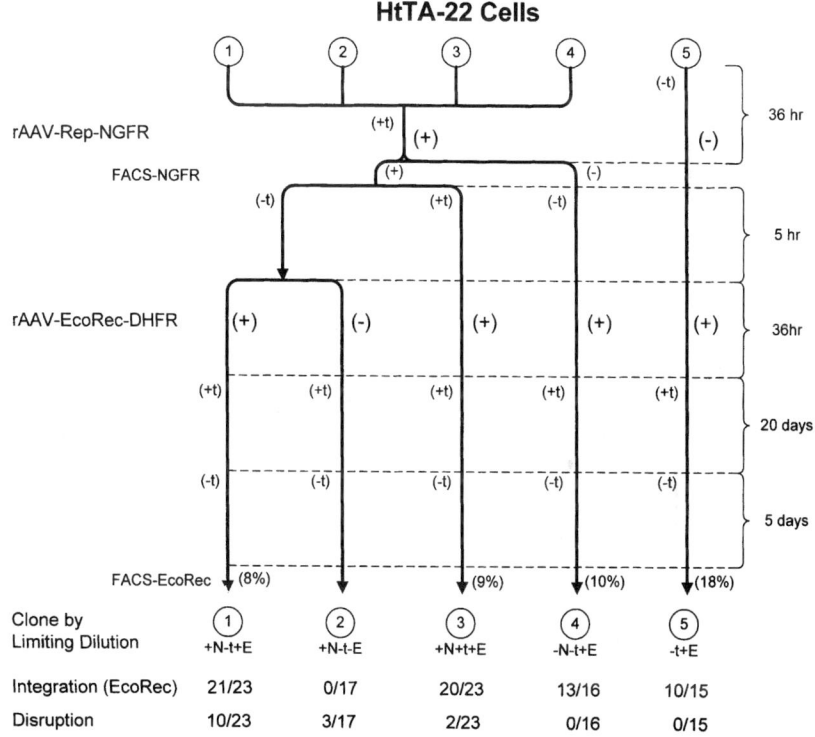

FIGURE 3. Experimental design to evaluate the influence of Rep expression from the rAAV-Rep-NGFR genome on integration of a "reporter" genome, rAAV-EcoRec-DHFR. Clones were isolated from 5 aliquots of HtTA-22 cells to evaluate integration of the rAAV-EcoRec-DHFR genome: 1) +N-t+E - Experimental cells which had been exposed to the rAAV-Rep-NGFR virus (+N), sorted to recover NGFR expressing cells, incubated in the absence of tetracycline (-t) to allow expression of the Rep protein and then exposed to rAAV-EcoRec-DHFR (MOI = 10^6); 2) +N-t-E - control cells processed identically to 1 except that exposure to rAAV-EcoRec-DHFR was omitted; 3) +N+t+E-control cells processed identical to 1 except that tetracycline was present prior to, and during transduction with rAAV-EcoRec-DHFR to suppress expression of the Rep gene; 4) -N-t+E-control cells recovered by FACS which lacked NGFR expression; and 5) -t+E - control cells which were not exposed to rAAV-Rep-NGFR virus provided another negative control for Rep expression. The experiment was initiated by exposing 10^6 HtTA-22 cells to rAAV-Rep-NGFR (MOI = 10^3) and then culturing these cells for 36 hours in the presence of tetracycline. At that time, FACS was performed to recover populations of NGFR positive and negative cells; 2×10^3 cells were processed to generate aliquots 1, 2, 3 and 4 as indicated. Separate aliquots (8×10^3) of sorted NGFR (+), incubated with or without tetracycline, or (-) cells were cultured for approximately 40 hours and then processed for Western blot analysis to evaluate Rep protein expression. Each of the five aliquots were cultured for 20 days in the presence of tetracycline and then for 5 days in medium lacking tetracycline to allow expression of the ecotropic receptor. FACS was performed to recover cells expressing EcoRec and these were plated at limiting dilution. At the appropriate time, individual clones were plucked and expanded to derive DNA for analysis of rAAV-EcoRec-DHFR integration, disruption of the AAVS1 locus on chromosome 19 and for the presence of co-migrating bands that hybridized to both the EcoRec and AAVS1 probes.

FACS. HtTA cells were initially transduced with rAAV-Rep-NGFR at an MOI of 10^3 and NGFR positive and negative cells were isolated. Tetracycline was then removed from the culture medium of the appropriate aliquots of cells after which the experimental and control aliquots were transduced with rAAV-EcoRec-DHFR at an MOI of 10^6. At this MOI, we anticipate that 100% of the HtTA-22 cells will be transduced by the rAAV-EcoRec-DHFR vector.[33] This experimental design had the advantage of validating transduction by rAAV-Rep-NGFR by virtue of NGFR expression, of allowing Rep expression to occur before the reporter vector was added and of achieving a ratio of reporter to Rep expressing vector particles of 10^3. The design was validated by demonstrating the presence of Rep expression in NGFR positive cells that were incubated without tetracycline and the absence of Rep proteins in the NGFR negative subset (data not shown). The vector preparations used in these experiments were free of detectable wild-type AAV as determined by both the particle and infectious center assays.

We found no influence of Rep expression on the proportion of cells expressing ecotropic receptor at three weeks; values ranged from 8–18% (FIG. 3). Fifteen to 23 clones were isolated by limiting dilution from each arm of the experiment; 90% of these were shown to contain the ecotropic receptor vector genome by Southern blot analysis. Rep expression did not appear to increase the copy number of the rAAV-EcoRec-DHFR genome as determined by comparing the signal intensities of the bands derived from the integrated rAAV-EcoRec-DHFR genome by phosphoimaging (data not shown).

Rep-Mediated Disruption of the Preferred Integration Site (AAVS1) on Chromosome 19

Several of the clones isolated from cells transduced with rAAV-EcoRec-DHFR in the presence of Rep expression (FIG. 3: Aliquot 1 +N-t+E) exhibited disruption of the AAVS1 site on chromosome 19 (FIG. 4). In the absence of Rep expression because tetracycline was added to the culture (FIG. 3: Aliquot 3 +N+t+E), because NGFR negative cells had been selected (FIG. 3: Aliquot 4 -N-t+E) or because rAAV-Rep-NGFR transduction was omitted (FIG. 2: Aliquot 5 -t+E), a lower frequency of disruption of the AAVS1 site was observed. Disruption of the AAVS1 site was also partially dependent on transduction with rAAV-EcoRec-DHFR; cells exposed only to rAAV-Rep-NGFR (FIG. 3: Aliquot 2 +N-t-E), showed a lower frequency of disruption of the AAVS1 integration site.

Rep-mediated Integration of a rAAV Genome into the AAVS1 Site on Chromosome 19

Southern blot analysis was performed on DNA restricted with an appropriate enzyme (NheI) to allow detection of a common band which, if present, hybridized to both AAVS1 and vector sequences (data not shown). A common migrating band was detected in 3 of 10 clones but each of these clones also contained other fragments which hybridized only to the vector probe suggesting multiple integration sites, only one of which was in chromosome 19. FISH analysis was used in an effort to confirm chromosome 19 integration site in several of the clones. Difficulties were encountered in these experiments in that rAAV-EcoRec-DHFR had integrated at multiple locations in the genome, as suggested by Southern blot analysis, usually as a single copy. Only in two clones were we able to confirm chromosome 19 specific integration by FISH analysis.

A second experiment was performed in which the HtTA cells were simultaneously transduced with rAAV-Rep-NGFR (MOI=10^4) and rAAV-EcoRec-DHFR (MOI=10^6) and similar results were obtained. Sixteen of 23 clones isolated from the population express-

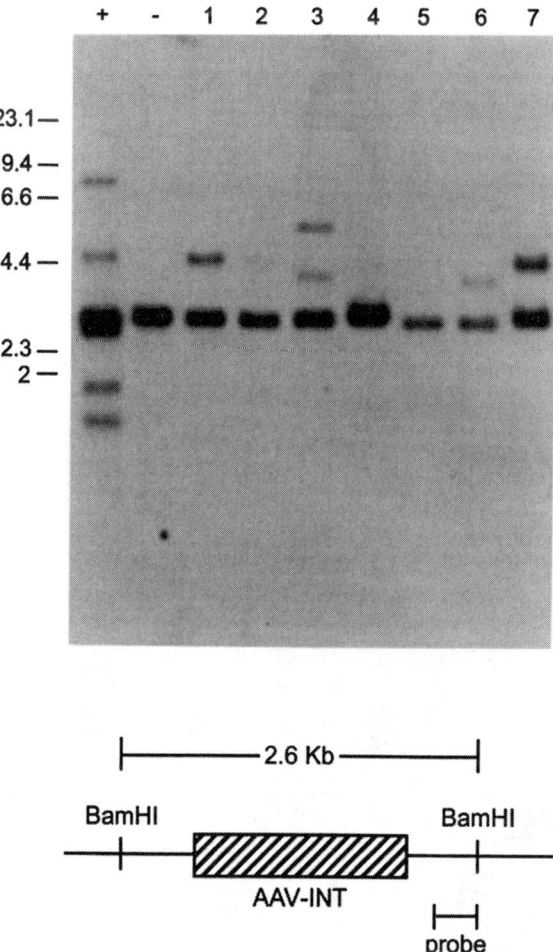

FIGURE 4. Disruption of the AAVS1 site on chromosome 19. DNAs isolated from seven individual clones that had been exposed to rAAV-Rep-NGFR, sorted to recover NGFR positive cells, cultured in the absence of tetracycline to allow Rep expression and exposed to rAAV-EcoRec-DHFR (MOI = 10^6) (FIG. 3: aliquot 1 +N-t+E) were analyzed by Southern blot analysis. The probe used flanked the preferred AAV integration site on chromosome 19. The negative control lane contains DNA derived from HtTA-22 cells whereas the positive control lane contains DNA derived from a mixed population of cells exposed to both rAAV-Rep-NGFR and rAAV-EcoRec-DHFR in a previous experiment.

ing Rep exhibited AAVS1 disruption, but integration of the rAAV-EcoRec-DHFR genome at this site was documented by co-migration or by FISH analysis in a minority of these clones. Furthermore, vector integration at other positions in these clones was also observed (data not shown).

A
23.1
9.4
6.6
4.4
2.3
2.0
2
1
ITR
rHS32^Aγ*3'RE
E
E
ITR
Probe
E
E
AAV-INT
Probe
ER'3*γ^A23SHr
E
E E
E E
E E
E
ITR
AAV-INT
γ Probe
ITR(s)
γ Probe
ITR(s)
γ Probe
ITR
AAVS1 Probe
B

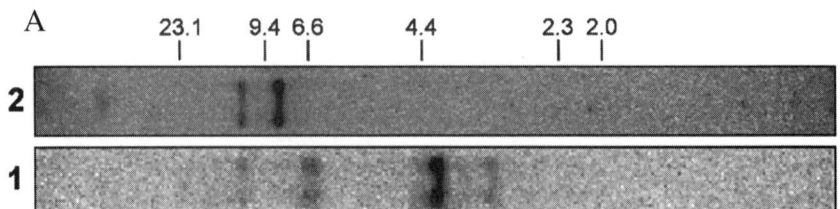

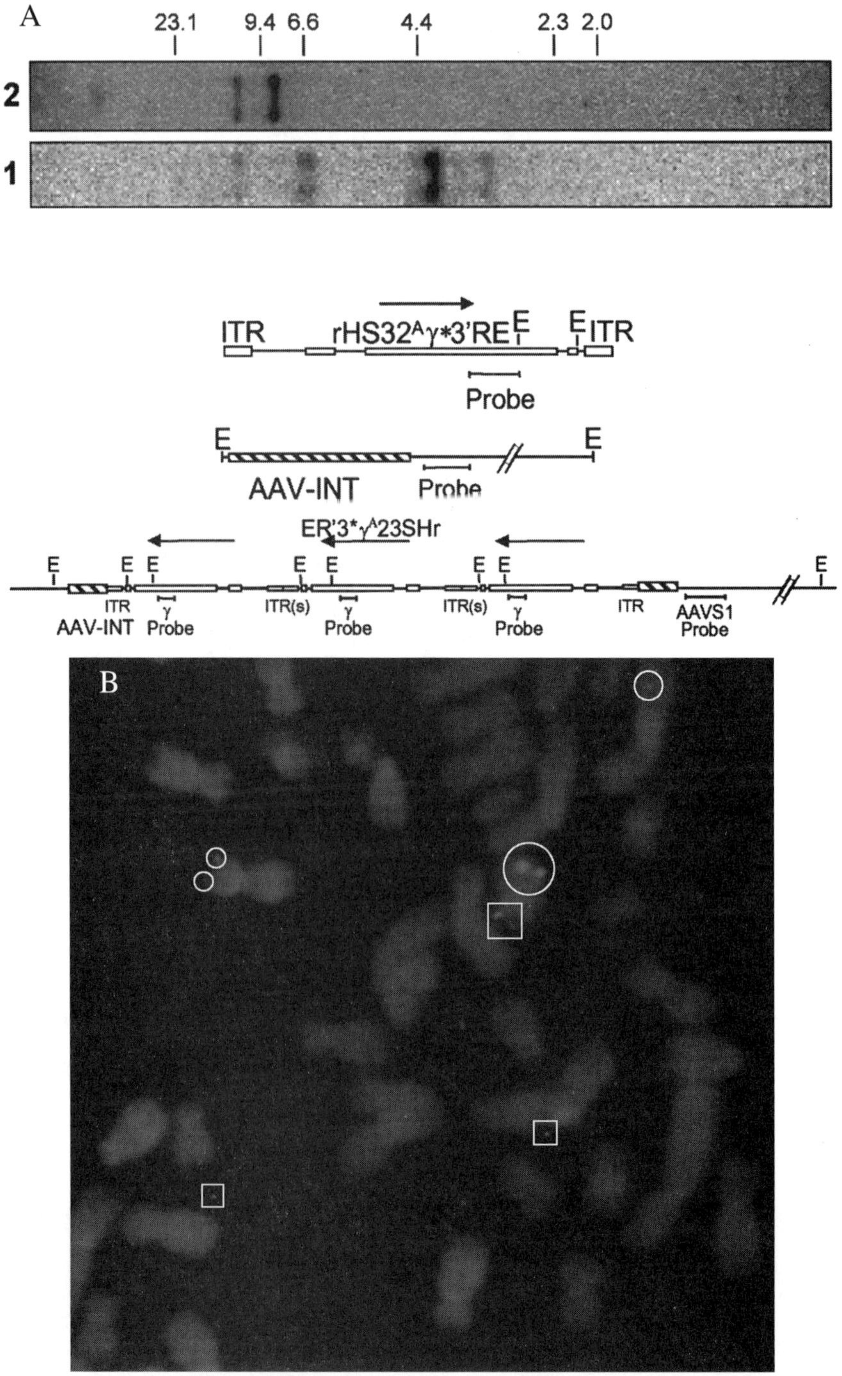

Targeted Integration of a rAAV Genome Containing a Human Globin Gene

Additional experiments were performed with the globin vector, HS32$^A\gamma^*$3'RE, which has been shown to commonly integrate as a tandem array[11] which is more readily detectable by FISH analysis. Sixteen clones that were derived from cells co-transduced with rAAV-Rep-NGFR (MOI = 10^4) and rHS32$^A\gamma^*$3'RE (MOI = 10^6) had integrated the globin vector genome. Six of these exhibited disruption of the AAVS1 site on chromosome 19 whereas zero out of fourteen clones isolated from cells transduced with HS32$^A\gamma^*$3'RE in the absence of Rep expression had chromosome 19 AAVS1 site disruption. Two of four clones studied by FISH analysis exhibited a rHS32$^A\gamma^*$3'RE signal on chromosome 19. In one clone, the site of integration of the vector genome on chromosome 19 was confirmed by demonstration of an integration junction fragment which hybridized to the AAVS1 and vector probes (FIG. 5A) and by FISH analysis (FIG. 5B).

DISCUSSION

Our experiments were undertaken to determine whether the AAV Rep proteins, when produced in *trans*, would facilitate the integration of a rAAV vector genome into the preferred AAV integration site (AAVS1). Chromosome 19–specific integration was documented with a vector, rHS32$^A\gamma^*$3'RE, containing a globin gene and associated regulatory elements which integrates as a head-to-tail tandem array but Rep proteins did not appear to increase the overall frequency of vector genome integration. Moreover, we found that Rep protein expression could lead to disruption of the AAVS1 site without integration of the vector genome at that position. Furthermore, the majority of vector integration events occurred at positions other than in AAVS1 even when Rep p78 was expressed at high levels.

Disruption of AAVS1 was documented in about 50% of the clones in which a vector genome had integrated while the Rep proteins were being expressed (FIGS. 3 and 4 and data not shown). This may represent a lower limit estimate of disruption frequency since major rearrangements as a consequence of Rep expression could remove the portion of AAVS1 which hybridizes to the probe used in these experiments. Only one half of the clones that exhibited AAVS1 disruption had a common sized band that hybridized to both the AAVS1 and vector specific probes when the DNA was restricted with an enzyme (NheI) which does not cut in either the vector genome or the AAVS1 integration site. These results are consistent with other recently published data in which Rep expression resulted in disruption of AAVS1 without evidence of vector integration in a proportion of

---

FIGURE 5. Targeted integration of rHS32$^A\gamma^*$ 3'RE to the AAV integration site on chromosome 19. (**A**) The clone studied was derived from HtTA-22 cells which had been co-transduced with rAAV-Rep-NGFR at a MOI of 10^4 and rHS32$^A\gamma^*$3'RE at a MOI of 10^6. Sixty hours after transduction, tetracycline (5 μg/ml) was added and cells were plated at limiting dilution. Individual clones were recovered and expanded to allow isolation of genomic DNA. *Lane 1* on the left contains DNA restricted with EcoRI and probed with a fragment hybridizing to the γ-globin genes (diagram below). Bands at 6.6 and 3.0kb represent the endogenous human γ-globin genes whereas the band at approximately 10kb and at 3.8kb represent the integrated $^A\gamma^*$ globin gene. The filter was stripped and rehybridized with a probe for the AAV integration site region; the band at 8.2kb is the native AAVS1 band whereas the hybridizing band at 10kb co-migrates with one detected with the γ-globin gene probe. The diagram below indicates the proposed pattern of integration including the derivation of the EcoRI band that hybridizes to both the AAVS1 and γ-globin gene probe. The 3.8kb band detected with the γ-globin gene probe is derived from a tandem head-to-tail array of the rHS32$^A\gamma^*$3'RE genome. (**B**) The integration of the vector genome on chromosome 19 was confirmed by FISH analysis. The red marker (indicated by *boxes*) is specific to chromosome 19 whereas the green marker (indicated by *circles*) detects the integrated rHS32$^A\gamma^*$3'RE genome on chromosome 19 as well as the native γ-globin gene locus on chromosome 11.

clones isolated after transfection of a Rep expression cassette in a plasmid containing AAV ITRs, as reflected by the detection of a common sized fragment by AAVS1 and vector probes[44] or by the detection of an integrated vector on chromosome 19 by FISH.[45] A current model for site-specific integration of an AAV genome involves DNA strand displacement during DNA replication initiated by Rep mediated cleavage at the AAVS1 terminal resolution site.[15,17,18] Cleavage by Rep with partial duplication of the AAVS1 region without strand displacement onto the AAV genome could result in modification of the AAVS1 region without AAV genome integration.

The relative inefficiency of Rep mediated site-specific integration of rAAV may be compared to the outcome of wild-type AAV infection with respect to integration position. In a survey of 22 AAV infected lines, the overall efficiency of chromosome 19 specific integration was 50% (11 of the original 22 clones) and AAVS1 disruption without evidence of viral genome integration at that site was documented in 14 clones.[15] Analysis of DNA from cell lines derived by transduction with a rAAV vector containing the native Rep genes revealed extra AAVS1 bands in 18 of 23; approximately 50% of these bands also hybridized to the vector probe.[46] A more recent survey[14] found the wild-type AAV genome in chromosome 19 by FISH analysis in 48 of 51 metaphase spreads among 86 in which a signal could be detected suggesting that under some conditions, site specific integration is quite efficient.

Site-specific integration of AAV is often cited as a desirable feature supporting the development of this vector system for gene therapy applications. Our data indicate that Rep mediated integration of a rAAV genome into chromosome 19 can be achieved, but that the process is inconsistent and accompanied by integration events into other sites in the genome. A better understanding and control of the variables which determine the site of AAV integration is needed to allow the relative site specificity of integration of AAV to be exploited for therapeutic purposes.

rAAV continue to hold promise as a vehicle for introducing globin genes into primary hematopoietic cells. Even without the benefit of Rep directed site specific integration, the rHS32$^A\gamma$'3'REgenome usually integrates as a stable, tandem, head-to-tail concatamer. High MOIs are required for transduction of primary hematopoietic progenitors with highly purified rAAV particles,[11] but lower MOIs were effective when crude preparations of virus were used.[10] These observations suggest that there are substances which influence transduction efficiency which, if identified, might be used to facilitate vector uptake. The growing understanding of the interaction of rAAV with target cells may ultimately allow this vector system to be developed for gene therapy of severe β-thalassemia.

ACKNOWLEDGMENTS

Joan Bertran was a recipient of a long-term fellowship from the European Molecular Biology Organization. We thank Dagmar Dilloo for a plasmid containing the gene for truncated NGFR, Derek Persons for help in constructing plasmid, pAAV-Rep-NGFR, and Jean Johnson for outstanding assistance in the preparation of this manuscript. We are grateful to John Chorini and Rob Kotin for introducing us to their methodology for making rAAV.[38] We thank Leonard Evans for providing monoclonal antibody 83A25 specific for retroviral envelope proteins, John Cunningham and Steve Jane for assistance in performing Western blot analysis, and Gary Kurtzman for providing a copy of his manuscript prior to publication.[45]

REFERENCES

1. DUNBAR, C. E. & R. V. EMMONS. 1994. Gene transfer into hematopoietic progenitor and stem cells: Progress and problems. Stem Cells **12**: 563–576.

2. WALSH, C. E., J. M. LIU, J. L. MILLER, A. W. NIENHUIS & R. J. SAMULSKI. 1993. Gene therapy for human hemoglobinopathies. Proc. Soc. Exp. Biol. Med. **204:** 289–300.
3. BRENNER, M. K., D. R. RILL, M. S. HOLLADAY, H. E. HESLOP, R. C. MOEN, M. BUSCHLE, R. A. KRANCE, V. M. SANTANA, W. F. ANDERSON & J. N. IHLE. 1993. Gene marking to determine whether autologous marrow infusion restores long-term haemopoiesis in cancer patients. Lancet **342:** 1134–1137.
4. DUNBAR, C. E., M. COTTLER-FOX, J. A. O'SHAUGHNESSY, S. DOREN, C. CARTER, R. BERENSON, S. BROWN, R. C. MOEN, J. GREENBLATT, F. M. STEWART, S. F. LEITMAN, W. H. WILSON, K. COWAN, N. S. YOUNG & A. W. NIENHUIS. 1995. Retrovirally marked, CD34-enriched peripheral blood and bone marrow cells contribute to long-term engraftment after autologous transplantation. Blood **85:** 3048–3057.
5. PLAVEC, I., T. PAPAYANNOPOULOU, C. MAURY & F. MEYER. 1993. A human beta-globin gene fused to the human beta-globin locus control region is expressed at high levels in erythroid cells of mice following engraftment with retrovirus-transduced hematopoietic stem cells. Blood **81:** 1384–1392.
6. LEBOULCH, P., G. M. HUANG, R. K. HUMPHRIES, Y. H. OH, C. J. EAVES, D. Y. TUAN & I. M. LONDON. 1994. Mutagenesis of retroviral vectors transducing human beta-globin gene and beta-globin locus control region derivatives results in stable transmission of an active transcriptional structure. EMBO J. **13:** 3065–3076.
7. SADELAIN, M., C. H. WANG, M. ANTONIOU, F. GROSVELD & R. C. MULLIGAN. 1995. Generation of a high-titer retroviral vector capable of expressing high levels of the human beta-globin gene. Proc. Natl. Acad. Sci. USA **92:** 6728–6732.
8. WALSH, C. E., J. M. LIU, X. XIAO, N. S. YOUNG, A. W. NIENHUIS & R. J. SAMULSKI. 1992. Regulated high level expression of a human gamma-globin gene introduced into erythroid cells by an adeno-associated virus vector. Proc. Natl. Acad. Sci. USA **89:** 7257–7261.
9. MILLER, J. L., C. E. WALSH, P. A. NEY, R. J. SAMULSKI & A. W. NIENHUIS. 1993. Single-copy transduction and expression of human γ-globin in K562 erythroleukemia cells using recombinant adeno-associated virus vectors: The effect of mutations in NF-E2 and GATA-1 binding motifs within the hypersensitivity site 2 enhancer. Blood **82:** 1900–1906.
10. MILLER, J. L., R. E. DONAHUE, S. E. SELLERS, R. J. SAMULSKI, N. S. YOUNG & A. W. NIENHUIS. 1994. Recombinant adeno-associated virus (rAAV) mediated expression of a human γ-globin gene in human progenitor derived erythroid cells. Proc. Natl. Acad. Sci. USA **91:** 10183–10187.
11. HARGROVE, P., E. F. VANIN, G. KURTZMAN & A. W. NIENHUIS. 1997. High level globin gene expression mediated by a recombinant adeno-associated virus genome which contains the 3'γ globin gene regulatory element and integrates as tandem copies in erythroid cells. Blood **89:** 2167–2175.
12. BERNS, K. I. & C. GIRAUD. 1996. Biology of adeno-associated virus. Curr. Top. Microbiol. Immunol. **218:** 1–23.
13. MUZYCZKA, N. 1992. Use of adeno-associated virus as a general transduction vector for mammalian cells. Curr. Top. Microbiol. Immunol. **158:** 97–129.
14. KEARNS, W. G., S. A. AFIONE, S. B. FULMER, M. C. PANG, D. ERIKSON, M. EGAN, M. J. LANDRUM, T. R. FLOTTE & G. R. CUTTING. 1996. Recombinant adeno-associated virus (AAV-CFTR) vectors do not integrate in a site-specific fashion in an immortalized epithelial cell line. Gene Ther. **3:** 748–755.
15. KOTIN, R. M., M. SINISCALCO, R. J. SAMULSKI, X. D. ZHU, L. HUNTER, C. A. LAUGHLIN, S. MCLAUGHLIN, N. MUZYCZKA, M. ROCCHI & K. I. BERNS. 1990. Site-specific integration by adeno-associated virus. Proc. Natl. Acad. Sci. USA **87:** 2211–2215.
16. CHIORINI, J. A., L. YANG, B. SAFER & R. M. KOTIN. 1995. Determination of adeno-associated virus Rep68 and Rep78 binding sites by random sequence oligonucleotide selection. J. Virol. **69:** 7334–7338.
17. LINDEN, R. M., P. WARD, C. GIRAUD, E. WINOCOUR & K. I. BERNS. 1996. Site-specific integration by adeno-associated virus. Proc. Natl. Acad. Sci. USA **93:** 11288–11294.
18. URCELAY, E., P. WARD, S. M. WIENER, B. SAFER & R. M. KOTIN. 1995. Asymmetric replication in vitro from a human sequence element is dependent on adeno-associated virus Rep protein. J. Virol. **69:** 2038–2046.

19. WEITZMAN, M. D., S. R. KYOSTIO, R. M. KOTIN & R. A. OWENS. 1994. Adeno-associated virus (AAV) Rep proteins mediate complex formation between AAV DNA and its integration site in human DNA. Proc. Natl. Acad. Sci. USA **91:** 5808–5812.
20. SAMULSKI, R. J., L. S. CHANG & T. SHENK. 1987. A recombinant plasmid from which an infectious adeno-associated virus genome can be excised in vitro and its use to study viral replication. J. Virol. **61:** 3096–3101.
21. XIAO, X., W. XIAO, J. LI & R. J. SAMULSKI. 1997. A novel 165-base-pair terminal repeat sequence is the sole cis requirement for the adeno-associated virus life cycle. J. Virol. **71:** 941–948.
22. FLOTTE, T. R. & B. J. CARTER. 1995. Adeno-associated virus vectors for gene therapy. Gene Ther. **2:** 357–362.
23. KOTIN, R. M. 1994. Prospects for use of adeno-associated virus as a vector for human gene therapy. Hum. Gene Ther. **5:** 793–801.
24. SAMULSKI, R. J., L. S. CHANG & T. SHENK. 1989. Helper-free stocks of recombinant adeno-associated viruses: normal integration does not require viral gene expression. J. Virol. **63:** 3822–3828.
25. FISHER, K. J., K. JOOSS, J. ALSTON, Y. YANG, S. E. HAECKER, K. HIGH, R. PATHAK, S. E. RAPER & J. M. WILSON. 1997. Recombinant adeno-associated virus for muscle directed gene therapy. Nat. Med. **3:** 306–312.
26. KAPLITT, M. G., P. LEONE, R. J. SAMULSKI, X. XIAO, D. W. PFAFF, K.L. O'MALLEY & M. J. DURING. 1994. Long-term gene expression and phenotypic correction using adeno-associated virus vectors in the mammalian brain. Nat. Genet. **8:** 148–154.
27. KOEBERL, D. D., I. F. ALEXANDER, C. L. HALBERT, D. W. RUSSELL & A. D. MILLER. 1997. Persistent expression of human clotting factor IX from mouse liver after intravenous injection of adeno-associated virus vectors. Proc. Natl. Acad. Sci. USA **94:** 1426–1431.
28. SNYDER, R. O., C. H. MIAO, G. A. PATIJN, S. K. SPRATT, O. DANOS, D. NAGY, A. M. GOWN, B. WINTHER, L. MEUSE, L. K. COHEN, A. R. THOMPSON & M. A. KAY. 1997. Persistent and therapeutic concentrations of human factor IX in mice after hepatic gene transfer of recombinant AAV vectors. Nat. Genet. **16:** 270–276.
29. XIAO, X., J. LI & R. J. SAMULSKI. 1996. Efficient long-term gene transfer into muscle tissue of immunocompetent mice by adeno-associated virus vector. J. Virol. **70:** 8098–8108.
30. CLARK, K. R., F. VOULGAROPOULOU, D. M. FRALEY & P. R. JOHNSON. 1995. Cell lines for the production of recombinant adeno-associated virus. Hum. Gene Ther. **6:** 1329–1341.
31. TAMAYOSE, K., Y. HIRAI & T. SHIMADA. 1996. A new strategy for large-scale preparation of high-titer recombinant adeno-associated virus vectors by using packaging cell lines and sulfonated cellulose column chromatography. Hum. Gene Ther. **7:** 507–513.
32. YANG, Y., J. BERTRAN, E. F. VANIN & A. W. NIENHUIS. 1997. Development of highly efficient producer cell clones for a recombinant AAV vector containing a human globin gene with regulatory elements. Submitted for publication.
33. BERTRAN, J., J. L. MILLER, Y. YANG, A. FENIMORE-JUSTMAN, F. RUEDA, E. F. VANIN & A. W. NIENHUIS. 1996. Recombinant adeno-associated virus-mediated high-efficiency, transient expression of the murine cationic amino acid transporter (ecotropic retroviral receptor) permits stable transduction of human HeLa cells by ecotropic retroviral vectors. J. Virol. **70:** 6759–6766.
34. GOSSEN, M. & H. BUJARD. 1992. Tight control of gene expression in mammalian cells by tetracycline-responsive promoters. Proc. Natl. Acad. Sci. USA **89:** 5547–5551.
35. HANENBERG, H., X. L. XIAO, D. DILLOO, K. HASHINO, I. KATO & D. A. WILLIAMS. 1996. Colocalization of retrovirus and target cells on specific fibronectin fragments increases genetic transduction of mammalian cells. Nat. Med. **2:** 876–882.
36. JOHNSON, D., A. LANAHAN, C. R. BUCK, A. SEHGAL, C. MORGAN, E. MERCER, M. BOTHWELL & M. CHAO. 1986. Expression and structure of the human NGF receptor. Cell **47:** 545–554.
37. SAMBROOK, J., E. F. FRITSCH & T. MANIATIS. 1989. Molecular Cloning: A Laboratory Manual. Cold Spring Harbor Laboratory. Cold Spring Harbor, NY.
38. CHIORINI, J. A., C. M. WENDTNER, E. URCELAY, B. SAFER, M. HALLEK & R. M. KOTIN. 1995. High-efficiency transfer of the T-cell co-stimulatory molecule B7-2 to lymphoid cells using high-titer recombinant adeno-associated virus vectors. Hum. Gene Ther. **6:** 1531–1541.
39. HIRT, B. 1967. Selective extraction of polyoma DNA from infected mouse cell cultures. J. Mol. Biol. **26:** 365–369.

40. GRAHAM, F. L. & L. PREVEC. 1992. Adenovirus-based expression vectors and recombinant vaccines. Biotechnology **20:** 363–390.
41. HÖLSCHER, C., M. HÖRER, J. A. KLEINSCHMIDT, H. ZENTGRAFT, BÜRKLE, R. HEILBRONN. 1994. Cell lines inducibly expressing the adeno-associated virus (AAV) *rep* gene: requirements for productive replication of *rep*-negative AAV mutants. J. Virol. **68:** 7169–7177.
42. EVANS, L. H., R. P. MORRISON, F. G. MALIK, J. PORTIS & W. J. BRITT. 1990. A neutralizable epitope common to the envelope glycoproteins of ecrotropic, polytropic, xenotropic, and amphotropic murine leukemia viruses. J. Virol. **64:** 6176–6183.
43. MELLENTIN, J. D., C. MURRE, T. A. DONLON, P. S. MCCAW, S. D. SMITH, A. D. CARROLL, M. MCDONALD, D. BALTIMORE & M. L. CLEARY. 1989. The gene for enhancer binding proteins E12/E47 lies at the (1, 19) breakpoint in acute leukemias. Science **246:** 379–382.
44. BALAGUE, C., M. KALLA & W.-W. ZHANG. 1997. Adeno-associated virus Rep78 protein and terminal repeats enhance integration of DNA sequences into the cellular genome. J. Virol. **71:** 3299–3306.
45. SUROSKY, R. T., M. URABE, S. G. GODWIN, S. A. MCQUISTON, G. J. KURTZMAN, K. OZAWA & G. NATSOULIS. 1997. The adeno-associated virus Rep proteins target DNA sequences to a unique locus in the human genome. J. Virol. **71:** 7951–7959.
46. SHELLING, A. N. & M. G. SMITH. 1994. Targeted integration of transfected and infected adeno-associated virus vectors containing the neomycin resistance gene. Gene Ther. **1:** 165–169.

High-Level Transfer and Long-Term Expression of the Human β-Globin Gene in a Mouse Transplant Model[a]

HARRY RAFTOPOULOS, MAUREEN WARD, AND
ARTHUR BANK[b]

*Department of Genetics and Development, Department of Medicine,
College of Physicians and Surgeons, Columbia University, New York,
New York 10032, USA*

ABSTRACT: Insertion of a normally functioning human β-globin gene into the hematopoietic stem cells (HSC) of patients with β-thalassemia may be an effective approach to the therapy of this disorder. Safe, efficient gene transfer and long-term, high-level expression of the transferred human β-globin gene in animal models are prerequisites for HSC somatic gene therapy. We have recently shown for the first time that, using a modified β-globin retroviral vector in a mouse transplant model, long-term, high-level expression of a transferred human β-globin gene is possible. The human β-globin gene continues to be detected up to eight months post-transplantation of β-globin–transduced hematopoietic cells into lethally irradiated mice. The transferred human β-globin gene is detected in three of five mice surviving long-term (>4 months) transplanted with bone marrow cells transduced with high-titer virus. The unrearranged 5.1 kb human β-globin gene–containing provirus is seen by Southern blotting in two of these mice. More importantly, long-term expression of the transferred gene is seen in two mice at levels of 5% and 20% that of endogenous murine β-globin. We document stem cell transduction by showing continued high-level expression of the human β-globin gene in secondarily transplanted recipient mice. These results provide evidence of HSC transduction with a human β-globin gene in animals and demonstrate that retroviral-mediated unrearranged human β-globin gene transfer leads to a high level of human β-globin gene expression in the long term for the first time. A gene therapy strategy may be a feasible therapeutic approach to the β-thalassemias if consistent human β-globin gene transfer and expression into HSC can be achieved.

Patients with β-thalassemia can be cured by allogeneic stem cell transplantation.[1,2] However, this treatment modality is associated with significant morbidity and mortality and is limited by the number of available HLA-compatible siblings.[3] Another potential approach to curing β-thalassemia is by the insertion of a normally functioning human β-globin gene into

---

[a]This work was supported by Public Health Service Grants from the National Institutes of Health (DK-25274, HL-28381, and HL-48345). Harry Raftopoulos was supported by a National Institutes of Health Hematology Training Grant (DK-07373).

[b]Address for correspondence: Dr. Arthur Bank, Columbia University, HHSC 16-1602, 701 West 168th Street, New York, NY 10032. Tel: 212-305-4186; Fax: 212-923-2090; e-mail: bank@cuccfa.ccc.columbia.edu.

the hematopoietic stem cells (HSC) of patients with the disorder. For this somatic gene therapy approach to be successful, safe and efficient gene transfer as well as long-term and high-level expression of the transferred gene are required. Retroviral vectors can be used to safely and efficiently transfer genes such as the human multiple drug resistance gene (MDR-1)[4–6] and the neomycin resistance gene (neo^R)[7] into HSC. Progress in successful β-globin gene transfer has been especially difficult, primarily due to the low titer vectors and poor expression of the transferred gene.[8–10] These problems have persisted even with incorporation of sequences from the β-globin locus control region (LCR).[11–17] Recently, several studies have shown more stable proviral transmission of human β-globin–containing constructs especially modified to remove splice signals.[18–20] We have recently shown for the first time that, using one of these modified β-globin retroviral vectors in a mouse transplant model, long-term, high-level expression of a transferred human β-globin gene is possible.[21,22] In addition, the transduced gene is capable of being transferred to secondary transplant recipients with continued expression, indicating HSC transduction. These results, therefore, represent progress towards the ultimate goal of somatic human β-globin gene therapy for β-thalassemia.

MATERIALS AND METHODS

Retroviral Vector

The retroviral vector p141 used in these studies is shown in FIGURE 1.[18] The vector contains an LXSN backbone and a deletion in the 3' LTR which results in self-inactivation. The neo^R gene, driven by the PGK promoter, is a selectable marker. The β-globin gene with deletions of the 3' enhancer and of a 372 bp region in intron 2 is inserted in reverse orientation. LCR elements HS2, HS3, and HS4 are included upstream of the β-globin gene.[23] Potential splicing and polyadenylation signals were mutated for increased stability of proviral transmission.[18]

Preparation of Viral Producer Lines

Retroviral producer lines containing the β-globin gene and/or the neo^R gene were prepared by transfecting GP+E86 ecotropic packaging cells[24] with the retroviral vectors p141 and N2, respectively, using calcium phosphate coprecipitation. Clones were then selected in medium containing 600 μg of G418 per ml, as described previously.[25] The producer lines were titered for viral production using G418 resistance of target 3T3 cells, as described by Markowitz and coworkers.[24,26]

Hematopoietic Cell Transduction and Transplantation

Femurs and tibias of 10–12 week old C57BL/6J male donor mice (Jackson Laboratories, Bar Harbor, Maine) were harvested to obtain bone marrow (BM) cells 48 hours after the animals had received one dose of 5-fluorouracil (150 mg/kg i.p.). Fetal liver (FL) cells were harvested from day 14.5 fetuses as described by Richardson and coworkers.[27] Cells were pre-incubated in T175 flasks (Nunc, Glostrup, Denmark) containing 80 ml α minimum essential medium (αMEM) with 20% fetal calf serum (FCS),

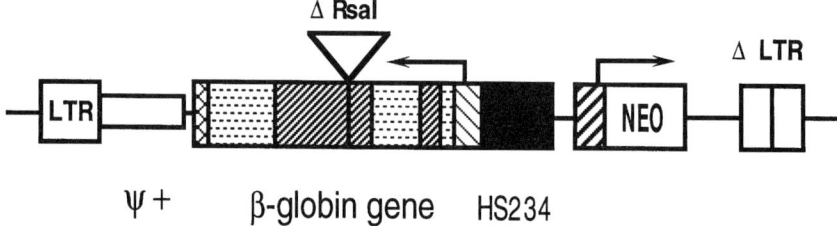

FIGURE 1. A diagram of the p141 vector. The vector is flanked by the 5' long terminal repeat (LTR) and 3' deleted long terminal repeat (Δ LTR). The extended packaging signal is represented by ψ+. The β-globin gene is in reverse orientation with exons (∴), introns (▨), the deleted 3' enhancer (✗) and the 372 bp deletion in intron 2 (Δ Rsa I). The LCR core sequences HS234 (■) and the neomycin resistance gene (NEO) with the PGK promoter (◐) are as indicated.

1% penicillin/streptomycin solution (GIBCO, Grand Island, NY), murine interleukin 3 (5–10 ng/ml; Intergen Company, Purchase, NY), human interleukin 6 (200 U/ml), and rat stem cell factor (100 ng/ml; a gift of Amgen, Thousand Oaks, CA) for 24 hours at 37°C. BM or FL (5×10^6–10^7 cells) were then co-cultured on 100-mm plates containing either semi-confluent GP+E86 β-producers or N2 producers. In co-culture, cells were incubated in αMEM with 20% FCS, 1% penicillin/streptomycin solution, murine interleukin 3 (5–10 ng/ml), interleukin 6 (200 U/ml), and stem cell factor (100 ng/ml) with the addition of polybrene 6 μg/ml or protamine 5 μg/ml (Sigma Chemical Co., St. Louis, Missouri) for 24–48 hours. Cells were harvested from the co-culture plates by gentle pipetting. Recipient C57BL/6J female mice were gamma-irradiated with 1,100 rad given in two doses 3 hours apart. Recipient mice were injected via tail vein with either 1–2×10^6 β-transduced cells or 1–2×10^6 N2-transduced cells.

Analysis of Transplanted Mice

Polymerase Chain Reaction

DNA for polymerase chain reaction (PCR) was prepared from Day 12 spleen colonies and peripheral blood at various time points post-transplantation using the Iso-Quick Kit (Microprobe, Garden Grove, CA), as described previously.[28] PCR reactions were performed to detect β-globin, neo^R, mouse platelet-derived growth factor (PDGF) B receptor, and Y chromosome sequences. The primers used for β-globin were 5'-TGGATCCTGAGAACTTCAGG-3' (sense) and 5'-CACTGGTGGGGTGAATTCTT-3' (antisense), which span the RsaI deletion in IVS-2 and result in a 564 bp amplification fragment from transferred human β-globin, and a 936 bp fragment from normal human DNA. PCR for PDGF B was used as a control for DNA loading, while Y chromosome analysis was used for reconstitution with donor cells (male donors to female recipients).[29]

Southern Blot Analysis

In some experiments, mice were sacrificed 9 months post-transplantation and chromosomal DNA extracted from blood, marrow, and spleens using a phenol extraction method. Approximately 10 µg of DNA was digested with SacI and XbaI and Southern blotting was performed using a ^{32}P-labeled neo^R probe.

Primer Extension Assays

RNA was extracted from 150 µl of peripheral blood at various time points post-transplantation using a Micro RNA Isolation Kit (Stratagene, La Jolla, CA). Primer extension assays were performed with ^{32}P end-labeled primers specific for human β-globin (5'-CTCCTCTTCAGGCGGCAATGAC-3') and mouse β^{maj} globin 5'-TGAT-GTCTGTTTCTGGGGTTGTG-3', with predicted extension products of 90 bp and 58 bp, respectively. RNA was also isolated from the blood of a transgenic mouse known to contain three copies of a human β-globin gene and to be expressing human β-globin.[30] This RNA was used as a positive control for primer extension. A phosphorimager was used to quantitate radioactive bands.

Secondary Transplantation

$1-2 \times 10^7$ unmanipulated marrow cells from sacrificed primary recipient mice were used to reconstitute lethally irradiated secondary recipients. Analyses for human β-globin gene transfer and expression were performed as for primary recipients.

RESULTS

Generation of Virus-Producing Lines

Two ecotropic producer clones containing vector p141 with titers of 1×10^4 and 1×10^5 G418 resistant 3T3 CFU/ml, respectively, were identified. Intact copies of the proviral construct were transferred into 3T3 cells as assessed by Southern blotting (data not shown). These lines were used for transplantation experiments. Producer lines containing the neo^R gene (N2) had titers of 1×10^6 to 1×10^7 G418 resistant 3T3 CFU/ml.

Gene Transfer

The majority of CFU-S assayed at Day 12 post-transplantation for the presence of the human β-globin gene by PCR were positive when a 10^5 titer β-globin gene–containing producer was used. Close to 100% transduction was observed in mice transplanted with N2-transduced hematopoietic cells (titer of producer 5×10^6), (data not shown).[21,22]

The human β-globin gene was detected by PCR of DNA from peripheral blood using human β-globin gene primers in 40–60% of transplanted mice at time points less than 4

TABLE 1. Human β-Globin Gene Transfer and Expression in Peripheral Blood

Experiment Number (titer, cell source, cation)	Total Mice	Short Term (< 4 months)			Long Term (> 4 months)		
		Mice PCR +	Mice RNA +	Hu β/ Mouse β	Mice PCR +	Mice RNA +	Hu β / Mouse β
1 (10^5, BM, PB)	5	3	—	—	3	2	20%[a] 5%[a]
2 (10^4, BM, PB)	9	1	0	—	1	0	—
3 (10^5, FL, PB)	10	4	1	3%	1	0	—
4 (10^5, BM, PT)	9	9	0	—	7	0	—

Hematopoietic cells were obtained, preincubated with growth factors, and then co-cultured with retroviral producer cells. Lethally irradiated recipient mice were injected with transduced cells and peripheral blood samples were analyzed for gene transfer by PCR and gene expression by primer extension at various time points as described in *Materials and Methods*.

Abbreviations: BM, bone marrow; FL, fetal liver; PB, polybrene; PT, protamine.

[a]Levels stable at 6 months and 8 months post-transplantation. These are Mice 3 and 4 in FIG. 4.

months post-transplantation when the 10^5 ecotropic producer was used (TABLE 1). There was virtually no short-term gene transfer when a lower titer producer (1/9) was used (TABLE 1). Long-term persistence of the transferred β-globin gene (assessed by PCR at time points from four to eight months post-transplantation) is seen in three of five (60%) of mice from Experiment 1 (FIG. 2, TABLE 1), all seven surviving mice from Experiment 4, and in a single

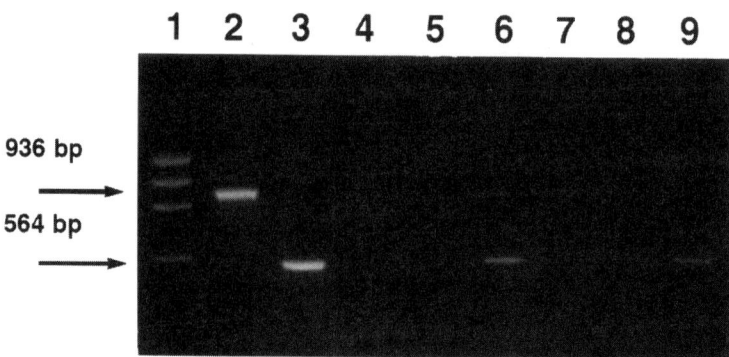

FIGURE 2. β IVS-2 PCR of 5-month peripheral blood samples. Peripheral blood samples from mice transplanted with human β-globin–transduced marrow (β-mice) and neomycin-resistance gene–transduced marrow (neo[R] mice), respectively, were analyzed by PCR using primers specific for the β-globin IVS-2 region. Lane 1 represents a size marker (φX); lane 2, a normal human DNA sample; lane 3, producer cell DNA; lane 4, a sample from a neo[R] mouse, and lanes 5–9 samples from β-mice. The predicted PCR bands for human β-globin (936 bp) and vector-derived human β-globin (564 bp) are indicated to the left of the figure. Three of five mice are positive.

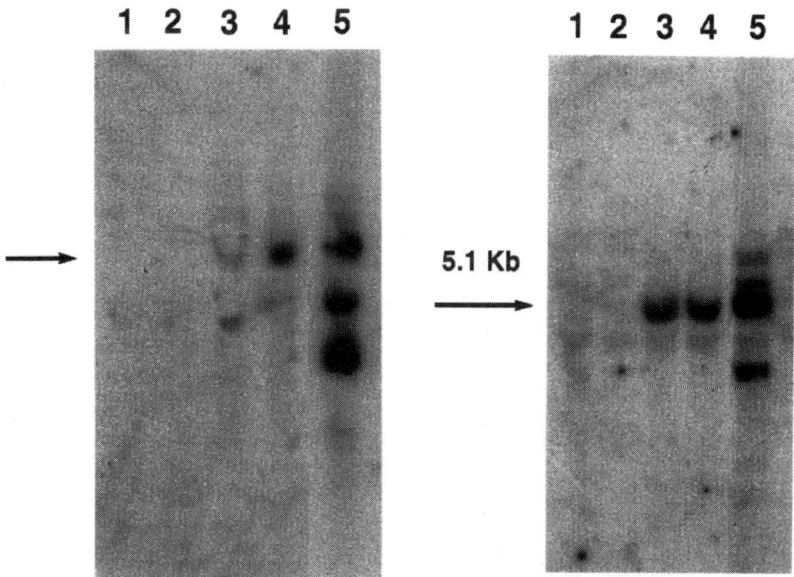

FIGURE 3. Southern blot analysis of mouse marrow. DNA obtained from marrow of Experiment 1 mice was digested with XbaI (*Left*) and SacI (*Right*) and probed with a neo[R] probe as described in *Materials and Methods*. In both panels, lanes 1–4 represent DNA samples obtained from bone marrow of Mice 1–4 and lane 5 represents producer cell DNA. The number of chromosomal integration sites was assessed using XbaI digestion, an enzyme which does not cut within the vector. Producer cells in lane 5 have four sites of proviral integration. There are no significant bands in Mice 1 and 2; while in Mouse 3 there at least two integration sites, and Mouse 4 shows a dominant integration site (indicated by the arrow on the left). (*Right*) The restriction enzyme SacI cuts the p141 vector within the LTR regions and was used to establish the integrity of the transferred β-globin gene. In producer cells, the intensity of the 5.1 kb band (by phosphorimager analysis) is three times that of the lower band in lane 5. We conclude that producer cells contain three intact copies and one truncated copy of the retroviral vector. There is no detectable band in Mice 1 and 2 bone marrow, while Mice 3 and 4 both have the intact 5.1 kb human β-globin gene–containing provirus (lanes 1–4). Twice as much DNA (10 μg) of marrow samples was loaded as was producer cell DNA (5 μg). The intensities of the 5.1 kb bands in Mice 3 and 4 (lanes 3 and 4) were compared by phosphorimaging to those of the single and the three copy bands from the producer line in lane 5; we calculate that there are 0.53 and 0.64 human β-globin gene copies per cell in the marrow cells of these mice.

mouse from Experiments 2 and 3 (TABLE 1). The persistence of a transduced gene in a mouse for more than four months post-transplantation is suggestive of stem cell transduction.

DNA from selected mice from Experiment 1 nine months post-transplantation were subjected to Southern blot analysis, which shows that Mouse 3 has at least two sites of chromosomal integration of the provirus; Mouse 4 appears to have a single dominant site, probably representing monoclonal reconstitution (FIG. 3, left). The presence of the intact 5.1

kb human β-globin gene–containing provirus in the two mice (Mice 3 and 4) expressing human β-globin is shown in the Southern blot in FIGURE 3, right using *Sac*I, which cuts in the β-globin retroviral LTRs. We calculate that there are 0.53 and 0.64 copies of the human β-globin gene per cell in these mice by comparing the intensities of bands from the producer line with those of the 5.1 kb bands in Mice 3 and 4 (lanes 3 and 4).

Human β-Globin Gene Expression

Human β-globin gene expression was assessed by primer extension assays performed on RNA extracted from peripheral blood samples at various time points post-transplantation. The results show that some of the PCR-positive mice express human β-globin at high levels (>3%, as much human β-globin mRNA as mouse β-globin mRNA) (FIG. 4, TABLE 1). Human β-globin RNA is present at a level 20% that of endogenous mouse β^{maj}-globin RNA at 6 and 8 months post-transplantation (TABLE 1) in one mouse from experiment 1. Another mouse from Experiment 1 using bone marrow cells showed 5% as much human β-globin as mouse expression at 8 months post-transplantation, while in Experiment 3, using fetal

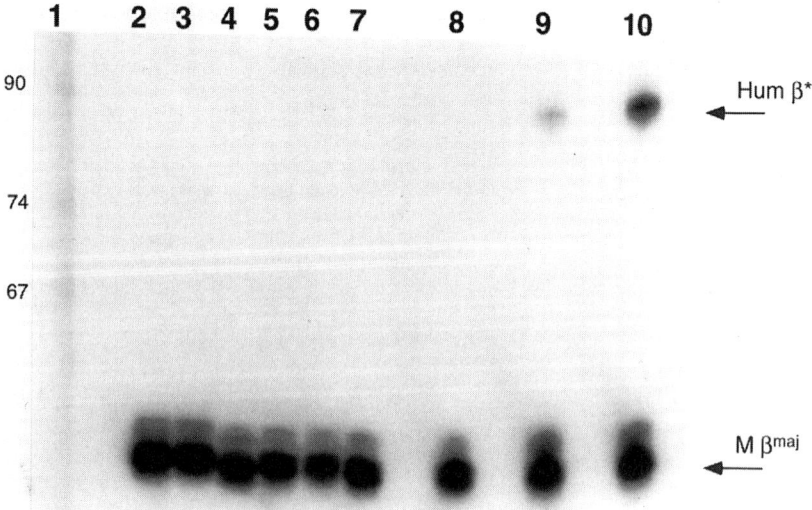

FIGURE 4. Primer extension analysis of RNA from peripheral blood samples. RNA samples were obtained from peripheral blood of mice 6 months after transplantation with human β-globin–transduced marrow. Primers specific for mouse β-globin major and human β-globin were used. Lane 1 represents a size marker; lanes 2 and 3, RNA from untransplanted mice; lanes 4 and 5, RNA from mice transplanted with N2-transduced marrow; lanes 6–10 are samples from mice transplanted with β-globin–transduced marrow. The arrows at the right of the figure indicate the position at 90 bp for human β-globin (Hum β) and at 58 bp for mouse β-globin (M β^{maj}). On the left of the figure, size markers are noted. Positive signals are seen in the mouse blood samples in lanes 9 and 10; these bands represent 5% and 20%, respectively, as much human β-globin as mouse β-globin (quantitation by phosphorimager analysis).

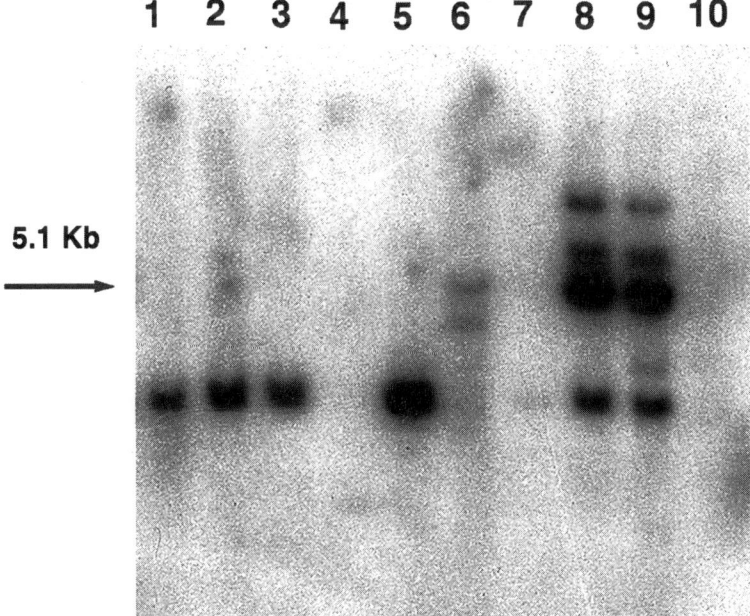

FIGURE 5. Southern blot analysis of mouse marrow. DNA obtained from marrow of Experiment 4 mice was digested with *Sac*I and probed with a neo^R probe as described in *Materials and Methods*. Lanes 1–5 represent DNA from five mice from Experiment 4; lane 6, DNA from a high-level human β-globin–expressing mouse (see FIG. 3B, lane 4); lanes 7 and 10, negative controls, and lanes 8 and 9, DNA from producer cells. The position of the 5.1 kb band (intact provirus) is indicated by the arrow at the left. Four of five mice from Experiment 4 have a truncated copy of the human β-globin provirus (± 4 kb).

liver cells, one mouse showed 3% as much expression at 3 months, which disappeared at 8 months.

In Experiment 4, the high-titer producer line was used, but only after several additional passages with G418 selection (TABLE 1). Each of the nine mice transduced with these producer cells was found to have a β-globin PCR signal but had no β-globin mRNA expression by primer extension (TABLE 1). On Southern blot analysis, four of five of these mice tested were found to have a truncated copy of the β-globin retrovirus, which was the same size in all samples (FIG. 5). This result was due to the presence of a smaller retrovirus containing an intact neo^R gene, but only part of the human β-globin gene. The truncated vector was also seen initially on Southern blot in the producer line in low amounts and was presumably selected by repeated growth in G418 (FIG. 5).

Secondary Transplants

Marrow cells from primary recipient mice from Experiment 1 sacrificed 9 months post-transplantation were used to reconstitute lethally irradiated secondary recipients (two recipients per primary mouse). Secondary recipients transplanted from primary mice expressing human β-globin RNA continued to retain and express the transferred gene 8 months post secondary transplantation (TABLE 2). This result provides strong evidence of stem cell transduction. By contrast, PCR-negative primary recipients result in PCR-negative secondary recipients.

DISCUSSION

The unique retroviral vector used in these experiments has a human β-globin gene modified to remove potential splicing and polyadenylation signals, incorporates locus control region core elements (HS2, HS3, and HS4), and has previously been shown to transduce mouse erythroleukemia cells and mouse marrow cells in culture without rearrangement.[18] We now demonstrate that this vector in an ecotropic producer line is capable of high-level unrearranged gene transfer in mice both short-term and long-term.

We show short-term gene transfer by both CFU-S assays and PCR from peripheral blood of mice (TABLE 1). We have previously reported a high level of stem cell transduction using the human MDR gene and a similar transduction protocol.[4,28] In TABLE 1, we show that the retroviral producer line with the higher titer, 10^5 as compared to 10^4, is more efficient in both the transfer and expression of the human β-globin gene in mice, as expected. Fetal liver cells appeared to be less transducible with the human β-globin gene than with the MDR gene in Experiment 3. When marrow cells and intact high-titer virus (Experiment 1) are used, three of five mice were transduced with the human β-globin gene

TABLE 2. Human β-Globin Gene Transfer and Expression in Peripheral Blood of Primary and Secondary Recipient Mice

Animal		Recipient	β-Globin PCR	Primer Extension	Human β/Mouse β^{maj} (%)
Mouse	1	Primary	+	−	−
	1A	Secondary	−	−	−
	1B	Secondary	−	−	−
Mouse	2	Primary	−	−	−
	2A	Secondary	−	−	−
	2B	Secondary	−	−	−
Mouse	3	Primary	+	+	5
	3A	Secondary	+	+	0.5
	3B	Secondary	+	+	2.8
Mouse	4	Primary	+	+	20
	4A	Secondary	+	+	9
	4B	Secondary	+	+	21

Four primary recipient mice from Experiment 1 were sacrificed 9 months post-transplantation and their marrow used to reconstitute secondary recipients. Peripheral blood samples of secondary recipients were analyzed for human β-globin gene transfer by PCR and gene expression by primer extension as described in *Materials and Methods*. Long-term data are shown for each of the primary and secondary recipients.

(+) indicates a signal for the human β-globin gene by PCR or mRNA by primer extension; (−) indicates no signal.

short-term and all three retained the gene long-term. In addition, we demonstrate long-term transfer of the intact human β-globin gene by Southern blot analysis 9 months post-transplantation (TABLE 1, FIGS. 2 and 3).

Stem cell transduction is a prerequisite for successful somatic gene therapy of β-thalassemia. At times longer than four months post-transplantation, it is presumed that persistent β-globin gene transfer is due to stem cell transduction as we have shown (TABLE 2, FIGS. 2 and 3). We have, additionally, documented stem cell transduction more definitively, by successful transfer of the human β-globin gene from mice transduced 9 months earlier into irradiated secondary recipient mice (TABLE 2). In a previous study, using a different vector, comparable short-term transfer of the human β-globin gene was obtained and some long-term gene transfer (>4 months) reported (4 of 51 mice).[17] However, no evidence for stem cell transduction was demonstrated in this study.[17]

In Experiment 4 (TABLE 1), failure to obtain human β-globin gene expression is probably due to the fact that G418 selection of producer cells leads to the preferential growth of cells containing a smaller retrovirus initially present in the calcium phosphate–selected clone. This results in the transfer of a truncated provirus containing only part of the human β-globin gene, which is not capable of expression (TABLE 1, FIG. 5). We have other producer clones now available for future use that do not contain this contaminant.

In addition to human β-globin gene transfer *in vivo,* most importantly, we now demonstrate both short- and long-term expression of the transferred human β-globin gene in mice, as assessed by primer extension (TABLE 1, FIG. 4). Long-term, high-level expression was achieved in two of three mice transduced using BM cells and high titer virus (Experiment 1, TABLE 1). One mouse shows 20% as high human β-globin expression as mouse β-globin expression. This high level of expression appears to be the result of high-level human β-globin gene expression of one stem cell clone that is predominantly represented in the marrow of this mouse at 8 months. This level of normal human β-globin gene expression, if achieved consistently in a patient with β-thalassemia, would be expected to ameliorate, if not cure, the disease.[31,32] In other studies, we show that marrow transferred from this and from another high β-globin–expressing mouse into irradiated secondary recipients also leads to persistence of human β-globin gene expression, confirming expression of the transferred gene in stem cells (TABLE 2).

SUMMARY

We have seen long-term expression of a human β-globin gene in mice transplanted with BM cells transduced with intact high titer virus in two of three mice. These experiments are the first to show the feasibility of high level, long-term expression of the human β-globin gene *in vivo.*

Even using the higher titer producer line, there is a great deal of variability in the level of human β-globin gene transfer and expression in these murine experiments. There is also no correlation between the copy numbers (0.53 and 0.64) (FIG. 3) and the levels of expression, which are 5% and 20% that of mouse β-globin in the two high human β-globin gene–expressing mice (FIG. 4). This lack of correlation between β-globin gene number and β-globin gene expression in our experiments is most likely due to differences in expression of the human β-globin gene inserted in different chromosomal positions (position effects), as well as to the small number of stem cell clones active in the oligoclonal reconstitution in this ablated mouse model. In addition, in our studies, unlike the data reported in transgenic mice,[12,33] β-globin LCR elements do not appear to confer site-independent chromosomal integration on the transferred human β-globin gene. Our results add to recent evidence that the β-LCR functions primarily as a strong erythroid-specific enhancer in retroviral constructs.[16,18,19] With single copies of the β-LCR, position independence of expression is variable.[34] In addition, the μ-LCR components HS 2, 3, and 4 used in our experiments may not be optimal for conferring consistent high-level expression on a single copy retroviral integrant; other β-LCR elements may be more optimal.

While our results demonstrate the feasibility of human β-globin gene transfer and expression, we recognize that before somatic human β-globin gene therapy can be attempted, it will be necessary to have more consistent high-level gene transfer and expression of the human β-globin gene in reconstituting stem cell clones. This may be achieved by (1) increasing the efficiency of gene transfer and expression, (2) constructing vectors that will permit position-independent expression, and/or (3) using a drug-resistance gene such as MDR either *in vivo* or *in vitro* to pre-select cells transduced with a cell surface marker such as MDR or CD24.[28,35] Constructs with (1) other LCR components, (2) nuclear localization signals to transduce non-dividing cells, (3) stem cell targeting strategies, (4) more effective cytokine combinations in transduction, and/or (5) other promoters and enhancers may be required to accomplish this. However, our finding that an unrearranged human β-globin gene transfer leads to the occasional high level of human β-globin gene expression long-term, as well as evidence of hematopoietic stem cell transduction for the first time in animals, provide the basis for using this and related β-globin retroviral producer lines to further improve this gene transfer system in pre-clinical studies. These studies also provide the impetus for considering that human globin retroviral gene transfer into human hematopoietic stem cells may eventually be a feasible approach to the treatment of β-thalassemia.

ACKNOWLEDGMENT

We thank Vivian Hayashi for her technical assistance.

REFERENCES

1. LUCARELLI, G. & C. GIARDINI. 1995. Bone marrow transplantation in thalassemia. Cancer Treat. Res. **76:** 43–58.
2. WALTERS, M. C., K. M. SULLIVAN, R. J. O'REILLY, F. BOULAD, J. BROCKSTEIN, K. BLUME, M. AMYLON, F. L. JOHNSON, M. KLEMPERER, J. GRAHAM-POLE, *et al.* 1994. Bone marrow transplantation for thalassemia. The USA experience. Am. J. Ped. Hematol.-Oncol. **16:** 11–17.
3. APPERLEY, J. F. 1993. Bone marrow transplant for the haemoglobinopathies: past, present and future. Baillieres Clin. Haematol. **6:** 299–325.
4. PODDA, S., M. WARD, A. HIMELSTEIN, C. RICHARDSON, E. DE LA FLOR-WEISS, L. SMITH, M. GOTTESMAN, I. PASTAN & A. BANK. 1992. Transfer and expression of the human multiple drug resistance gene into live mice. Proc. Nat. Acad. Sci. USA **89:** 9676–9680.
5. SORRENTINO, B. P., S. J. BRANDT, G. BODINO, M. GOTTESMAN, I. PASTAN, A. CLINE & A. W. NIENHUIS. 1992. Selection of drug-resistant bone marrow cells *in vivo* after retroviral transfer of human MDR1. Science **257:** 99–103.
6. BANK, A. 1996. Human somatic cell gene therapy. Bioessays **18:** 999–1007.
7. BRENNER, M. K. 1996. Gene transfer to hematopoietic cells. N. Engl. J. Med. **335:** 337–340.
8. KARLSSON, S., D. M. BODINE, L. PERRY, T. PAPAYANNOPOULOU & A. NIENHUIS. 1988. Expression of the human β globin gene following retroviral-mediated transfer into multipotential hematopoietic progenitors of mice. Proc. Natl. Acad. Sci. USA **85:** 6062–6066.
9. DZIERZAK, E. A., T. PAPAYANNOPOULOU & R. C. MULLIGAN. 1988. Lineage-specific expression of a human beta-globin gene in murine bone marrow transplant recipients reconstituted with retrovirus-transduced stem cells. Nature **331:** 35–41.

10. BENDER, M. A., R. E. GELINAS & A. D. MILLER. 1989. A majority of mice show long-term expression of a human beta-globin gene after retrovirus transfer into hematopoietic stem cells. Mol. Cell. Biol. **9:** 1426–1434.
11. TUAN, D., W. SOLOMON, O. LI & I. M. LONDON. 1985. The "beta-like-globin" gene domain in human erythroid cells. Proc. Natl. Acad. Sci. USA **82:** 6384–6388.
12. GROSVELD, F., G. B. VAN ASSENDELFT, D. R. GREAVES & G. KOLLIAS. 1987. Position-independent, high-level expression of the human beta-globin gene in transgenic mice. Cell **51:** 975–985.
13. FORRESTER, W. C., U. NOVAK, R. GELINAS & M. GROUDINE. 1989. Molecular analysis of the human beta-globin locus activation region. Proc. Natl. Acad. Sci. USA **86:** 5439–5443.
14. STROUBOULIS, J., N. DILLON & F. GROSVELD. 1992. Developmental regulation of a complete 70-kb beta globin locus in transgenic mice. Genes & Dev. **6:** 1857–1864.
15. TUAN, D. Y. H., W. B. SOLOMON, I. M. LONDON & D. P. LEE. 1989. An erythroid-specific, developmental-stage-independent enhancer far upstream of the human "beta-like globin" genes. Proc. Natl. Acad. Sci. USA **86:** 2554–2558.
16. NOVAK, U., E. HARRIS, W. FORRESTER, M. GROUDINE & R. GELINAS. 1990. High-level β globin expression after retroviral transfer of locus activation region-containing human β globin gene derivatives into murine erythroleukemia cells. Proc. Natl. Acad. Sci. USA **87:** 3386–3390.
17. PLAVEC, I., T. PAPAYANNOPOULOU, C. MAURY & F. MEYER. 1993. A human beta-globin gene fused to the human beta-globin locus control region is expressed at high levels in erythroid cells of mice engrafted with retrovirus-transduced hematopoietic stem cells. Blood **81:** 1384–1392.
18. LEBOULCH, P., G. M. HUANG, R. K. HUMPHRIES, Y. H. OH, C. J. EAVES, D. Y. TUAN & I. M. LONDON. 1994. Mutagenesis of retroviral vectors transducing human beta-globin gene and beta-globin locus control region derivatives results in stable transmission of an active transcriptional structure. EMBO J. **13:** 3065–3076.
19. SADELAIN, M., C. H. WANG, M. ANTONIOU, F. GROSVELD & R. C. MULLIGAN. 1995. Generation of a high-titer retroviral vector capable of expressing high levels of the human beta-globin gene. Proc. Natl. Acad. Sci. USA **92:** 6728–6732.
20. TAKEKOSHI, K. J., Y. H. OH, K. W. WESTERMAN, I. M. LONDON & P. LEBOULCH. 1995. Retroviral transfer of a human beta-globin/delta-globin hybrid gene linked to beta locus control region hypersensitive site 2 aimed at the gene therapy of sickle cell disease. Proc. Natl. Acad. Sci. USA **92:** 3014–3018.
21. RAFTOPOULOS, H., M. WARD, P. LEBOULCH & A. BANK. 1997. Long-term transfer and expression of the human beta-globin gene in a mouse transplant model. Blood **90:** 3414–3422.
22. RAFTOPOULOS, H., M. WARD, P. LEBOULCH & A. BANK. 1996. Long-term transfer and expression of the human beta-globin gene in a mouse transplant model. Blood (Suppl) **88:** 273a.
23. MILLER, A. D., M. A. BENDER, E. A. S. HARRIS, M. KALEKO & R. E. GELINAS. 1988. Design of retrovirus vectors for transfer and expression of the human β globin gene. J. Virol. **62:** 4337–4345.
24. MARKOWITZ, D., S. GOFF & A. BANK. 1988. A safe packaging line for gene transfer: Separating viral genes on two different plasmids. J. Virol. **62:** 1120–1125.
25. WIGLER, M., A. PELLICER, S. SILVERSTEIN, R. AXEL, G. URLAUB & L. CHASIN. 1979. DNA-mediated transfer of the adenine phosphoribosyltransferase locus into mammalian cells. Proc. Natl. Acad. Sci. USA **76:** 1373–1376.
26. MARKOWITZ, D., S. GOFF & A. BANK. 1988. Construction and use of a safe and efficient amphotropic packaging cell line. Virology **167:** 400–405.
27. RICHARDSON, C., M. WARD, S. PODDA & A. BANK. 1994. Mouse fetal liver cells lack functional amphotropic retroviral receptors. Blood **84:** 433–439.
28. RICHARDSON, C. & A. BANK. 1995. Preselection of transduced murine hematopoietic stem cell populations leads to increased long-term stability and expression of the human multiple drug resistance gene. Blood **86:** 2579–2589.
29. YAN, X. Q., R. BRIDDELL, C. HARTLEY, G. STONEY, B. SAMAL & I. MCNIECE. 1994. Mobilization of long-term hematopoietic reconstituting cells in mice by the combination of stem cell factor plus granulocyte colony-stimulating factor. Blood **84:** 795–799.
30. O'NEILL, D., J. YANG, K. BORNSCHLEGEL & A. BANK. 1995. Delayed human gamma- to beta-globin gene switching in a transgenic mouse line by deletion of a nuclear protein binding site. Blood (Suppl) **86:** 7a.

31. BANK, A., L. W. DOW, M. G. FARACE, J. V. O'DONNELL, S. FORD & C. NATTA. 1973. Changes in globin synthesis with erythroid cell maturation in sickle thalassemia. Blood **41:** 353–357.
32. PLATT, O. S. 1995. The Sickle Syndromes. *In* Blood: Principles and Practice of Hematology. R. Handin, S. Lux & T. Stossel, Eds.: 1645–1650. Lippincott. Philadelphia.
33. PETERSON, K. R., Q. L. LI, C. H. CLEGG, T. FURUKAWA, P. A. NAVAS, E. J. NORTON, T. G. KIMBROUGH & G. STAMATOYANNOPOULOS. 1995. Use of yeast artificial chromosomes (YACs) in studies of mammalian development: Production of beta locus YAC mice carrying human globin developmental mutants. Proc. Natl. Acad. Sci. USA **92:** 5655–5659.
34. ELLIS, J., K. C. TAN-UN, A. HARPER, D. MICHALOVICH, N. YANNOUTSOS, S. PHILIPSEN & F. GROSVELD. 1996. A dominant chromatin-opening activity in 5' hypersensitive site 3 of the human beta-globin locus control region. EMBO J. **15:** 562–568.
35. PAWLIUK, R., R. KAY, P. LANSDORP & R. K. HUMPHRIES. 1994. Selection of retrovirally transduced hematopoietic cells using CD24 as a marker of gene transfer. Blood **84:** 2868–2877.

Pathophysiology of Iron Overload[a]

CHAIM HERSHKO,[b-d] GABRIELA LINK,[d] AND
IOAV CABANTCHIK[e]

[c]*Department of Medicine, Shaare Zedek Medical Center, [d]Department of Human Nutrition and Metabolism, Hebrew University Hadassah Medical School, and [e]Department of Biological Chemistry, Institute of Life Sciences, The Hebrew University, Jerusalem, Israel*

> ABSTRACT: In thalassemia, iron overload is the joint outcome of excessive iron absorption and transfusional siderosis. While iron absorption is limited by a physiologic ceiling of about 3 mg/d, plasma iron turnover in thalassemia may be 10 to 15 times normal, caused by the wasteful, ineffective erythropoiesis of an enormously expanded erythroid marrow. This outpouring of catabolic iron exceeds the iron-binding capacity of transferrin and appears in plasma as non-transferrin-plasma iron (NTPI). The toxicity of NTPI is much higher than of transferrin-iron as judged by its ability to promote hydroxyl radical formation resulting in peroxidative damage to membrane lipids and proteins. In the heart, this results in impaired function of the mitochrondrial respiratory chain and abnormal energy metabolism manifested clinically in fatal hemosiderotic cardiomyopathy. Ascorbate increases the efficacy of iron chelators by expanding the intracellular chelatable iron pool, but, at suboptimal concentrations is a pro-oxidant, enhancing the catalytic effect of iron in free radical formation. NTPI is removed by i.v. DFO in a biphasic manner and reappears rapidly upon cessation of DFO, lending support to the continuous, rather than intermittent, use of chelators. Unlike DFO and other hexadentate chelators, bidentate chelators such as L1 may produce incomplete intermediate iron complexes at suboptimal drug concentrations.

As an introduction to this session dedicated to iron-chelating therapy in thalassemia, it may be useful to review the reasons why this treatment is necessary and the mechanisms of tissue damage caused by the excessive accumulation of iron. Accordingly, I would like to focus on the following points related to the pathophysiology of iron overload in thalassemia: (1) the anomalous pathways of iron exchange in thalassemic patients; (2) the nature of non–transferrin-bound plasma iron (NTBI); (3) the role of NTBI in organ damage in thalassemia; and (4) the mechanism of iron mobilization by iron-chelating drugs and its consequences.

IRON BALANCE IN THALASSEMIA

Normal iron balance is characterized by a very efficient reprocessing of catabolic iron derived from senescent red blood cells and its reutilization for the production of new erythrocytes. This cycle represents about 85% of the plasma iron turnover (PIT), which is

---

[a]This work was supported by the Israel Science Foundation administered by the Israel Academy of Sciences and Humanities.

[b]Address for correspondence: C. Hershko, Dept. of Medicine, Shaare Zedek Medical Center, Jerusalem, Israel, P.O. Box 293.

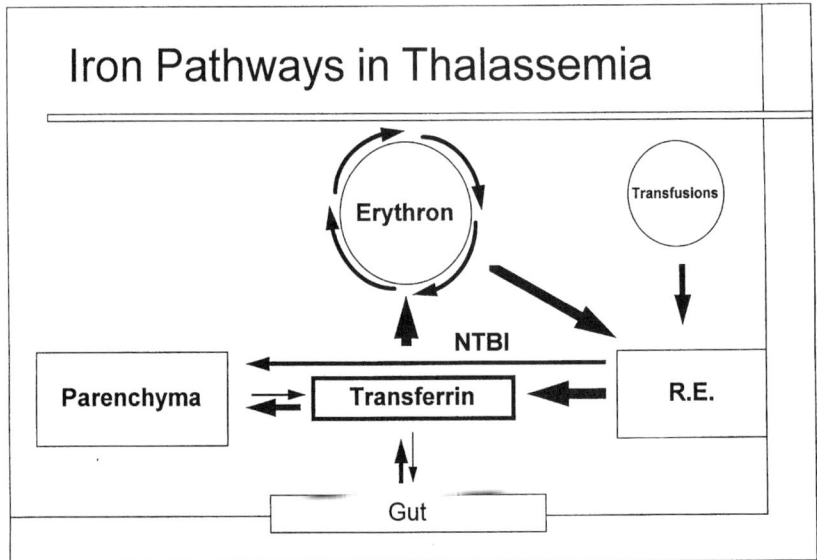

FIGURE 1. Schematic description of the anomalous metabolism of iron in thalassemia. Because of an emormously increased rate of ineffective erythropoiesis, hemoglobin breakdown in RE cells results in the outpouring of catabolic iron and a 10–15-times increase in plasma iron turnover. This results in complete saturation of transferrin and the emergence of an anomalous non-transferrin–bound plasma iron (NTBI) fraction.[2,5] The net increase in iron stores is caused by increased intestinal absorption and transfusions.

normally about 0.7 mg/kg/d. Only about 3% of the PIT is contributed by intestinal aborption.[1] By contrast, in thalassemia, ineffective erythropoiesis results in a drastic increase in PIT, 10 to 15 times that in normal subjects.[2] This wasteful production of non-viable RBC stimulates iron absorption, but most of the iron released to the circulation is derived from RBC catabolism (FIG. 1). Since the capacity of transferrin to carry iron is limited, some of this catabolic iron emerges in the plasma in the form of non–transferrin-bound plasma iron or NTBI.

NON-TRANSFERRIN PLASMA IRON

The concept of an anomalous plasma iron fraction in severe iron overload when transferrin is completely saturated originated from our studies on the mechanism of *in vivo* iron chelation. We have found that diethylenetriamine pentaacetic acid (DTPA), a hydrophilic chelator unable to penetrate cells, promotes urinary iron excretion of catabolic RBC iron with an efficiency equal to that of deferoxamine (DF).[3] Accordingly, we have concluded that iron chelation does not necessarily require the intracellular presence of a chelator, raising the possibility that chelatable iron may exist in the plasma.

Studying serum samples from thalassemic patients with severe iron overload, we have found that transferrin in such patients is completely saturated.[4] In order to examine whether all iron in the plasma was transferrin-bound, we used two methods: First, we employed a Sephadex adsorption column in which all iron bound to transferrin was eluted, but low molecular iron complexes were retained. Second, we used Amicon filters, which retained transferrin and all proteins above a molecular weight of 25,000 daltons.

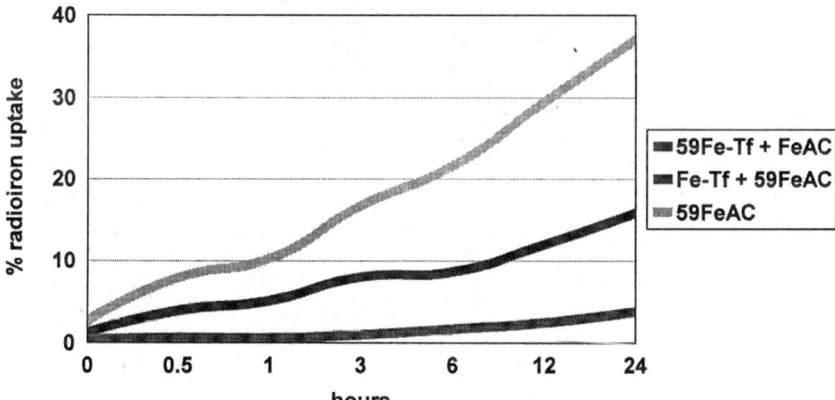

FIGURE 2. Iron uptake (transferrin-bound and NTBI radioiron) by cultured heart cells. The iron-loading solution contained 20 μg/ml of elemental iron (NTBI) supplied as ferric ammonium citrate.[14] Radioiron was either bound to transferrin first and then followed by NTBI (^{59}Fe-Tf +FeAC) or transferrin was first saturated with cold iron followed by NTBI labeled with radioiron (Fe-Tf +^{59}FeAC); or radioiron mixed with NTBI in serum-free medium (^{59}FeAC). As the iron-binding capacity of transferrin represented only 3.1% of the total iron in the culture medium, NTBI uptake was several hundredfold higher than that of transferrin iron.

Measurements employing both methods have been in close agreement, indicating the presence of low molecular weight iron at a concentration ranging from 1 to 11 μmol/L.[5] In addition, we have shown that the NTPI fraction disappeared following the addition of unsaturated transferrin, confirming its availability for transferrin binding. We have also shown that the addition of ferritin to normal plasma did not result in the production of NTPI. Finally, we have shown a close correlation between the magnitude of NTPI and the amount of DTPA-induced urinary iron excretion in the same patients, implying a direct participation of NTPI in the chelatable extracelullar iron pool. We have proposed that "in view of the known toxicity of unbound iron, its identification in thalassemic sera might be of relevance to the pathogenesis of tissue damage and the protective effect of iron-chelating therapy in this disease."[5]

Our original description of the existence of a chelatable, low molecular weight plasma iron fraction in patients with severe iron overload has been greeted with considerable skepticism. However, subsequent studies have confirmed the existence of NTPI using a variety of methods.[6–13] NTPI was shown to promote the formation of free hydroxyl radicals and to accelerate the peroxidation of membrane lipids *in vitro*.[11] Improved methods for the direct quantitation of NTPI in patients undergoing chelation therapy with DF, using nitriloacetic acid ultrafiltration and UV detection with high-performance liquid chromatography,[6] have been developed. Studies by Al-Rafaie and coworkers in thalassemic patients have shown that long-term treatment with DF or Deferiprone (L1) results in a marked decrease of their NTPI measurements.[12] More recent studies by Porter and coworkers[13] have clearly demonstrated that plasma NTPI is removed by intravenous DF therapy in a biphasic manner and that upon cessation of DF infusion it reappears rapidly, lending support to the continuous, rather than intermittent, use of DF in high-risk patients. The rate of low molecular weight iron uptake by cultured rat heart cells is over 300-times greater than that of transferrin iron (FIG. 2).[14] Moreover, unlike transferrin-iron uptake, which is inhibited at high tissue iron concentrations by down-regulation of transferrin receptor production, non-transferrin iron uptake is increased by high tissue iron content.[15] Such uptake was shown to result in increased myocardial lipid peroxidation and abnormal contractility, and these effects were reversed by *in vitro* treatment with DF.[16] Recognition of NTPI as a potentially toxic component of plasma iron in thalassemic siderosis has important practical implications for designing better strategies for the effective administration of DF and other iron-chelating drugs.

ROLE OF NTPI IN MYOCARDIAL DISEASE

The failure to produce a satisfactory animal model of hemochromatosis has greatly hindered research on the pathogenesis of iron toxicity. Consequently, we have developed an experimental model of rat myocardial cells in culture for studying the harmful effects of iron and the protective effects of iron chelation.[16–22] A unique feature of these cultures is their ability to differentiate into spontaneously contracting cells, offering an opportunity to study simultaneously the biochemical and functional effects of iron toxicity in heart cells.[14] We have used ferric ammonium citrate at concentrations ranging from 5 to 40 µg/ml to simulate the effect of NTPI on cultured heart cells. Employing iron-loading for 24 h, this method resulted in the uptake of 20 to 30% of NTPI from the culture medium. It also resulted in marked aberrations in heart cell function expressed in decreased rates and amplitude of contractility and in severe arrhythmia resembling ventricular fibrillation.[16]

The role of iron in promoting the conversion of superoxide and hydrogen peroxide into the highly toxic free hydroxyl radicals through the Haber-Weiss reaction is well documented.[23] Increased lipid peroxidation is the most easily measurable effect and is usually regarded as the most significant event in the pathogenesis of cellular damage. Increased *in vivo* lipid peroxidation may be measured by the increased formation and tissue concentrations of malonyldialdehyde (MDA), of conjugated dienes in tissues, or increased respiratory excretion of low molecular weight alkanes,[24,25] all of which represent products of lipid peroxidation. The peroxidation of polyunsaturated fatty acids results in the formation of highly reactive aldehydes such as malonyldialdehyde and 4-hydroxynonenal, leading to the formation of covalent links to proteins or protein adducts.[26]

A number of cellular lipid membrane structures have been considered as possible targets for iron-induced peroxidative damage. Decreased latent activity of *lysosomal* enzymes, implying increased fragility of the lysosomal membrane, has been demonstrated in biopsies obtained from the livers of patients with primary and transfusional hemosiderosis.[27] Disruption of lysosomal membranes resulting in the release of hydrolytic enzymes into the cytosol may result in significant damage to other subcellular organelles and ultimately in cell death.[28] Our own studies, employing lysosomal β-hexosaminidase as an indicator of iron-induced lysosomal damage, have shown that *in vitro* iron loading of cultured heart cells is associated with a marked increase in total β-hexosaminidase activity, and that this may be attributed to increased lysosomal fragility as evidenced by the loss of lysosomal latency and increased free enzyme activity.[29]

Another organelle implicated in iron toxicity is the cytoplasmic or, in the case of heart cells, sarcolemmal membrane. Disruption of the sarcolemmal membrane in cultured mouse myocardial cells has been demonstrated following exposure to increased concentrations of environmental oxygen and iron.[30] Our studies of sarcolemmal thiolic enzymes in iron-loaded heart cells have shown a loss of 5'-nucleotidase and Na,K-ATPase activity attributed to the direct, or indirect (via lipid peroxidation products) effects of increased oxidative stress on sarcolemmal thiolic enzymes.[31] Since Na,K-ATPase plays a significant role in cellular calcium homeostasis through the Na/Ca exchange mechanism, inactivation of Na,K-ATPase by iron toxicity may provide a direct link between the structural and functional abnormalities observed in iron-loaded cells.

Finally, mitochondrial injury has been implicated by Bacon and coworkers in rats with chronic iron overload, with a progressive reduction in ADP-stimulated respiration and res-

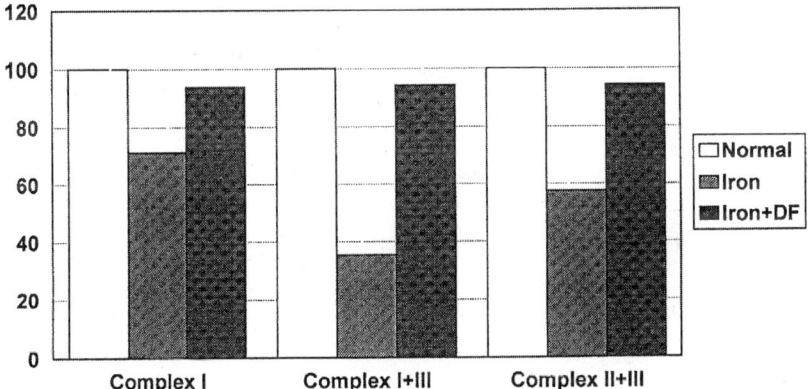

FIGURE 3. Effect of iron and deferoxamine on heart cell mitochondrial respiratory complex activity. Results are expressed as percent of control activity. Note the marked decrease in mitochondrial inner membrane respiratory complex activity after 24 h iron-loading as described in FIGURE 2, and its restoration by subsequent 24 h treatment with 0.3 mM DF. Complex I, NADH-ferricyanide reductase; Complex I+III, NADH-cytochrome c oxidoreductase; Complex II+III, Succinate cytochrome c oxidoreductase.[34]

piratory control rates at hepatic iron concentrations exceeding 1,000 μg/g together with increased conjugated diene formation, suggesting a cause-and-effect relation between iron-induced lipid peroxidation and impaired mitochondrial function.[32] These authors have also shown a 70% reduction in cytochrome c oxidase activity and a loss of hepatic ATP and ADP levels.[33] Our own studies in cultured, iron-loaded rat heart cells have shown a marked inhibition in the function of segments II to III of the mitochondrial inner membrane respiratory chain, monitored by measuring the activity of succinate-cytochrome c oxidoreductase.[34] This was completely reversed by *in vitro* DF treatment of the cultured heart cells (FIG. 3).

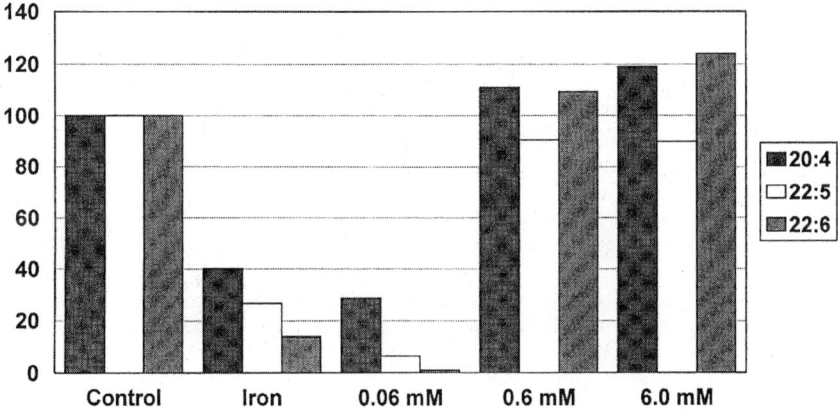

FIGURE 4. Biphasic effect of ascorbate on polyunsaturated fatty acid (PUFA) composition in iron-loaded heart cell membranes. 20:4, arachidonic acid; 22:5, docosapentaenoic acid; 22:6, docosahexaenoic acid. Note the sharp decrease in PUFA indicating increased lipid peroxidation caused by 24 h iron-loading, the aggravation of peroxidative damage at low ascorbate (0.06 mM) concentrations, and the prevention of peroxidative damage at high ascorbate concentrations.[20]

The toxicity of iron to heart cells is not a simple function of iron concentrations. It may be aggravated or inhibited by a number of coexistent variables: Reduction of ferric to ferrous iron promotes hydroxyl radical formation via the iron-driven Haber-Weiss reaction. Ascorbic acid, a natural reducing agent accelerates iron-induced lipid peroxidation in biological systems at low concentrations, but acts as an antioxidant at high concentrations (FIG. 4).[20,35,36] Moreover, clinical observations indicate that ascorbate supplementation may aggravate or accelerate the development of cardiac disease in patients with iron overload.[37] Conversely, α-tocopherol, a natural lipid-soluble antioxidant, is able to interrupt the chain reaction of membrane lipid peroxidation initiated by free radicals and to interfere with iron-induced lipid peroxidation in liposomes.[19,20,36] Finally, as shown in our heart cell culture studies, deferoxamine removes iron directly from iron-loaded heart cells, inhibits lipid peroxidation,[16–19] and reverses the abnormalities in cellular contractility and rhythmicity induced by iron.

PRINCIPLES OF IRON CHELATION

The Intracellular Labile Iron Pool

Current models of iron acquisition, sequestration, and storage by mammalian cells are based on a regulated adjustment of membrane transferrin receptor and cytosolic ferritin levels. Iron in transit between these two iron-binding proteins is believed to exist in a weakly bound low molecular weight complex,[38–40] which is also available for interaction with iron-chelating drugs.[41–44] This chelatable labile iron pool (LIP) is assumed to be sensed by a cytosolic iron-responsive protein (IRP), which coordinately represses ferritin mRNA translation and increases transferrin receptor mRNA stability.[45]

Measurement of the intracellular chelatable iron pool has been associated with major technical difficulties.[40] Analytical techniques relying on cell-disruptive steps are of limited use due to the dynamic nature of the cytosolic iron pool. Likewise, uncertainty exists regarding the relative levels of di- and trivalent iron in the cytosolic chelatable pool. Physicochemical measurements of tissue iron implicated Fe^{2+} as the dominant low molecular weight form in the cytosol,[46] but chemical determinations of iron in tissue extracts yielded variable results reflecting the propensity of Fe^{2+} for oxidation.[47]

Study of the LIP has been greatly facilitated by the recent development of a method allowing the continuous monitoring of intracellular fluorescence associated with the metal-sensitive probe calcein.[48] The fluorescence of calcein is quenched by its binding to Fe^{2+} and recovers when it yields iron to more potent iron chelators capable of penetrating the cell. Using this method, it was shown that in K562 cells the cytoplasmic concentration of Fe^{2+} ranges from 0.3 to 0.5 μM, and its mean transit time through the chelatable pool is 1–2 h. Further studies in K562 cells have shown the existence of efficient regulatory mechanisms preventing fluctuations in the size of the labile iron pool under conditions of moderate iron deprivation and iron loading. However, massive iron loading (100–200 μM ferric ammonium citrate) at concentrations similar to those used in our previous studies of iron-loaded heart cells, causes an apparently uncontrollable expansion in the chelatable pool, which fails to be matched by the sequestrating capacity of cellular ferritin.[49] This expanded LIP is an obvious target of intracellular iron chelation by drugs that are able to cross the barrier of the cytoplasmic membrane.

Role of Iron Stores in Reticuloendothelial and Parenchymal Cells

In iron overload, excess iron may be deposited in almost all tissues, but the bulk of iron is found in association with two cell types: reticuloendothelial (RE) cells, found in the spleen, liver, and bone marrow, and parenchymal tissues, represented by hepatocytes, endocrine cells, and myocytes. In contrast to RE cells, in which iron accumulation is relatively harmless, parenchymal siderosis, may result in significant organ damage. It is quite important therefore to determine whether DF or any other chelating drug may or may not interact preferentially with one of these two cellular storage compartments.

The source of iron and the proportion of iron retained in ferritin stores or recycled into the circulation from the two cell types are quite different. Reticuloendothelial cells have a limited ability to assimilate transferrin iron and they derive iron from the catabolism of hemoglobin in non-viable erythrocytes.[50] Most of this catabolic iron is recycled to plasma transferrin or NTPI within a few hours. In contrast, hepatic parenchymal cells maintain a dynamic equilibrium with plasma transferrin, with iron uptake predominating when transferrin saturation is high and release when serum iron and transferrin saturation are low.[1] In contrast to RE cells, the turnover of parenchymal iron stores is extremely low. In general, iron overload associated with increased intestinal absorption, such as hereditary hemochromatosis, results in predominant parenchymal siderosis, whereas in conditions wherein iron overload is caused by multiple blood transfusions, the primary site of siderosis is the RE cells. Considerable redistribution of iron may take place subsequently.

A number of experimental and clinical observations support the assumption that the urinary excretion of chelated iron is derived mainly from RE cells. Studies in hypertransfused rats using continuous DF infusion to capture all chelatable iron have shown that in contrast to hepatocellular radioiron excretion, which is confined entirely to the bile, most of the radioiron excretion derived from the RE label is recovered in the urine.[3,51,52] Moreover, when DTPA or IRC11, water-soluble synthetic chelators that do not enter cells easily, are employed in the same experimental model, there is no enhancement at all of hepatocellular iron excretion, but the enhancement of urinary RE radioiron excretion is similar or higher than that observed previously with DF.[53] Hence, DF obtains iron for chelation by one of two alternative mechanisms (1) *in situ* interaction with hepatocellular iron and subsequent biliary excretion and (2) chelation of iron derived from RBC catabolism in the RE system with subsequent urinary excretion. The observations described do not permit a firm conclusion as to whether RE-derived iron is chelated by DF within the RE cell or following its release into the plasma in the form of NTPI.[13]

Current Issues in Chelator Development

The introduction of effective long-term iron-chelating therapy by deferoxamine (DF) has changed the life expectancy of thalassemic patients.[54] This may be attributed mainly to the drastic decrease in cardiac mortality in well-chelated patients. DF is able to prevent cardiac disease and even reverse symptomatic myocardiopathy by aggressive, high-dose, continuous intravenous administration. Undoubtedly, DF remains the drug of choice for the management of transfusional siderosis in thalassemic patients. However, its high cost and the inconvenience of its parenteral administration by portable pumps are major limitations underlying the need for developing alternative orally effective new iron-chelating drugs. In the search for new and improved chelators it is useful to remember the following basic principles determining the safety and efficacy of iron chelators.

(1) The first principle is the stability of the chelator-iron complex. Stability is determined not only by the affinity of the drug to ferric iron, but also by the nature of their interaction. DF is a hexadentate chelator interacting with iron at a 1:1 ratio and forming of a neutral, stable complex preventing iron from participating in harmful chemical reactions, such as hydroxyl radical formation through the Haber-Weiss reaction. By contrast, deferiprone (L1) is a bidentate chelator. Three molecules of L1 and one ferric iron molecule are required to form a stable, neutral complex.[55] Hence, at suboptimal concentrations

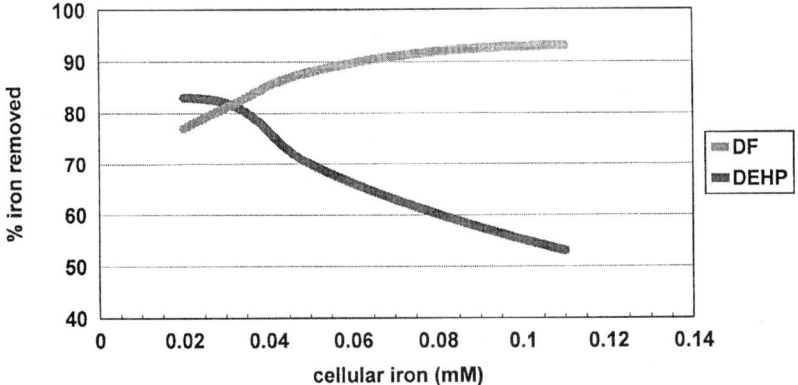

0.25 mM chelator / 24 h

FIGURE 5. Effect of cellular iron concentration on chelating efficiency. Comparison of the chelating efficiency in iron-loaded heart cells of a hexadentate (deferoxamine, DF) and bidentate (diethylhydroxypyrid-4-one, DEHP) chelator. Note the steady effect of 0.25 mM DF on the removal (80–90%) of cellular iron at all tissue iron concentrations. By contrast, DEHP has a diminishing effect with increasing tissue iron concentrations.[21]

of L1, when either tissue iron concentrations are very high or drug concentrations too low, incomplete 1:1 or 2:1 complexes may be formed resulting in impaired chelating efficiency on the one hand (FIG. 5) and the formation of potentially toxic intermediate iron complexes on the other. Thus, hexadentate chelators would, on theoretical grounds, always be preferable to bidentate or tridentate chelators in the quest for improved new medications.

(2) The partition coefficient of a chelator, its relative solubility in water and lipids, determines its ability to cross lipid membranes. Lipophilic compounds penetrate cells with relative ease and improve the ability of a chelator to interact with intracellular iron stores. Unfortunately, as shown by the experience with the family of hydroxypyrid-4-ones (of which L1 is the dimethyl derivative), increased lipophilicity may also increase drug toxicity.[56]

(3) Molecular weight is a critical feature in designing new chelators with improved oral efficacy and also important in determining the handling of iron following its chelation. Macromolecular complexes of iron chelators may be effective in binding iron but may also interfere with its subsequent urinary excretion. Likewise, new chelators with excellent *in vitro* interaction with chelatable iron in cell cultures or following their parenteral administration may be ineffective if their size interferes with their intestinal absorption.

(4) Prodrugs are an excellent solution for a number of requirements in the development of oral chelators. An outstanding example is the improvement of the hexadentate chelator N,N'-bis(2-hydroxybenzoyl) ethylenediamine-N,N'-diacetic acid (HBED) by converting its carboxylic groups into methyl esters.[57] By comparison with HBED, the prodrug dimethylHBED is less polar and its intestinal absorption is improved dramatically. Following its absoption it is converted into HBED. However, because of its gradual absorption, its overall effect in enhancing iron excretion is several-fold higher than that of HBED. Other hexadentate prodrugs of HBED-derivatives are presently under intensive evaluation.[58] As emphasized earlier, protection against the harmful effects of circulating NTBI is optimal when the chelator is permanently present in the plasma. Similar to continuous sub-

cutaneous or intravenous drug infusion, this effect may be achieved conveniently by employing orally effective prodrugs in slow-release tablets.

SUMMARY

Ineffective erythropoiesis and polytransfusion in thalassemic patients results in severe aberrations in iron homeostasis leading to severe iron overload and the emergence of an anomalous non-transferrin-bound plasma iron (NTBI) compartment.

NTBI deposition in parenchymatous tissues accelerates the development of myocardial and hepatic siderosis, induces peroxidative injury to membrane lipids and proteins, and terminates in severe damage to vital organs.

Myocardial disease is the leading cause of mortality related to iron overload in thalassemia. It is both preventible and reversible by effective iron-chelating therapy.

Better understanding of the pathophysiology of iron toxicity and the mechanism of iron chelation is vital for the development of improved strategies of iron-chelating therapy.

REFERENCES

1. COOK, J. D., G. MARSAGLIA, J. W. ESCHBACH et al. 1970. Ferrokinetics: A biologic model for plasma iron exchange in man. J. Clin. Invest. **49**: 197–205.
2. HERSHKO, C. & E. A. RACHMILEWITZ. 1979. Mechanism of desferrioxamine-induced iron excretion in thalassaemia. Br. J. Haematol. **42**: 125–132.
3. HERSHKO, C. 1975. A study of the chelating agent diethylenetriamine pentaacetic acid using selective radioiron probes of reticuloendothelial and parenchymal iron stores. J. Lab. Clin. Med. **85**: 913–921.
4. HERSHKO, C. & E.A. RACHMILEWITZ. 1975. Non transferrin plasma iron in patients with transfusional iron overload. In Proteins of Iron Storage and Transport in Biochemistry and Medicine. R. R. Crichton, Ed.: 437–433. Amersham. The Netherlands.
5. HERSHKO, C., G. GRAHAM, G. W. BATES & E. A. RACHMILEWITZ. 1978. Non-specific serum iron in thalassaemia: an abnormal serum iron fraction of potential toxicity. Br. J. Haematol. **40**: 255–263.
6. SINGH, S., R. C. HIDER & J. B. PORTER. 1990. A direct method for quantification of non-transferrin bound iron (NTBPI). Anal. Biochem. **186**: 320–323.
7. BATEY, R. G., P. LAI CHUNG FONG & S. SHERLOCK. 1978. The nature of serum iron in primary haemochromatosis. Clin. Sci. **55**: 24–28.
8. ANUWATANAKULCHAI, M., P. POOTRAKUL, P. THUVASETHAKUL & P. WASI. 1984. Non-transferrin plasma iron in β-thalassaemia/HbE and haemoglobin H diseases. Scand. J. Haematol. **32**: 153–158.
9. WANG, W. C., N. AHMED & M. HANNA. 1986. Non-transferrin-bound iron in long-term transfusion in children with congenital anemias. J. Pediatr. **108**: 552–557.
10. WAGSTAFF, M., S. W. PETERS, B. M. JONES & A. JACOBS. 1985. Free iron and iron toxicity in iron overload. Br. J. Haematol. **61**: 566–567.
11. GUTTERIDGE, J. M. C., D. A. ROWLEY, E. GRIFFITHS & B. HALLIWELL. 1985. Low-molecular-weight iron complexes and oxygen radical reactions in idiopathic haemochromatosis. Clin. Sci. **68**: 463–467.
12. AL-REFAIE, F. N., D. G. WICKENS, B. WONKE, G. J. KONTOGHIORGHES & A. V. HOFFBRAND. 1992. Serum non-transferrin-bound iron in beta-thalassaemia major patients treated with desferrioxamine and L1. Br. J Haematol. **82**: 431–436.
13. PORTER, J. B., R. D. ABEYSINGHE, L. MARSHALL, R. C. HIDER & S. SINGH. 1996. Kinetics of removal and reappearance of non-transferrin-bound plasma iron with deferoxamine therapy. Blood **88**: 705–713.
14. LINK, G., A. PINSON & C. HERSHKO. 1985. Heart cells in culture: a model of myocardial iron overload and chelation. J. Lab. Clin. Med. **106**: 147–153.

15. RANDELL, E. W., J. G. PARKES, N. F. OLIVIERI & D. M. TEMPLETON. 1994. Uptake of non-transferrin-bound iron by both reductive and nonreductive processes is modulated by intracellular iron. J. Biol. Chem. **269**: 16046–16053.
16. LINK, G., P. ATHIAS, A. GRYNBERG, A. PINSON & C. HERSHKO. 1989. Effect of iron loading on transmembrane potential, contraction and automaticity of rat ventricular muscle cells in culture. J. Lab. Clin. Med. **113**: 103–111.
17. MOREB, J., C. HERSHKO & Y. HASIN. 1988. Effects of acute iron loading on contractility and spontaneous beating rate of cultured rat myocardial cells. Basic Res. Cardiol. **83**: 360–368.
18. LINK, G., A. PINSON & C. HERSHKO. 1985. Heart cells in culture: a model of myocardial iron overload and chelation. J. Lab. Clin. Med. **106**: 147–153.
19. HERSHKO, C., G. LINK & A. PINSON. 1987. Modification of iron uptake and lipid peroxidation by hypoxia, ascorbic acid, and a-tocopherol in iron-loaded rat myocardial cell cultures. J. Lab. Clin. Med. **110**: 355–361.
20. LINK, G., A. PINSON, I. KAHANE & C. HERSHKO. 1989. Iron loading modifies the fatty acid composition of cultured rat myocardial cells and liposomal vesicles: Effect of ascorbate and a-tocopherol on myocardial lipid peroxidation. J. Lab. Clin. Med. **114**: 243–249.
21. HERSHKO, C., G. LINK, A. PINSON, H. H. PETER, P. DOBBIN & R. C. HIDER. 1991. Iron mobilization from myocardial cells by 3-hydroxypyridin-4-one chelators: Studies in rat heart cells in culture. Blood **77**: 2049–2053.
22. LINK, G., P. ATHIAS, A. GRYNBERG, C. HERSHKO & A. PINSON. 1991. Iron loading modifies β-adrenergic responsiveness of cultured ventricular myocytes. Cardioscience **2**: 27–30.
23. HALLIWELL, B. & J. M. C. GUTTERIDGE. 1990. Role of free radicals and catalytic metal ions in human disease: an overview. Methods Enzymol. **186**: 1–85.
24. GODDARD, J. G. & G. D. SWEENEY. 1983. Ferric nitriloacetate: a potent stimulant of in vivo lipid peroxidation in mice. Biochem. Pharmacol. **32**: 3879–3882.
25. DILLARD, C. J., J. E. DOWNEY & A. L. TAPPEL. 1984. Effect of antioxidants on lipid peroxidation in iron-loaded rats. Lipids **19**: 127–133.
26. HOUGLUM, K., M. FILIP, J. L. WITZTUM & M. CHOIKIER. 1990. Malondialdehyde and 4-hydroxynonenal protein adducts in plasma and liver of rats with iron overload. J. Clin. Invest. **86**: 1991–1998.
27. SEYMOUR, C. A. & T. J. PETERS. 1978. Organelle pathology in primary and secondary hemochromatosis with special reference to lysosomal changes. Br. J. Haematol. **40**: 239–253.
28. WEIR, M. P., J. F. GIBSON & T.J. PETERS. 1984. Haemosiderin and tissue damage. Cell Biochem. Funct. **2**: 186–194.
29. LINK, G., A. PINSON & C. HERSHKO. 1993. Iron loading of cultured cardiac myocytes modifies sarcolemmal structure and increases lysosomal fragility. J. Lab. Clin. Med. **121**: 127–134.
30. SCOTT, J. A., B. ANKHAW, E. LOCKE, E. HABER & C. HOMNEY. 1985. The role of free radical-mediated processes in oxygen-related damage in cultured murine myocardial cells. Circ. Res. **56**: 72–77.
31. LINK, G., A. PINSON & C. HERSHKO. 1994. The ability of orally effective iron chelators dimethyl- and diethyl-hydroxypyrid-4-one and of deferoxamine to restore sarcolemmal thiolic enzyme activity in iron-loaded heart cells. Blood **83**: 2692–2697.
32. BACON, B. R., C. H. PARK, G. M. BRITTENHAM, R. O'NEILL & A. S. TAVILL. 1985. Hepatic mitochondrial oxidative metabolism in rats with chronic dietary iron overload. Hepatology **5**: 789–797.
33. BACON, B. R., R. O'NEILL & R. S. BRITTON. 1993. Hepatic mitochondrial energy production in rats with chronic iron overload. Gastroenterology **105**: 1134–1140.
34. LINK, G., R. TIROSH, A. PINSON & C. HERSHKO. 1996. Role of iron in the potentiation of anthracycline toxicity: Identification of heart cell mitochondria as the site of iron-anthracycline interaction. J. Lab. Clin. Med. **127**: 272–278.
35. HEYS, A. D. & T. L. DORMANDY. 1981. Lipid peroxidation in iron loaded spleens. Clin. Sci. **60**: 295–301.
36. O'CONNELL, M. J., R. J. WARD, H. BAUM & T. J. PETERS. 1985. The role of iron in ferritin- and haemosiderin-mediated lipid peroxidation in liposomes. Biochem. J. **229**: 135–139.
37. NIENHUIS, A. W. 1981. Vitamin C and iron. N. Engl. J. Med. **304**: 170–171.
38. JACOBS, A. 1977. Low molecular weight intracellular iron transport compartments. Blood **50**: 433–436.

39. CRICHTON, R. R. & R. J. WARD. 1992. *In* Iron and Human Diseases, R. B. Laufer, Ed.: 23–76. CRC Press. Boca Raton, FL.
40. BREUER, W., S. EPSZTEIN & Z. I. CABANTCHIK. 1995. Iron acquired from transferrin by K562 cells is delivered into a cytoplasmic pool of chelatable iron(II). J Biol. Chem. **270**: 24209–24215.
41. HERSHKO, C. & D. J. WEATHERALL. 1988. Iron chelating therapy. Crit. Rev. Clin. Lab. Sci. **26**: 303–345.
42. ROTHMAN, R. J., A. SERRONI & J. L. FARBER. 1992. Cellular pool of transient ferric iron, chelatable by deferoxamine and distinct from ferritin, that is involved in oxidative cell injury. Molec. Pharmacol. **42**: 703–710.
43. PONKA, P., R. W. GRADY, A. WILCZYNSKA & H. M. SCHULMAN. 1984. The effect of various chelating agents on the mobilization of iron from reticulocytes in the presence and absence of pyridoxal isonicotinoyl hydrazone. Biochim. Biophys. Acta **802**: 477–489.
44. BAKER, E., D. RICHARDSON, S. GROSS & P. PONKA P. 1992. Evaluation of the iron chelation potential of hydrazones of pyridoxal, salicylaldehyde and 2-hydroxy-1-naphthylaldehyde using the hepatocyte in culture. Hepatology **15**: 492–501.
45. KLAUSNER, R. D., T. A. ROUAULT & J. B. HARFORD. 1993. Regulating the fate of mRNA: The control of cellular iron metabolism. Cell **72**: 19–28.
46. ST. PIERRE, T. G., D. R. RICHARDSON, E. BAKER & J. WEBB. 1992. A low-spin iron complex in human melanoma and rat hepatoma cells and a high-spin iron(II) complex in rat hepatoma cells. Biochim. Biophys. Acta **1135**: 154–158.
47. POLLACK, S. 1992. Receptor mediated iron uptake and intracellular iron transport. Am. J Hematol. **39**: 113–117.
48. BREUER, W., S. EPSZTEJN, P. MILLGRAM & Z. I. CABANTCHIK. 1995. Transport of iron and other transition metals into cells as revealed by a fluorescent probe. Am. J. Physiol. **268**: C1354–1361.
49. BREUER, W., S. EPSZTEJN & Z. I. CABANTCHIK. 1997. Dynamics of the cytosolic chelatable iron pool of K562 cells. FEBS Lett. **382**: 304–308.
50. HERSHKO, C. 1977. Storage iron regulation. Progr. Hematol. **10**: 105–148.
51. HERSHKO, C. 1978. Determinants of fecal and urinary iron excretion in desferrioxamine treated rats. Blood **51**: 415–424.
52. HERSHKO, C., R. W. GRADY & A. CERAMI. 1978. Mechanism of iron chelation in the hypertransfused rat: definition of the two alternative pathways of iron mobilization. J. Lab. Clin. Med. **92**, 144–151.
53. HERSHKO, C, G. RIVKIN, G. LINK, E. SIMHON, R. L. CYJON & J. Y. KLEIN. 1996. IRC11, a new synthetic chelator with selective interaction with catabolic red cell iron. Blood **88** (Suppl. 1): abstract 1951.
54. GABUTTI, V. & C. BORGNA-PIGNATTI. 1994. Clinical manifestations and therapy of transfusional haemosiderosis. Clin. Haematol. **7**: 919–940.
55. PORTER, J. B., E. R. HUEHNS & R. C. HIDER. 1989. The development of iron chelating drugs. Clin. Haematol. **2**: 257–292.
56. PORTER, J. B., K. P. HOYES, R. D. ABEYSINGHE, P. N. BROOKS, E. R. HUEHNS & R. C. HIDER. 1991. Comparison of subacute toxicity and efficacy of orally active 3-hydroxypyridin-4-one iron chelators. Blood **78**: 2727–2734.
57. HERSHKO, C., R. W. GRADY & G. LINK. 1984. Phenolic ethylenediamine derivatives: A study of orally effective iron chelators. J. Lab. Clin. Med. **103**: 337–346.
58. SCHNEBLI, H. P., P. ACKLIN, P. BUHLMAYER *et al.* 1997. Progress towards new, orally active iron chelators. Presented at Sixth International Conference on Thalassaemia and the Haemoglobinopathies. St. Pauls's Bay, Malta. April 5–10, 1997. Abstract # 216.

The Origin of the Differences in (R)- and (S)-Desmethyldesferrithiocin

Iron-Clearing Properties[a]

RAYMOND J. BERGERON,[b] JAN WIEGAND, KATIE RATLIFF-THOMPSON, AND WILLIAM R. WEIMAR

Department of Medicinal Chemistry, University of Florida, Gainesville, Florida 32610, USA

ABSTRACT: The iron clearance properties, toxicity, and pharmacokinetics of (R)- and (S)-desmethyldesferrithiocin (DMDFT) are described. The studies were performed in rodent and primate models. While both enantiomers were found to be effective iron chelators with minimal toxicity in the rodents, only (S)-DMDFT was able to induce the clearance of any iron in the primates. In addition, two out of nine of the monkeys given (R)-DMDFT died within 24 h of drug administration. The reason for the differences in iron clearance properties and the apparent toxicity of the (R)-enantiomer in the primates is likely related to the disparities in the pharmacokinetics of the two analogues. The pharmacokinetic data suggest enantioselectivity in renal clearance of the desferrithiocins and their iron complexes with (S)-DMDFT clearance 3.5 times greater than that of (R)-DMDFT, and Fe^{III} [(S)-DMDFT]$_2$ clearance 6.8 times greater than that of Fe^{III} [R-DMDFT]$_2$. In all primates studied Fe^{III} [(R)-DMDFT]$_2$ in the plasma exceeded 25 mg/L (50 µM) for several hours and remained above 10 mg/L (20 µM) at 8 h while levels of Fe^{III} [(S)-DMDFT]$_2$ never exceeded 50 µM and were at or below the limits of detection 8 h post-injection.

The commercial introduction of Desferrioxamine B (DFO) 30 years ago[1] provided a life-saving treatment for iron overload in chronically transfused thalassemia patients. The subcutaneous infusion of DFO is still regarded as the method of choice for handling transfusional iron overload.[2–4] Although the drug's efficacy and long-term tolerability are well documented, it still suffers from a number of shortcomings associated with its high cost of production, poor to moderate efficiency, and its marginal oral activity. This situation is further complicated by the fact that DFO has a very short half-life in the body and must therefore be administered by continuous subcutaneous infusion over long periods of time and can be very immunogenic.[5–7] This translates at the clinical level into poor patient compliance.[8] In order to alleviate these problems, the development of an orally effective iron chelator has been a therapeutic strategy for many years.

Although a substantial number of synthetic iron chelators have been studied in recent years as potential orally active therapeutics, *e.g.*, pyridoxal isonicotinic hydrazone,[9] hydroxypyridones,[10,11] and bis(*o*-hydroxybenzyl) ethylenediaminediacetic acid analogues,[12] none has yet proven to be completely satisfactory. Interestingly, the siderophores, microbial iron

---

[a]Financial support was provided by National Institutes of Health Grant No. RO1DK49108.

[b]Correspondence and reprint requests should be sent to: Raymond J. Bergeron, Department of Medicinal Chemistry, P.O. Box 100485 JHMHC, University of Florida, Gainesville, FL 32610; Tel: (352) 846-1956; Fax: (352) 392-8406; E-mail: bergeron@mc.cop.ufl.edu

chelators, have remained relatively untouched in this search. Their evaluation as iron clearing agents has not at all paralleled the rate of their isolation and structural elucidation.

While most siderophores fall primarily into two structural classes, hydroxamates or catecholamides,[13–19] there are a number of compounds which do not belong to either family, e.g., pyochelin,[20] rhizobactin,[21] and 2-(3′-hydroxypyrid-2′-yl)-4-methylthiazoline-4(S)-carboxylic acid (desferrithiocin, DFT).[22–27] DFT, isolated from *Streptomyces antibioticus*,[28] was shown to form a stable 2:1 complex with iron (III), ($K^f = 4 \times 10^{29}$ M^{-1}).[29] Studies in rodents have demonstrated mobilization of iron from liver ferritin by DFT,[30] and a preliminary investigation in primates[31] suggested that it was indeed an orally active iron chelator. A more comprehensive investigation in our laboratory carried out in a bile duct-cannulated rat model[22–24,32] as well as in a *Cebus* monkey model[22,24,27,33–35] has supported these findings and quantified the drug's effectiveness.[22–24,34] Unfortunately, animals chronically exposed to DFT presented with nephrotoxicity.[24,35]

We have demonstrated that small structural changes in the desferrithiocin molecule can have a profound effect on the compound's iron clearance and toxic properties.[24–27] For example, formal reduction of the desazadesmethyl DFT thiazoline to a thiazolidine, expansion of the desmethyl DFT thiazoline ring to a thiazine, or substitution of the thiazoline sulfur of desazadesmethyl DFT with an oxygen all led to a substantial loss of activity,[25] while the conversion of (S)-DFT to (S)-desmethyl DFT (DMDFT) resulted in an analogue with acceptable iron clearance properties and substantially reduced toxic effects.[24] The iron clearance properties and the toxicity of (S)-DMDFT have been reported,[23,24] but until now, little was known about the properties of its (R)-enantiomer.[23] Because the starting material for (R)-DMDFT is the common naturally occurring amino acid L-cysteine,[23] (R)-DMDFT offers an enormous advantage in terms of synthesis as compared to the (S)-DMDFT analogue, whose starting material is D-cysteine. We now present a comparison of the iron-clearing efficiency and toxicity of (R)- versus (S)-DMDFT in a rodent model and in an iron-loaded *Cebus* monkey model. We also report a marked enantiospecific difference in the plasma and urine pharmacokinetics of (R)- and (S)-DMDFT and the corresponding Fe^{III} complexes following oral administration of (R)- vs. (S)-DMDFT to primates. The differences in toxicity between the two enantiomers is likely related to their pharmacokinetic behavior.

MATERIALS AND METHODS

Materials

DFO (desferrioxamine B mesylate salt, trade name: Desferal) was purchased from the hospital pharmacy. The (R)- and (S)-DMDFT analogues were synthesized as previously described,[23] except that the starting material for the (S)-DMDFT was D-cysteine. *Cebus apella* monkeys were purchased from World Wide Primates (Miami, FL). All reagents and standard iron solutions were obtained from Aldrich Chemical Co. (Milwaukee, WI). Atomic absorption (AA) measurements were made on a Perkin-Elmer model 5100 PC spectrophotometer (Norwalk, CT). Ultrapure salts were obtained from Johnson Matthey Electronics (Royston, England). Imferon, an iron dextran solution, was obtained from Fisons (Bedford, MA). Nalgene metabolic cages, rat jackets, and fluid swivels were purchased from Harvard Bioscience (South Natick, MA). Intramedic polyethylene tubing was obtained from Fisher Scientific (Pittsburgh, PA). All hematological and serum chemical tests were carried out by Allied Clinical Laboratories (Gainesville, FL). Cremophor RH-40 was obtained from BASF (Parsippany, NJ); Multistix 10 SG reagent strips for urinalysis were obtained from Miles Inc., Diagnostics Division (Elkhart, IN).

Noniron-Overloaded Bile Duct-cannulated Rat

Male Sprague-Dawley rats averaging 400 g were housed in Nalgene plastic metabolic cages during the experimental period and were provided free access to water. The animals were anesthetized using sodium pentobarbital (50 mg/kg) given intraperitoneally (i.p.). The bile duct was cannulated, using 22-gauge polyethylene tubing, about 1 cm from the duodenum. The cannula was inserted about 2 cm into the duct, and once bile flow was established, the cannula was tied snugly in place. A skin tunneling needle was inserted from the shoulder area around to the abdominal incision. The cannula was threaded through the needle until it emerged from the shoulder opening.

The cannula was then passed from the rat to the swivel inside a metal torque-transmitting tether, which was attached to a rodent jacket around the animal's chest. The cannula was directed from the rat to a Gilson micro fraction collector by a fluid swivel mounted above the metabolic cage. This system allowed the animal to move freely in the cage while continuous bile samples were being collected. Bile samples were collected at 3-h intervals. Urine samples were taken every 24 h. Sample handling was as previously described.[24,33]

Rodent Toxicity Studies

Male or female Sprague-Dawley rats averaging 400 g were housed in individual metabolic cages and fasted overnight. Prior to drug administration, the animals were weighed and evaluated for their general condition, and a baseline urine sample was obtained. The rats were then given the drugs once daily, following an overnight fast, for ten days. The compounds were administered by gavage at a dose of 384 µmol/kg (equivalent to 100 mg/kg of (S)-DFT sodium salt) in a 40% (v/v) Cremophor/water solution. The rats were allowed access to food 3 h after drug administration and for 5 h thereafter. The amount of food and water consumed and the volume of urine produced were recorded daily. The urine samples were analyzed each morning by dip-stick (Multistix 10 SG) for pH and specific gravity as well as for the presence of white blood cells, nitrite, urobilinogen, protein, blood, ketones, bilirubin, and glucose. In addition, the animals were weighed and their activity level and general condition were noted each day prior to the administration of the drug. A necropsy was performed whenever an animal died or at the conclusion of the experiment. Control animals were given an equivalent amount of the Cremophor/water solution and were maintained on the same diet schedule as the test animals.

Drug Preparation and Administration

DFO was given s.c. to rats at a dose of 150 µmol/kg in 40% (v/v) Cremophor RH-40/water and was given s.c. to primates at the same dose in sterile water. The desferrithiocin analogues were solubilized in 40% (v/v) Cremophor RH-40/water and were administered orally to rats and monkeys at a dose of 150 and 300 µmol/kg, respectively. Prior to chelator administration, monkeys were sedated with ketamine, 7–10 mg/kg administered intramuscularly (i.m.), and given scopolamine, 0.03–0.05 mg/kg i.m. to prevent ketamine-related salivation and vomiting. Both rats and monkeys were fasted for 24 h before dosing.

Primate Iron Loading

After i.m. anestheshia with ketamine, an intravenous (i.v.) infusion was started in a leg vein.[33] The iron dextran was added to approximately 90 ml of sterile normal saline and administered to the animals at a dose of 200 to 300 mg/kg. The iron solution was infused over 45 to 60 min. Two to three infusions separated by 10 to 14 days were necessary to load the monkeys to a level of 500 mg/kg of iron. This brought the serum transferrin iron saturation to 70 to 80%. The serum half-life of iron dextran in humans is 2.5 to 3 days. We waited 20 half-lives, or 60 days, before using any of the animals in iron-clearing experiments.

Primate Iron Balance Studies

Animals were maintained on a low-iron liquid diet[33] for seven days prior to drug administration. The animals were allotted food according to their body weight, and intake was carefully monitored. Three days before drug administration (day –2 to day 0), baseline iron intake and output values were measured. These same measurements were made for days +1 through +3 following drug administration. Iron balance status was determined by subtracting the iron output from the iron input.

Primate Fecal and Urine Samples

Twenty-four hour fecal and urine collections were initiated four days prior to the administration of the test drug. Fecal samples were assayed for the presence of occult blood, weighed, mixed with distilled deionized water, and autoclaved. The mixture was then homogenized and lyophilized; a sample of the resulting powder was digested by refluxing with low-iron nitric acid for 48 h. Monkey urine samples were sterilized, acidified and reconstituted to initial volume after sterilization. Iron concentrations were determined by flame AA.

Efficiency Calculations

The efficiency of each ligand was calculated assuming a 1:1 desferrioxamine-iron complex, or a 2:1 ligand-iron complex for the desferrithiocin analogues. Thus, in theory, 150 µmol/kg DFO or 300 µmol/kg DMDFT could induce an output of 150 µg-atoms Fe/kg, and efficiency = (actual total induced Fe/theoretical output) × 100%. For each individual monkey, total drug-induced iron excretion was calculated by averaging the iron output for three days prior to the administration of the drug and subtracting this baseline from the total iron excretion during the three days following the administration of the drug. Most of the induced Fe excretion occurred on day +1, with a return to baseline by day +2. The total drug-induced Fe excretion in the rodent model was calculated by subtracting the iron excretion of control animals from the iron excretion of treated animals.

Primate Hematological Screen

Animals were placed in metabolic cages[22,24] seven days prior to the administration of the drug and started on the low-iron liquid diet. Blood samples were taken at this time for testing. Due to the diurnal variability in some of the measurements, *i.e.,* UIBC, plasma iron, *etc.,* the blood samples were always drawn at the same time of day. The assays performed included: iron profile (iron, UIBC, TIBC, % saturation), CBC (white blood cells, red blood cells, hemoglobin, hematocrit, MCV, MCH, MCHC, platelet count), differential, and chemistry profile (glucose, sodium, potassium, chloride, CO_2, BUN, creatinine, calcium, phosphorous, total protein, albumin, alkaline phosphatase, SGOT, SGPT, total cholesterol, total bilirubin, globulin, gamma-glutamyl transpeptidase). Evaluation of these parameters allowed us to assess the health of the animals going into the experiment and to evaluate any subtle changes which the test drug may induce. Finally, a post-drug blood sample was taken from each animal on the last day of the experiment.

Collection of Pharmacokinetic Samples in Monkeys

Monkeys were fasted for approximately 16 h prior to a pharmacokinetic experiment and a fasting weight obtained. Animals were sedated with ketamine and scopolamine as described above and maintained with additional ketamine as needed. A 5 Fr., 16 inch urethral catheter was lubricated with K-Y Jelly and inserted into the bladder to allow for urine withdrawal. The compounds were solubilized in 40% (v/v) Cremophor RH-40/water and administered orally by gavage at a dose of 300 µmol/kg via an 8 Fr. feeding tube. It is important to point out that the pharmacokinetic studies for (R)- and (S)-DMDFT were carried out in the same *individual* animals, with a four-week resting period between experiments.

At times t = 0, 0.5, 1, 2, 3, 4, 6, and 8 h post-drug, blood samples (1.8 ml) were taken from a leg vein, mixed with 0.2 ml sodium citrate buffer, and centrifuged immediately. The separated plasma was stored on dry ice during the experiment. Urine was collected prior to drug administration and at 1/2-h intervals for four hours thereafter. At each designated time, the urine was aspirated and the bladder was rinsed two times with 5 ml of sterile normal saline. The volume of the combined urine-saline washes was recorded, and the urine mix was stored on dry ice. At the conclusion of the experiment, the plasma and urine samples were stored at –20 °C until HPLC analysis.

Plasma and Urine Analytical Methods

Plasma and urine pharmacokinetic samples were prepared for HPLC analysis by the following procedure: Samples were treated with an equal volume of methanol (1:1 v/v) at 4 °C for 30 minutes and centrifuged at $3000 \times g$ for 15 minutes to remove precipitated proteins. The methanolic supernatant was filtered through a 0.2-µm filter prior to injection. Calibration standards were prepared by the addition of known amounts of DMDFT or $Fe^{III}(DMDFT)_2$ to control plasma or urine, and the samples were then treated in the same manner as described above.

Analytical separation was performed on a Polymer Laboratories PLRP-S column (4.6 mm × 150 mm, 5 µm, 100 Å) using a Rainin Instrument Company HPLC system and UV detection at 310 nm by a Linear UVIS-206 Multiple Wavelength detector (Linear Instruments Corporation). The solvent gradient program consisted of an initial 5-min isocratic portion with 5% aqueous CH_3CN, followed by a linear gradient increase to 80% aqueous CH_3CN at 15 min, and ramping back to 5% CH_3CN for 3 min. The mobile phase was pumped at a flow rate of 1.0 ml/min.

The concentrations of DMDFT and Fe^{III} $(DMDFT)_2$ were calculated from the peak area fitted to calibration curves by nonweighted least squares linear regression with Rainin Dynamax HPLC Method Manager software (Rainin Instrument Co.). The method had a detection limit of 0.5 mg/L, and was reproducible and linear over a range of 1–500 mg/L.

Pharmacokinetic Analyses

Model-independent and model-dependent pharmacokinetic parameters were estimated from DMDFT and Fe^{III} $(DMDFT)_2$ plasma concentration-time data with the aid of PCNONLIN (SCI Software, Lexington, KY). The terminal elimination rate constant (k_{el}) was estimated by linear regression of the terminal concentration-time data; the terminal elimination half-life ($t_{1/2}$) was calculated from $0.693/k_{el}$. The area under the time-concentration curve from time zero to the time of the last measured plasma concentration (8 h) was calculated by the trapezoidal method. The AUC to the time infinity ($AUC_{0-\infty}$) was extrapolated by adding AUC_{0-8h} to the quotient of Cp/k_{el} where Cp is the last measured concentration (*i.e.,* at t = 8 h). The mean residence time (MRT) was obtained from $AUMC_{0-\infty}/AUC_{0-\infty}$ where AUMC is the area under the first moment curve (Cp*t vs. t). The renal clearance (CL_R) was calculated U_{0-4}/AUC_{0-4} where U_{0-4} is the amount of DMDFT or Fe^{III} $(DMDFT)_2$ excreted in the urine over a 4-hour collection interval (0–4 h), divided by the plasma AUC over the same interval, and normalized to adjust for the differences in body weights.

D-Amino Acid Oxidase Assay

(*S*)-DMDFT, (*R*)-DMDFT, Fe^{III} [(*S*)-DMDFT]$_2$, and Fe^{III} [(*R*)-DMDFT]$_2$ were examined for their effects on the activity of D-amino acid oxidase (D-AAO), both as potential substrates in comparison to D-phenylalanine (D-Phe) and as inhibitors in comparison to kojate. For both determinations, crystalline hog kidney D-AAO (Sigma A 1789), beef liver catalase (C 3155), flavin adenine dinucleotide (FAD, F 6625), kojic acid, and D-Phe were obtained from Sigma Chemical Co., St. Louis, MO. Rates of oxygen consumption in the air-saturated assay mixture were measured polarographically at 37 °C with an oxygen electrode (Yellow Spring Instruments) and chart recorder. The substrate activity assay mixture contained D-Phe or presumed D-AAO substrate (10 mM), FAD (20 µM), and catalase (2.5 µg) in a volume of 2.5 ml. The reaction was initiated by the addition of 2.5 µg D-AAO in 50 µl to the incubated, stirred assay mixture[36] resulting in a rapid rate of oxygen consumption when the substrate was 10 mM D-Phe. The ability to inhibit the D-AAO catalyzed reaction was examined by the addition of one of the above chelators or iron complexes (250 µM) to such a complete reaction mixture with D-Phe as substrate. Addition of 50 µl 2.5 mM kojate (final concentration of 100 µM), a known substrate-competitive D-AAO inhibitor (K_i = 15 µM), resulted in almost complete cessation of oxygen consumption and was a positive control for inhibition experiments.

RESULTS

Chelator-Induced Iron Clearance in Rodents

Three iron chelators (FIG. 1) were evaluated: Desferrioxamine (DFO), (*S*)-DMDFT (**1**), and (*R*)-DMDFT (**2**). The efficiency of orally (p.o.) administered desferrithiocin analogues was compared with subcutaneously (s.c.) administered DFO as a positive control. The efficiencies of the drugs were calculated based on the assumption that DFO and the desferrithiocin analogues form a 1:1 or a 2:1 complex, respectively, with the metal. At a dose of 150 µmol/kg, DFO induced a net excretion of 207 ± 37 µg Fe/kg (FIG. 2), with an efficiency of 2.5 ± 0.7%. Desmethyl DFT in the (*S*)-configuration given p.o. at the same dose induced 101 ± 20 µg Fe/kg, with an efficiency of 2.4 ± 0.6%. The (*R*)-enantiomer at the same dose was slightly more effective than the (*S*)-enantiomer (p > 0.12, *t*-test), generating 166 ± 37 µg Fe/kg (FIG. 2) with an efficiency of 3.9 ± 1.8%.

Rodent Drug Toxicity

We have reported that when (*S*)-DMDFT was evaluated in male Sprague-Dawley rats, no significant toxic side effects were found.[24] We have now completed the assessment of

Desferrioxamine B (DFO)

1 2

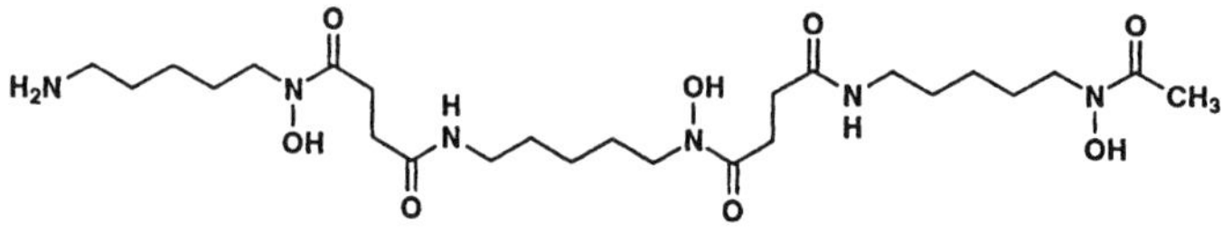

FIGURE 1. Structures of the iron chelators chosen for evaluation: Desferrioxamine (DFO), (*S*)-desmethyl DFT (**1**), and (*R*)-desmethyl DFT (**2**).

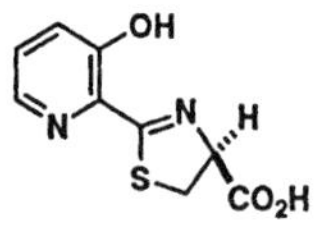

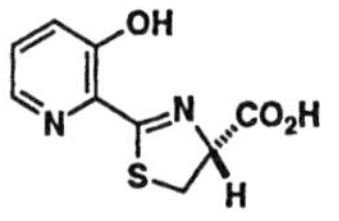

the (*R*)-enantiomer in both male and female rats. Once again, all of the rodents survived the 10-day exposure to the drug. The animals ate well and had normal urine and fecal production throughout the experiment. In addition, white blood cell counts, differentials, and urinalysis values were comparable to those obtained from control animals. Postmortem examination and kidney histology revealed no significant abnormalities and no notable differences between the enantiomers. The compounds thus emerged as promising analogues and were evaluated in the iron-loaded *Cebus* monkey model.

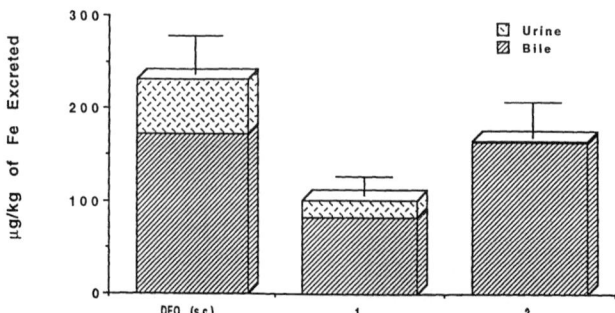

FIGURE 2. Response of the bile-duct cannulated rats to DFO, **1** and **2**. DFO was administered s.c. to the rats at a dose of 150 µmol/kg. The desferrithiocin analogues **1** and **2** were given orally by gavage at a dose of 150 µmol/kg. All of the compounds were solubilized in 40% (v/v) Cremophor RH-40/water.

Chelator-Induced Iron Clearance in Primates

While the variability in ligand-induced iron clearance was higher in the monkeys than in the rats, with each primate serving as its own control, effective chelators were readily identified. *Cebus* monkeys responded differently to the ligands than did rats (FIG. 3). We have demonstrated[33] that DFO administered s.c. to the monkeys at a dose of 150 µmol/kg cleared 471 ± 73 µg Fe/kg, an efficiency of 5.5 ± 0.9%, nearly twice that seen with the rodents. Oral administration of (*S*)-DMDFT to monkeys at a dose of 150 µmol/kg (1A) induced a net excretion of 203 ± 111 µg Fe/kg, an efficiency of 4.8 ± 2.7%. Furthermore, an excellent dose response relationship was observed.[24] The p.o. administration of 300 µmol/kg of the drug (1B) resulted in an excretion of 668 ± 206 µg Fe/kg (FIG. 3), an efficiency of 8.0 ± 2.5%, while p.o. administration of 450 µmol/kg of the drug (1C) induced elimination of 1358 ± 404 µg Fe/kg of iron, an efficiency of 10.8 ± 3.2%. Finally, (*S*)-DMDFT administered at a dose of 150, 300 or 450 µmol/kg was able to hold monkeys in negative iron balance.[24]

In contrast, at a dose of 300 µmol/kg in 40% (v/v) Cremophor/water, the (*R*)-enantiomer (**2**) had an induced iron clearance of only 46 ± 144 µg Fe/kg (FIG. 3), an efficiency of 0.5 ± 2%. Not surprisingly, the compound was not able to hold monkeys in negative iron balance. Owing to the death of one of the animals given (*R*)-DMDFT at a dose of 300 µmol/kg, higher dosages and parenteral administration were not attempted. The difference in the behavior of (*S*)-DMDFT versus (*R*)-DMDFT in the primates was noteworthy in view of the similarities seen in the rodents. Since the death of the monkey could not be definitively linked to the drug, we decided to perform pharmacokinetic studies in an attempt to explain the basis of the enantiomeric differences observed in primates.

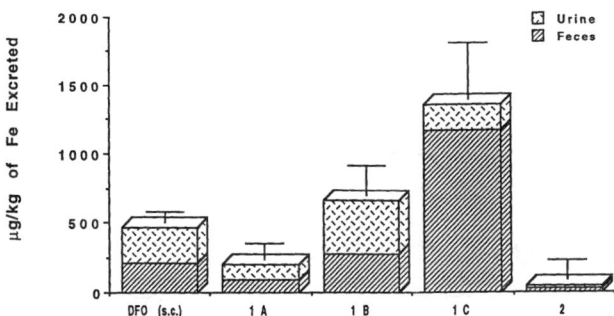

FIGURE 3. Response of the iron-loaded *Cebus* monkeys to DFO, **1** and **2**. DFO was administered s.c. to the monkeys at a dose of 150 µmol/kg in sterile water. (*S*)-DMDFT (**1**) was given orally to the primates at doses of 150, 300, and 450 µmol/kg (1A, 1B, and 1C, respectively). The two lower doses were solubilized in 40% (v/v) Cremophor RH-40/water and given by gavage, while the highest dose tested was given in capsules. (*R*)-DMDFT (**2**) was given orally by gavage in 40% (v/v) Cremophor RH-40/water at a dose of 300 µmol/kg.

Pharmacokinetics of (S)- and (R)-Desmethyldesferrithiocin in Primates

Inspection of the plasma concentration-time curves for (S)- vs. (R)-DMDFT (FIG. 4–*top*) and for Fe^{III} [(S)-DMDFT]$_2$ vs. Fe^{III} [(R)-DMDFT]$_2$ (FIG. 4–*bottom*) reveals several striking features. Note that, to avoid inter-individual differences, these experiments used the same four monkeys (2A4, 2A6, 2A12, and IC2). The peak plasma concentrations as well as AUC's of (R)-DMDFT and Fe^{III} [(R)-DMDFT]$_2$ curves (*dashed lines*) equal or exceed those of the corresponding (S)-DMDFT and Fe^{III} [(S)-DMDFT]$_2$ curves (*solid lines*). At 8 h post-treatment, the plasma concentrations of (S)-DMDFT and Fe^{III} [(S)-DMDFT]$_2$ had declined

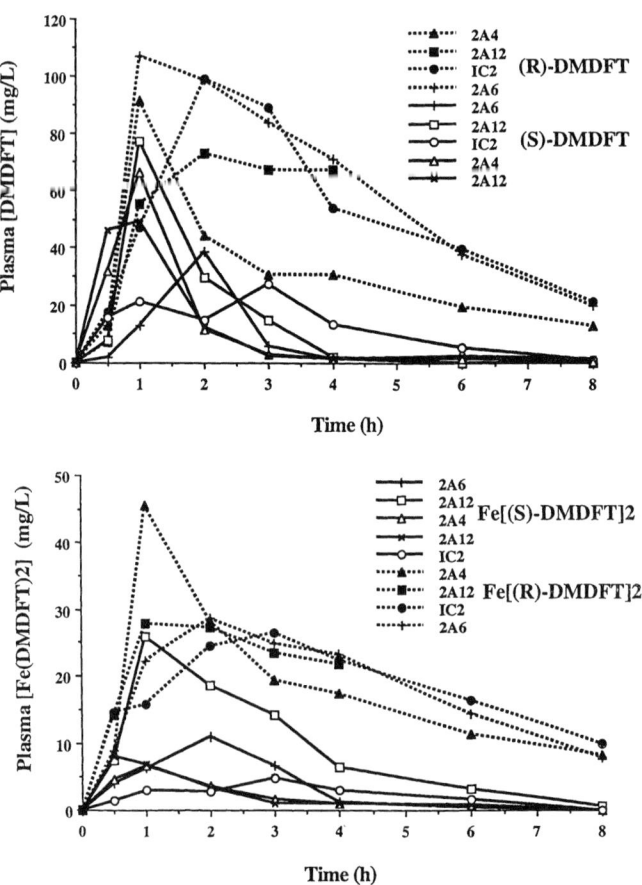

FIGURE 4. Plasma concentration vs. time curves for *Cebus* monkeys treated with (S)-DMDFT or (R)-DMDFT. (S)-DMDFT (**1**) or (R)-DMDFT (**2**) was given orally by gavage in 40% (v/v) Cremophor RH-40/water at a dose of 300 µmol/kg. *Top*: (S)- and (R)- DMDFT plasma concentrations vs. time; *Bottom*:: Fe[(S)- and (R)-DMDFT]$_2$ plasma concentrations vs. time.

to levels approaching the limits of detection, whereas substantial plasma concentrations of (R)-DMDFT and Fe^{III} [(R)-DMDFT]$_2$ still remained. Perhaps of special significance is that in every instance Fe^{III} [(R)-DMDFT]$_2$ in the plasma exceeded 25 mg/L (50 µM) for several hours and remained above 10 mg/L (20 µM) at 8 h. The quantitative pharmacokinetic information derived from these data is summarized in TABLE 1. The ratios for $AUC_{0-4}/AUC_{0-\infty}$ are 0.89 and 0.81 for (S)-DMDFT and Fe^{III} [(S)-DMDFT]$_2$, respectively, compared to 0.50 and 0.44 for (R)-DMDFT and Fe^{III} [(R)-DMDFT]$_2$, reflecting the prolonged residence times of the latter enantiomer. The most remarkable and revealing finding from the pharmacokinetic experiments was the marked enantioselectivity of the renal clearance observed with (S)-DMDFT, a clearance that was *3.5 times* greater than that of (R)-DMDFT, (FIG. 5–*top*) and a Fe^{III} [(S)-DMDFT]$_2$ clearance that was *6.8 times* greater than that of Fe^{III} [(R)-DMDFT]$_2$ (FIG. 5–*bottom*). Owing to the death of one of the animals given the (R)-DMDFT, we were unwilling to perform intravenous pharmacokinetic studies.

Drug Toxicity in Primates

Complete blood counts and kidney and liver profiles fell within the accepted normal range of the human values at the outset of all of the experiments. Monkey ferritin could not be determined utilizing the commercially available human ferritin antibody assay. Although a formal toxicity study was not performed in the primates, animals treated with a single dose of (S)-DMDFT were alert, active, ate well, and had normal urine and feces production both before and after drug administration. Unfortunately, animals treated with (R)-DMDFT did not fare as well. Two out of nine primates treated with (R)-DMDFT died within 24 h of drug administration, one during an iron clearance study and another in the course of a pharmacokinetic experiment. The animals that died were subjected to a complete necropsy, but no specific pathology was identified. However, it is important to point out that the animal that died in the pharmacokinetic study had been given the (S)-enantiomer at the same dose in an earlier pharmacokinetic experiment and had no difficulties. Thus, it does seem likely that the death of this animal was related to the stereochemistry of the drug.

DISCUSSION

As a family of iron chelators, the desferrithiocins are very effective when given orally. Nevertheless, their toxicity still remains somewhat of a concern. In a systematic

TABLE 1. Pharmacokinetic Parameters for *Cebus* Monkeys Treated with (S)- vs. (R)-DMDFT and Respective Ferric Chelates

N	(S)-DMDFT 5	(R)-DMDFT 4	R/S	Fe[(S)-DMDFT]$_2$ 5	Fe[(R)-DMDFT]$_2$ 4	R/S
$t_{1/2}$ (Elimination) (h)	0.89 ± 0.25*	3.00 ± 0.35	3.37	1.30 ± 0.42*	3.86 ± 0.60	2.97
MRT (AUMC/AUC) (h)	1.94 ± 0.55	4.87 ± 0.33	2.51	2.52 ± 0.42	5.78 ± 0.64	2.29
AUC (0-4 h) (mg-h/L)	78.1 ± 16.9	236.9 ± 51.2	3.03	24.74 ± 17.8	88.0 ± 4.8	3.56
AUC (0-∞) (mg-h/L)	88.1 ± 17	472 ± 97.9	5.36	30.6 ± 21.8	199.3 ± 16.6	6.51
AUMC (0-4 h) (mg-h^2/L)	121.2 ± 34.7	531.3 ± 136.3		46.6 ± 35.4	191.2 ± 4.5	
AUMC (0-∞) (mg-h^2/L)	171.7 ± 64.3	2301.5 ± 522		77.7 ± 57.3	1161.6 ± 215.2	
Urinary Excretion (0-4 h)						
(% Total Dose)	50.7% ± 4.2%	37.8% ± 6.1%		0.51% ± 0.09%	0.42% ± 0.11%	
CL(Renal) (mL/h-kg)	492 ± 55	140 ± 56	3.51	47 ± 12	7 ± 2	6.78

(S)-DMDFT (**1**) or (R)-DMDFT (**2**) was given orally by gavage in 40% (v/v) Cremophor RH-40/water at a dose of 300 µmol/kg.

structure–activity study, we were able to identify both the structural fragments requisite for iron clearance[23–25] and which fragments, on alteration, would reduce side effects without compromising iron clearance.[24] Prior to the study described herein, we had identified at least two desferrithiocin analogues which are now moving forward in preclinical trials; however, the pressing question as to the origin of the toxicity of the desferrithiocins still remained to be answered.

In an attempt to determine if metabolic products were responsible for the observed toxicity, we examined the rate of hydrolysis and the hydrolysis products of DFT, (*R*)-DMDFT, and (*R*)-desazadesmethyl DFT.[26] The rate of hydrolysis of these compounds was measured

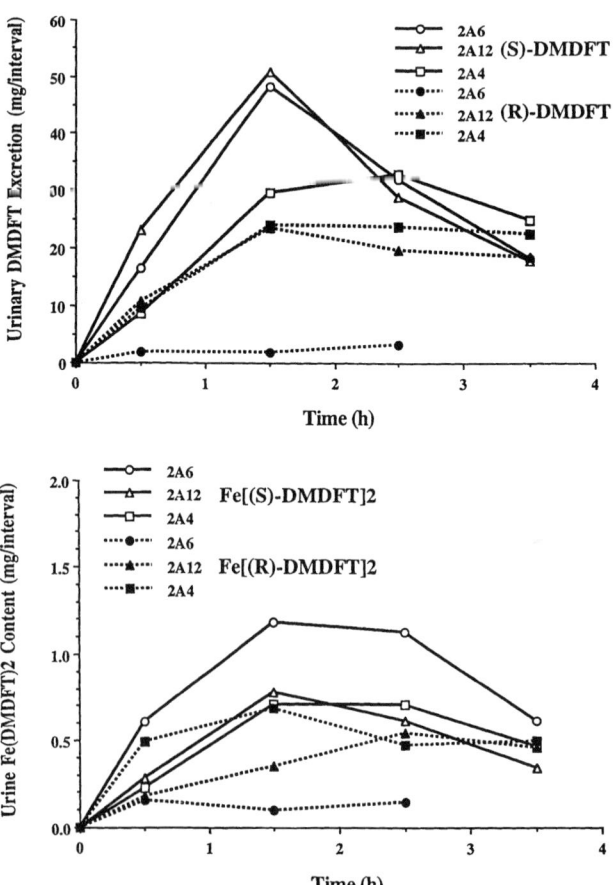

FIGURE 5. Urinary excretion data for *Cebus* monkeys treated with (*S*)-DMDFT or (*R*)-DMDFT. (*S*)-DMDFT (**1**) or (*R*)-DMDFT (**2**) was given orally by gavage in 40% (v/v) Cremophor RH-40/water at a dose of 300 µmol/kg. *Top*: urinary excretion of (*S*)- and (*R*)- DMDFT; *Bottom*: urinary excretion of ferric (*S*)- and (*R*)- DMDFT.

at both gastric (2.5) and blood (7.2) pH. The actual hydrolysis products of (*R*)-desazadesmethyl DFT (**3**), the thioester (**4**) and the thiol amide (**5**), FIGURE 6, were also synthesized and assessed for toxicity in rodents. Finally, the iron complex of **3** was prepared and evaluated for toxicity in mice.

The results were consistent with the hypothesis that simple hydrolysis was not the basis for the toxicity observed. The level of hydrolysis of the desferrithiocins at pH 2.5, while easily measured *in situ*, did not seem likely to be a significant factor considering the residence time of the ligands in the stomach.[26] The $t_{1/2}$ for hydrolysis of DFT, DMDFT, and desazadesmethyl DFT at pH 2.5 were 18.6 h, 8.74 h, and 31.7 h, respectively. The compounds were virtually unhydrolyzed at pH 7.2, even at times > 48 h. Furthermore, the diastereomeric iron complexes of **3** were even more resistant to hydrolysis than the parent drugs. In order to be certain that the thioester and thiol amide did not represent a significant component of the compounds' toxicity, even though they were produced only in small quantities, rodents were subjected to intraperitoneal (i.p.) injections of the thioester, the thiol amide, or the parent molecule.[26] After five days, all of the animals given the parent drug i.p. died; however, none of the animals given either the thioester or the thiol amide died, even after 10 days of treatment. Interestingly, all of the rodents administered the iron complex of desazadesmethyl DFT at the same molar concentration as the parent drug died after only two days. This finding is in keeping with the idea that the iron complex itself may be the toxic factor with the desferrithiocins.

In the present series of experiments we found that (*R*)- and (*S*)-DMDFT were nearly identical in both their iron-clearing and toxicity profiles in rodents. In the primates, however, the (*R*)- enantiomer was both ineffective as an iron chelator and possibly toxic. Given the results of the earlier experiments, along with the observation that (*R*)- and (*S*)-desmethyldesferrithiocin behave so differently in terms of their iron clearing properties in primates, we elected to compare the level of free drug and iron complex of these compounds in the plasma of test animals. It is important to point out that structurally the only difference between (*R*)- and (*S*)-DMDFT is the configuration at C-4 of the thiazoline ring.

Surprisingly, in the course of the pharmacokinetic studies, one out of four primates given (*R*)-DMDFT at 300 μmol/kg died; administration of the (*S*)- enantiomer did not elicit side effects even at 450 μmol/kg.[24] When we looked at the pharmacokinetics of the iron complexes, in contrast to Fe^{III} [(*S*)-DMDFT]$_2$, Fe^{III} [(*R*)-DMDFT]$_2$ in the plasma exceeded 25 mg/L (50 μM) for several hours (FIG. 4). Thus, with (*R*)-DMDFT, unlike with (*S*)-DMDFT, a substantial amount of ferric ion is mobilized into the plasma, where it persists at very high concentrations over a prolonged period of time. It has been reported that the presence of 50 μM ferrithiocin in cell culture medium is toxic to hepatocytes *in vitro*.[35] Furthermore, the redistribution of iron into the plasma may expose vulnerable tissues, such as the myocardium and certain CNS regions,[37] to toxic levels of ferric ion capable of catalyzing Fenton chemistry oxidative damage.

It has been demonstrated that (*R*)-Δ^2-thiazoline-4-carboxylic acid is converted to formic acid and cysteine in hog liver homogenates.[38-39] We therefore elected to examine whether DMDFT, a thiazoline carboxylic acid, or its ferric chelates might affect the activity of D-amino acid oxidase (D-AAO). Thiazolidine carboxylates have been reported to be excellent substrates of D-AAO,[40-41] a peroxide-producing enzyme present in high concentrations in the peroxisomes of mammalian liver and kidney proximal tubules.[36] Moreover, D-AAO-catalyzed metabolism of a D-cysteine derivative has been implicated in acute nephrotoxicity in the dog and results in selective ultrastructural changes in the S1 and S2 cells of the proximal tubules and decreased renal clearance.[42] As expected, incubation of D-AAO with a known substrate, 10 mM D-Phe, resulted in a rapid rate of oxygen consumption which was almost totally suppressed immediately upon introduction of a competitive inhibitor, kojate (100 μM), into the assay mixture. However, when present at a concentration of 10 mM in place of D-Phe, the (*R*)- or (*S*)-DMDFT and the corresponding ferric chelates were

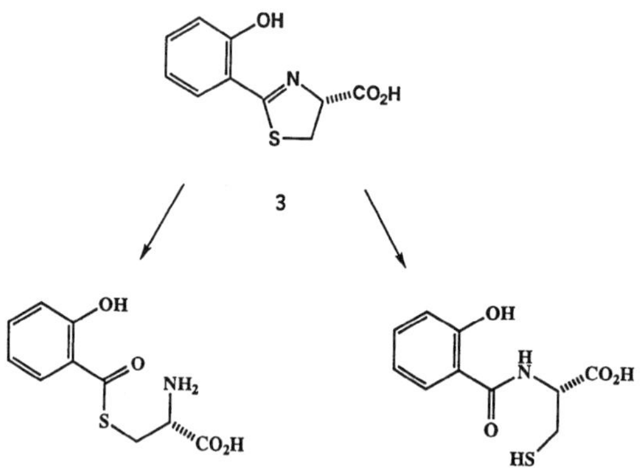

FIGURE 6. Hydrolysis products of (*R*)-desazadesmethyl DFT (**3**): the thioester *S*-(2'-hydroxybenzoyl)-L-cysteine (**4**) and the thiol amide *N*-(2'-hydroxybenzoyl)-L-cysteine (**5**).

not substrates of the oxidase; furthermore, no inhibitory activity was observed at 250 μM. Thus, interaction with this enzyme does not appear to provide an explanation for chiral differences in the activity or toxicity of these compounds.

While a complete explanation of the mechanism of chiral recognition of desferrithiocin analogues is not readily apparent based on these experiments, the plasma pharmacokinetic results do provide a basis to explain the *selective toxicity* of (*R*)-DMDFT in the primates. It seems that the plasma level and clearance properties of the metal chelate is of some concern when appraising a given ligand's potential toxicity.

ACKNOWLEDGMENTS

We would like to thank Hristina Dimova and Curt Zimmerman for their expert technical assistance, and Dr. Eileen Hughes for her editorial comments.

REFERENCES

1. BICKEL, H., G. E. HALL, W. KELLER-SCHIERLEIN, V. PRELOG, E. VISCHER & A. WETTSTEIN. 1960. Metabolic products of actinomycetes. Ferrioxamine B. Helv. Chim. Acta. **43:** 2129–2138.
2. PIPPARD, M. J. & S. T. CALLENDER. 1983. The management of iron chelation therapy. Br. J. Haematol. **54:** 503–507.
3. GRAZIANO, J. H., A. MARKENSON, D. R. MILLER, A. CHANG, M. BESTAK, P. MEYERS, P. PISCIOTTO & A. RIFKIND. 1978. Chelation therapy in beta-thalassemia major. 1. Intravenous and subcutaneous deferoxamine. J. Pediatr. **92:** 648–652.
4. BRITTENHAM, G. M., P. M. GRIFFITH, A. W. NIENHUIS, C. E. MCLAREN, N. S. YOUNG, E. E. TUCKER, C. J. ALLEN, D. E. FARRELL & J. W. HARRIS. 1994. Efficacy of deferoxamine in preventing complications of iron overload in patients with thalassemia major. N. Engl. J. Med. **331:** 567–573.
5. SHALIT, M., A. TEDESCHI, A. MIADONNA & F. LEVI-SCHAFFER. 1991. Desferal (desferrioxamine)- A novel activator of connective tissue-type mast cells. J. Allergy Clin. Immunol. **88:** 854–860.

6. BOUSQUET, J., M. NAVARRO, G. ROBERT, P. AYE & F. B. MICHEL. 1983. Rapid desensitization for desferrioxamine anaphylactoid reactions. Lancet **2:** 859–860.
7. MILLER, K. B., L. J. ROSENWASSER, J. A. M. BESSETTE, D. J. BEER & R. E. ROCKLIN. 1981. Rapid desensitization for desferrioxamine anaphylactic reactions. Lancet **1:** 1059.
8. KIRKING, M. H. 1991. Treatment of chronic iron overload. Clin. Pharm. **10:** 775–783.
9. PONKA, P., J. BOROVA, J. NEUWIRT & O. FUCHS. 1979. Mobilization of iron from reticulocytes: Identification of pyridoxal isonicotinoyl hydrazone as a new iron chelating agent. FEBS Lett. **97:** 317–321.
10. UHLIR, L. C., P. W. DURBIN, N. JEUNG & K. N. RAYMOND. 1993. Specific sequestering agents for the actinides. 21. Synthesis and initial biological testing of octadentate mixed catecholate-hydroxypyridinonate ligands. J. Med. Chem. **36:** 504–509.
11. KONTOGHIORGHES, G. J., M. A. ALDOURI, L. SHEPPARD & A. V. HOFFBRAND. 1987. 1,2-Dimethyl-3-hydroxypyrid-4-one, an orally active chelator for the treatment of iron overload. Lancet **1:** 1294–1295.
12. GRADY, R. W. & C. HERSHKO. 1990. HBED: A potential oral iron chelator. Ann. N.Y. Acad. Sci. **612:** 361–368.
13. BERGERON, R. J. 1984. Synthesis and solution structure of microbial siderophores. Chem. Rev. **84:** 587–602.
14. BERGERON, R. J. & J. S. MCMANIS. 1991. Synthesis of catecholamide and hydroxamate siderophores. *In* Handbook of Microbial Iron Chelates. G. Winkelmann, Ed.: 271–307. CRC Press. Boca Raton, Fl.
15. BERGERON, R. J., K. A. MCGOVERN, M. A. CHANNING & P. S. BURTON. 1980. Synthesis of N^1-acylated N^1,N^8-bis(acyl)spermidines: An approach to the synthesis of siderophores. J. Org. Chem. **45:** 1589–1592.
16. BERGERON, R. J. & J. S. MCMANIS. 1989. The total synthesis of Bisucaberin. Tetrahedron **45:** 4939–4944.
17. BERGERON, R. J., J. S. MCMANIS, P. T. PERUMAL & S. E. ALGEE. 1991. The total synthesis of Alcaligin. J. Org. Chem. **56:** 5560–5563.
18. BERGERON, R. J. & O. PHANSTIEL, IV. 1992. The total synthesis of Nannochelin: A novel cinnamoyl hydroxamate-containing siderophore. J. Org. Chem. **57:** 7140–7143.
19. BERGERON, R. J. & J. S. MCMANIS. 1993. Synthesis and biological activity of hydroxamate-based iron chelators. *In* The Development of Iron Chelators for Clinical Use. R. J. Bergeron & G. M. Brittenham, Eds.: 237–273. CRC Press. Boca Raton, Fl.
20. COX, C. D., K. L. RINEHART, JR., M. L. MOORE & J. C. COOK, JR. 1981. Pyochelin: Novel structure of an iron-chelating growth promoter for *Pseudomonas aeruginosa*. Proc. Natl. Acad. Sci. USA **78:** 4256–4260.
21. SMITH, M. J. 1989. Total synthesis and absolute configuration of rhizobactin, a structurally novel siderophore. Tetrahedron Lett. **30:** 313–316.
22. BERGERON, R. J., R. R. STREIFF, J. WIEGAND, J. R. T. VINSON, G. LUCHETTA, K. M. EVANS, H. PETER & H-B. JENNY. 1990. A comparative evaluation of iron clearance models. Ann. N. Y. Acad. Sci. **612:** 378–393.
23. BERGERON, R. J., J. WIEGAND, J. B. DIONIS, M. EGLI-KARMAKKA, J. FREI, A. HUXLEY-TENCER & H. H. PETER. 1991. Evaluation of desferrithiocin and its synthetic analogues as orally effective iron chelators. J. Med. Chem. **34:** 2072–2078.
24. BERGERON, R. J., R. R. STREIFF, E. A. CREARY, R. D. DANIELS, JR., W. KING, G. LUCHETTA, J. WIEGAND, T. MOERKER & H. H. PETER. 1993. A comparative study of the iron-clearing properties of desferrithiocin analogues with desferrioxamine B in a *Cebus* monkey model. Blood **81:** 2166–2173.
25. BERGERON, R. J., C. Z. LIU, J. S. MCMANIS, M. X. B. XIA, S. E. ALGEE & J. WIEGAND. 1994. The desferrithiocin pharmacophore. J. Med. Chem. **37:** 1411–1417.
26. BERGERON, R. J., M. WOLLENWEBER & J. WIEGAND. 1994. An investigation of desferrithiocin metabolism. J. Med. Chem. **37:** 2889–2895.
27. BERGERON, R. J., J. WIEGAND, M. WOLLENWEBER, J. S. MCMANIS, S. E. ALGEE & K. RATLIFF-THOMPSON. 1996. Synthesis and biological evaluation of naphthyldesferrithiocin iron chelators. J. Med. Chem. **39:** 1575–1581.
28. NAEGELI, H. U. & H. ZAEHNER. 1980. Metabolites of microorganisms. Part 193. Ferrithiocin. Helv. Chim. Acta. **63:** 1400–1406.

29. ANDEREGG, G. & M. RAEBER. 1990. Metal complex formation of a new siderophore desferrithiocin and of three related ligands. J. Chem. Soc., Chem. Commun.: 1194–1196.
30. LONGUEVILLE, A. & R. R. CRICHTON. 1986. An animal model of iron overload and its application to study hepatic ferritin iron mobilization by chelators. Biochem. Pharmacol. **35:** 3669–3678.
31. WOLFE, L. C., R. J. NICOLOSI, M. M. RENAUD, J. FINGER, M. HEGSTED, H. PETER & D. G. NATHAN. 1989. A non-human primate model for the study of oral iron chelators. Br. J. Haematol. **72:** 456–461.
32. BERGERON, R. J., Z. R. LIU, J. S. MCMANIS & J. WIEGAND. 1992. Structural alterations in desferrioxamine compatible with iron clearance in animals. J. Med. Chem. **35:** 4739–4744.
33. BERGERON, R. J., R. R. STREIFF, J. WIEGAND, G. LUCHETTA, E. A. CREARY & H. H. PETER. 1992. A comparison of the iron-clearing properties of 1,2-dimethyl-3-hydroxypyrid-4-one, 1,2-diethyl-3-hydroxypyrid-4-one and deferoxamine. Blood **79:** 1882–1890.
34. BERGERON, R. J., R. R. STREIFF, W. KING, R. D. DANIELS, JR. & J. WIEGAND. 1993. A comparison of the iron clearing properties of parabactin and desferrioxamine. Blood **82:** 2552–2557.
35. BAKER, E., A. WONG, H. PETER & A. JACOBS. 1992. Desferrithiocin is an effective iron chelator in vivo and in vitro but ferrithiocin is toxic. Br. J. Haematol. **81:** 424–431.
36. WEIMAR, W. R. & A. H. NEIMS. 1976. Hog cerebellar D-amino acid oxidase and its histochemical and immunofluorescent localization. J. Neurochem. **28:** 559–572.
37. LIU, D., R. YANG, X. YAN & D. J. MCADOO. 1994. Hydroxyl radicals generated in vivo kill neurons in the rat spinal cord: Electrophysiological, histological, and neurochemical results. J. Neurochem. **62:** 37–44.
38. MACKENZIE, C. M. & J. HARRIS. 1957. N-Formylcysteine synthesis in mitochondria from formaldehyde and L-cysteine via thiazolidinecarboxylic acid. J. Biol. Chem. **227:** 393–406.
39. CAVALLINI, D., C. DE MARCO, B. MONDOVI & F. TRASARTI. 1956. Studies of the metabolism of thiazolidine carboxylic acid by rat liver homogenate. Biochim. Biophys. Acta. **22:** 558–564.
40. ST.-JULES, R., J. KENNARD, W. SETLIK & E. HOLTZMAN. 1991. Peroxisomal oxidation of thiazolidine carboxylates in firefly fat body, frog retina, and rat liver and kidney. Eur. J. Cell Biol. **55:** 94–103.
41. FREDERIKS, W. M., C. J. VAN-NOORDEN, F. MARX, P. T. GALLAGHER & B. P. SWANN. 1993. *In situ* kinetic measurements of D-amino acid oxidase in rat liver with respect to its substrate specificity. Histochem. J. **25:** 578–582.
42. KREJCI, M. E., R. E. RIDGEWELL & D. A. KOECHEL. 1991. Acute effects of the D-isomer of S-(1,2-dichlorovinyl) cysteine on renal function and ultrastructure in the pentobarbital-anesthetized dog: Site-specific toxicity involving the S1 and S2 cells of the proximal tubule. Toxicol. **69:** 151–164.

Long-Term Trials of Deferiprone in Cooley's Anemia[a]

NANCY F. OLIVIERI,[b,d,e] AND GARY M. BRITTENHAM[c]

[b]*Departments of Medicine and Pediatrics, University of Toronto, Canada*

[c]*Department of Medicine, MetroHealth Medical Center, Case Western Reserve University, Cleveland, USA*

> ABSTRACT: Deferoxamine is the currently available agent for the iron-chelation therapy required by Cooley's anemia patients. The difficulties associated with parenteral administration have mandated a search for alternative therapies, especially orally active iron chelators, to remove excess iron that results in damage to the liver, endocrine organs, and heart. Four orally active agents have reached clinical trials in the last decade. The agent under consideration in this paper, deferiprone (1,2-dimethyl-3-hydroxypyridin-4-one), has shown some promise, but, according to the studies discussed here, may not provide adequate sustained control of body iron in a substantial proportion of Cooley's anemia patients.

In patients with Cooley's anemia and hereditary hemochromatosis, excess iron acquired through transfusions or absorption results in damage to the liver, endocrine organs and heart.[1] Several studies have highlighted the importance of sustained reduction of body iron burden as the principal determinant of clinical outcome in these disorders.[2-5] While venesection can effectively and safely reduce body iron in individuals homozygous for hereditary hemochromatosis,[2] patients with Cooley's anemia require life-long chelating therapy to promote the excretion of iron accumulated from transfusions.[6] The only iron-chelating agent available for clinical use is deferoxamine, long-term compliance which with prevents the complications of iron overload, and improves survival, in Cooley's anemia.[4,7] The difficulties associated with parenteral administration of deferoxamine have mandated a search for safe and effective therapeutic alternatives, including orally active iron chelators,[1] four of which have reached clinical teals in the past decade. The compounds N,N'-bis (2-hydroxybenzoyl) ethylenediamine N,N'-diacetic acid (HBED), the aryl hydrazone pyridoxal isonicotinoyl hydrazone (PIH), and the diethyl hydroxypyridinone CP94, have all been evaluated in short-term trials over the last five years, but are not under clinical development at this time.[6] The orally active iron-chelating agent most extensively evaluated to date is 1,2-dimethyl-3-hydroxypyridin-4-one (deferiprone; L1),

---

[a]Supported in part by research grants from: The Medical Research Council of Canada, The Ontario Heart and Stroke Foundation, The Ontario Thalassemia Foundation, APOTEX Inc., The United States Cooley's Anemia Foundation, The National Institutes of Health Grants #HL 42824 and AI 35827, and The Food and Drug Administration Orphan Products Grant FD-R-000532.

[d]Address correspondence and reprint requests to Dr. N.F. Olivieri, The Hospital for Sick Children, Division of Hematology, University Of Toronto, 555 University Avenue, Toronto, Ontario, Canada M5G 1X8; Tel: (416) 813-6823; Fax: (416) 813-5346; E-mail: noliv@sickkids.on.ca

[e]Dr. Olivieri is a recipient of a Scientist Award from the Medical Research Council of Canada.

one of the 3-hydroxypyridin-4-one iron chelators patented in 1982 as an potential alternative to deferoxamine for the treatment of chronic iron overload.[8]

Animal studies of deferiprone have reported variable efficacy in rodents and rabbits, and insufficient efficacy for maintenance of negative iron balance in iron-loaded primates.[6] In transfused patients with Cooley's anemia, 75 milligrams of deferiprone per kilogram body weight induces urinary iron excretion approximately equivalent to that achieved with 30–40 milligrams of deferoxamine per kilogram.[1,9,10] Because fecal iron excretion induced by deferiprone is much less than that by deferoxamine,[9,10] the short-term efficacy of deferiprone is acknowledged to be inferior to that of deferoxamine.

Effectiveness of Deferiprone as Estimated by Serum Ferritin Concentration

While the earliest studies reported no sustained decrease in serum ferritin concentration over one to 15 months of deferiprone therapy,[11,12] two short-term trials subsequently reported statistically significant reductions in mean serum ferritin concentration in patients with Cooley's anemia, with the most substantial declines observed in patients whose pre-study ferritin concentrations exceeded 5000 µg/L.[13,14] As previously noted, reliance on changes in the concentration of serum ferritin alone may lead to inaccurate assessment of body iron burden in individual patients; direct assessment of tissue iron is crucial in the evaluation of any new potential iron-chelating agent.[6] Such studies therefore could not establish convincingly the efficacy of deferiprone in the reduction of body iron burden.

Effectiveness of Deferiprone as Estimated by Hepatic Iron Concentration

Reduction in hepatic iron stores during deferiprone therapy was first demonstrated in a patient with thalassemia "intermedia."[15] In a subsequent study in patients with Cooley's anemia unable or unwilling to use deferoxamine, short-term deferiprone treatment was shown to reduce hepatic storage iron in many patients over three years.[16] As emphasized at the time of that report, the long-term effectiveness of this agent remained undetermined.[17]

To assess the effectiveness of deferiprone in the long-term control of body iron in Cooley's anemia we have continued to determine hepatic iron concentration in these patients, in whom results through June 1994 were reported previously.[16] As of June 1996, 18 of 21 patients remain evaluable; one patient interrupted deferiprone for 0.7 years, and two patients stopped deferiprone after one year. These 18 patients constitute the only group worldwide to receive long-term deferiprone in conjunction with serial measurements of hepatic iron concentration to accurately determine body iron. As in our previously reported analysis,[16] hepatic iron concentration, determined in tissue obtained at biopsy or by magnetic susceptometry,[4] was the primary endpoint of effectiveness. The criteria used are those derived from long-term studies of morbidity and mortality associated with increasing concentrations of hepatic storage iron *in vivo*.[2-5,18] These will be briefly reviewed.

Information about the risks associated with lower levels of body iron arises from experience in patients heterozygous for the iron-loading disorder hereditary hemochromatosis, in a proportion of whom maintenance of modestly elevated concentrations of hepatic iron (approximately 3.2 to 7 milligrams iron per gram liver, dry weight) is associated with normal life expectancy and no evidence of iron-induced toxicity.[18] Individuals with body iron burdens above this range, and up to about 15 milligrams iron per gram liver, dry weight, are at an increased risk of hepatic fibrosis and other complications of iron overload.[2,3,5]

Patients who sustain hepatic storage iron concentrations exceeding 15 milligrams iron per gram liver, dry weight have a greatly heightened risk of cardiac disease and early death.[4] Accordingly, patients who reduce and maintain hepatic storage iron concentrations within the range of 3.2 to 7 milligrams iron per gram liver, dry weight are considered to have maintained body storage iron within optimal range while receiving deferiprone. Patients in whom long-term chelating therapy fails to maintain hepatic storage iron in this range are considered to be at risk for iron-induced complications of iron overload. Finally, those patients in whom therapy fails to maintain hepatic storage iron below 15 milligrams iron per gram liver, dry weight, are considered to be at risk of cardiac disease and early death.[4]

Although support for Toronto's long-term trial was terminated prematurely in 1996 by the corporate sponsor, continued follow-up of hepatic storage iron concentrations has provided information regarding the long-term effectiveness of deferiprone in Cooley's anemia. Our most recent analysis of this cohort shows that, in one-third of patients, hepatic iron concentrations presently exceed the threshold associated with increased risk of heart disease and early death in Cooley's anemia.[4] Of the 16 patients with a hepatic iron concentration below this threshold when previously reported,[16] the hepatic iron concentration now exceeds the threshold in four patients ($p = 0.05$); in the two other patients, the hepatic iron concentration has continued to exceed the threshold during 2.3 and 3.9 years of deferiprone, respectively. In these six patients. mean compliance with deferiprone exceeding 90% drug taken of that prescribed.[19] Another interpretation of these data has recently been presented.[20,21]

In parallel, investigators in the United Kingdom reported the results of deferiprone therapy over 42.5 months (range, 8 to 56 months) in 42 patients with Cooley's anemia aged 29.9 years (range, 20 to 58 years).[22,23] No significant declines in serum ferritin concentration were reported in these patients over this period of therapy. In the 17 patients in whom hepatic iron concentrations were determined after therapy, concentrations exceeded the threshold for cardiac disease and early death[4] in ten patients. The conclusion of this analysis is similar to those in the Canadian study:[19] the U.K. investigators have now concluded that "long-term therapy with deferiprone may not provide adequate control of body iron in a substantial proportion of patients with thalassemia major."[22,23]

In summary, two interpretation of the results obtained from the only centers to quantitatively determine body iron burden in patients receiving long-term deferiprone therapy raise concerns that long-term deferiprone may not provide adequate sustained control of body iron in a substantial proportion of patients with Cooley's anemia.[19,22,23]

Toxicity Studies

As detailed previously,[6] deferiprone did not receive full formal toxicologic evaluation before being given to humans; permission to administer the drug in early studies in the United Kingdom, India, Europe and Canada was granted on the basis of limited toxicity studies in rodents. Adrenal hypertrophy, gonadal and thymic atrophy, bone marrow atrophy and pancytopenia, growth retardation, and embryotoxicity have also been reported in animals. In humans, the most common adverse effect associated with administration of deferiprone has been arthralgias, primarily of the large joints, the etiology of which remains elusive.[6] The most serious adverse effect associated with the administration of deferiprone has been severe neutropenia or agranulocytosis, first reported in 1989.[24] To date, this complication has been reported in several patients, most with Cooley's anemia, as early as six weeks and up to 21 months after the initiation of deferiprone. The mechanism of deferiprone-induced neutropenia is unknown; this adverse effect appears not to be dose-dependent, but idiosyncratic and unpredictable.[6]

No study of long-term toxicity of deferiprone has been conducted. Monitoring of the safety of deferiprone in most prospective studies continues to be directed to abnormalities reported in animal studies.[23-29] Treatment of iron-loaded Mongolian gerbils with a hydroxypyridinone closely related to deferiprone (1,2-di*ethyl*-3-hydroxypyridin-4-one) has been associated with the acceleration of hepatic fibrosis and the development of cardiac fibrosis in these animals, the only species which develops hemochromatosis of the liver and heart in the same manner as patients with Cooley's anemia.[29] While hepatic iron accumulation was inhibited during co-administration of 1,2-diethyl-3-hydroxypyridin-4-one over the short-term in the gerbils, hepatic iron increased significantly during extended drug administration.[29] Of further concern, accelerated fibrosis was noted in both the livers and hearts of animals in which 1,2-diethyl-3-hydroxypyridin-4-one was co-administered with iron, compared to animals treated with iron alone. These observations, and the theoretical concerns with respect to the toxicity of a bidentate ligand, discussed elsewhere in this volume, have raised concerns as to whether long-term deferiprone therapy may be associated with worsening of hepatic fibrosis, and cardiac iron loading and fibrosis, in humans.

By oversight, in this and all other trials of deferiprone worldwide, hepatic histology has never been evaluated prospectively in patients receiving long-term therapy. As well, the effect of deferiprone on cardiac iron loading and fibrosis has not been been the primary endpoint of any prospective trial. Nevertheless, the studies by the group in the United Kingdom have provided indirect information regarding cardiac disease in patients with Cooley's anemia treated with long-term deferiprone. In this long-term treatment cohort,[23] 18 of 42 patients left the study, a dropout rate of 43 percent. Review of these 18 patients shows that five dropouts had died, four of cardiac disease, while on deferiprone therapy, while another patient withdrew from treatment because of tachycardia. In all the study dropouts, mean initial serum ferritin concentration, which exceeded 4,500 μg/L, reportedly did not change significantly during deferiprone therapy.[23] These data underscore the concerns that long-term deferiprone may not adequately reduce body iron burden below concentrations that are associated with an increased risk of cardiac disease and early death in Cooley's anemia,[4] confirming the findings summarized above.[19,22,23]

In summary, data from two centers conducting long-term trials of deferiprone support our previous conclusion that "long-term therapy with deferiprone may not provide adequate control of body iron in a substantial proportion of patients with thalassemia major."[19] Further prospective trials may be indicated to address these potential toxicities of deferiprone.

REFERENCES

1. BRITTENHAM, G. M. 1992. Development of iron-chelating agents for clinical use. Blood **80:** 569–574.
2. NIEDERAU, C., R. FISCHER, A. SONNENBERG *et al.* 1985. Survival and causes of death in cirrhotic and in noncirrhotic patients with primary hemochromatosis. N. Engl. J. Med. **313:** 1256–1262.
3. LOREAL, O., Y. DEUGNIER, R. MOIRAND *et al.* 1992. Liver fibrosis in genetic hemochromatosis. Respective roles of iron and non-iron related factors in 127 homozygous patients. J. Hepatol. **16:** 122–127.
4. BRITTENHAM, G. M., P. M. GRIFFITH, A. W. NIENHUIS *et al.* 1994. Efficacy of deforoxamine in preventing complications of iron overload in patients with thalassemia major. N. Engl. J. Med. **331:** 567–573.
5. NIEDERAU, C., R. FISCHER, W. STREMMEL *et al.* 1996. Long-term survival in patients with hereditary hemochromatosis. Gastroenterology **110:** 1107–1119.

6. OLIVIERI, N. F. & G. M. BRITTENHAM. 1997. Iron-chelating therapy and the treatment of thalassemia. Blood **89:** 739–761.
7. OLIVIERI, N. F., D. G. NATHAN, J. H. MACMILLAN et al. 1994. Survival in medically treated patients with homozygous β thalassemia. N. Engl. J. Med. **331:** 574–578.
8. HIDER, R. C., G. J. KONTOGHIORGHES, J. SILVER. 1982. U.K. patent GB-2118176.
9. OLIVIERI, N. F., G. KOREN, C. HERMANN et al. 1990. Comparison of oral iron chelator L1. and desferrioxamine in iron-loaded patients. Lancet **336:** 1275–1279.
10. COLLINS, A. F., F. F. FASSOS, S. S. STOBIE et al. 1994. Iron balance and dose response studies of the oral iron chelator 1,2-dimethyl-3-hydroxypyrid-4-one (L1) in iron-loaded patients with sickle cell disease. Blood **83:** 2329–2333.
11. KONTOGHIORGHES, G. J., A. N. BARTLETT, A. V. HOFFBRAND et al. 1990. Long-term trial with the oral iron chelator 1,2-dimethyl-3-hydroxypyrid-4-one (L1). Br. J. Haematol. **76:** 295–304.
12. TONDURY, P., G. J. KONTOGHIORGHES, A. R. RIDOLFI-LUTHY et al. 1990. L1. (1,2-dimethyl-3-hydroxypyrd-4-one) for oral iron chelation in patients with beta-thalassaemia major. Br. J. Haematol. **76:** 550–553.
13. AL-REFAIE, F. N., B. WONKE, A. V. HOFFBRAND et al. 1992. Efficacy and possible adverse effects of the oral iron chelator 1,2-dimethyl-3-hydroxypyrid-4-one (L1) in Cooley's anemia. Blood **80:** 592–599.
14. AGARWAL, M. B., S. S. GUPTE, C. VISWANATHAN et al. 1992. Long-term assessment of efficacy and safety of L1, an oral iron chelator, in transfusion-dependent thalassemia: Indian trial. Br. J. Haematol. **82:** 460–466.
15 OLIVIERI, N. F., D. MATSUI, G. KOREN et al. 1992. Reduction of tissue iron stores and normalization of serum ferritin during treatment with the oral iron chelator L1 in thalassemia intermedia. Blood **79:** 2741-2748.
16. OLIVIERI, N. F., G. M. BRITTENHAM, D. MATSUI et al. 1995. Iron chelation therapy with oral deferiprone in patients with thalassemia major. N. Engl. J. Med. **332:** 918–922.
17. NATHAN, D. G. An orally active iron chelator. 1995. N. Engl. J. Med. **332:** 953–954.
18. CARTWRIGHT, G. E., C. Q. EDWARDS, K. KRAVITZ et al. 1979. Hereditary hemochromatosis: Phenotypic expression of the disease. N. Engl. J. Med. **301:** 175–179.
19. OLIVIERI, N. F., Iron Chelation Research Group. 1996. Long-term follow-up of body iron in patients with thalassemia major during therapy with the orally active iron chelator deferiprone (L1) [abstract]. Blood **88:** 310a.
20. TRICTA, F., G. SHER, R. LOEBSTEIN et al. 1997. Long-term chelation therapy with the orally active iron chelator deferiprone (L1) in patients with thalassemia major [abstract]. Presented at the Sixth International Conference on Thalassaemia and the Haemoglobinopathies & Eight Annual Thalassaemia Parent and Thalassaemics International Conference. St. Paul's Bay, Malta, April 5–10, 1997.
21. DOGHERTY, P., T. EINARSON, G. KOREN & G. SHER. 1997. The effectiveness of deferiprone in thalassemia [letter]. Blood **90:** 894.
22. HOFFBRAND, A.V., B. WONKE, F. AL-REFAIE et al. 1996. Over 3 year follow up of 56 transfusion dependent patients receiving oral iron chelation [abstract]. Blood **88:** 651a.
23. HOFFBRAND, A.V. & B. WONKE. 1997. Long term follow-up of 42 regularly transfused thalassaemia patients treated with deferiprone [abstract]. Presented at the Sixth International Conference on Thalassaemia and the Haemoglobinopathies & Eight Annual Thalassaemia Parent and Thalassaemics International Conference. St. Paul's Bay, Malta, April 5–10, 1997.
24. HOFFBRAND, A. V., A. N. BARTLETT, P. P. VEYS et al. 1989. Agranulocytosis and thrombocytopenia in patients with Blackfan-Diamond anaemia during oral chelator trial [letter]. Lancet **2:** 457–458.
25. PORTER, J. B., J. MORGAN, K. P. HOYES et al. 1990. Relative oral efficacy and acute toxicity of hydroxypyridin-4-one iron chelators in mice. Blood **76:** 2389–2396.
26. PORTER, J. B., K. P. HOYES, R. D. ABEYSINGHE et al. 1991. Comparison of the subacute toxicity and efficacy of 3-hydroxypyridin-4-one iron chelators in overloaded and nonoverloaded mice. Blood **78:** 2727–2734.
27. BIESEMEIER, J. A. & J. LAVEGLIA. 1991. 14-day oral toxicity study in dogs with 1.2-dimethyl-3-hydroxypyrid-4-one (DMHP, L1). Food and Drug Research Laboratories, Waverly, NY, Contract No. N01-DK-4-2255, NIDDK, NIH, USA.

28. BERGERON, R. J., R. R. STREIFF, J. WEIGAND *et al.* 1992. A comparison of the iron-clearing properties of 1,2-dimethyl-3-hydroxypyrid-4-one. 1,2-diethyl-3-hydroxypyrid-4-one, and deferoxamine. Blood **79:** 1882–1890.
29. SCHNEBLI, H. P. 1993. Final Report, Pre-clinical evaluation of CGP 37–391 (L1). Pharmaceutical Division, Ciba-Geigy Biology Report ERS 62/93; 30 pp.
30. CARTHEW, P., A. G. SMITH, R. C. HIDER *et al.* 1994. Potentiation of iron accumulation in cardiac myocytes during the treatment of iron overload with the hydroxypyridinone iron chelator CP94. BioMetals **7:** 267–271.

A Multi-Center Safety Trial of the Oral Iron Chelator Deferiprone

ALAN COHEN,[a,e] RENZO GALANELLO,[b] ANTONIO PIGA,[c] CALOGERO VULLO,[d] AND FERNANDO TRICTA[c,f]

[a]*Childrens Hospital of Philadelphia, Philadelphia, Pennsylvania 19104, USA*
[b]*Istituto di Clinica e Biologia Dell'Eta' Evolutiva, Cagliari, Italy*
[c]*University of Torino, Torino, Italy*
[d]*Azienda Ospedaliera "Archispedale S. Anna," Ferrara, Italy*

ABSTRACT: Deferiprone, also known as L1, is an orally active iron chelator that has been studied extensively in clinical trials. The sporadic occurrence of agranulocytosis in association with deferiprone and the highly variable frequency of other possible side effects such as arthralgia have created uncertainty about the true incidence of deferiprone-related complications. A multi-center, 1-year trial was initiated to determine the safety profile of deferiprone. Using the Apotex formulation of deferiprone, 187 patients with thalassemia who were unable or unwilling to use deferoxamine were enrolled in four centers; 162 patients completed one year of therapy. Agranulocytosis (ANC < 500/mm^3) occurred in one patient after 15 weeks of treatment, was not accompanied by infection and resolved following treatment with G-CSF. Nine other subjects developed less severe neutropenia (ANC 500-1500/mm^3) with the lowest absolute neutrophil count reaching 500-1250/mm^3. The neutropenia in these patients developed after 1-50 weeks of therapy, frequently accompanied febrile illnesses, and occurred predominantly in non-splenectomized patients. Reasons other than neutropenia for discontinuing use of deferiprone included nausea (4), voluntary withdrawal (3), high ALT (2), platelet count <100,000/mm3 (2), low but unconfirmed ANC (1), protocol violation (1) fatigue (1), and depression (1). Mean ALT levels rose within three months of therapy and stabilized thereafter. Arthralgia and nausea and/or vomiting occurred in 6% and 24% of subjects, respectively. In this multi-center trial with weekly monitoring of blood counts, the incidence of agranulocytosis was 0.58 per 100 patient-years, and the frequency of agranulocytosis after one year was 0.5%. These findings support the safety of this formulation of deferiprone, using the careful monitoring system employed in this trial.

Deferiprone, also known as L1, is the first orally active iron chelator to enter extensive human trials.[1] In the course of these studies, investigators have reported complications such as agranulocytosis and arthritis.[2] However, the differing designs of these trials and the use of deferiprone from different sources have made it difficult to establish an accurate safety profile for the chelator. Following discussions with the Food and Drug Administration in 1993, a formal safety study of deferiprone was conceived and implemented. This multi-center study was designed to include sufficient patients to assess the incidence of agranulocytosis and other drug-related complications, using drug produced by a single manufacturer.

PATIENTS AND METHODS

One hundred and eighty-seven patients with thalassemia major were enrolled in the study. The mean age at entry was 18.4 years with a range of 10 to 41 years. The patients were equally divided between males and females, and the majority of patients were of

[e]Corresponding Author: Alan Cohen, M.D., Division of Hematology, Childrens Hospital of Philadelphia, 34th Street and Civic Center Boulevard, Philadelphia, PA 19104; Tel: (215) 590-3438; Fax: (215) 590-3525; E-mail: cohen@email.chop.edu

[f]Approximately 1 month before the conclusion of the trial, Dr. Tricta assumed his current position as Medical Advisor, Apotex, Inc., Weston, Ontario, Canada.

Italian origin. Most patients had received previous therapy with deferoxamine. The major inclusion criteria for enrollment included, in addition to transfusion-dependent thalassemia, a serum ferritin level greater than 2,000 µg/L or liver iron concentration greater than 4 mg/g dry weight, an inability or unwillingness to continue treatment with deferoxamine, and age greater than 10 years. Patients were excluded if they had a history of neutropenia within two years prior to the trial, chronic active hepatitis, cirrhosis or hepatic failure, if they were pregnant or breast feeding, if taking other investigational drugs, or if receiving drugs associated with neutropenia.

Patients received deferiprone at a dose of 75 mg/kg/day, divided into three doses. Blood counts with differentials were obtained weekly. Neutropenia was defined as an absolute neutrophil count of less than $1500/mm^3$ with confirmation within 24 hours. Agranulocytosis or severe neutropenia, the major outcome of interest, was defined as a confirmed absolute neutrophil count of less than $500/mm^3$. The threshold for thrombocytopenia, defined initially as a platelet count less than $100,000/mm^3$, was subsequently lowered to $50,000/mm^3$. The occurrence of confirmed neutropenia or thrombocytopenia required discontinuation of deferiprone; re-challenge was prohibited.

Serum alanine aminotransferase (ALT) levels, anti-nuclear antibody, rheumatoid factor, anti-double stranded DNA, and anti-histone antibody were measured at entry and every three months thereafter. Subjects were interviewed weekly regarding potential adverse events, and underwent complete physical examinations at entry, three months, six months, nine months and twelve months, or at the time of early termination.

RESULTS

Of 187 patients initially enrolled in the trial, deferiprone was discontinued in 25 (13%) (TABLE 1) and 162 (87%) completed one year. The mean number of patient-days of therapy with deferiprone was 334. One subject developed agranulocytosis, defined as an absolute neutrophil count less than $500/mm^3$. This episode in a non-splenectomized patient occurred after fifteen weeks of treatment with deferiprone and was unassociated with recent infection. The nadir of the absolute neutrophil count was $180/mm^3$, and resolution of the neutropenia, defined as two consecutive absolute neutrophil counts greater than $2000/mm^3$, occurred in eight days. The patient received G-CSF for six days.

Nine other subjects in the trial developed neutropenia with the lowest absolute neutrophil count reaching $500-1250/mm^3$. The episodes of neutropenia in these subjects occurred within one to fifty weeks of beginning deferiprone. Six had a history of a recent viral infection. Resolution of neutropenia occurred in 4–84 days. These nine patients had lower average neutrophil counts prior to treatment with deferiprone than the other subjects. Only one (11%) of the nine patients was splenectomized. In contrast, 72 (40%) of the remaining 178 patients had previously undergone splenectomy ($p = 0.08$ by Fishers exact test).

Adverse reactions, defined as occurrences that are possibly, probably or definitely related to the study drug, are shown in TABLE 2. The most common reaction, an orange color in the urine, was due to the drug itself. Nausea and/or vomiting occurred in 24% of subjects, and 13% of subjects developed abdominal pain. Arthralgia occurred in 6% of

TABLE 1. Reasons for Discontinuation

Abnormal Laboratory Values		Others	
Neutropenia	10 patients	Nausea	4 patients
ANC < $500/mm^3$ (agranulocytosis)	1 patient	Voluntary withdrawal	3 patients
		Unconfirmed low ANC	1 patient
ANC $500-1500/mm^3$	9 patients	Fatigue	1 patient
PLT < $100,000/mm^3$	2 patients	Depression	1 patient
High ALT	2 patients	Protocol violation	1 patient

Abbreviations: ALT, alanine amino transferase; PLT, platelet count; ANC, absolute neutrophil count.

subjects. Only one patient developed symptoms or clinical findings compatible with arthritis. Five percent of subjects reported an increase in appetite, and, as noted above, 5% developed neutropenia.

The mean ALT value, already elevated at 61 U/L at entry, increased to 76 U/L at three months and decreased slightly from six months to termination. ALT levels increased to twice the baseline value on at least one measurement in 48% of subjects. This change was independent of hepatitis C serostatus. The rise in ALT level was most commonly first noted at three months. In two subjects, deferiprone was discontinued because of persistently elevated ALT levels.

Sustained immunologic abnormalities were defined as newly appearing positive tests that remained positive on at least one subsequent measurement. No patient had a sustained positive ANA, six patients had sustained positive rheumatoid factor, two patients had a sustained positive anti-double stranded DNA and no patient had a sustained antihistone antibody. All positive antibodies were at low titers of 1:20 or 1:40. None of the patients with sustained positive rheumatoid factor had positive anti-double stranded DNA antibody. One of the patients with sustained positive rheumatoid factor complained of recurrent knee and ankle pain, but none of the other patients with positive immunologic studies complained of joint pain.

Although this study was designed primarily to assess the safety of deferiprone, a secondary objective was assessment of iron stores as measured by serum ferritin level. The mean ferritin level did not change significantly between baseline and termination ($p = 0.38$). Patients who entered the study with more severe iron overload, as indicated by ferritin levels greater than 2500 µg/L, showed a decline in mean ferritin level from 4181 to 3780 µg/L ($p = 0.002$). For patients who entered the study with ferritin levels less than 2500 µg/L, the mean ferritin level rose from 1632 µg/L at entry to 1823 µg/L at termination ($p = 0.05$).

DISCUSSION

In this multi-center, one-year safety study of deferiprone, treatment was generally well tolerated; 87% of the subjects completed the study and 13% withdrew or discontinued therapy. Weekly monitoring of blood counts identified agranulocytosis (absolute neutrophil count less than 500/mm^3) in one (0.5%) and less severe neutropenia (absolute neutrophil count 500–1500/mm^3) in 9 (5%) of 187 subjects. The incidence of agranulocytosis, the most serious side effect previously associated with deferiprone,[2–6] was 0.58 per 100 patient-years. Less severe neutropenia usually occurred in non-splenectomized patients who had lower average neutrophil counts prior to therapy with deferiprone, and this may be due to hypersplenism, perhaps aggravated by a viral infection, rather than deferiprone. However, it remains possible that neutropenia might have progressed to agranulocytosis in some subjects if neutrophil counts had not been measured weekly and if deferiprone had not been promptly withdrawn when indicated. This one-year trial could not determine the cumulative incidence of neutropenia over a longer time period. A continuation study addressing this question is currently underway.

TABLE 2. Adverse Reactions Occurring in 5% or More Subjects

Reaction	Affected Subjects
Urine abnormality	74 (40%)
Nausea and/or vomiting	45 (24%)
Abdominal pain	25 (13%)
Arthralgia	12 (6%)
Increased appetite	10 (5%)
Neutropenia	10 (5%)

Increased ALT levels occurred commonly during the initial months of treatment with deferiprone, and usually stabilized or regressed after three to six months. Similar findings have previously been reported.[2,7] Two patients discontinued therapy because of high ALT levels. In the remaining patients, the increased ALT values were not associated with clinical or biochemical evidence of progressive liver disease despite continued treatment with deferiprone.

Arthralgia and arthritis occurred less frequently than in previous studies.[7–9] Immunologic abnormalities were uncommon, and no evidence of drug-induced lupus or other significant immunologic problems was found.[10–12]

Overall, mean ferritin levels did not change significantly during this one-year study. Deferiprone was more effective in reducing iron stores, as measured by serum ferritin levels, in patients who began with more severe iron overload. A similar effect of degree of iron overload on subsequent changes in iron stores during deferiprone therapy has been noted by other investigators.[13] Other factors, such as the rate of transfusional iron loading, that might influence the effectiveness of deferiprone therapy in the current study are being investigated.

In summary, these findings support the safety of this formulation of deferiprone as an orally active iron chelating agent, using the careful monitoring system employed in this trial.

ACKNOWLEDGMENTS

This study was sponsored by Apotex, Inc., Weston, Ontario, Canada. Doctors Nancy Olivieri and Gary Brittenham participated in the organization and conduct of this trial but did not take part in the data analyses and manuscript preparation and do not agree with the conclusions.

REFERENCES

1. BRITTENHAM, G. M. 1992. Development of iron-chelating agents for clinical use. Blood **80**: 569–574.
2. AL-REFAIE, F. N., C. HERSHKO, A. V. HOFFBRAND, et al. 1995. Results of long-term deferiprone (L1) therapy: A report by the International Study Group on Oral Iron Chelators. Br. J. Haematol. **91**: 224–229.
3. HOFFBRAND, A. V., A. N. BARTLETT, P. A. VEYRS, et al. 1989. Agranulocytosis and thrombocytopenia in patients with Blackfan-Diamond anaemia during oral chelator trial. Lancet **2**: 437.
4. BARTLETT, A. N., A. V. HOFFBRAND & G. J. KONTOGHIORGHES. 1990. Long-term trial with the oral iron chelator 1,2-dimethyl-3-hydroxypyrid-4-one (L1). II. Clinical observations. Br. J. Haematol. **76**: 301–304.
5. AL-REFAIE, F. N., B. WONKE & A. V. HOFFBRAND. 1994. Deferiprone-associated myelotoxicity. Eur. J. Haematol. **53**: 293–301.
6. OLIVIERI, N. F. 1996. Long-term therapy with deferiprone. Acta Haematol. **95**: 37–48.
7. AL-REFAIE, F. N., B. WONKE, A. V. HOFFBRAND, et al. 1992. Efficacy and possible adverse effects of the oral iron chelator 1,2-dimethyl-3-hydroxypyrid-4-one (L1) in thalassemia major. Blood **80**: 593–599.
8. AGARWAL, M. B., S. S. GUPTE, C. VISWANATHAN, et al. 1992. Long-term assessment of efficacy and safety of L1, an oral iron chelator, in transfusion-dependent thalassaemia: Indian trial. Br. J. Haematol. **82**: 460–466.
9. BERKOVITCH, M., R. M. LAXER, R. INMAN, et al. 1994. Arthropathy in thalassaemia patients receiving deferiprone. Lancet **343**: 1471–1472.
10. MEHTA, J., S. SINGHAL, R. REVANKAR, et al. 1991. Fatal systemic lupus erythematosus in patient taking oral iron chelator L1. Lancet **337**: 298.
11. BERDOUKAS, V. A. 1991. Anti-nuclear antibodies in patients taking L1. Lancet **337**: 672.
12. CASTRIOTA-SCANDERBEG, A. & M. SACCO. 1997. Agranulocytosis, arthritis and systemic vasculitis in a patient receiving the oral iron chelator L1 (deferiprone). Br. J. Haematol. **96**: 254–255.
13. OLIVIERI, N. F., G. M. BRITTENHAM, D. MATSUI, et al. 1995. Iron-chelation therapy with oral deferiprone in patients with thalassemia major. N. Engl. J. Med. **332**: 918–922.

Survival and Disease Complications in Thalassemia Major

CATERINA BORGNA-PIGNATTI,[a,b] SIMONE RUGOLOTTO,[c] PIERO DE STEFANO,[d] ANTONIO PIGA,[e] FELICIA DI GREGORIO,[f] MARIA RITA GAMBERINI,[g] VINCENZO SABATO,[h] CATERINA MELEVENDI,[i] MARIA DOMENICA CAPPELLINI,[j] AND GIUSEPPE VERLATO[k]

[b]*Department of Clinical and Experimental Medicine, University of Ferrara*

[c]*Department of Pediatrics, University of Verona*

[d]*Department of Pediatrics, IRCCS "San Matteo," Pavia*

[e]*Department of Pediatrics, University of Turin*

[f]*Department of Pediatrics, University of Catania*

[g]*Annunziata Di Palma, Division of Pediatrics, Ospedale Sant'Anna;*
[h]*Department of Pediatrics, University of Bari*

[i]*Division of Pediatrics, Ospedale Galliera, Genova*

[j]*Department of Internal Medicine, University of Milan*

[k]*Institute of Medical Statistics, University of Verona*

ABSTRACT: We studied survival and disease complications in 1,146 patients with thalassemia major, born from January 1, 1960 to December 31, 1987. At last follow-up, in March 1997, probability of survival to age 20 years was 89% and to age 25 years was 82% for patients born in the years 1970–1974. Patients who died had a serum ferritin level, measured the year before death, significantly higher than those who survived. Diabetes was present in 5.4% of the patients; heart failure in 6.4%; arrhythmias in 5.0%, thrombosis in 1.1%, hypothyroidism in 11.6%, HIV infection in 1.8%. Hypogonadism was diagnosed in 55% of 578 patients who had reached pubertal age: 83.5% of hypogonadic females and 78.6% of males were receiving substitutive hormonal therapy. In conclusion, the survival of patients with thalassemia major is good and improving, but the prevalence of severe complications is still high.

Organ damage and early death used to be inevitable consequences of thalassemia major. The prognosis of the disease, however, has been improved by regular transfusions and iron chelation.

In the last 14 years, as a part of a cooperative study, we followed a large number of patients with thalassemia major treated at seven Italian hospitals, and we confirmed that the survival of transfusion-dependent patients has been steadily and significantly increasing.[1] Unfortunately, the prevalence of complications due to iron overload is still high.

[a]Address for correspondence: C. Borgna-Pignatti, Department of Clinical and Experimental Medicine, Pediatrics, University of Ferrara, Via Savonarola 9, 44100 Ferrara, Italy. Fax: 39-532-202 103; E-mail: bre@dns.unife.it

PATIENTS AND METHODS

Seven Italian teaching hospitals contributed their patients with thalassemia major to this study. Inclusion criteria required that the patients be born after January 1, 1960 and be alive at the time since when, at each center, clinical records were complete and reliable. The first data collection took place in 1983. Latest follow-up was March 1997.

The patients notified by the participating centers were 1,146 (614 males and 532 females). The distribution by calendar period of birth is shown in FIGURE 1.

The Kaplan-Meier method[2] and log-rank test[3] were used to estimate and compare survival and appearance of complications. Since, for older patients, no information could be drawn on mortality in the first decade of life, overall survival was evaluated only for patients born in or after 1970, while survival after the first decade of life was evaluated for all patients. In addition we collected, by means of specially prepared forms, data on complications potentially affecting the quality of life of the patients. Complications considered were: insulin-dependent diabetes, hypothyroidism requiring substitutive therapy, thrombosis, heart failure or arrhythmias requiring therapy, absence of signs of puberty at age 15 years for females and at age 17 for males, and HIV positivity. Mean yearly serum ferritin was available for the years 1991–1996. Since it was not normally distributed, a preliminary logarithmic transformation was required for subsequent analysis. Comparison of ferritin levels between groups was performed by Student's t test.

RESULTS

At last follow-up, 769 patients of 1,146 were alive with thalassemia, 26 had been lost to observation, and 248 had died. One hundred and three had undergone bone marrow transplantation; 13 of them had died as a consequence of the procedure. Crude death rates ranged from 67% for patients born before 1965 to 2.5% for those born after 1979.

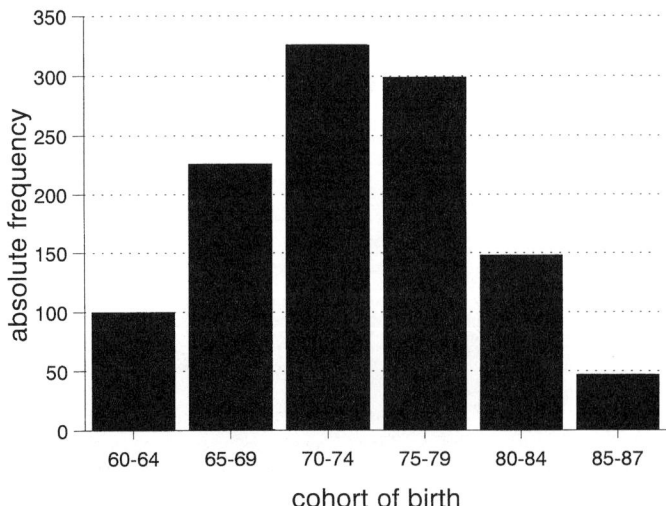

FIGURE 1. Distribution by cohort of birth of patients with thalassemia major who entered the study.

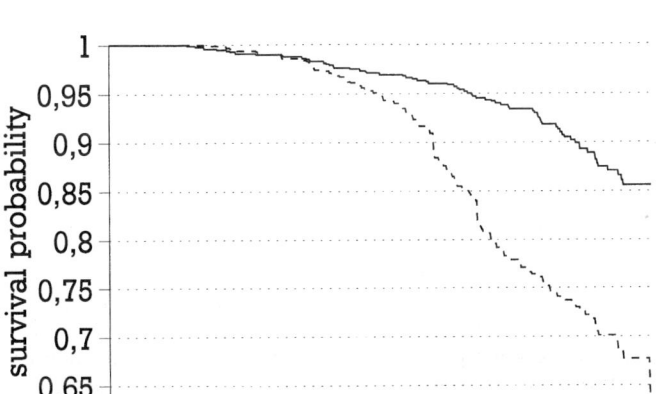

FIGURE 2. Probability of survival and of disease-free survival (excluding hypothyroidism and treated hypogonadism) of patients with thalassemia major born in 1970–1987.

Survival and complications appearance were evaluated for the whole population born after 1970 (FIG. 2) and for the birth cohorts 1970–1974, 1975–1979, 1980–1984, and 1985–1987. The probability of survival at different ages are presented in TABLE 1.

The serum ferritin level of the year before death was, for patients who died between 1991 and 1996, significantly higher than for patients who survived (3,314 ± 2,468 versus 2,002 ± 1,455, $p < 0.001$).

When data for males and females were analyzed separately, we found that females have a significantly better survival than males, both for the whole group born between 1960–1974 ($p = 0.0242$) and for the older patients (1960–1969) alone ($p = 0.039$).

Heart disease was the most frequent cause of death, being directly responsible for the death of 71% of the patients. Infection directly caused the death of 12% of the patients. Liver disease represented the third most frequent cause of death being directly responsible for the death of 6% of them. Other causes of death are reported in TABLE 2.

The risk of developing complications was evaluated only for patients born after 1970 (718). The prevalence of heart failure at age 15 was found to have decreased from 5% in patients from the cohort 1970–1974 to 2% in patients born in 1980–1984. Corresponding values for diabetes are 2.6% and zero. On the contrary, hypothyroidism is apparently becoming more frequent, being present, at age 15 years, in 4.8% of the patients born between 1970 and 1974, but in 8% of those born between 1980 and 1984. Overall, diabetes was present in 5.4%, heart failure 6.4%, arrhythmias 5.0%, thrombosis 1.1%, hypothyroidism 11.6%, and HIV infection 1.8%. Hypogonadism was diagnosed in 55% of 578 patients who had reached pubertal age: 83.5% of hypogonadic females and 78.6% of males were receiving substitutive hormonal therapy.

TABLE 1. Survival by Birth Cohort at Different Ages of Patients with Transfusion-Dependent Thalassemia

Age (years)	1970–1974	1975–1979	1980–1984
10	98% (96–99)	98% (96–99)	99% (95–100)
15	95% (92–97)	97% (94–98)	98% (93–100)
20	89% (85–92)	96% (93–98)	
25	82% (77–86)		

DISCUSSION

In the last three decades, the treatment of thalassemia major has changed in many ways. Administration of deferoxamine by the intramuscular route became available to the majority of Italian patients in 1975, while regular subcutaneous infusion was started between 1979 and 1981. In the same years the transfusion regimen evolved from correction of symptomatic anemia to the so-called hypertransfusion or supertransfusion regimens, aimed at maintaining a minimum hemoglobin level from 9–10 g/dl to above 12 g/dl. The impression that the supertransfusion regimen had increased the iron overload and its consequences has recently induced most centers to return to hypertransfusion. In addition, the early detection of complications has been actively pursued and their aggressive treatment has become the rule. A major pivotal point in the history of thalassemia treatment has been the introduction in 1981 of bone marrow transplantation from an HLA-identical sibling.[4] This progress has made information about survival and complications with conventional therapy particularly important.

Not many data have been reported so far on survival of transfusion-dependent patients with thalassemia. Economidou reported in 1982[5] that at age 28 only 24% of Greek patients with thalassemia major and intermedia were alive. In 1982, Modell and coworkers[6] found that the probability of reaching age 25 years was 25%. There is convincing evidence from several reports that iron chelation improves organ function,[7–9] and that it is capable of preventing the development of cardiac disease.[10] More recently, Brittenham and coworkers observed that the risk of dying and of developing diabetes and cardiac disease were decreased by the early use of deferoxamine.[11] Data from Olivieri and coworkers, who studied 97 patients born before 1976, demonstrate that after 15 years of chelation therapy, the probability of being free from cardiac disease is 91%, provided that less than one third of serum ferritin values exceeded 2,500 ng/ml.[12] In our study we found that serum ferritin, and therefore, presumably, the iron burden, was higher in patients who died than in patients who survive.

TABLE 2. Causes of Death Reported in Patients with Thalassemia, Born between 1960 and 1984

Cardiac causes	171	71%
Liver	15	6%
Endocrine	6	3%
Infections	28	12%
Thrombosis	3	1%
Anemia	2	1%
Tumors	7	3%
Unknown	3	1%
Other	5	2%

We reported in 1989 the fatality rate and the causes of death in a group of patients with thalassemia major born since 1960.[1] A remarkable improvement in life expectancy was observed when different birth cohorts were compared. This improvement was mainly due to the decrease in mortality for cardiac causes. Conversely, mortality due to causes other than heart disease had not decreased. The results have not changed at subsequent follow-ups. At the latest data collection the difference in survival between cohorts is still striking (TABLE 1). Moreover, the study of complications has confirmed that patients born in more recent years have a lower risk of developing heart disease, diabetes and hypogonadism, than patients born earlier. The trend is not so clear for hypothyroidism, which, in the past, was probably underdiagnosed.

With modern therapy, complications and death should be unusual in the first ten years of life. This expectation is confirmed by our data. Only four patients out of 283 from the cohort 1970–1974, and none from the subsequent cohorts, have developed heart failure in the first decade of life. However, diabetes developed in the first decade of life in two children from the cohort 1975–1979.

In conclusion, the favorable trend that we observed in the past seems to continue for patients who had the advantage of early chelation therapy. Despite the fact, however, that thalassemia is no longer a rapidly fatal disease and that the majority of the patients will reach the age of employment and of marriage, the prevalence of complications is still high. Research should therefore be aimed at containing as much as possible the complications of the disease that could make the life of these patients unsatisfactory and not productive. Less invasive methods of chelation, such as oral or intermittent chelation could also contribute to making the life of these patients easier.

REFERENCES

1. ZURLO, M. G., P. DE STEFANO, C. BORGNA-PIGNATTI *et al.* 1989. Survival and causes of death in thalassemia major. Lancet **2**: 27–30.
2. KAPLAN, E. L., P. MEIER. 1958. Nonparametric estimations from incomplete observations. J. Am. Stat. Assoc. **53**: 457–481.
3. PETO, R., M. C. PIKE, P. ARMITAGE *et al.* 1977. Design and analysis of randomized clinical trials requiring prolonged observation of each patient. II Analysis and examples. Br. J. Cancer **35**: 1–39.
4. THOMAS, E. D., C. D. BUCKNER, J. E. SANDERS *et al.* 1982. Marrow transplantation for thalassemia. Lancet **ii**: 227–229.
5. ECONOMIDOU, J. 1982. Problems related to treatment of beta-thalassemia major. Paediatrician **11**: 157–177.
6. MODELL, B., E. A. LETSKY, D. M. FLYNN *et al.* 1982. Survival and desferrioxamine in thalassaemia major. Br. Med. J. **284**: 1081–1084.
7. COHEN, A., M. MARTIN & E. SCHWARTZ. 1984. Depletion of excessive liver iron stores with desferrioxamine. Br. J. Haematol. **58**: 369–373.
8. KAYE, S. B., M. OWEN. 1978. Cardiac arrhythmias in thalassaemia major: Evaluation of chelation treatment using ambulatory monitoring. Br. Med. J. **1**: 342.
9. DAVIES, S. C., J. L. HUNGERFORD, G. B. ARDEN, *et al.* 1983. Ocular toxicity of high-dose intravenous desferrioxamine. Lancet **ii**: 181–184.
10. WOLFE, L., N. OLIVIERI, D. SALLAN *et al.* 1985. Prevention of cardiac disease by subcutaneous deferoxamine in patients with thalassemia major. N. Engl. J. Med. **312**: 1600–1603.
11. BRITTENHAM, G. T. M., P. M. GRIFFITH, A.W. NIENHUIS *et al.* 1994. Efficacy of deferoxamine in preventing complications of iron overload in patients with thalassemia major. N. Engl. J. Med. **331**: 567–573
12. OLIVIERI, N. F., D. G. NATHAN, J. H. MACMILLAN *et al.* 1994. Survival in medically treated patients with homozygous beta-thalassemia. N. Engl. J. Med. **331**: 574–577.

New Approaches to the Management of Hepatitis and Endocrine Disorders in Cooley's Anemia

BEATRIX WONKE,[a,e] A. V. HOFFBRAND,[b] P. BOULOUX,[c]
C. JENSEN,[d] AND P. TELFER[a]

[a]*Department of Haematology, Whittington Hospital, London*

[b]*The Royal Free Hospital, Academic Department of Hematology*

[c]*Department of Endocrinology, The Royal Free Hospital*

[d]*Department of Obstetrics and Gynaecology, The Whittington Hospital*

ABSTRACT: Hepatitis C infection is common in patients receiving life-long blood transfusion therapy. Interferon-α induces long term viral clearance in 25–30% of patients suffering from Cooley's anemia. Ribavirin, an orally active guanoside analogue together with interferon-α produces a sustained response in up to 40% of patients with cirrhosis, who had previously failed single agent treatment. Growth retardation in iron-overloaded patients is the result of growth hormone deficiency in up to 30% of patients. Height gain can be sucessfully achieved in these patients with growth hormone treatment. Pregnancy in women with Cooley's anemia is now a reality, and over 100 pregnancies have been documented. Conception may be spontaneous or the result of ovulation induction. Cardiomyopathy and diabetes require careful assessment in these patients before a decision is made to treat with gonadotrophins to induce ovulation.

With optimal treatment, life expectancy of patients with thalassemia (TM) is open ended. However, longevity depends on good clinical management, which includes the treatment of transfusional transmitted viruses, in particular hepatitis C. To ensure good quality of life, patients should be given the opportunity to have normal growth, sexual development, normal reproduction, and normal bone metabolism. In this paper we wish to discuss some of these issues in which we have a particular interest. Our experience is based on more than 200 multi-ethnic TM patients resident in the United Kingdom.

HEPATITIS C

Hepatitis C virus (HCV) infection is common in patients with TM on life long transfusions. In the United Kingdom, 23% of patients have antibodies to HCV[1] and in other parts of the world the prevalence is much greater (FIG. 1).[2–5]

In the majority of cases, HCV infection gives rise to chronic hepatitis with risk of progression to cirrhosis and hepatocellular carcinoma.[6] In the case of patients with TM, the hepatic damage due to HCV infection is exacerbated by transfusional iron overload lead-

---

[e]Address for correspondence: Beatrix Wonke, Department of Haematology, Whittington Hospital, Highgate Hill, London N19 5NF. Tel: 0171 288 5034; Fax: 0171 288 3485.

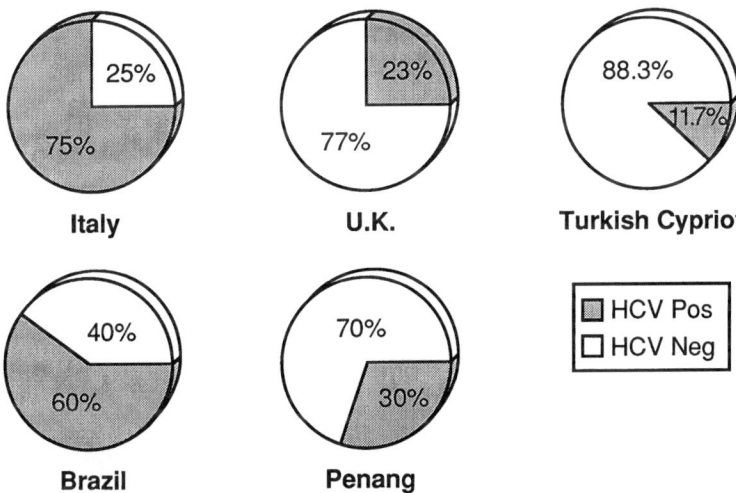

FIGURE 1. Prevalence of hepatitis C in thalassemia major. Anti-HCV positive thalassemia major patients.

ing to the development of early cirrhosis. Liver disease indeed is a well recognized cause of mortality in TM patients.[7]

The therapeutic goal in TM patients with HCV is the early eradication of the virus in order to prevent long-term clinical complications. Interferon-alpha (IFN), the only agent currently licensed for therapy, induces sustained viral clearance in about 25–30% of thalassemia patients.[2,8] Sustained response to IFN is most likely to occur in young patients with a histological picture of chronic active hepatitis and with low liver iron content.[2,9]

First line management strategy for thalassemia patients with chronic hepatitis C is described in FIGURE 2. Side effects of IFN treatment are listed in TABLE 1. The incidence of primary hypothyroidism in iron overloaded thalassemia patients is 6.2%.[10] Many patients, however, have pre-clinical or mild hypothyroidism and during treatment with IFN overt hypothyroidism can develop, requiring treatment with L-thyroxine. The pathophysiology of this complication is not well understood. Severe depression is a common problem during IFN treatment. Very close supervision of these patients is mandatory and the use of antidepressants may be necessary. TM patients who fail to attain sustained response to IFN treatment or relapse after cessation of therapy may benefit from ribavirin

TABLE 1. Side Effects of Interferon Treatment

Pyrexia, rigors, fatigue
Depression
Marrow suppression
Hypothyroidism
    Myalgia
    Hair loss
Weight loss
    Cardiac effects
        Glucose intolerance

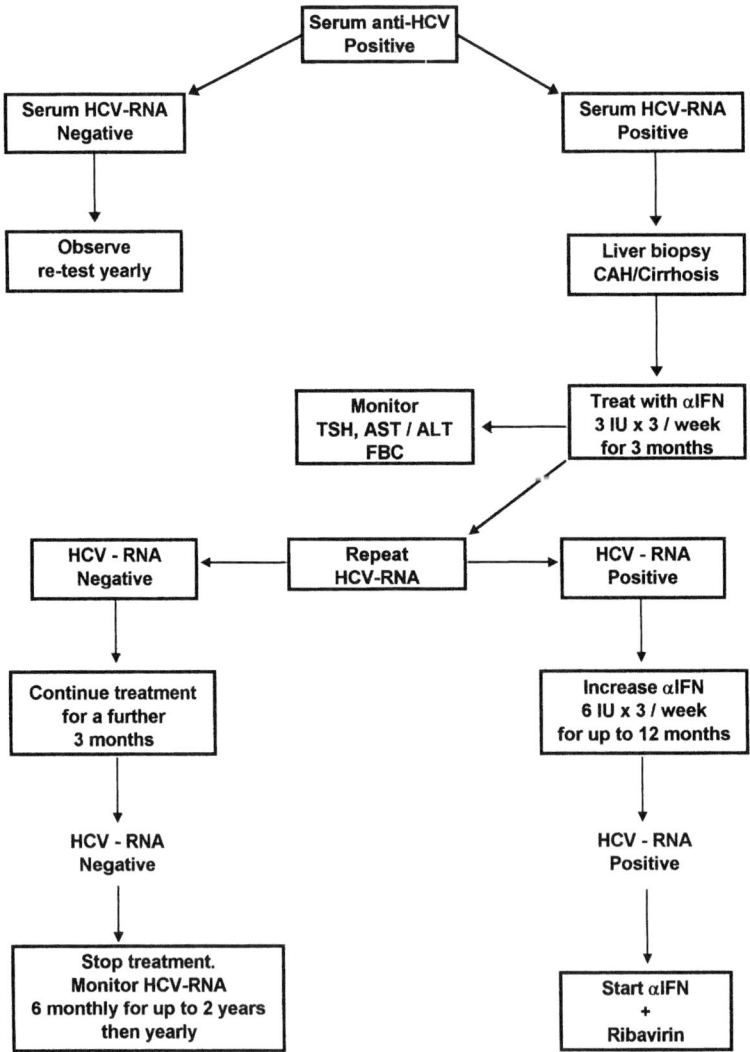

FIGURE 2. Algorithm for first line management of thalassemia in patients with chronic active hepatitis C.

in combination with IFN. Ribavirin is an orally active guanoside analogue with an *in vitro* activity against a wide range of DNA and RNA viruses.[11] When used as a single agent for HCV infection, the response rate with ribavirin has been disappointing. Furthermore, there is evidence of increased hemolysis in most patients, and some cases of reversible hemolytic anemia while on therapy.[12,13] Ribavirin in combination with IFN has, however, produced sustained responses of 45–60% in several recent pilot studies.[14–16] Good

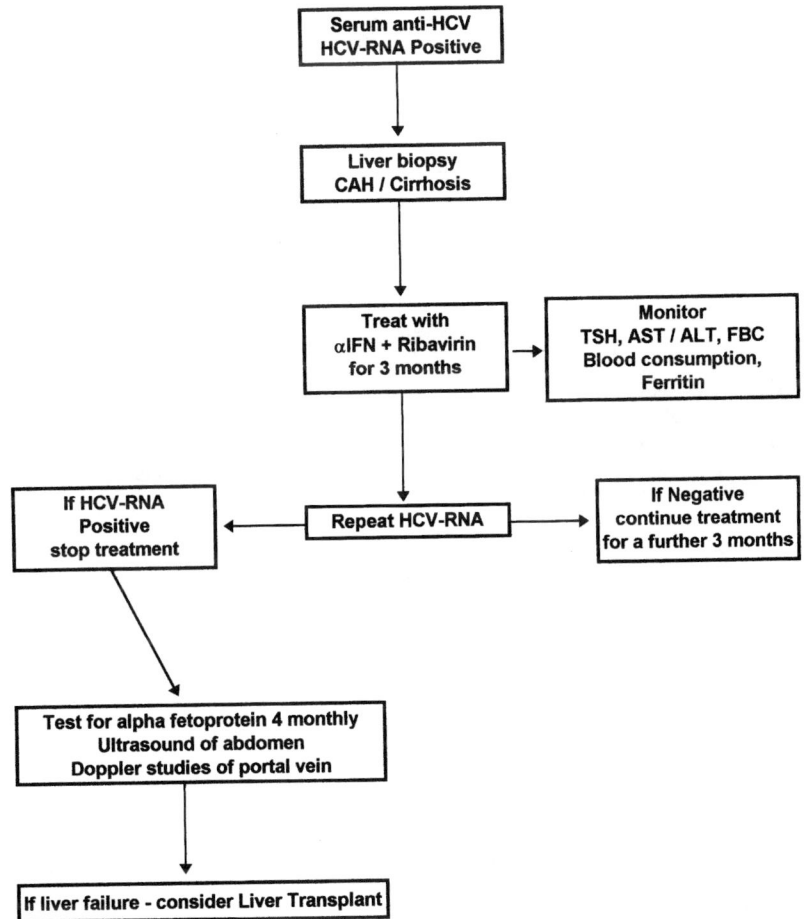

FIGURE 3. Algorithm for second line management of thalassemia patients with chronic active hepatitis C.

responses have been obtained even in patients with cirrhosis, who had previously failed on IFN alone. IFN, three mega units thrice weekly, self-administered subcutaneously (s.c) together with ribavirin (Viratek, California), 1 gram per day orally in two divided doses, is the recommended protocol for TM patients. Second line management of TM patients with chronic hepatitis C is proposed in FIGURE 3. Adverse affects observed during combination therapy are similar to those mentioned in TABLE 1 but in addition, transfusion requirements increase significantly during the treatment period. Ribavirin therapy is almost invariable associated with hemolysis, the mechanism of which is related to the accumulation of the drug within erythrocytes by ribavirin competing with adenosine nucleotides and causing deficiency of intracellular ATP, with consequent reduction of red cell survival.[17] The hemolysis is more marked in patients who are undergoing regular transfusions. The degree of increased transfusion necessitates the intensification of iron chelation therapy. The presence of HCV-RNA at week 12 of combination treatment predicts a lack of sustained response and therefore we suggest discontinuation of treatment at this stage (FIG. 3). Stopping therapy after 12 weeks in non-responders will avoid unnecessary prolongation of therapy, increased transfusions, and iron load. The use of serum clearance of HCV-RNA as a criterion of treatment response in mono and in combination therapy[2,3] is essential, since serum transaminase levels may be elevated in TM due to the

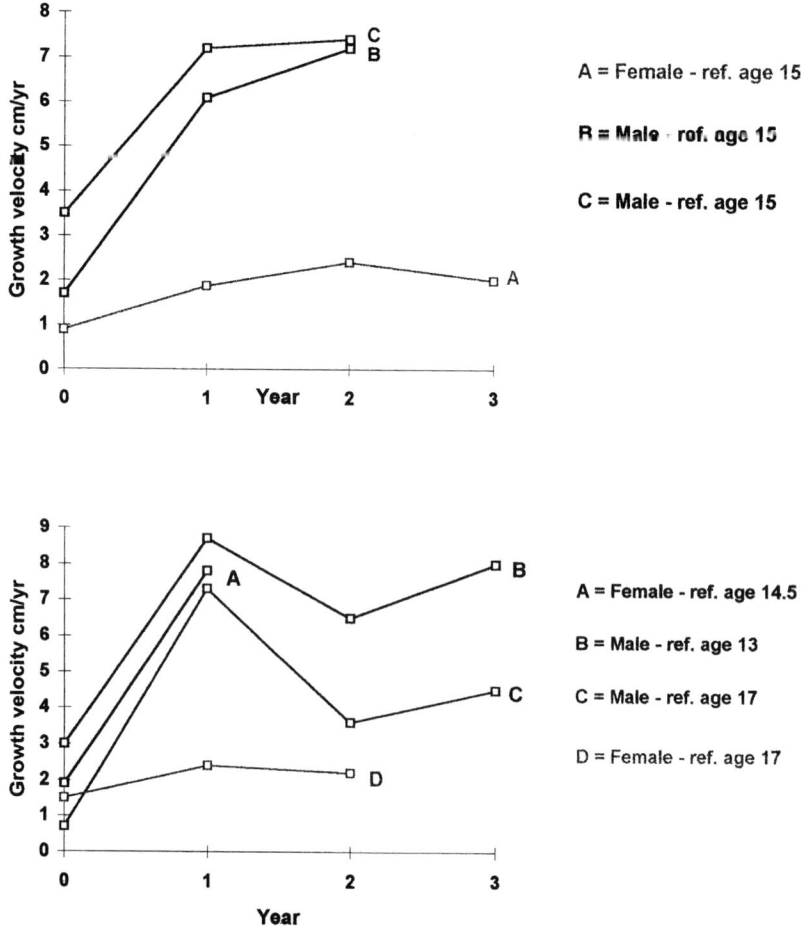

FIGURE 4. (Top) Hypogonadotrophic hypogonadism on sex steriods only. Growth velocity of TM patients on sex steroid treatment. (Bottom) Hypogonadotrophic hypogonadism and GH deficiency on sex steroids and GH. Growth velocity of TM patients on sex steroids and rhGH treatment.

concomitant toxic effect of iron in the liver. TM patients who do not respond to mono or combination therapy are at risk of hepatic failure or hepatocellular carcinoma. This risk is increased in those who have severe iron overload. Careful monitoring of these patients' progress is recommended with intensification of iron chelation, monitoring liver function, and assessment for liver transplantation (FIG. 3).

GROWTH IN THALASSAEMIA MAJOR

Many thalassemic children of both sexes show reduced growth around the age of 10–11 years. This results in a final height below the predicted mid-parental height. The causes of short stature in TM patients are complex and multi-factorial. Chronic hypoxia secondary to anemia when pre-transfusion Hb is below 8.5 g/l,[18] growth hormone insufficiency,[19] defective hepatic biosynthesis of somatomedin insulin-like growth factor 1 (IGF 1),[20] and sex steroid deficiency are the principal responsible factors. High doses or hypersensitivity to deferoxamine (DF) in therapeutic doses may also result in growth retardation. It is known that DF inhibits DNA synthesis, fibroblast proliferation, collagen formation, and may also cause zinc deficiency.[21] The toxic effects of DF may result in painful hips, lower back, wrists, and sometimes, walking difficulties. The body measurement of children and adults are disproportionate with short trunk, long extremities and short stature. Swelling of the wrists and knees and genu valgum of variable severity is often found. The patients invariably have a normal onset of puberty and pubertal development.

Treatment

The treatment of anemia consists of regular transfusions, maintaining an overall mean hemoglobin (Hb) concentration of 12 g/dl. The overall mean pre-transfusion Hb should be kept not lower than 9 g/dl.

Growth Hormone Insufficiency

This condition is treated with recombinant human growth hormone (rhGH) given as self-administered daily subcutaneous doses varying from 0.6–0.9 IU/kg body weight/week. **Good-responders** to rhGH treatment are those whose growth velocity increment equals, or is greater than, 4 cm above the previous year. **Partial-responder's** growth velocity increment equals, or is 2–4 cm above, the previous year, **non-responder's** growth velocity is less than 2 cm per year above the previous year.[22]

Growth Hormone Resistance

Patients are investigated by injection of rhGH (0.1 unit/kg body weight/day s.c for four days) followed by measurements of IGF1, and insulin-like growth factor and their binding protein (IGFBP3) levels in the serum. *Low levels* of increments indicate some degree of growth hormone resistance. *The treatment* of these patients is with increased rhGH 1 unit/kg body weight/week. In our experience the response to growth hormone treatment is variable. Half the patients have good response, others may require larger doses of rhGH in case of growth hormone resistance. Chronic liver disease may contribute to this. Glucose tolerance must be controlled in these patients as they are prone to develop an abnormality in glucose homeostasis. *In DF toxicity,* deferiprone the orally active iron-chelating agent

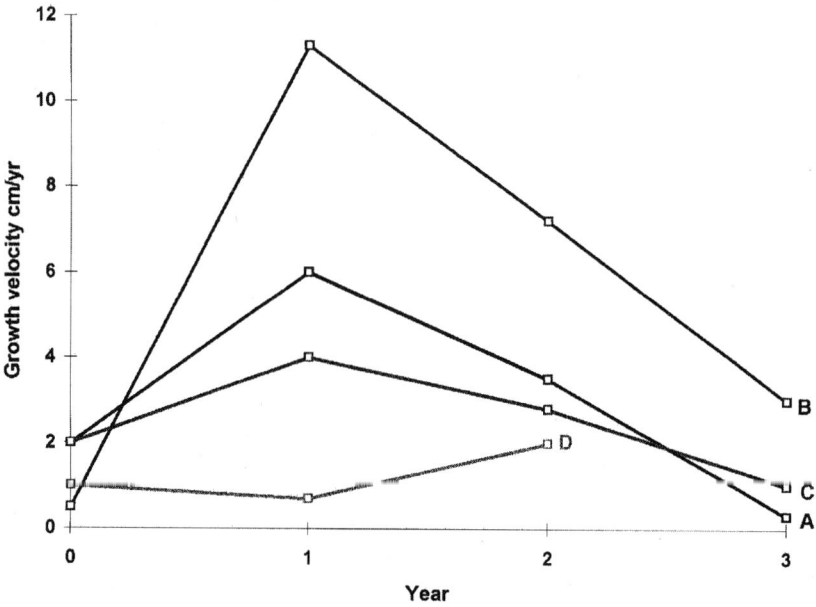

FIGURE 5. Growth velocity of TM patients with growth hormone resistance. (A) Male-ref. age 16, (B) Male-ref. age 12.5, (c) Female-ref age 13.5, (D) Male-ref. age 12.5.

should be tried. In conclusion, multiple factors contribute to growth retardation, not all are operative in every child at any one time, but several of the factors can be inter-related, requiring careful investigation and the appropriate treatment (FIGS. 4 and 5).

OSTEOPOROSIS

Osteoporosis associated morbidity has become a major problem in the aging thalassemia population. Backache, cord compression, nerve route lesions, fractures on minimal trauma, followed by slow healing are common occurrence. Historically, severe bone deformities with marked facial and limb changes were originally described by Cooley and colleagues in 1927[23] in untreated TM patients. The presence of osteopenia in the well treated TM patients has been described by Giardina[24] and Goni[25] and their colleagues in 1995,[24-25] however the high incidence and severity of osteoporosis in these patients have only recently been appreciated.[26] Jensen and colleagues investigated 82 TM patients of both sexes with a mean age of 27 (range 12–43) years. The incidence of osteoporosis was 51% (FIGS. 6 and 7). Multi-variant analysis showed that hypogonadotrophic-hypogonadism, gender, and diabetes were significant risk factors for developing severe osteoporosis. No association was found between ethnicity, smoking, exercise, calcium supplementation, age of the patient, age at starting DF chelation therapy, number of years on chelation, the number of units of blood per year, the overall mean pre-transfusion Hb, and the current serum ferritin concentration. Jensen's study shows that in spite of optimal management, the majority of TM patients of both sexes develop severe osteoporosis. Most surprising is the finding of low

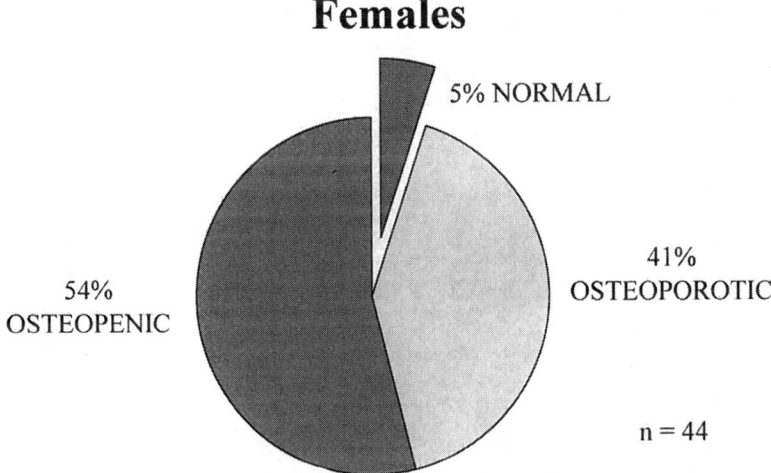

FIGURE 6. Incidence of osteoporosis in 44 female thalassemia major patients.

bone mineral density at ages as young as twelve years, which indicate that the peak bone mass is also adversely affected. Another observation unique to the TM population is the importance of the gender in developing osteoporosis. In TM, men are more commonly and more severely affected than females. In men, both lumbar vertebrae and neck of femur are involved, whilst in women the osteoporosis mainly involves the spine. This is despite the fact that all the hypogonadal men and 97% of hypogonadal women in this group were on hormone replacement therapy (HRT). Osteoporosis is a progressive disease, prevention and early diagnosis are more important than attempting to treat the established disease. We treat

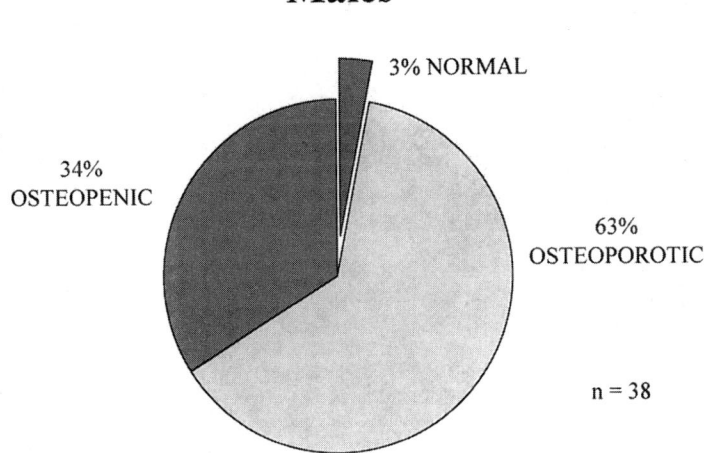

FIGURE 7. Incidence of osteoporosis in 38 male thalassemia major patients.

osteopenic patients with oral calcium and vitamin D supplementation (Calcichew D_3) and encourage active exercise, give dietary advice, promote non-smoking, and treat hypogonadal patients with HRT. Patients with osteoporosis in addition receive pamidronate (15 mg, i.v.) monthly prior to the routine blood transfusion. Bisphosphonates are potent inhibitors of bone resorption[27] and have been successfully used in the treatment of postmenopausal osteoporosis.[28] We have selected to use intravenous pamidronate to overcome the poor oral absorption of these drugs and to ensure that patient compliance with this treatment modality can be accurately assessed.

Our preliminary data suggest increase in bone density in some of our patients but a longer term follow-up is necessary to evaluate the beneficial affects of this treatment protocol.

REFERENCES

1. WONKE, B., A. V. HOFFBRAND, D. BROWN et al. 1990. Antibody to hepatitis C virus in multiply transfused patients with thalassemia major. J. Clin. Pathol. **43**: 638–640.
2. CAO, A., R. GALANELLO, M. C. ROSATELLI et al. 1996. Clinical experience of management of thalassaemia; The Sardinian experience. Sem. Hematol. **1**: 66-75.
3. BOZKURT, G., T. DIKENGIL, O. ALIMOGLU et al. 1993. Hepatitis C among Turkish Cypriot Thalassemic Patients. Presented at Fifth International Conference on Thalassemias and Hemaglobinopathies. Nicosia, Cyprus, 1993. p. 176.
4. CANCADO, R. D. I., G. M. GUERRA, M. O. J. A. ROSENFELD et al. 1993. Prevalence of hepatitis C virus antibody in beta thalassaemic patients. Presented at Fifth International Conference on Thalassemias and Hemoglobinopathies. Nicosia, Cyprus, 1993. p. 176
5. KAUR, P. & B. KAUR. 1995. Thalassemia in Penang. Presented at First Asian Congress on Thalassemia. Penang, Malaysia. p. 70–72.
6. ALTER, H. J. 1995. To C or not to C. These are the questions. Blood **85**: 1681–1695.
7. ZURLO, M. G., P. DE STEFANO, C. BORGNA-PIGNATI et al. 1989. Survival and causes of death in thalassemia major. Lancet **ii**: 27–30.
8. DONOHUE, S. M., B. WONKE, A. V. HOFFBRAND et al. 1993. Alpha interferon in the treatment of chronic hepatitis C virus in multiply transfused patients with thalassaemia major. Br. J. Haematol. **83**: 491–497.
9. ROWNTREE, C., P. T. TELFER, B. WONKE et al. 1995. Long-term follow up of alpha interferon therapy for chronic hepatitis C infection in thalassemic patients. Br. J. Haematol. (Supplement 1) Abstract 199: 55.
10. Italian Working Groups on Endocrine Complications in Non-endocrine Diseases. 1995. Multicentre study on prevalence of endocrine complications in thalassemia major. Clin. Endocrinol. **42**: 581–586.
11. PATTERSON, J. L. & R. FERNANDEZ-LARSSON. 1990. Molcecular mechanisms of action of ribavirin. Rev. Infect. Dis. **12**: 1139–1146.
12. DI BISCEGLIE, A. M., M. SHINDO, T. L. FONG. 1992. A pilot study of ribavirin therapy for chronic hepatitis C. Hepatol. **16**: 649–654.
13. REICHARD, O., Z. YUN, A. SONNERBORG. 1993. Hepatitis C viral RNA titres in serum prior to during and after oral treatment with ribavirin for chronic hepatitis C. J. Med. Virol. **41**: 99–102.
14. TELFER, P. T., J. A. GARSON, K. WHITBY et al. 1997. Combination therapy with interferon alpha and ribavirin for chronic hepatitis C virus infection in thalassemic patients. Br. J. Haematol. **98**: 850–855.
15. BRILLIANTI, S., J. A. GARSON, M. FOLI et al. 1994. A pilot study of combination therapy with ribavirin plus inteferon alpha for interferon alpha-resistant chronic hepatits C. Gastroenterology **107**: 812–817.
16. SCHWARCZ, R., Z. B. YUN, A. SONNERBORG. 1995. Combined treatment with interferon alpha-2b and ribavirin for chronic hepatitis C in patients with a previous non-response or non-sustained response to interferon alone. J. Med. Virol. **46**: 43–47.
17. SHULMAN, N. R. 1984. Assessment of hematologic effects of ribavirin in humans. *In*: Clinical Applications of Ribavirin. R. Smith & V. Knight, Eds.: 79–92. Academic Press. New York.
18. DE SANCTIS, V., M. KATZ, C. VULLO et al. 1994. Effect of different treatment regimes on linear growth and final height is ß thalassemia major. Clin. Endocrinol. **40**: 791–798.

19. PINTOR, C., S. G. CELLA, P. MANSO et al. 1986. Impaired growth hormone response to GH-releasing hormone in thalassemia major. J.Clin Endocrinol Metab, **62**: 263–267.
20. SAENGER, P., E. SCHWARTZ, A. L. MARKENSON et al. 1980. Depressed serum somatomedin in ß thalassaemia. J. Pediatr. **96**: 214–218.
21. DE VIRGILIIS, S., M. CONGIA, F. FRAU et al. 1988. Deferoxamine-induced growth retardation in patients with thalassemia major. J. Pediatr. **113**: 661–669.
22. DE SANCTIS, V. & B. WONKE.1994. Growth in Thalassemia. Mediprint. Rome.
23. COOLEY, T. B., E. R. WITWER & P. LEE. 1927. Anemia in children with splenomegaly and peculiar changes in the bones. Am. J. Dis. Child. **34**: 347–363.
24. GIARDINA, P. J., R. SCHNEIDER, M. LESSER et al. 1995. Abnormal bone metabolism in thalassemia. *In* Endocrine Disorders in Thalassemia (pp. 38–46). Springer-Verlag.
25. GONI, M. H., V. MARKUSSIS & G. TOLIS. 1995. Bone mineral content by single and dual-photon absorptionmetry in thalassemic patients. *In* Endocrine Disorders in Thalassemia (pp. 47–51). Springer-Verlag.
26. JENSEN, C. E., S. M. TUCK, J. E. AGNEW et al. 1997. Osteoporosis in young adults with transfusion dependent β thalassemia major. Br. J. Haematol. (Submitted for publication.)
27. FLEISCH, H., R. G. G. RUSSEL & M. D. FRANCIS. 1969. Bisphosphonates inhibit hydroxyapatite dissolution in vitro and bone resorption in tissue culture and in vivo. Science **165**: 1261–1264.
28. WATTS, N. B., S. T. HARRIS, H. K. GENANT et al. 1990. Intermittent cyclical etidronate treatment of post-menopausal osteoporosis. N. Eng. J. Med. **323**: 73–79.

Diagnosis and Management of Iron-induced Heart Disease in Cooley's Anemia

MARIELL JESSUP[a] AND CATHERINE S. MANNO

Heart Failure/Transplant Center, Allegheny University Hospitals, Philadelphia, Pennsylvania 19129, USA

Children's Hospital of Philadelphia, Philadelphia, Pennsylvania 19104, USA

ABSTRACT: Patients with homozygous β-thalassemia are chronically transfused and, if not assiduously chelated, are at risk for cardiac dysfunction. Available data suggest that even in optimally chelated patients, cardiac pathology is abnormal secondary to iron deposition, fibrosis, hypertrophy, and the structural effects of chronic anemia. Evidence of myopericarditis may also be found. Cardiac performance is usually only subtly affected, primarily with diastolic abnormalities not routinely detected on echocardiograms or nuclear scan. In poorly chelated patients, severe heart failure occurs and is easily predictable but invariably fatal, despite treatment with diuretics, vasodilators, inotropes, and antiarrhythmics. Based on successful prevention of heart failure with ACE inhibitors in other forms of cardiomyopathy, we suggest multicenter trials to explore methods to stabilize cardiac function in patients at risk for iron-induced heart disease. Long-term adverse effects of iron deposition, diastolic dysfunction, and abnormal hormone regulation need to be quantitated in patients reaching their third and fourth decades when the potential for ischemic cardiac disease could compound cardiac dysfunction.

Patients with β-thalassemia major, or Cooley's anemia, develop severe anemia and require routine red blood cell transfusions. Transfusional iron deposits in multiple tissue sites, including the liver and heart. The resultant hemochromatosis prompts cardiac dysfunction, which remains the leading cause of death in β-thalassemia, despite advances in treatment.[1-3] Therapeutic maneuvers have primarily focused on chelation of excessive iron by the subcutaneous or intravenous infusion of deferoxamine. Chelation therapy clearly benefits many patients, prevents cardiac dysfunction, and enhances survival, but is not uniformly successful.[4-6] Accordingly, interest continues in efforts to detect early cardiac deterioration so that intensified chelation may be instituted or alternative regimens considered. These diagnostic possibilities have often lead to more unanswered questions than helpful insights into management. One source of potential confusion is the variability of cardiac pathology in patients with thalassemia major.

The classic description of end-stage iron-induced cardiomyopathy is a combination of left ventricular diastolic dysfunction, pulmonary hypertension, and right ventricular dilatation.[1,2,7] Symptoms include breathlessness, ascites, pulmonary and peripheral edema, arrhythmias, and rapid progression to death. Fortunately, this clinical presentation is becoming less frequent as chelation is widely and continuously applied. Indeed, older patients dying from this symptom complex have almost always been either non-compliant with their deferoxamine regimen or unable to comply (unpublished personal data).[4-6,8]

---

[a]Address for correspondence: Mariell Jessup, M.D., Heart Failure/Transplant Center, Allegheny University Hospitals, 3300 Henry Avenue, Philadelphia, Pennsylvania 19129. Tel: (215) 842-7607; Fax: (215) 991-4884; E-mail: jessup@AUHS.edu

More commonly, older, adequately chelated patients are frequently asymptomatic and may have subtle abnormalities of both systolic and diastolic function that are multifactorial in etiology.[8–10]

CARDIAC PATHOPHYSIOLOGY

Important factors which contribute to cardiac dysfunction include the following.

(1) *Consequences of chronic hemolytic anemia.* In patients with severe chronic anemia of other causes, Bahl and coworkers have described a number of significant differences in echocardiographic indices compared to normals.[11] They found elevated cardiac outputs, larger left ventricles, an increased mitral annular size, and enhanced left ventricular contractility. There was no evidence of diastolic dysfunction. Whether some of these structural changes also occur in Cooley's anemia independently of abnormal iron storage is not clear.

(2) *Iron-induced cardiomyopathy.* The relationship of iron deposition within the myocytes to the development of myocardial dysfunction remains controversial.[12] Some patients with evidence of excessive tissue iron storage in the liver will have little cardiac iron deposition.[13] Conduction/rhythm abnormalities correlate poorly with conduction tissue infiltration in autopsy sections of patients who have died of cardiac arrhythmias.[14] Moreover, subendocardial iron concentration is half that found in the epicardial layer, so that endomyocardial biopsy techniques may underestimate the degree of iron deposition.[12] Iron may cause a reactive fibrosis or hypertrophy within the myocardium to account for the variable responses observed.

(3) *Myocarditis and pericarditis.* Early reports noted that as many as half of all patients with thalassemia major and transfusional iron overload develop acute pericarditis at some point in their lives.[1,2] More recently, the clinical manifestations and sequelae of myocarditis have been documented. Kremastinos and colleagues followed 1,048 patients, 47 (4.5%) of whom were diagnosed as having acute myocarditis.[15] Serum ferritin was used as a measurement of the effectiveness of chelation. After 8 months, serum ferritin was similar in those patients who did and did not acquire myocarditis. Of these, 11 patients (23.4%) developed acute heart failure (CHF) accompanied by left ventricular systolic dysfunction; mortality was high. Thirteen (27.6%) patients developed chronic CHF with left ventricular systolic dysfunction. Thus, it is possible that at least some of the cardiac deaths attributed to iron deposition in earlier series were related to acute myocarditis.

(4) *Miscellaneous problems.* A number of other illnesses or acquired disorders can result in symptoms mimicking cardiac dysfunction, cause cardiac dysfunction or intensify cardiac decompensation. These include mitral valve prolapse (unpublished personal data), systemic infections, pulmonary embolus, arrhythmias and thyroid disease.[16]

DIAGNOSTIC POSSIBILITIES

In general, diagnostic modalities have not been very useful in detecting early iron-induced cardiac dysfunction. Evaluation of these patients is complicated.

(1) *Symptoms*. Unfortunately, the symptoms of iron-induced cardiomyopathy parallel that of left ventricular function, remaining normal at rest until the development of overt CHF. In addition, many symptoms that may indicate early cardiac disease are non-specific. Palpitations could be related to mitral valve prolapse or anemia (prior to a transfusion); poor exercise tolerance might be secondary to deconditioning, or anemia.

(2) *Electrocardiograms.* Abnormal electrocardiograms have either been used in the past as indicative of cardiac disease [6,12] or ignored entirely in the noninvasive assessment of patients.[8,9] Data are lacking about any particular electrocardiographic finding that would suggest iron-induced cardiac dysfunction, *e.g.,* very abnormal EKGs can remain stable as long as chelation is ongoing (FIGS. 1 and 2). Serial tracings are probably therefore useful. Changes in tracings are usually indicative of a process other than increased iron deposition.

(3) *Echocardiograms*. The ultrasonic characteristics of patients with thalassemia major have been extensively studied and debated.[8,9,11] In general, with increased iron loading, indices of systolic function, cardiac dimensions, and myocardial wall thickness are normal until unequivocal symptoms of CHF are apparent. A standardized quantitation of diastolic function in patients is more accurate but difficult to obtain, as it is not routinely done in

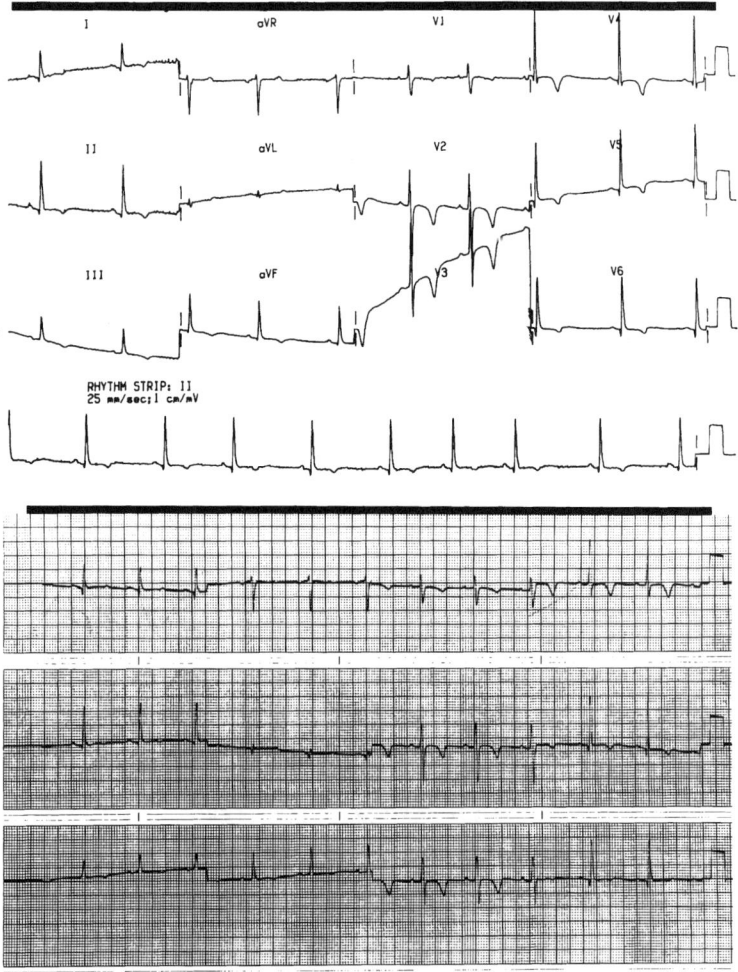

FIGURE 1. (*Top*) Tracing from a 24-year-old woman with thalassemia major who had been chelated poorly and required a pericardial window two months earlier. Her serum ferritin was 5,000 mg/ml, but left ventricular and right ventricular ejection fractions were normal. (*Bottom*) Four years later, the tracing is still abnormal but unchanged, despite effective chelation and unchanged ejection fraction.

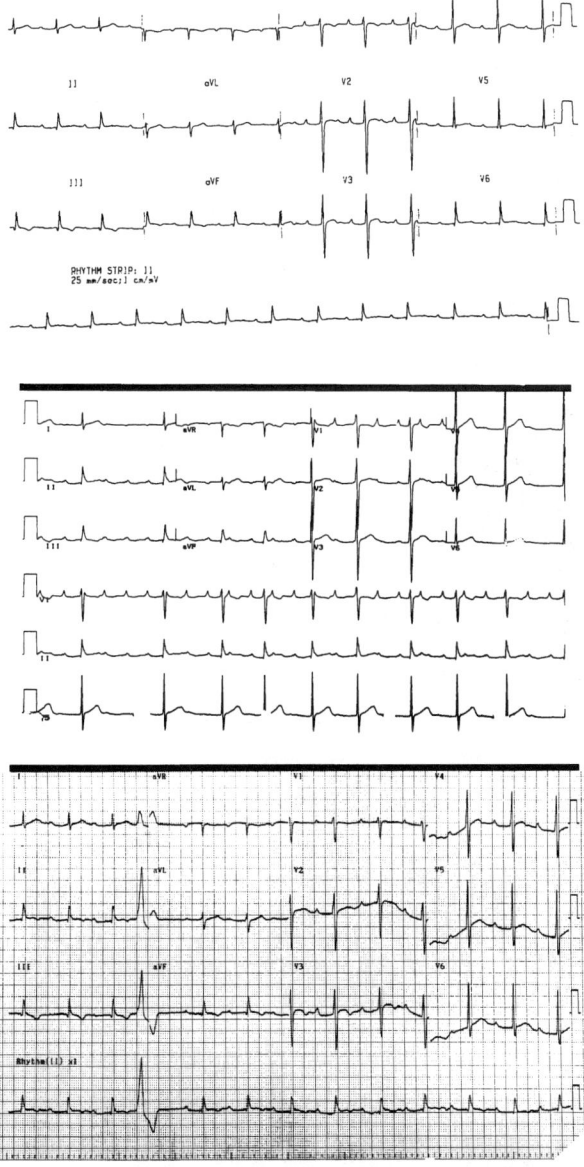

FIGURE 2. (*Top*) Tracing from a 33-year-old male with thalassemia major who started chelation as an adolescent. His serum ferritin is 500 mg/ml, left ventricular ejection fraction 46%. He has marked first degree A-V block, and diffuse T-wave abnormalities. (*Middle*) Now 35, he develops a low grade fever, some backache, and a slow atrial tachycardia. His ferritin is 500 mg/ml, and his ejection fraction is unchanged. (*Bottom*) Two months later, his symptoms have resolved and his tracing is identical to that of 1995. Radiofrequency ablation of the atrial tachycardia was unsuccessful, but the arrhythmia has not recurred.

most echo labs, and is time consuming. Non-specific diastolic dysfunction is usually only seen in the oldest patients with highly elevated serum ferritin values,[8] making it less useful as a prognostic tool. Progressive diastolic dysfunction is a normal consequence of age and must be corrected for body habitus as well. Abnormalities in myocardial acoustic properties have been detected but do not correlate well with the number of transfusions or ferritin value.[9] The left ventricular end-systolic pressure-dimension (LV P_{ES}-D_{ES}) relation is a noninvasive method of assessing contractility independent of ventricular loading. This method has been used to assess 20 thalassemia patients (ages 7–25 years).[17] Six patients had abnormal systolic function determined by percent fractional shortening on routine echocardiogram and all had abnormal P_{ES}–D_{ES} slopes. However, all seven patients 15 years or older had abnormal values as well. On follow-up, 2 of 10 patients with abnormal slopes developed overt signs of CHF, but there is no information about adequacy of chelation in these patients. Thus this technique may be of some value in the early detection of cardiac dysfunction but it needs to be evaluated in a larger group of patients.

(4) *Nuclear studies*. The determination of resting left and right ventricular ejection fraction (EF) by nuclear first pass or gated techniques has been no more successful than resting echocardiography in identifying patients with subsequent cardiac problems. However, Leon and colleagues described the measurement of left ventricular EF during exercise in 24 patients, with a mean ferritin of 4,083 ± 625.[18] Although exercise LVEF did prove to be abnormal in some patients with normal resting echocardiograms, a history of the number of transfusions also predicted abnormal exercise LVEF by first pass. Only 3 of 16 patients who had received over 100 RBC units had a normal response to exercise. In our center, patients have found the study unpleasant and have been unwilling to return for serial studies. Subsequent studies of exercise EF have also shown that normal subjects, particularly women, do not always increase their EF with dynamic exercise.[19]

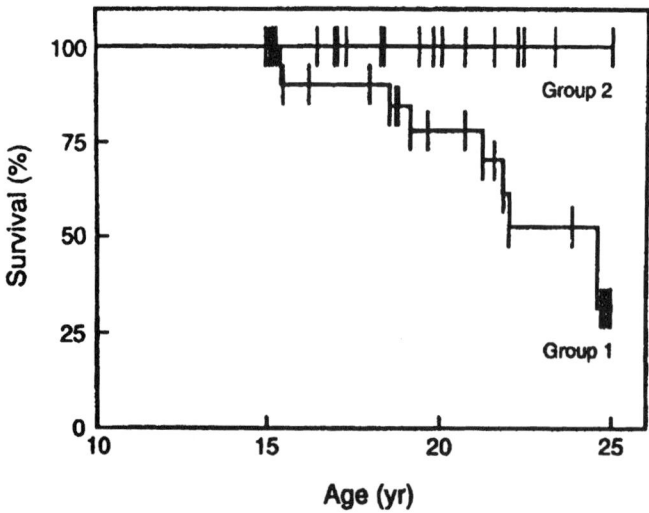

FIGURE 3. Life-table analysis of the survival of 38 patients with thalassemia major aged 15 years or older. Group 1 had the highest transfusional iron load and the lowest deferoxamine use while Group 2 patients were the remaining patients. Survival in Group 2 was significantly better over the 10 years of the study than in Group 1. (From Brittenham *et al.*[4] Reproduced by permission.)

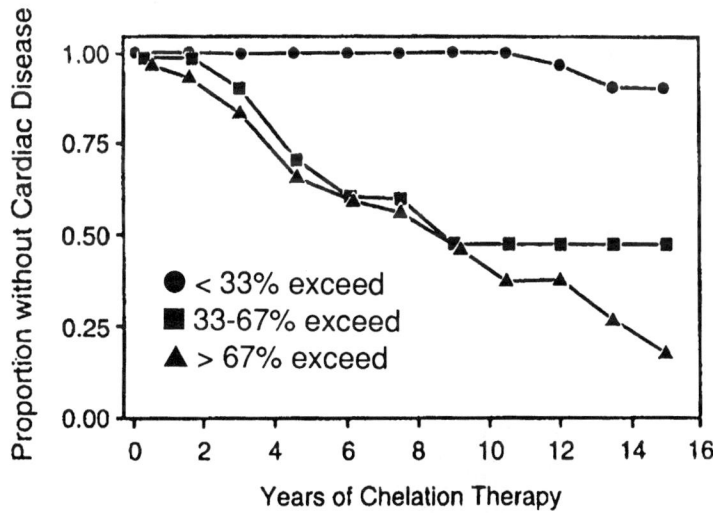

FIGURE 4. Survival without cardiac disease according to the proportion of serum ferritin measurements greater than 2,500 mg/ml. (From Olivieri et al.[5] Reproduced with permission.)

(5) *Endomyocardial biopsy*. Serial heart biopsies are routinely done in patients post cardiac transplant with low risk to the patient. Biopsy could easily be done in patients with Cooley's anemia so that intensified regimens could be initiated in patients with increasing cardiac iron stores. However, as mentioned earlier, subendocardial iron concentration is less than that found in the epicardial layer and neither has been well correlated with myocardial dysfunction.[12] Also, there is a well acknowledged variability of biopsy sampling so that a significant increase in iron deposits might be missed. In addition, the amount of iron may not be the critical determinant of cardiac function, but rather the degree of tissue reaction to the iron with subsequent proliferation of fibrosis and/or hypertrophy. Finally, serial endomyocardial biopsies are life-saving in transplant patients but are certainly not in thalassemia patients, so that the small risk of biopsy may not be justified.

None of the above methods to assess early myocardial impairment in thalassemia has been rigorously tested in a prospective manner. Indeed, the combined information of a patient's transfusion record, serial serum ferritin levels, and details of their adherence to a chelation regimen provides as much predictive power as any of the non-invasive tests outlined above (FIGS. 3 and 4).[4,5] It is also unwise to expect any single diagnostic test to be highly predictive of subsequent cardiac events because it has not been the case in many other cardiac diseases. Patients with idiopathic or ischemic dilated cardiomyopathy and congestive heart failure are routinely triaged to medical therapy or cardiac transplant on the basis of the results of several assessments, including left ventricular ejection fraction, intracardiac pressures, and maximum oxygen uptake obtained during exercise.[20,21] Complications from coronary artery disease are best predicted from an analysis of a patients' risk profile in combination with myocardial perfusion studies during exercise.

THERAPY OF ESTABLISHED DISEASE

When patients with β-thalassemia major develop symptoms of breathlessness, ascites, or edema consistent with CHF, they are in danger of imminent death. There are scattered reports about successful treatments in a handful of such end-stage patients. An intensified chelation regimen can occasionally reverse symptoms of CHF and improve abnormal echocardiographic findings.[22,23] However, CHF secondary to myocarditis will not respond predictably to an escalated chelation regimen, and the distinction between myocarditis and non-induced cardiomyopathy might be clinically difficult. Ultrafiltration may be useful to aid in the removal of excessive fluid while the underlying cardiac dysfunction is being treated.[24] Increasingly, cardiac or combined heart-liver transplantation has been undertaken, with initial promising results.[25,26] Pharmacologic therapy of CHF from other causes has improved remarkably over the past decade with an increased understanding of the pathophysiologic consequences of neurohormonal activation and the development of the angiotensin converting enzyme inhibitors.[16,27] However, early cardiac dysfunction in thalassemia is most accurately characterized as secondary to diastolic abnormalities, and there is no universally accepted treatment for diastolic dysfunction and very few studies. Preliminary reports about one ACE-inhibitor, lisinopril, in the treatment of CHF and diastolic dysfunction have not been promising.[28]

The treatment of arrhythmias in thalassemia major can be treacherous. If arrhythmias are related to active inflammation, antiarrhythmic agents may not be effective. Moreover, all antiarrhythmic drugs have the potential to cause proarrhythmia or other toxicities in the setting of CHF.[30,31] Cardiac electrophysiologists should be involved early in the care of these patients.

SUMMARY AND RECOMMENDATIONS

The pathophysiology of cardiac dysfunction in Cooley's anemia is poorly understood and multifactorial in etiology. The long-term consequences of chronic anemia, abnormal iron-deposition within the myocardium, reactive fibrosis, and hypertrophy all contribute to the disease spectrum. Diagnostic tools used to detect early cardiac dysfunction have not been routinely applied or significantly predictive of subsequent cardiac events. At present the most powerful predictive information includes a patients' transfusion record, serial serum ferritin levels, and compliance to a chelation regimen. Treatment of significant CHF in the setting of classic restrictive left ventricular dysfunction and right ventricular dilatation is extremely limited and has forced transplantation to be seriously considered as a reasonable option. Ultimately gene therapy of this disease will eradicate its devastating consequences.[32]

REFERENCES

1. ENGLE, M. A., M. ERLANDSON & C. H. SMITH. 1964. Late cardiac complications of chronic, severe refractory anemia with hemochromatosis. Circulation **30**: 698–705.
2. EHLERS, K. H., A. R. LEVIN, A. L. MARKENSON *et al.* 1980. Longitudinal study of cardiac function in thalassemia major. Ann. N.Y. Acad. Sci. **344**: 397–404.
3. ZURLO, M. G., P. DESTEFANO, C. BORGNA-PIGNATTI *et al.* 1989. Survival and causes of death in thalassemia major. Lancet **2**: 27–30.
4. BRITTENHAM, G. M., P. M. GRIFFITH, A. W. NIENHUIS *et al.* 1994. Efficacy of deferoxamine in preventing complications of iron overload in patients with thalassemia major. N. Engl. J. Med. **331**: 567–73.
5. OLIVIERI, N. F., D. G. NATHAN, J. H. MACMILLAN *et al.* 1994. Survival in medically treated patients with homozygous β-Thalassemia. N. Engl. J. Med. **331**: 574–578.

6. RICHARDSON, M. E., R. N. MATTHEWS, J. F. ALISON et al. 1993. Prevention of heart disease by subcutaneous deferoxamine in patients with thalassemia major. Aust. N.Z. J. Med. **23**: 656–661.
7. CRISARU, D., E. A. RACHMILEWITZ, M. MOSSERI et al. 1990. Cardiopulmonary assessment in β-thalassemia major. Chest **98**: 1138–1142.
8. KREMASTINOS, D. T., D. P. TSIAPRAS, G. A. TSETSOS et al. 1993. Left ventricular diastolic doppler characteristics in β-Thalassemia major. Circulation **88**: 1127–1135.
9. LATTANZI, F., P. BELLOTTI, E. PICANO et al. 1993. Quantitative ultrasonic analysis of myocardium in patients with thalassemia major and iron overload. Circulation **87**: 748–754.
10. DESIDERI, A., G. SCATTOLIN, A. GABELLINI et al. 1994. Left ventricular function in thalassemia major: Protective effect of deferoxamine. Can. J. Cardiol. **10**: 93–96.
11. BAHL, V. K., O. P. MALHOTRA, D. KUMAR et al. 1992. Noninvasive assessment of systolic and diastolic left ventricular function in patients with chronic severe anemia: A combined M-mode, two-dimensional, and Doppler echocardiographic study. Am. Heart J. **124**: 1516–1523.
12. FITCHETT, D. H., D. J. COLTART, W. A. LITTLER et al. 1980. Cardiac involvement in secondary hemochromatosis: a catheter biopsy study and analysis of myocardium. Cardiovasc. Res. **14**: 719–724.
13. BUJA, C. M. & W. C. ROBERTS. 1971. Iron in the heart. Am. J. Med. **51**: 209–219.
14. SCHELLHAMMER, P. F., M. A. ENGLE & T. W. HAGSTROM. 1967. Histochemical studies of the myocardium and conduction tissue in acquired iron storage disease. Circulation **35**: 631–637.
15. KREMASTINOS, D. T., G. TINIAKOS, G. N. THEODORAKIS et al. 1995. Myocarditis in β-thalassemia major. A cause of heart failure. Circulation **91**: 66–71.
16. VECCHIO, C. & G. DERCHI. 1995. Management of cardiac complications in patients with thalassemia major. Sem. Hematol. **32**: 288–296.
17. BOROW, K. M., R. PROPPER, F. Z. BIERMAN et al. 1982. The left ventricular end-systolic pressure-dimension relation in patients with thalassemia major. A new non-invasive method for assessing contractile state. Circulation **66**: 980–985.
18. LEON, M. B., J. S. BORER, S. L. BACHARACH et al. 1979. Detection of early cardiac dysfunction in patients with severe beta-thalassemia and chronic iron-overload N. Engl. J. Med. **301**: 1143–1148.
19. GIBBONS, R. J., K. L. LEE, F. COBB et al. 1981. Ejection fraction response to exercise in patients with chest pain and normal coronary arteriograms. Circulation **64**: 952–958.
20. MANCINI, D. M., H. EISEN, W. KUSSMAUL et al. 1991. Value of peak oxygen consumption for optimal timing of cardiac transplantation in ambulatory patients with heart failure. Circulation **83**: 778–783.
21. O'CONNELL, J. B., R. C. BOURGE, M. R. COSTANZO-NORDIN et al. 1992. Cardiac transplantation: Recipient selection, donor procurement, and medical follow-up: A statement for health professionals from the Committee on Cardiac Transplantation of the Council on Clinical Cardiology. American Heart Association. Circulation **86**: 1061–1079.
22. MARCUS, R. E., S. C. DAVIES, H. M. BANTOCK et al. 1984. Deferoxamine to improve cardiac function in iron-overloaded patients with thalassemia major. Lancet **1**: 392–393.
23. POLITI, A., M. STICCA & M. GALL. 1995. Reversal of haemochromatic cardiomyopathy in β-Thalassemia by chelation therapy. Br. Heart J. **73**: 486–487.
24. MELONI, C., M. MOROSETTI, L. MESCHINI et al. 1994. Isolated ultrafiltration in refractory heart failure on patients with Cooley's anemia. Artific. Cells Blood Subst. Immobil. Biotech. **22**: 109–113.
25. OLIVIERI, N. F., P. P. LIU, G. D. SHER et al. 1994. Brief report: Combined liver and heart transplantation for end-stage iron-induced organ failure in an adult with homozygous beta-thalassemia. N. Engl. J. Med. **330**: 1125–1127.
26. KOERNER, M. M., G. TENDRERICH, K. MINAMI et al. 1997. Heart transplantation for end-stage heart failure caused by iron overload. Br. J. Haematol. **97**: 293–296.
27. PACKER, M. 1995. Evolution of the neurohormonal hypothesis to explain the progression of chronic heart failure. Eur. Heart J. **16** (Supplement F): 4–6.
28. LANG, C. C., H. M. MCALPINE & N. KENNEDY. 1995. Effects of lisinopril on congestive heart failure in normotensive patients with diastolic dysfunction but intact systolic function. Eur. J. Clin. Pharmacol. **49**: 15–19.

29. PEARSON, H. A., A. R. COHEN, P. V. J. GIARDINA *et al.* 1996. The changing profile of homozygous β-thalassemia: Demography, ethnicity, and age distribution of current North American patients and changes in two decades. Pediatrics **97**: 352–356.
30. FRANCIS, G. S. 1986. Development of arrhythmias in the patient with congestive heart failure: Pathophysiology, prevalence and prognosis. Am. J. Cardiol **57**: 3B–7B.
31. GOTTLIEB, S. S. 1989. The use of antiarrhythmic agents in heart failure: Implications of CAST. Am. Heart J. **118**: 1074–1077.
32. RUND, D. & E. RACHMILEWITZ. 1995. Thalassemia Major 1995: Older patients, new therapies. Blood Rev. **9**: 25–32.

Global Epidemiology of Hemoglobin Disorders

MICHAEL ANGASTINIOTIS[a] AND BERNADETTE MODELL[b]

[a]Thalassemia Centre, Arch Makarios III Hospital, 1474 Nicosia, Cyprus
[b]Royal Free Hospital School of Medicine, University College London Medical School, Department of Primary Care and Population Sciences, Whittington Hospital-Archway Site, Highgate Hill, London N19 5NF, United Kingdom

ABSTRACT: Thalassemias and the hemoglobinopathies such as Hemoglobins S, C and E, are now a global problem. They have spread through migration from their native areas in the Mediterranean, Africa and Asia and are now endemic throughout Europe, the Americas and Australia. Comprehensive control programs in recent years have succeeded in limiting the numbers of new births and prolonging life in affected individuals. Such programs have been successful in a minority of countries and have little global impact. Over 300,000 infants with major syndromes are born every year and the majority die undiagnosed, untreated or under-treated.

Countries may be divided into three general categories according to the services available: A. Endemic Mediterranean countries. In these long-established prevention programs have succeeded in achieving 80%–100% prevention. Specialized clinics able to provide optimum treatment. B. Areas of the developed, industrialized world where prevalence is increasing because of migration. These countries have the means to provide adequate control but have problems in reaching immigrant groups with different cultural background. C. Countries of the developing world where the provision of services is hampered by economic difficulties, other health priorities due to high infant mortality from infectious diseases, and religious/cultural constraints.

Hemoglobin disorders are unusual among genetic conditions, because survey data is available for most parts of the world and frequency estimates can be made for almost every country. Global data has been accumulating since the 1980s through the Hereditary Diseases Program of the WHO Division of Noncommunicable diseases. A working group on the control of hereditary disease was responsible for initiating the collection of data and Prof. B. Modell undertook to record and update the data over the years.[1–6]

The reported figures are the best estimates based on local surveys, reports by visiting experts and personal communications. Over the years more accurate data have allowed a more clear picture to emerge concerning the global situation. However, until now, all information concerned the size of the problem and its distribution. More countries are now offering programs for the control of hemoglobin disorders and many more are planning to develop services. We propose that the time has come to revise and upgrade available epidemiological information on a global scale in terms of service indicators.

[a]Tel: 00357 2 305090; (Direct Line) 653186; Fax: 00357 2 314552; E-mail: Thalassemia @cytanet.com.cy
[b]Tel: 0044 171 288 3597; Fax: 0044 171 281 8004; E-mail: b.modell@ucl.ac.uk

Control programs have been developed and applied in several countries, which include the provision of optimum treatment for those affected by major syndromes, coupled with prevention with the aim of limiting the number of affected births.

Carrier screening, genetic counseling and prenatal diagnosis are feasible for all these conditions. There is an increasing world-wide demand for these services and comprehensive control programs are being incorporated in the health policies of many countries. Epidemiological data should be used to develop service indicators for each country, in a standardized format appropriate for health service planning.

BASIC SERVICE INDICATORS

The basic service indicators selected in this study are listed in TABLE 1.

Epidemiological information on the hemoglobin disorders should be analysed by administrative borders (country and administrative regions within each country). Most countries have an uneven distribution of carriers. One example is Italy, where frequency varies from 1–2% in much of the North, reaching 12% in Sardinia and Ferrara. The average for the whole country is 5%. Even in a small country like Cyprus, regional differences can be recognized, e.g., the south-east of Cyprus has a higher frequency of α^0-thalassemia genes, while sickle cell disease was more prevalent on the Northern coast (M. Angastiniotis-personal communication). Recognizing regional differences will assist in targeting services to areas where these are most needed.

In many countries, several ethnic groups coexist. This is especially so in countries where the hemoglobin disorders have been imported by immigrants. The main examples of the latter situation are Northern Europe and the USA. Another example is Oman,[7] where the Belushi tribe, which settled there 200 years ago from Iran and Pakistan (Beluchistan), has a very high carrier rate (10%) compared to the indigenous Arab population (1–2%). This form of micromapping is also important since it helps to direct services to the at-risk group.

Infant mortality is an important indicator because of the observation that countries come to recognize the need for genetic services when the rate falls below 40-50/1000. At higher rates public health concerns give priority to infectious diseases and malnutrition. Using this criterion, genetic services are not likely to be considered a priority in three WHO Regions, (FIG. 1).

However, the large-scale view obscures individual country differences. All developing countries include a social spectrum ranging from professionals with a health level comparable to that in developed countries, to the rural poor. Infant mortality can fall quite rapidly, (FIGS. 2 and 3). In reality, in every country where hemoglobin disorders are common, there is a demand for treatment and prevention among at least a section of the population. The total births per year are an indicator for neonatal screening, especially where sickle cell disorders are prominent (FIG. 4).

Health education and counseling services are key elements in any national control program. In planning and directing such services to the target populations which need them most, it is useful to know the carrier frequency and the estimated total number of carriers (FIGS. 5 and 6). In many countries, the ante-natal clinic is the focus for carrier detection and

TABLE 1. Basic Service Indicators

• Population	• Annual at risk pregnancies
• Infant Mortality	• Annual Births/Birth Rate
• Carriers/Carrier rates	• Affected births per year
• Pregnant Carriers/year	

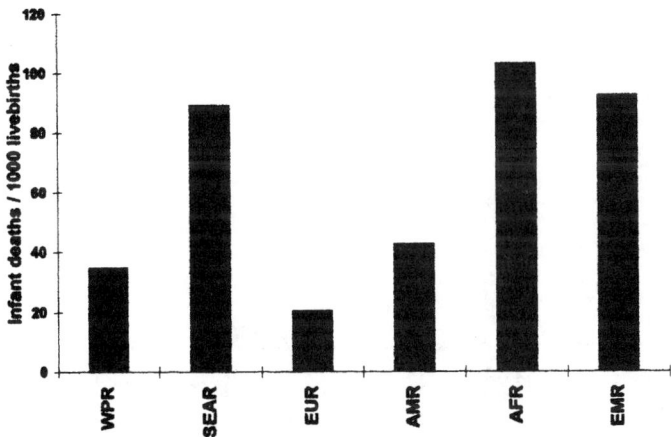

FIGURE 1. WHO Regions: Infant mortality/1000.

counseling. In this respect, it is important to have figures such as the annual pregnant carriers (FIG. 7). This will assist in deciding the number of counsellors that will be needed, their language and culture and where they should be located. The annual at-risk pregnancies (FIG. 8) will indicate where there is a need not only for ante-natal screening laboratories but also for more specialist counseling because from this group the candidates for prenatal diagnosis will be recruited. Prenatal diagnosis was initially by foetal blood sampling at 18–20 weeks gestation. By the application of molecular technology, first trimester diagnosis has

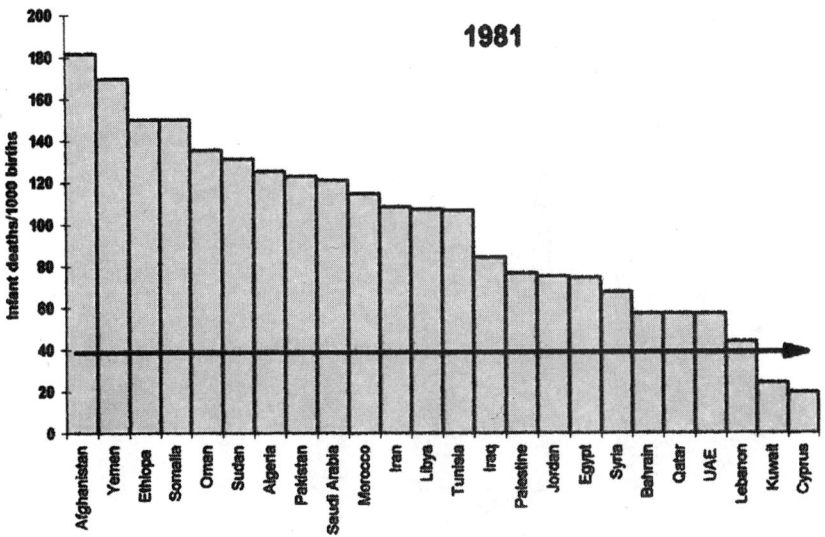

FIGURE 2. Infant mortality in countries of the WHO Eastern Mediterranean Region.

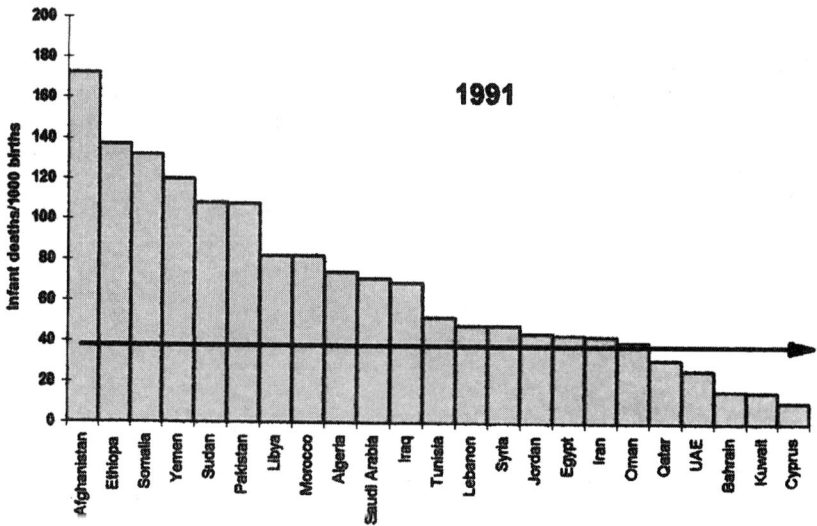

FIGURE 3. Infant mortality in countries of the WHO Eastern Mediterranean Region.

become the more acceptable method. Planning this service requires not only introducing the appropriate laboratory technology but also addressing the religious, ethical, legal and cultural issues which affect its acceptability in various ethnic and religious groups.

The need for clinical services and their location will be assessed more accurately by knowing the birth rate of affected births (births/1000/year) and the total affected births per year (FIG. 9). This indicator is also useful as a means of monitoring the prevention program comparing the actual annual homozygote births to the expected births according to carrier frequency and birth rate (see FIG. 18).

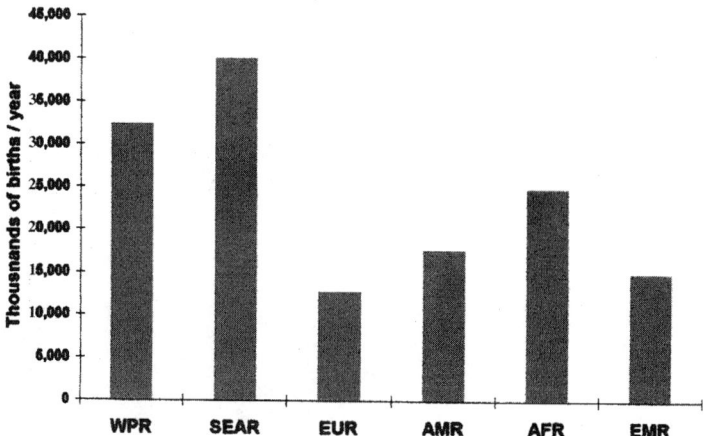

FIGURE 4. WHO Regions: Thousands of births/yr.

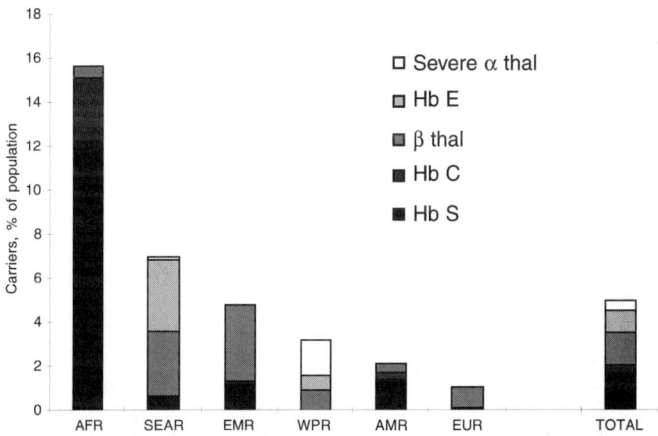

FIGURE 5. WHO Regions: % of the population carrying an Hb disorder.

THE GLOBAL SCENE

Accurate epidemiological data is not available for all parts of the world and micromapping has been carried out in only a minority of countries. The best estimates that could be obtained have, therefore, been used for some areas. WHO regions are used to describe the global picture. These regions are listed in TABLE 2. Even though AFR and EMR have the smallest populations (FIG. 10), they have the highest birth rate (FIG. 11), and the highest infant mortality (FIG. 4). World-wide, the carriers of hemoglobin disorders are estimated to total 269 million. Most of them live in the South-east Asian region (FIG. 6), where the thalassemias (β-thalassemia, α-thalassemia and hemoglobin E) predominate. AFR comes next with the sickle cell genes and Hemoglobin C.

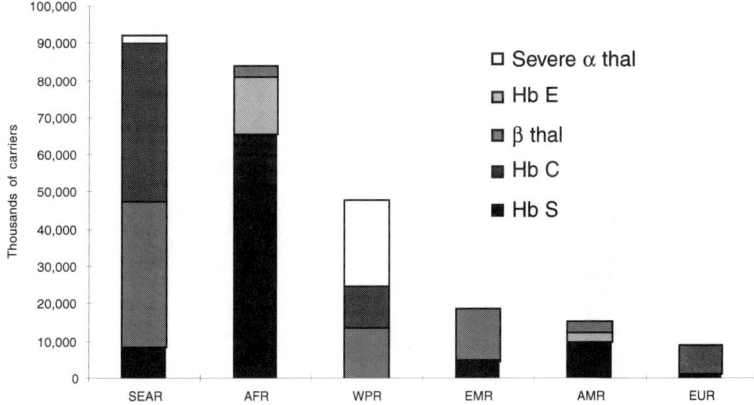

FIGURE 6. WHO Regions: Carriers of Hb disorders (thousands) (Total = 269 million).

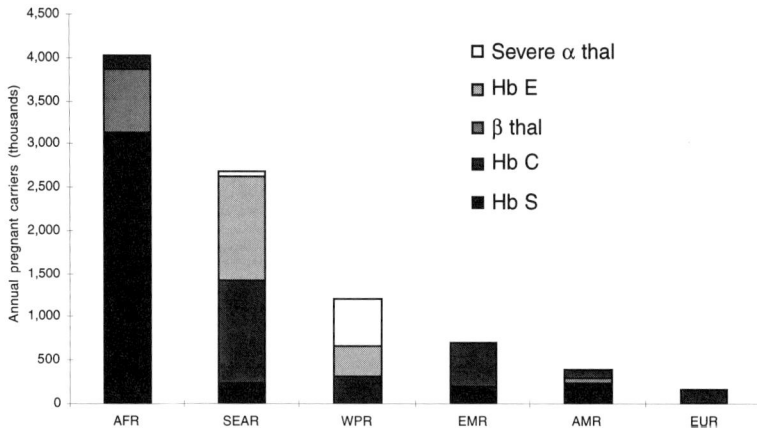

FIGURE 7. WHO Regions: Annual carriers born (thousands), = annual pregnant carriers (Total = 9.2 million/yr.).

Because of the high birth rate, Africa has the highest number of at-risk pregnancies per year—almost 1 million out of a total of 1.47 million world-wide (FIG. 8), while there are 9.2 million pregnant carriers annually (FIG. 7). It is estimated that 365,100 infants are born each year with major hemoglobin disorders, (FIG. 9).

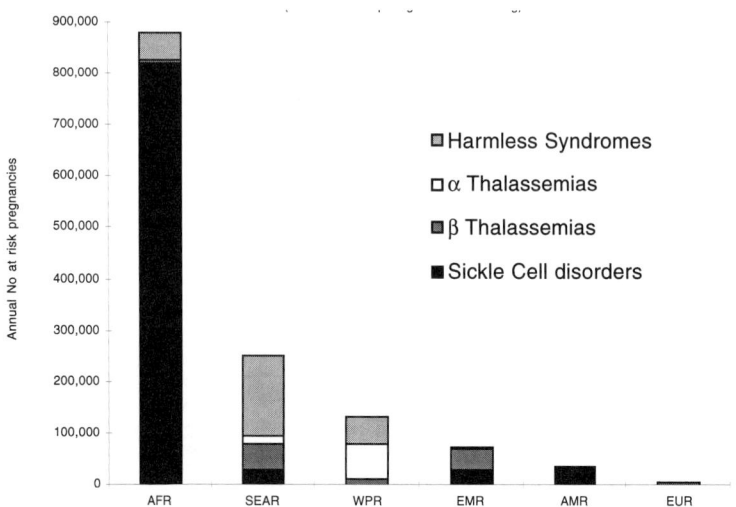

FIGURE 8. WHO Regions: Annual pregnancies at risk for Hb disorders (Total = 1.47 million).

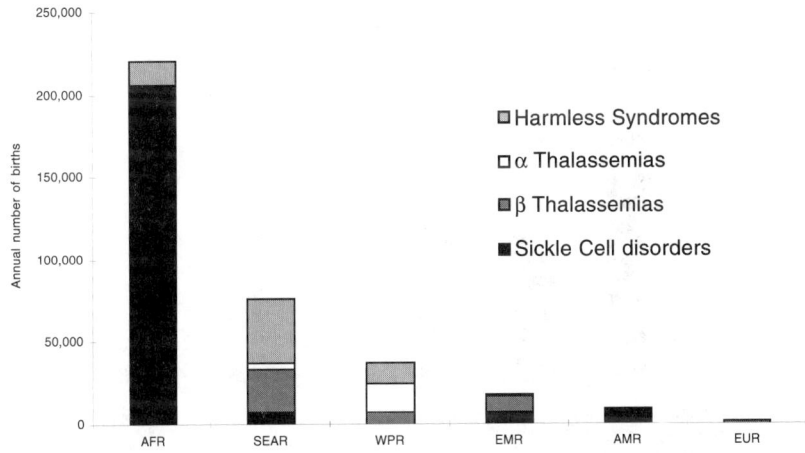

FIGURE 9. WHO Regions: Annual number of infants born with Hb disorders (Total = 365100).

SERVICES

According to the services available, both for treatment and prevention, countries may be described according to three general categories:

1. In some endemic countries, mostly, but not only, in the Mediterranean, long-established control programs have achieved 80–100% prevention of new affected births and the provision of optimum treatment in specialized clinics.[8–11]

2. Countries of the developing world where the provision of services is hampered by economic difficulties and other health priorities. In this group, services vary from non-existent to very good in either isolated countries or part of a country.

3. Areas of the developed, industrialized world where prevalence is increasing mainly because of migration from endemic areas. These countries have the means to provide adequate control, but have problems in reaching immigrant groups, scattered throughout the host country, often ignorant of the problem and with significant cultural differences.[4,12–14]

As an example of the first category, the island of Cyprus[8] is characteristic and shares the overall success of its program with Greece and Italy. It is a small country with a very high frequency of β-thalassemia genes (TABLE 3). It belongs to the EMR and is one of the smallest countries in the region (FIG. 12). In the EMR, all countries have a high frequency of carriers with Cyprus leading (FIGS. 13 and 14). However, the much larger countries with

TABLE 2. WHO Regions

• AFR: Sub-Saharan Africa	• EUR: Europe
• AMR: The Americas	• SEAR: South East Asian Region
• EMR: East Mediterranean Region	• WPR: West Pacific Region

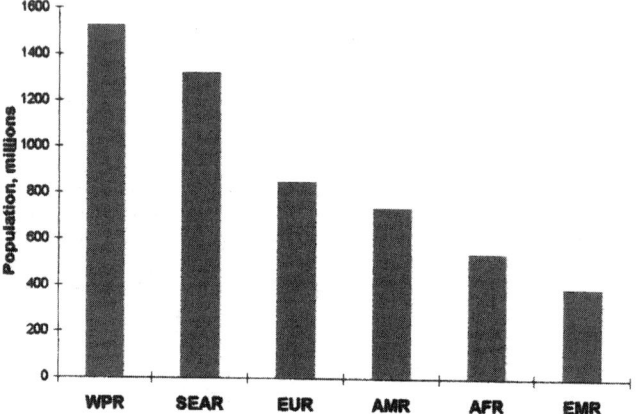

FIGURE 10. WHO Regions: Population, millions.

much higher birth rates account for many more affected births per year (FIG. 15). In Cyprus, there are about 200 pregnancies per year needing prenatal diagnosis and practically all who need it take advantage of the service. If Pakistan were to start a similar comprehensive service, it would need to program for over 12000 such tests per year (FIG. 16). Iran, which has already introduced prenatal diagnosis, will have to expand its services to accommodate almost 8000 at-risk pregnancies per year. This it must do, otherwise it will not be able to maintain the standard of care it has already initiated, since the addition of 2000 new cases annually (FIG. 17) will expand the homozygote population, now surviving because of treatment, national resources will be strained and regression to inadequate treatment will result.

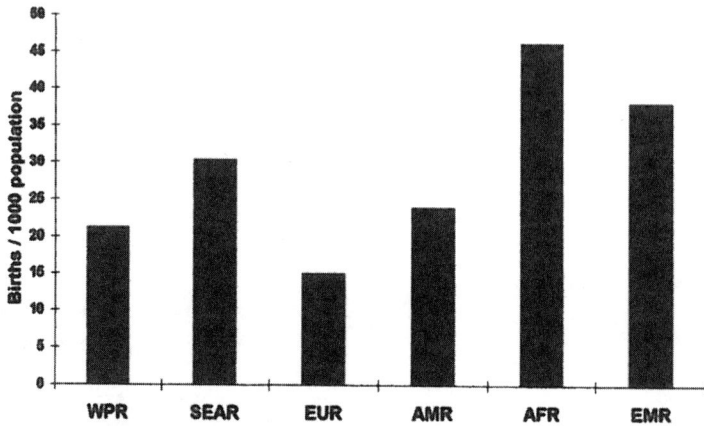

FIGURE 11. WHO Regions: Birth rate/1000.

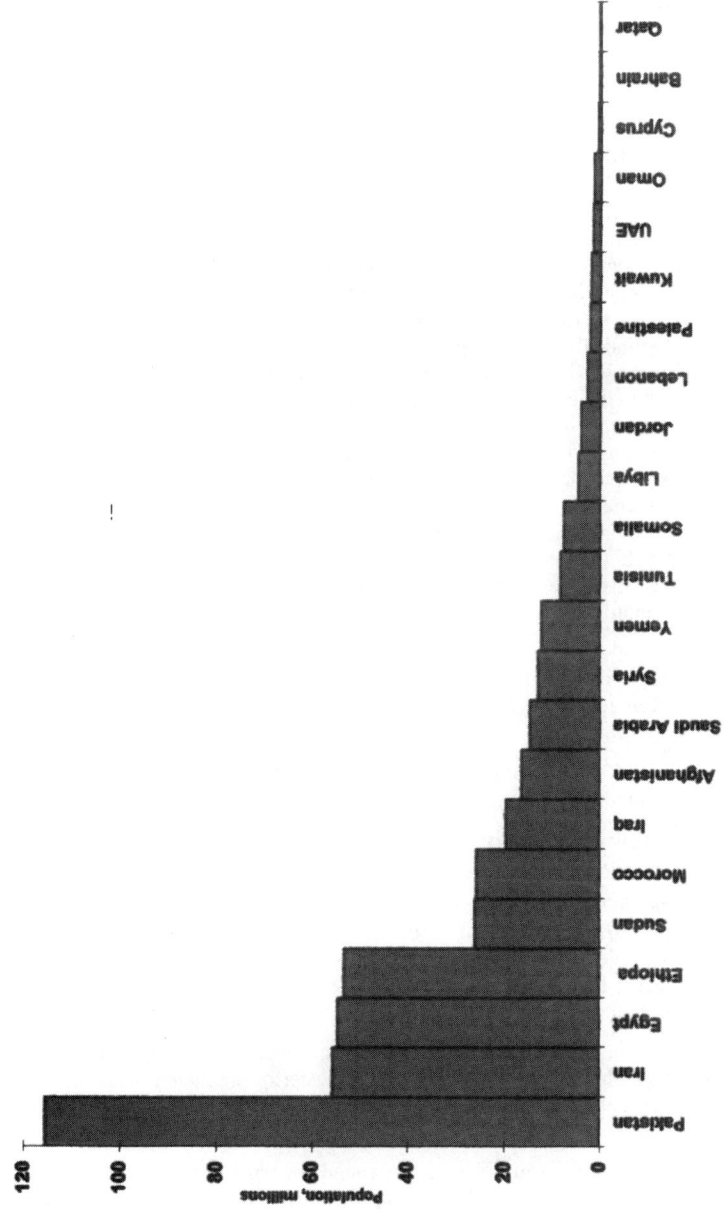

FIGURE 12. Population of the countries of the WHO Eastern Mediterranean Region, 1991 (Total 443 million).

TABLE 3. β-Thalassemia in Cyprus

- 1:7 is a carrier of β-Thalassemia
- 1:49 couples are both carriers
- 1:158 newborns are expected to be affected
- 1:1000 of the population is currently homozygous

The smaller, homogeneous population of Cyprus has fully responded to the program. For the last 12 years (since 1985) the annual births of homozygotes has been 0–2% of the expected births (FIG. 18).

In the SEAR and WPR, many countries belong to the second category, in which no services have developed. Some countries, however, are steadily achieving the range of health indicators where genetic and congenital disorders are recognized as important. Many are developing an interest in the hemoglobin disorders. The main examples are Thailand[15] and Malaysia. In this region, there is a complex picture with a very high incidence of milder mutations (HbE and α + - thalassemia) leading to a high proportion of milder syndromes, (HbE/β-thalassemia and HbH disease) (FIG. 19). Long-term survival is possible even in the absence of appropriate services. There is lack of information about many countries such as Bhutan and Nepal and the larger parts of Indonesia.

Prenatal diagnosis is now available in Thailand, India, Singapore, and Malaysia. Carrier screening and counseling programs, however, have not been conducted in a systematic way. Owing to the large populations of certain countries, new and efficient approaches will be needed, *e.g.*, the dissemination of information using electronic pathways.

The UK represents the group of countries of Northern Europe and North America where massive south to north migration has introduced thalassemias and hemoglobinopathies in areas where the indigenous population was free or relatively free from these disorders. These countries face a series of problems in dealing with health problems that arise, for example:

1. The ethnic minority groups are often of a lower socio-economic status and educational level. Language problems often exist. They, therefore, have difficulty using the services.[14,15]

2. The birth rate in these communities is often higher than in the indigenous population, and the annual homozygote birth rate is high.

3. Often, there is no epidemiological information since data are difficult to gather in population subgroups scattered geographically.

4. Language and cultural differences with the host population make it difficult to effectively establish screening and counseling programs. Prenatal diagnosis is often unacceptable in the 2nd trimester of pregnancy, though it may be acceptable if offered early.[13] Ideally, counselors from the same linguistic and ethnic group should be recruited and trained.[14,15]

5. It is difficult to provide for premarital screening. Most at-risk couples are picked up by antenatal clinic screening in the 2nd trimester of pregnancy. This limits their choices to either terminating the pregnancy after midtrimester prenatal diagnosis or keeping the child. Termination may be contrary to religious belief.

6. Although the minority groups are usually found concentrated in few main cities, many settle in various parts of the country in smaller groups. It can be difficult to provide adequate prevention programs for a few families or medical expertise in treating patients, when only small numbers are treated.

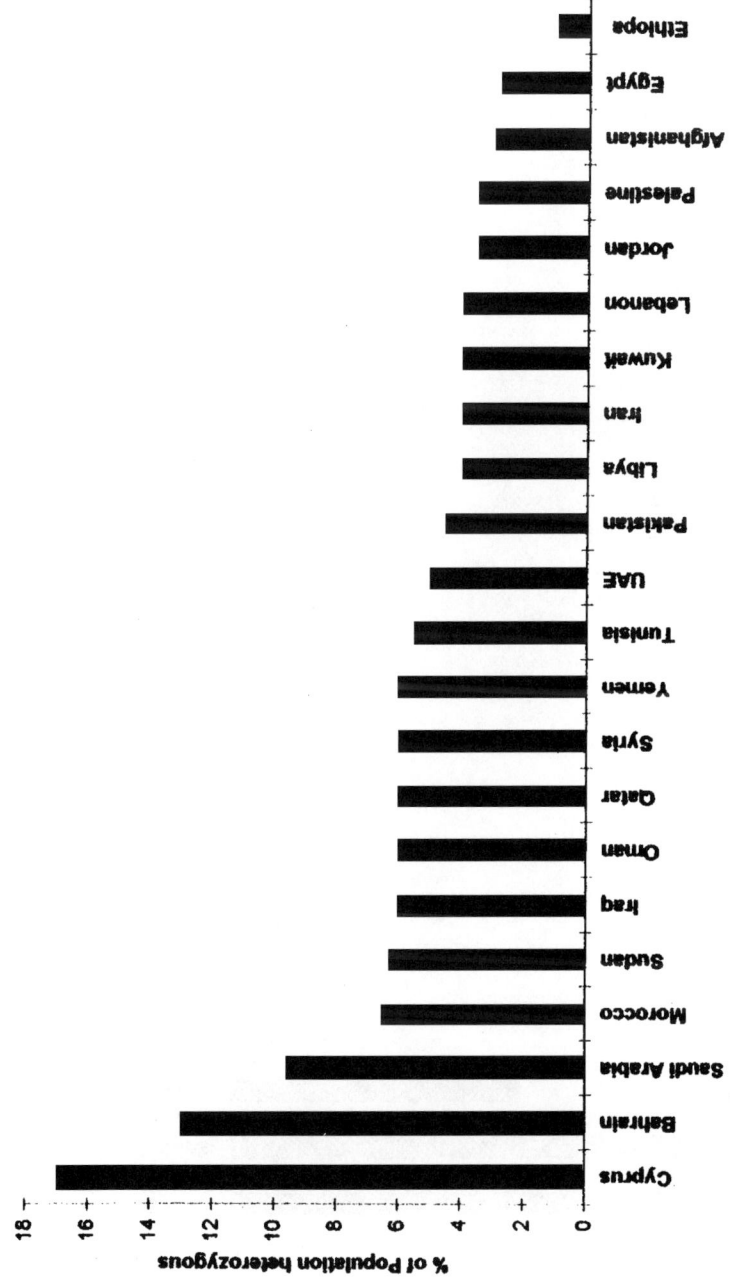

FIGURE 13. EMR countries: % of the population carrying a hemoglobin disorder.

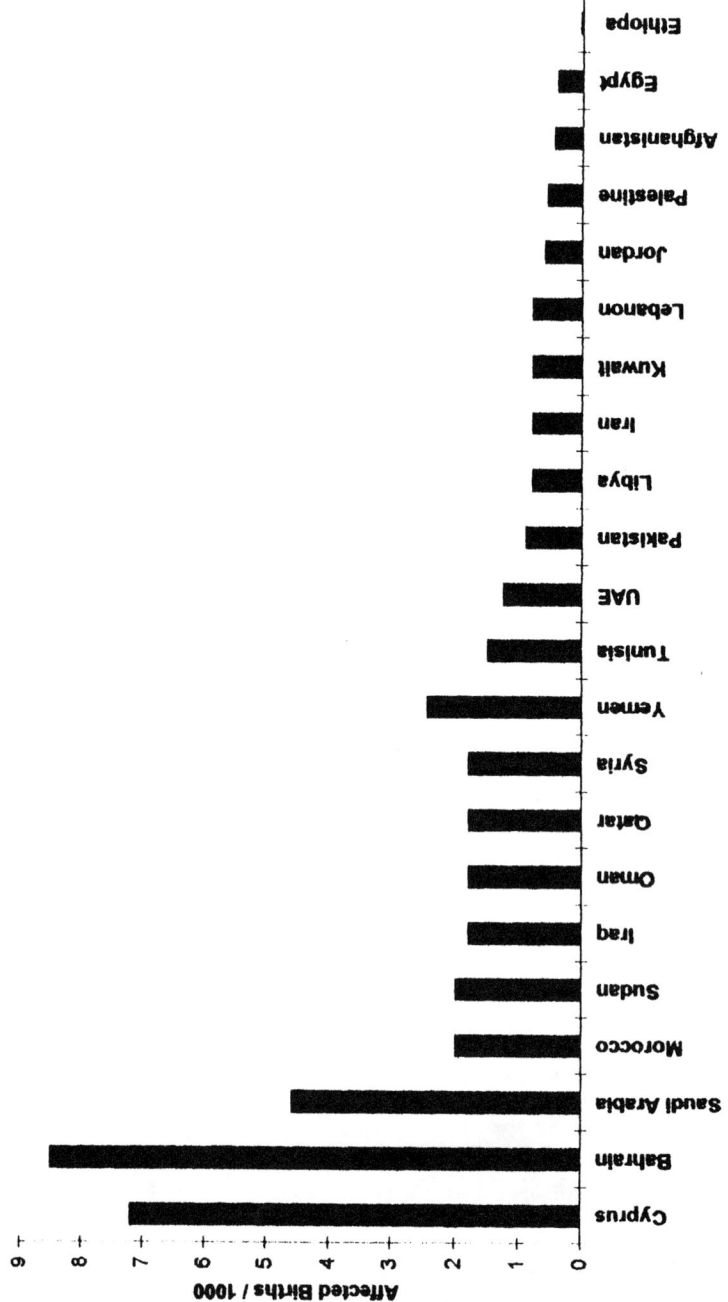

FIGURE 14. EMR countries: Birth rate/1000 of children with a major hemoglobin disorder.

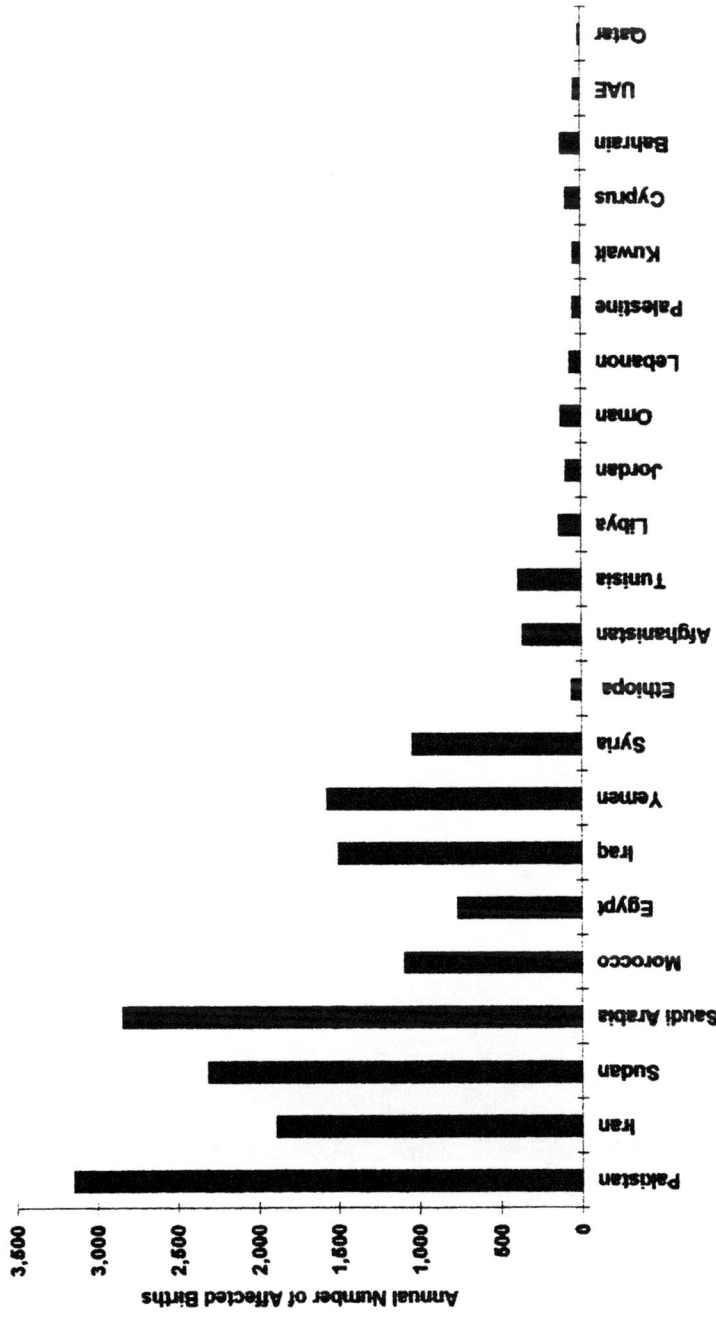

FIGURE 15. Annual number of children born with major Hb disorders in EMR countries.

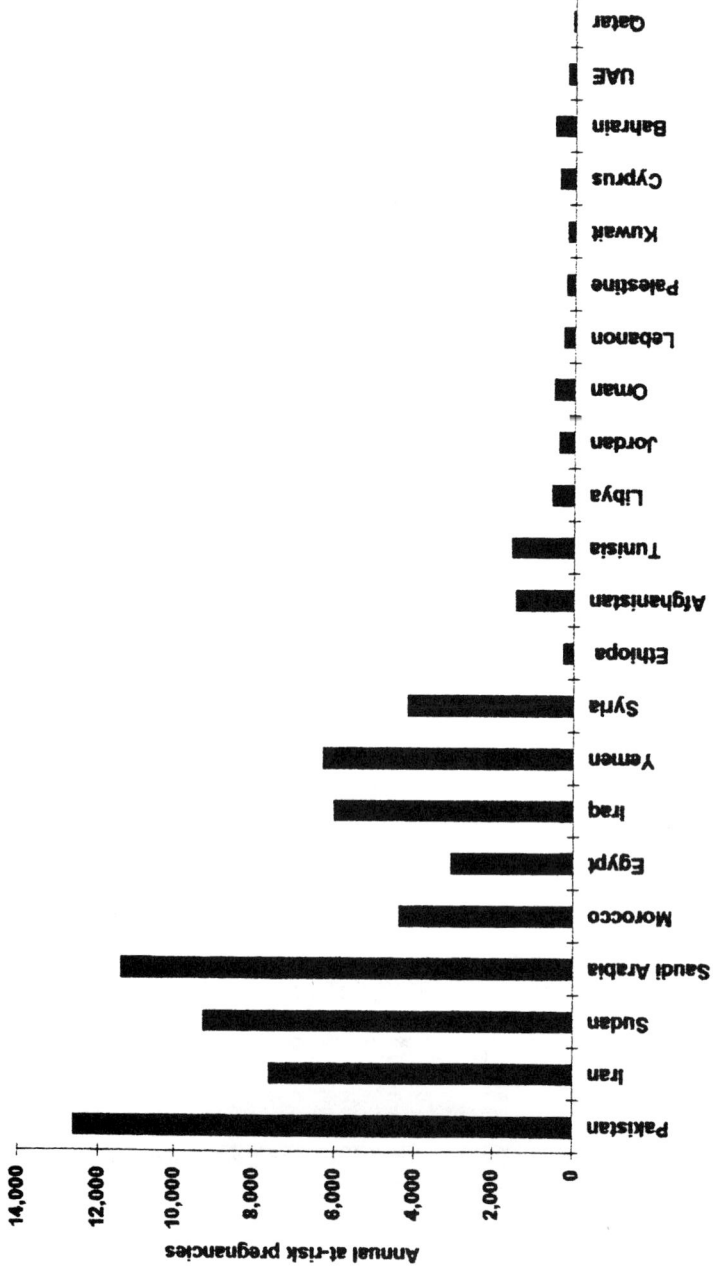

FIGURE 16. Annual number of pregnancies at risk for Hb disorders, EMR countries.

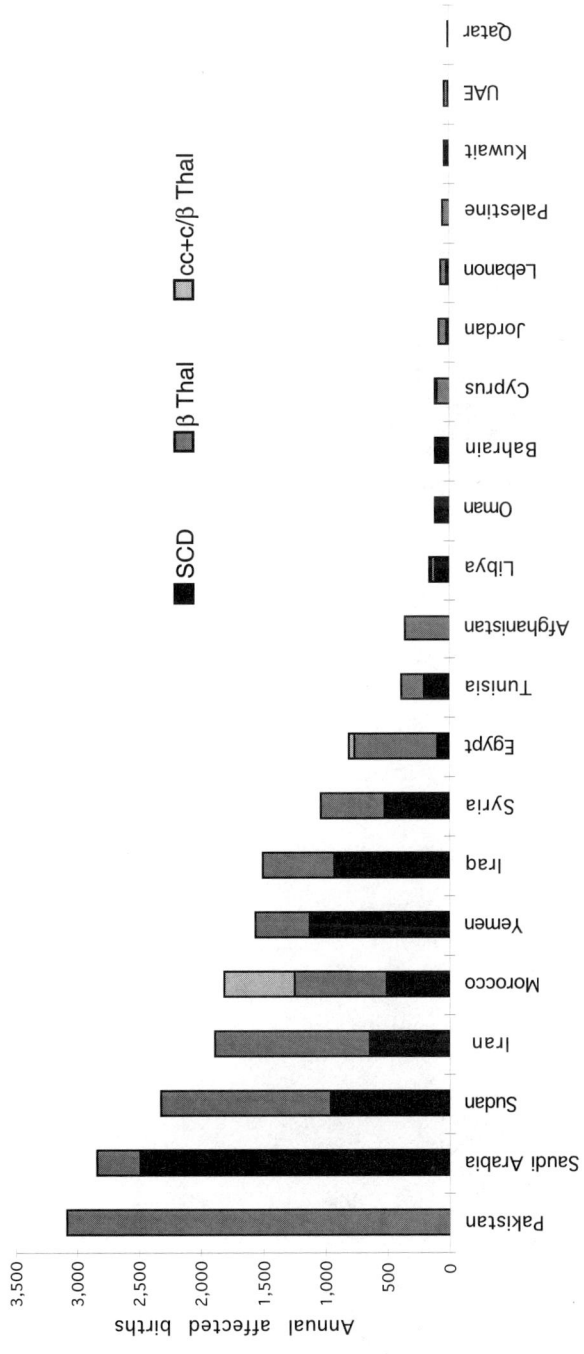

FIGURE 17. Eastern Mediterranean Region: Annual number of infants born with Hb disorders (Total = 18,600).

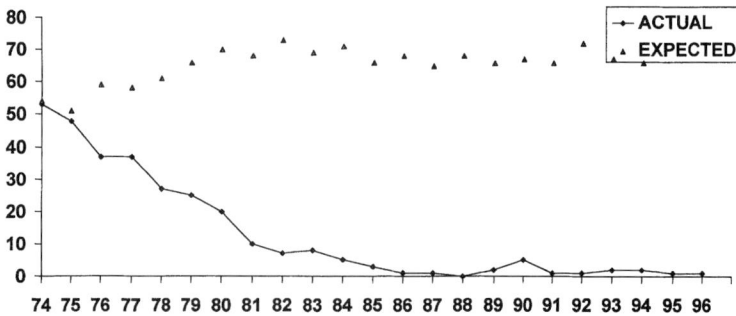

FIGURE 18. Actual affected births vs. expected.

7. For the UK, all data are presented by ethnic group (TABLE 4) based on 1991 census data.[17–19] These figures have been combined with estimates for the proportion of each ethnic group carrying a hemoglobin disorder to produce indicators for screening, counseling and prenatal diagnosis. In this paper, we do not examine all service indicators. The purpose is to demonstrate the complexity of the problem.

The 11 main ethnic minorities are carriers of at least four groups of hemoglobin disorders (AS/AC, β-thalassemia, α-thalassemia and HbE) (FIG. 20). The largest contribution is from the black population so that sickle cell disorders are by far the commonest problem in the UK. There have been few surveys of carrier frequency by ethnic group in the UK. However, surveys have been conducted in most relevant countries; the results, collected by Lingstone (1985) and by the author for WHO (Modell, 1985[1]), may be applied to equivalent groups in the UK.

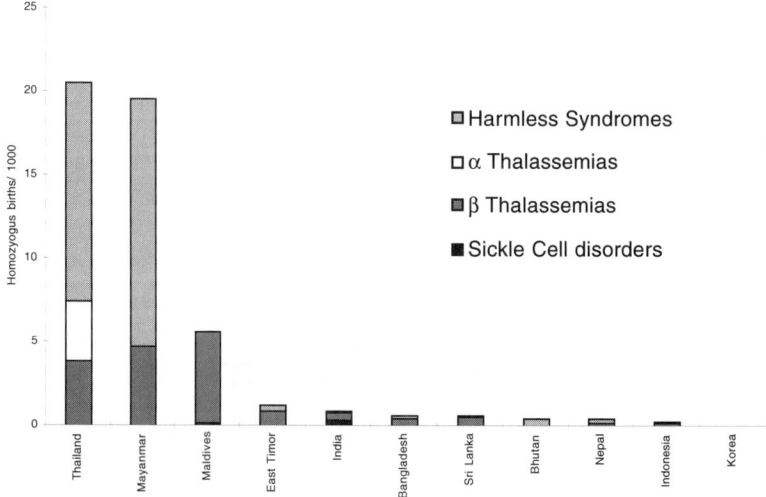

FIGURE 19. South East Asian Region. Main groups of major Hb disorders, births/1000.

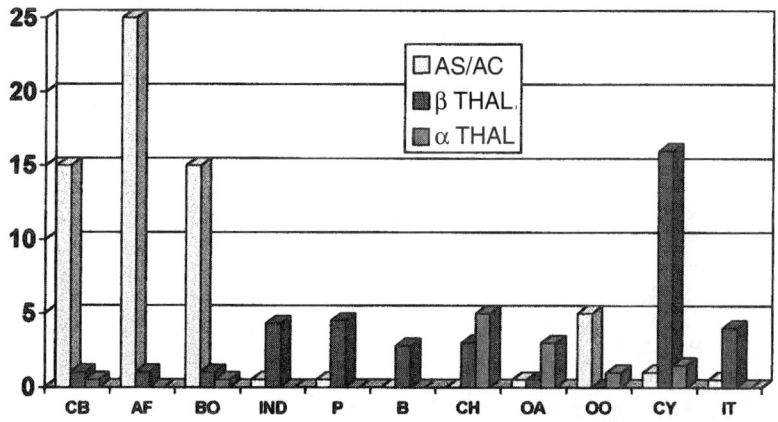

FIGURE 20. Carriers of Hb disorders in UK ethnic minorities.

The affected births per year (FIG. 21) indicate that both SCD and β-thalassemia births are increasing the homozygote population which is already surviving because of the centers of excellence which have been providing treatment for many years, especially in the London area. Prevention programs are, therefore, essential. The effectiveness of prevention, measured ultimately by a reduction in homozygote births, may be estimated by measuring service utilization. An example is the proportion of at-risk pregnancies actually coming to prenatal diagnosis (from the Register of Prenatal Diagnosis—Mary Petrou 1994). There is marked variation in utilization of this service in the various ethnic groups as well as in the regions of the health service.

The variation is not due to the uneven distribution of ethnic groups with different attitudes to prenatal diagnosis, *e.g.,* the Pakistani group have most difficulty with the concept

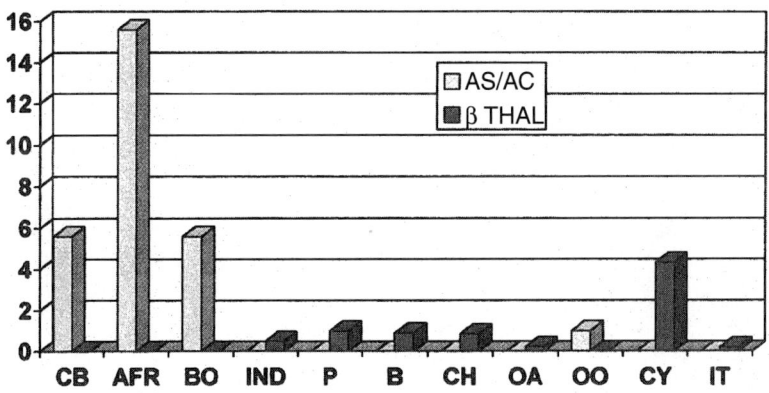

FIGURE 21. Affected births/1000 in ethnic minorities in the UK.

TABLE 4. Ethnic Groups in UK

- Black: Caribbean, African, Other
- Asian: Indian, Pakistani, Bangladeshi, Chinese, Other
- Other Other: Various mixed parentage, North African, Middle Eastern *etc.*
- Mediterranean: Cypriots, Italians

of prenatal diagnosis, but 60% of at-risk couples in London use prenatal diagnosis compared with less than 20% living in other parts of the country. The underlying reasons are now being investigated but preliminary results show delays in antenatal screening, lack of own-language counseling, and poor follow-up of at-risk couples. Another example concerns the prenatal diagnosis of α^0-thalassemia for Chinese couples (the commonest genetic risk among this ethnic group). Data strongly suggests under-utilization because over 50% of at-risk couples are missed in screening and can be missed even when a hydropic baby is born.[15,21]

Identification of these problems should lead to improvements. Monitoring of the national effort by means of national registers of patients and of prenatal diagnosis, coupled with the service indicators, will help to achieve these improvements.

REFERENCES

1. WHO 1985. Update of the Progress of Hemoglobinopathies Control. Report of the Third and Fourth Annual Meetings of the WHO Working Group for the Community Control of Hereditary Anaemias. Unpublished report of the WHO: HMG/WG/85.8. May be obtained free of charge from: The Hereditary Diseases Program, WHO, Geneva, Switzerland.
2. MODELL, B. & V. BOULYJENKOV. 1988. Distribution and control of some genetic disorders. World Health Statistics Quarterly **41:** 209–218.
3. WHO 1989. Report of the VIth Annual Meeting of the WHO Working Group on the Feasibility Study on Hereditary Disease Community Control Programs (Hereditary Anaemias). Cagliari, Sardinia, Italy, 8–9 April 1989 (WHO/HDP/WG/HA/89.2).
4. WHO 1987. The Hemoglobinopathies in Europe. WHO Regional Office for Europe, unpublished document IPC/MCH 110. (May be obtained from: WHO Regional Office for Europe, 8 Scherfigsvej, DK-2100, Copenhagen, Denmark).
5. WHO 1993. Joint WHO/TIF meeting on the prevention and control of hemoglobinopathies (7th meeting of the WHO Working Group on the Control of Hereditary Anaemias). Nicosia, Cyprus 3–4 April 1993. Unpublished report WHO/HDP/TIF/HA/93.1.
6. WHO 1994. Guidelines for control of hemoglobin disorders. Unpublished document of the WHO. WHO/HDP/HB/GL/94.1. Obtainable free of charge from the Hereditary Diseases Program, WHO, Geneva, Switzerland.
7. WHITE, J. M. *et al.* 1993. Frequency and clinical significance of erythrocyte genetic abnormalities in Oman. J. Med. Genet. **30:** 396–400.
8. ANGASTINIOTIS, M. A., S. KYRIAKIDOU & M. HADJIMINAS. 1986. How thalassemia was controlled in Cyprus. World Health Forum 7: 291–297.
9. KULIEV, A. 1986. Thalassemia can be prevented. World Health Forum **7:** 286–90.
10. CAO, A. 1987. Results of programs for antenatal detection of thalassemia in reducing the incidence of the disorder. Blood Rev. **1:** 169–76.
11. GRANDA, H., S. GISPERT, A. DORTICOS, M. MARTIN, Y. CUADRAS, M. CALVO, G. MARTINEZ, M. A. ZAYAS, J. A OLIVA & L. HEREDERO. 1991. Cuban program for prevention of sickle cell disease. Lancet **337:** 152.
12. ANIONWU, E. N., N. PATEL, G. KANJI, H. RENGES & M. BROSOVIC. 1987. Counseling for prenatal diagnosis of sickle cell disease and β-Thalassemia major: A four year experience. J. Med. Genet. **25:** 769.
13. PETROU, M., M. BRUGIATELLI, R. H. T. WARD & B. MODELL. 1992. Factors affecting the uptake of prenatal diagnosis for sickle cell disease. J. Med. Genet. **29:** 820–23.
14. DARR, A. 1990. The social implications of thalassemia among Muslims of Pakistani origin in England—family experience and service delivery. Ph.D. Thesis. University of London.

15. WINICHAGOON, P., S. FUCHAROEN, V. THONGLAIROAM, V. TANAPOTIWIRAI & P. WASI. 1990. Thalassemia in Thailand. Ann. N. Y. Acad. Sci. **612:** 31–42.
16. MODELL, B., A. BENSON & C. R. PAYLING-WRIGHT. 1972. Incidence of Beta Thalassemia trait among Cypriots in London. British Medical Journal **ii:** 737.
17. BULMER, M. 1996. The ethnic question in the 1991 census of population. *In* OPCS. Ethnicity in the 1991 Census. Vol. 1. Demographic characteristics of the ethnic minority populations. Coleman, D. & J. Salt, Eds.: OPCS, London.
18. AL-RASHEED, M. 1996. The Other-Others: Hidden Arabs? OPCS. Ethnicity in the 1991 Census. Vol. 2. The ethnic minority populations of Great Britain. Ed Ceri Peach. OPCS, London.
19. OPCS. 1996. Ethnicity in the 1991 Census. Vol. 1. Demographic characteristics of the ethnic minority populations. D. Coleman & J. Salt, Eds.: OPCS, London.
20. LIVINGSTONE, F. A. 1985. Frequencies of hemoglobin variants. Oxford University Press. New York and Oxford.
21. PETROU, M., M. BRUGIATELLI, J. OLD, P. HURLEY, R. H. T. WARD, K. P. WONG *et al.* 1992. Alpha Thalassemia hydrops fetalis in the UK: The importance of screening pregnant women of Chinese, other South East Asian and Mediterranean extraction for alpha Thalassemia trait. Br. J. Obstet. Gynaecol. **99:** 985–89.

Bone Marrow Transplantation in Thalassemia

The Experience of Pesaro

GUIDO LUCARELLI,[a] MARIA GALIMBERTI, CLAUDIO GIARDINI, PAOLA POLCHI, EMANUELE ANGELUCCI, DONATELLA BARONCIANI, BUKET ERER, AND DJAVID GAZIEV

Divisione Ematologica e Centro Trapianto Midollo Osseo di Muraglia, Azienda Ospedale S. Salvatore di Pesaro, 6110 Pesaro, Italy

ABSTRACT: Early trials of allogenic bone marrow transplantation (BMT) for homozygous β thalassemia and the analyses of results of transplantation in patients under 17 years of age have allowed us to identify 3 classes of risk using the criteria of degree of hepatomegaly, the degree of portal fibrosis, and the quality of the chelation treatment given before the transplant. Patients for whom all 3 criteria were adverse constituted Class 3, patients with none of the adverse criteria constituted Class 1, and patients with 1 or various associations of 2 of the adverse criteria formed Class 2. Most patients older than 16 years have disease characteristics that place them in Class 3, with very few in Class 2. For all the patients with an HLA identical donor we are actually using 2 protocols to which the patient is assigned on the basis of the Class he belongs to at the time of BMT and independently from the age of the patient. For 104 patients in Class 1 and for 262 patients in Class 2 prepared for the transplant with busulfan 14mg/kg, cyclophosphamide 200mg/kg and cyclosporine alone, the probabilities of survival and of event-free survival are 95% and 90% for Class 1 and 87% and 84% for Class 2. For 33 Class 3 patients prepared for the transplant with busulfan 14 mg/kg, cyclophosphamide reduced to 160 mg/kg, cyclosporine, and "short" methotrexate, the probabilities of survival and event-free survival are 89% and 64%. For 57 adult patients (17 to 35 years), who underwent the transplant after preparation with the same protocol used for Class 3, the probabilities of survival and of event-free survival are 70% and 68%, respectively. BMT remains the only form of radical treatment for thalassemia in those patients with an HLA-identical donor.

Patients with homozygous thalassemia are dependent on red blood cell transfusions. They are sick mainly because of complications arising from the unavoidable organ iron overload (even if reduced by the adequate chelation treatment), from hepatitis due to blood-borne viral infections, or from a combination of both liver iron overload and hepatitis. Because of these complications, thalassemia major is a progressive disease.

BONE MARROW TRANSPLANTATION

On December 5, 1981 a one-year-old untransfused thalassemic patient was transplanted in Seattle from his HLA-identical sister. After more than 15 years, he is alive and well and is the first ex-thalassemic after bone marrow transplantation.[1] On December 17, 1981 a 14-year-old thalassemic patient who had received 150 red cell transfusions was transplanted

[a]E-mail: g.lucarelli@wnt.it

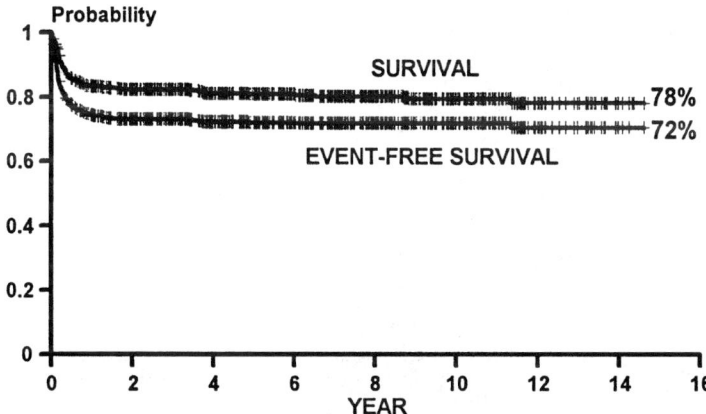

FIGURE 1. Kaplan-Meier probabilities of survival, event-free survival, rejection, and non-rejection mortality for 826 thalassemic patients, age 1 through 35 years, transplanted in Pesaro from December 17, 1981 through April 10, 1997 and calculated on May 15,1997.

in Pesaro but he had recurrence of thalassemia and returned to the pre-transplant condition.[2] This patient is the first of a consecutive series of bone marrow transplantation in thalassemia cases done in Pesaro that has reached 826 transplants at April 10, 1997.

The ages of the patients at the time of the transplant ranged between 1 and 35 years. Eight hundred patients received the marrow from a HLA-identical donor (25 parents and 775 siblings), 25 from a HLA–partially matched donor, and one from a HLA-identical unrelated donor. Overall results on 826 patients calculated on May 15, 1997 are reported in FIGURE 1.

In March 1989, statistical analyses were performed on a group of 222 patients aged 1 through 15 years consecutively treated in our center with the same preparative regimen that had been adopted in June 1985.[3] The analysis of potential risk factors for the outcome of transplantation indicated that poor quality of previous iron chelation therapy, marked hepatomegaly, and portal fibrosis were factors associated with a reduced probability of survival and of disease-free survival. Using these factors as criteria, we were able to categorize patients into three classes of risk for the outcome of marrow transplantation. Patients with none of these risk factors were categorized as Class 1, patients with all three factors were categorized as Class 3, and all other patients were Class 2. All had been treated with a regimen that included busulfan (14 mg/kg) and cyclophosphamide (200 mg/kg) and cyclosporine alone. Results of the transplants, analyzed in March 1989, were good for both Class 1 and for Class 2, but were poor for Class 3 as a consequence of intolerable cardiac and liver toxicity. This led us to adopt new preparative regimens for transplants in Class 3.[4] Since the adoption of new and less toxic preparative protocols for the transplant of patients in Class 3, patients older than 16 years of age have no longer been excluded from the transplant program and they form the group of adult thalassemia patients.

RESULTS

We report here the results of bone marrow transplantation in thalassemia from HLA-identical family member donors and performed with the protocols actually in use at our center and updated at May 15, 1997.

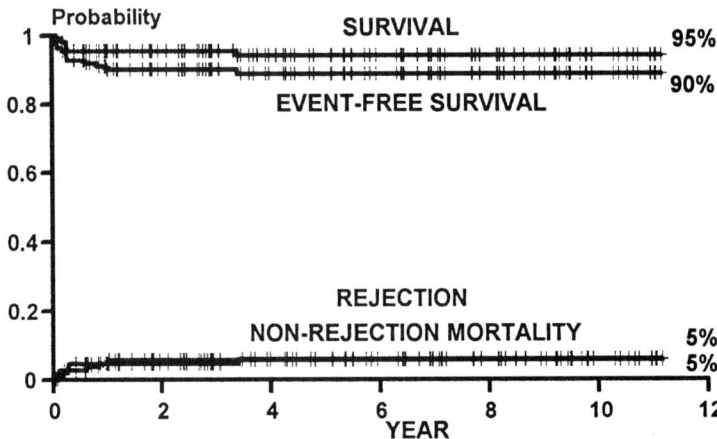

FIGURE 2. Kaplan-Meier probabilities of survival, event-free survival, rejection, and non-rejection mortality for 121 Class 1 thalassemic patients aged less than 17 years, transplanted from HLA-identical donors after preparation with busulfan (14 mg/kg), cyclophosphamide (200 mg/kg), and cyclosporine alone from January 2, 1986 through April 10, 1997 and calculated on May 15, 1997.

Starting on January 1986, 121 thalassemic patients aged less than 16 years in Class 1 and 272 patients in Class 2, were prepared for the transplant with busulfan (14 mg/kg), cyclophosphamide (200 mg/kg), and cyclosporine alone for prophylaxis of graft-versus-host disease (GVHD) (FIG. 2 and FIG. 3).

Starting on March 1989, 125 thalassemic patients less than 16 years old included in Class 3, received busulfan (14mg/kg), cyclophosphamide (120–160 mg/kg), and cyclosporine plus short methotrexate as prophylaxis for GVHD (FIG. 4).

Starting on November 1989, 19 thalassemic patients older than 16 years of age and included in Class 2 received busulfan (14mg/kg) and cyclophosphamide (200 mg/kg). Another group of 90 patients older than 16 years of age in Class 3, received busulfan (14 mg/kg) and cyclophosphamide (120–160 mg/kg) (FIG. 5).

The Ex-thalassemic after Bone Marrow Transplantation

At present only myeloablative regimens followed by marrow transplantation can eradicate hematologic thalassemia. For the thalassemic patients who have acquired normal bone marrows as a result of transplantation the term "ex-thalassemic after transplant" has been proposed by us because there is uncertainty about the reversibility of the various lesions suffered by different organs as a result of the thalassemia and its treatment.

In particular, we do not yet know how effectively excess iron deposits can be mobilized and excreted from the body once the patient's marrow is functioning normally and transfusions are no longer needed. Some of the pre-existing lesions, such as persistent and aggressive chronic hepatitis initiated by the hepatitis C virus, may progress or may not readily be reversed. After successful transplantation the body is left with a severe iron overload. Even under the best of circumstances, normal homeostatic mechanisms would take a long time to return the iron load and distribution to normal.

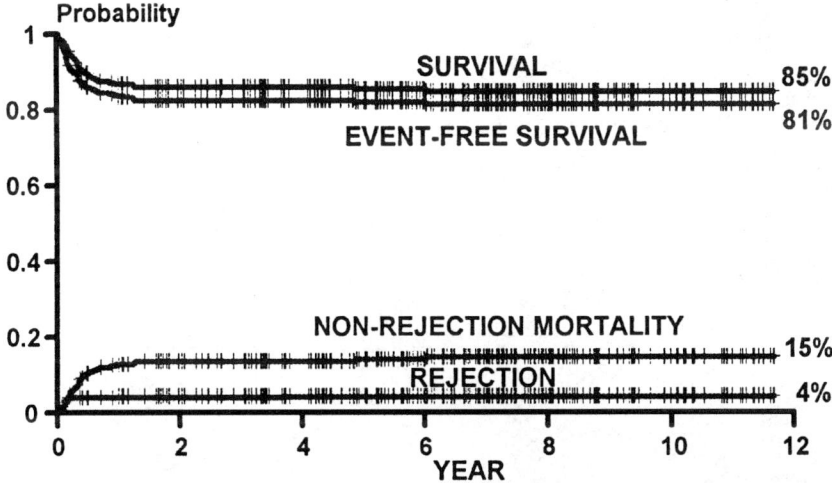

FIGURE 3. Kaplan-Meier probabilities of survival, event-free survival, rejection, and non-rejection mortality for 272 Class 2 thalassemic patients aged less than 17 years, transplanted from HLA-identical donors after preparation with busulfan (14 mg/kg), cyclophosphamide (200 mg/kg), and cyclosporine alone from June 6, 1985 through April 10, 1997 and calculated on May 15, 1997.

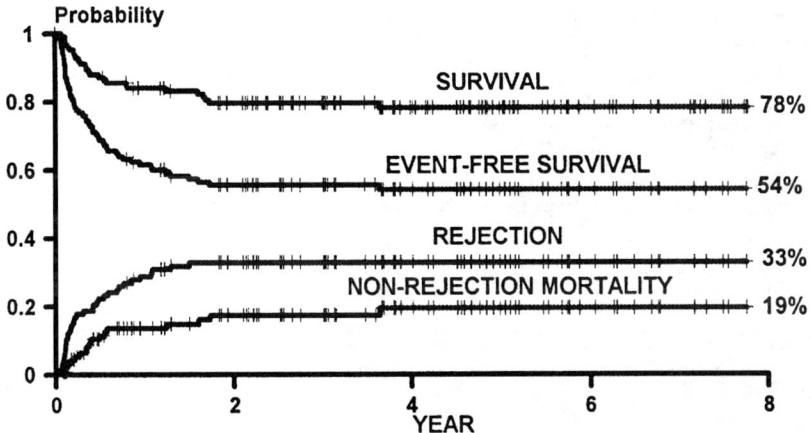

FIGURE 4. Kaplan-Meier probabilities of survival, event-free survival, rejection, and non-rejection mortality for 125 Class 3 thalassemic patients aged less than 17 years, transplanted from HLA-identical siblings after preparation with busulfan (14 mg/kg), cyclophosphamide (120–160 mg/kg), and cyclosporine plus "short" methotrexate from March 1989 through April 10, 1997 and calculated on May 15, 1997.

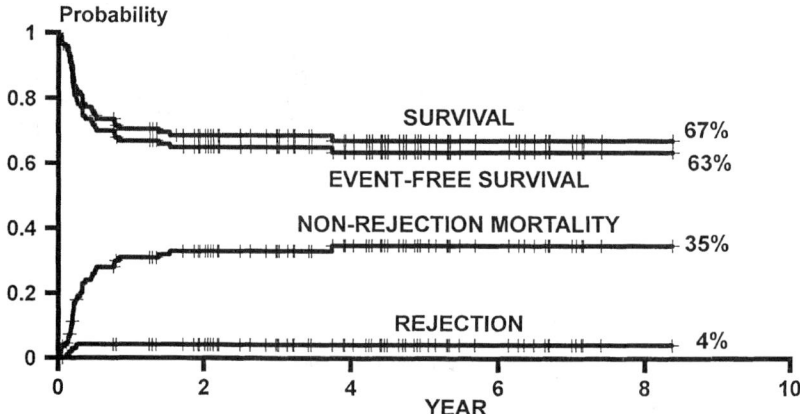

FIGURE 5. Kaplan-Meier probabilities of survival, event-free survival, rejection, and non-rejection mortality calculated on May 15, 1997 for 109 adult thalassemic patients aged more than 16 years (17 through 35 years of age), transplanted from HLA-identical sibling. Nineteen patients were in Class 2 and received the transplant after preparation with the protocol used for the Class 2 from October 13, 1988 through April 10, 1997 [Busulfan (14 mg/kg) and cyclophosphamide (200 mg/kg)]. Ninety patients, who were in Class 3, received the transplant after preparation with the protocol actually in use for the Class 3, from November 26, 1993 through April 10, 1997 [Busulfan 14 mg/kg and cyclophosphamide (120–160 mg/kg)].

The use of chelating agents to hasten clearance in the ex-thalassemic after transplant has been proved to be very effective in young patients[5] while periodic bleeding has been found to be the treatment of choice for the older of the ex-thalassemic who maintain high levels of iron overload.[6] There is some evidence that Class 1 patients will achieve relatively normal iron distribution within a year or two, but early indications are that this will be more difficult to achieve in patients with advanced disease. The need to retain the option for reversing thalassemia-induced lesions to organs other than the marrow is one of the factors that favor early rather than late transplantation.

There are long-term complications that arise from the allogeneic transplant itself. Thus a small proportion of patients develop chronic GVHD, which may be occasionally be severely disabling . There are indications that gonadal function of some patients who have undergone

TABLE 1. Reported Transplants for Thalassemia and Kaplan and Meier Probabilities of Survival and Disease-Free Survival in Various International Transplant Centers[8]

Center	Patients	Survival (%)	Disease-free survival (%)
Pescara	102	91	87
Cagliari 1	25	80	72
Cagliari 2	37	88	88
U.S.A.	68	87	70
U.K.	50	90	76
Teheran	60	83	73
Vellore	50	76	68
Malaysia	28	86	75
Hong Kong	25	86	83
Bangkok	21	76	53

marrow transplantation for thalassemia is impaired, but it is not clear how much of this effect is a result of previous iron overload or a consequence of the preparatory regimen.[7]

CONCLUSION

The results of transplantation from HLA-identical family members are clear. Class 1 patients have a very high probability of cure with a very low early and late morbidity and mortality. There is no reason for denying these patients the advantages of a life free from daily tedious, expensive, and uncomfortable therapy. We do not know the probability that a patient receiving conventional therapy will deteriorate into a worse risk category, but the fact is that every day transplant centers are confronted with patients in risk classes 2 and 3 who represent failures of conventional treatment. Delay of transplantation until the patient is in a risk category beyond Class 1 substantially reduces the probability of transplant success and jeopardizes the reversibility of liver and cardiac damage. We therefore believe that patients with β-thalassemia who have HLA-identical donors should be transplanted as soon as possible. Analyses on bone marrow transplantation in thalassemia performed in many other centers around the world have been reported at the Third International Symposium on Bone Marrow Transplantation in Thalassemia held in Pesaro in September 1996.[8]

Approximately 60% of thalassemic children do not have HLA-identical family members. The use of family member donors genotypically identical for one HLA haplotype with minimal mismatching on the other haplotype has not been very rewarding, with only 3 successes in 11 patients mismatched for one antigen and only one success out of 7 patients mismatched for more than one antigen. Clearly more studies are needed of partially matched transplants, but they are not at present an attractive option in the early management of patients who can obtain and tolerate conventional therapy.

There is no extensive experience of the use of unrelated donors, but the results in the first three such transplants and the results of transplants from partially matched related donors indicate that unrelated donor transplants should not be performed except in the context of a well-defined research environment.

REFERENCES

1. THOMAS, E. D., C. D. BUCKNER, J. E. SANDERS et al. 1982. Marrow transplantation for thalassaemia. Lancet **ii:** 227–229.
2. LUCARELLI, G., T. IZZI, P. POLCHI et al. 1983. Bone marrow transplantation in thalassemia. J. Exp. Clin. Cancer Res. **3:** 313–315.
3. LUCARELLI, G., M. GALIMBERTI, P. POLCHI et al. 1990. Bone marrow transplantation in patients with thalassemia. N. Engl. J. Med. **322:** 417–421.
4. LUCARELLI, G., R. A. CLIFT, M. GALIMBERTI et al. 1996. Marrow transplantation for patients with thalassemia: results in Class 3 patients. Blood. **87:** 2082–2088.
5. GIARDINI, C., M. GALIMBERTI, G. LUCARELLI, P. POLCHI et al. 1994. Desferrioxamine therapy accelerates clearance of iron deposits after bone marrow transplantation. Br. J. Haematol. **89:** 868–873.
6. ANGELUCCI, E., P. MURETTO, G. LUCARELLI et al. 1997. Phlebotomy to reduce iron overload in patients cured of thalassemia by bone marrow transplantation. **90:** 30.
7. DE SANCTIS, V., M. GALIMBERTI, G. LUCARELLI & P. POLCHI. 1991. Gonadal function after allogeneic bone marrow transplantation for thalassaemia. Arch. Dis. Child. **66:** 517–520.
8. Proceedings of the 3rd International Symposium on Bone Marrow Transplantation in Thalassemia. 1997. G. Lucarelli, Ed., Bone Marrow Transplantation. **19,** Supplement 2.

Current and Future Preparative Regimens for Bone Marrow Transplantation in Thalassemia[a]

RAINER STORB,[b-d] CONG YU,[c] H. JOACHIM DEEG,[c,d] GEORGE GEORGES,[c] HANS-PETER KIEM,[c] PETER A. MCSWEENEY,[c,d] RICHARD A. NASH,[c,d] BRENDA M. SANDMAIER,[c,d] KEITH M. SULLIVAN,[c,d] JOHN L. WAGNER,[c] AND MARK C. WALTERS[c,e]

Transplantation Biology Program, [c]Clinical Research Division, Fred Hutchinson Cancer Research Center

[d]Departments of Medicine and [e]Pediatrics, University of Washington School of Medicine, Seattle, Washington 98109, USA

> ABSTRACT: Preparative regimens for marrow allografts in thalassemia have two objectives. One is eradication of diseased marrow and the other suppression of host-versus-graft (HVG) reactions so that the allograft survives. A common regimen to accomplish these goals has combined high-dose busulfan with cyclophosphamide. Postgrafting immunosuppression with cyclosporine/methotrexate has been used for GVHD prevention. Some patients may die from regimen-related toxicity. Overall event-free survival is 75%. Occasional patients have become mixed donor/host hematopoietic chimeras and, yet, disease symptoms have abated. This has raised the possibility of developing safer and less toxic transplant programs that result in stable mixed hematopoietic chimerism. We have devised such a program in dogs consisting of a nonlethal dose of total body irradiation (200 cGy) before and a novel combination of mycophenolate mofetil and cyclosporine after transplant. Mixed donor/host chimerism (≥ 50% donor cells in all lineages) has persisted for > 80 weeks, even though immunosuppression was discontinued after five weeks.

Marrow allografts are currently the only definitive therapy for thalassemia.[1-4] For allografts to be successful, a double immunological barrier, composed of host-versus-graft (HVG) and graft-versus-host (GVH) reactions, must be crossed. In the setting of major histocompatibility complex (MHC) identical related grafts, both reactions are mediated by T cells. Given the role T cells play in maintaining both barriers, pre- and posttransplant immunosuppression have been integral parts of transplant regimens for thalassemia. Currently used regimens, summarized in TABLE 1, have their origin in the first successful transplant done for thalassemia in 1981 at the Fred Hutchinson Cancer Research Center (FHCRC).[1] The hematological changes and the drug regimen in this

---

[a]Supported in part by grants HL36444, CA18221, DK42716, CA15704, HL 03701 awarded by the National Institutes of Health. Support was also received from a prize awarded to R.S. by the Josef Steiner Krebsstiftung, Bern, Switzerland. H.J.D. is supported by an award from the National Marrow Donor Program/Baxter Health Care Division.

[b]Address for correspondence: Rainer Storb, M.D., Fred Hutchinson Cancer Research Center, 1100 Fairview Ave. North D1-100, P.O. Box 19024, Seattle, WA 98109-1024; Tel: 206/667-4407; Fax: 206/667-6124; E-mail: rstorb@fhcrc.org

TABLE 1. Current Allogeneic Transplant Program for Thalassemia Major

Components	Purpose
1. BU (14–16 mg/kg) + CY (200 mg/kg) ± ATG (90 mg/kg)	Host immunosuppression and eradication of underlying disease, "creation of marrow space"
2. Stem Cell Graft	"Rescue" from regimen-related myelosuppression and establishment of normal hematopoiesis.
3. MTX/CSP ± CY ± Pred.	Immunosuppression for the prevention of GVHD and induction of graft-host tolerance

Abbreviations: BU = busulfan; CY = cyclophosphamide; ATG = antithymocyte globulin; MTX = methotrexate; CSP = cyclosporine; Pred. = prednisolone; GVHD = graft-versus-host disease.

patient are shown in FIGURE 1. The first component of the transplant, the conditioning regimen, consisted of intravenously administered dimethylbusulfan or dimethylmyleran (DMM) and was given with the aim of eliminating thalassemia and creating marrow space for the donor cells to home. Additionally, canine studies had shown that DMM provided some degree of host immunosuppression.[5] In current regimens, oral busulfan (BU) has been substituted for DMM since DMM is no longer available. Another integral part of the regimen's first component was pretransplant cyclophosphamide (CY) for host immunosuppression.[6–9] The second component was the stem cell graft, which ultimately established normal hematopoiesis, and whose immediate role was to "rescue" the patient

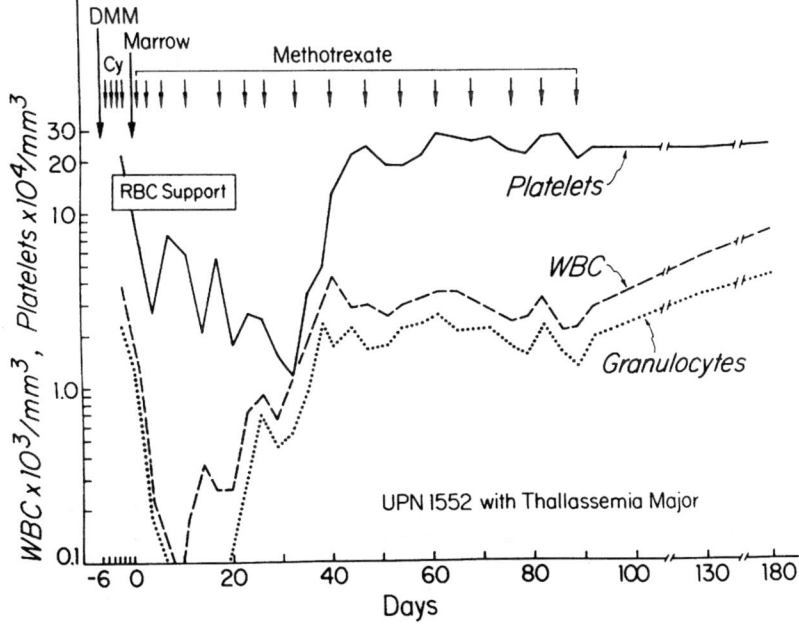

FIGURE 1. Transplant regimen and hematological changes in a patient with thalassemia major given an HLA-identical marrow transplant in December 1981.[1] Abbreviations: DMM=dimethylbusulfan; CY=cyclophosphamide; WBC=white blood cell count; RBC=red blood cells.

TABLE 2. Toxicities of Busulfan and Cyclophosphamide Conditioning

Obligatory	Potential
Nausea, vomiting, mucositis, diarrhea, alopecia, pancytopenia (and associated risk of infections), infertility, retardation of growth and development	Seizures, hemorrhagic cystitis, idiopathic interstitial pneumonia, veno-occlusive disease of the liver, cardiomyopathy, secondary cancer, cataracts

from regimen-related myelosuppression and, thereby, reduce the risk of infections. The third component was postgrafting immunosuppression, which commonly consisted of methotrexate (MTX) and cyclosporine (CSP),[10,11] but might also include other agents, and was aimed at preventing graft-versus-host disease (GVHD) and inducing stable graft-host tolerance.

The conditioning regimen's toxicities are severe, and patients are placed in a hospital setting for their transplants. TABLE 2 shows obligatory and potential toxicities of BU and CY conditioning. Given these toxicities, patients with advanced class 3 thalassemia, per Pesaro criteria, tolerated the conditioning regimens poorly, compared to class 1 and 2 patients, and experienced significant mortality. Lucarelli and colleagues reported a 24–39% nonrejection mortality in patients with class 3 disease who were <17 years of age and 35% in those age ≥17.[12,13] The risks from regimen-related toxicities versus benefits from transplantation have been at the center of the controversy as to the role of transplantation versus supportive management of thalassemia.

In order to reduce the risks due to toxicities from the transplant programs and, thereby, to help resolve the controversy of how best to manage patients with thalassemia, we have utilized a preclinical canine model of marrow transplantation. With this canine model we have developed novel transplant programs that are safer than current regimens and potentially can be administered in the ambulatory care setting rather than on intensive care wards. The novel programs, if effective, also offer potential for significant cost savings.

TABLE 3 summarizes our working hypotheses which have guided the design of the canine studies. We postulated, firstly, that cytotoxic agents were not needed for creation of marrow space; secondly, that allogeneic stem cell grafts could be established solely through suppression of HVG; thirdly, that grafts could "create" their own marrow space through an allogeneic effect that is accomplished by transient GVH reactions; fourthly, that HVG reactions could be suppressed through the same agents that were used to prevent GVHD; and finally that to effectively treat thalassemia, complete eradication of the underlying disease was not required; rather, stable mixed donor-host hematopoietic chimerism was sufficient.

Given that BU is not only very toxic but, at equitoxic doses, significantly less immunosuppressive than total body irradiation (TBI) we elected to carry out the canine studies with TBI conditioning delivered as a single dose from two opposing 60-Cobalt sources at a dose rate of 7 cGy/min. TABLE 4 illustrates the marrow toxicity of TBI in dogs not "res-

TABLE 3. Hypotheses Underlying Novel Low-Risk Allogeneic Transplant Programs

1. Cytotoxic agents, e.g., BU and CY, are not needed for "creation of marrow space."
2. Stem cell grafts can be established solely through suppression of HVG.
3. Grafts "create" marrow space through an allogeneic effect that is accomplished by transient GVH reactions.
4. HVG reactions can be suppressed through agents used for GVHD prevention.
5. Complete eradication of thalassemia is not required, and mixed donor-host hematopoietic chimerism is effective treatment.

Abbreviations: BU = busulfan; CY = cyclophosphamide; HVG = host-versus-graft; GVH = graft-versus-host; GVHD = graft-versus-host disease.

cued" by subsequent marrow infusion. With best supportive care including transfusions, 200 cGy TBI was sublethal, 300 cGy represented the "LD_{75}," and 400 cGy the "LD_{99}."[14]

TABLE 5 shows that a very high dose of TBI was needed for successful engraftment of marrow from dog lymphocyte antigen (DLA)-identical littermates given no postgrafting immunosuppression. Consistent engraftment was seen only at 920 cGy TBI while rejection rates gradually increased as TBI doses were decreased to the still supralethal range of 450 cGy.[15,16]

We then asked whether allogeneic engraftment could be improved in dogs given 450 cGy TBI by administering immunosuppression with CSP either before or after transplantation (TABLE 6).[17] All nine dogs given CSP before transplant rejected while all seven dogs given CSP after transplant (Day –1 to Day 35) engrafted. Engraftment was manifested either as all-donor type or mixed donor-host type hematopoietic chimerism. Chimerism was assessed on the basis of microsatellite marker polymorphisms using a polymerase chain reaction (PCR)-based assay.[18] In this and all subsequent canine studies that addressed the role of postgrafting immunosuppression on engraftment, the last dose of CSP was given on Day 35, and no further immunosuppression was given thereafter.

In the next experiment, we decreased the TBI dose to a sublethal range of 200 cGy (TABLE 7).[19] Four dogs were given CSP only. All four rejected their allografts at 4 weeks and they survived with complete autologous recovery. Six dogs were given a combination of MTX and CSP, a drug combination that was previously shown to be synergistic with regard to GVHD prevention both in humans and in dogs.[10,11] Three of the six dogs became stable mixed chimeras, and three rejected their grafts at 2, 7, and 11 weeks after transplant, respectively. One of the stable chimeras was euthanized shortly after Week 8 because of severe papilloma virus infection on all paws, owing to CSP-induced immunosuppression. Two mixed chimeras are alive >82 weeks after transplant. Next, we studied mycophenolate mofetil (MMF), a drug that blocks the *de novo* purine synthesis pathway by binding to a key enzyme, inosine monophosphate dehydrogenase, thereby blocking lymphocyte replication. We chose this agent because previous studies had shown MMF and CSP to be synergistic and superior to MTX/CSP with regard to GVHD prevention.[20] Ten dogs were transplanted. One rejected the allograft beyond Week 12, while nine have remained stable mixed chimeras for up to 78 weeks after transplant. Dogs did not experience severe toxicities. They did not require parenteral fluid and electrolyte support, and they did not require blood product transfusions. The dogs did not show clinical manifestations of GVHD. FIGURE 2 also illustrates the blood cell changes in one of the dogs along with the results of microsatellite marker studies, which showed persistence of both the donor and host-specific bands in peripheral blood and marrow cells after transplantation, consistent with mixed chimerism. FIGURE 3 illustrates stable mixed chimerism in nucleated peripheral blood cells from six of seven transplanted dogs up to Week 75. One dog lost donor cell engraftment after Week 13. The percent donor cells in the remaining dogs ranged from 45–85%. TABLE 8 compares marker study results in marrow to those in peripheral blood mononuclear cells and granulocytes, as well as lymph node lymphocytes. The highest proportions of donor cells were seen among peripheral blood granulocytes and the lowest among mononuclear cells.

These findings provided evidence in a large random bred animal species that the goal of establishing stable mixed hematopoietic chimerism following a nonmyeloablative and nontoxic conditioning program can be achieved through the use of pharmacological immunosuppression after transplant. This immunosuppressive approach both contained HVG reactions and prevented clinical manifestations of GVHD.

We next reduced the dose of TBI further (TABLE 9).[19] All six dogs given 100 cGy of TBI rejected their grafts, and donor cells had disappeared 3–12 weeks after transplant. Similarly, both dogs given no TBI lost their mixed chimerism 2 weeks after transplant. As yet unpublished preliminary observations in five dogs given canine recombinant

TABLE 4. Marrow Toxicity of Total Body Irradiation in Dogs Not Given Marrow Transplants[14]

Total Body Irradiation Dose (cGy)	Number of Dogs Surviving / Number of Dogs Studied
200	18/19
300	7/21
400	1/28

TABLE 5. Marrow Grafts from DLA-Identical Littermates in Dogs Given Single Doses of TBI From Dual ^{60}Co Sources at 7 cGy/Min and No Postgrafting Immunosuppression[15,16]

Total Body Irradiation Dose (cGy)	Number of Dogs	Rejection	Percent Survival With Autologous Recovery	Percent Survival With Successful Allograft[a]
920	21	5	0	95
800	3	20	0	80
700	5	40	0	60
600	23	48	17	52
450	39	59	36	41

[a]Includes both dogs with complete and mixed donor-host hematopoietic chimerism.

TABLE 6. Dogs Given 450 cGy TBI and Marrow Grafts from DLA-Identical Littermates[17]

Additional Immunosuppression	Number of Dogs Studied	Graft Rejection	Successful Allograft Mixed Chimerism	Successful Allograft All Donor Cells
None	17	11	3	3
CSP[a] before transplant	9	9	0	0
CSP[b] after transplant	7	0	2	5

[a]Cyclosporine, 10 mg/kg BID i.v. Days –7 to –1;
[b]Cyclosporine, 15 mg/kg BID p.o. Days –1 to 35.

TABLE 7. Dogs Given 200 cGy TBI and Marrow Grafts From DLA-Identical Littermates[19]

Postgrafting Immunosuppression	Number of Dogs with Rejection/ Number of Dogs Studied	Duration of Mixed Chimerism (Weeks)
CSP[a]	4/4	4,4,4,4
MTX[b]/CSP[a]	3/6	2, 7, 11, >8, >82, >82
MMF[c]/CSP[a]	1/10	12, >10, >14, >28, >28, >28, >57, >77, >77, >78

[a]Cyclosporine, 15 mg/kg BID p.o. Days –1 to 35
[b]Methotrexate, 0.4 mg/kg/ i.v. Days 1,3,6,11
[c]Mycophenolate mofetil , 10 mg/kg BID s.c. Days 0–27.

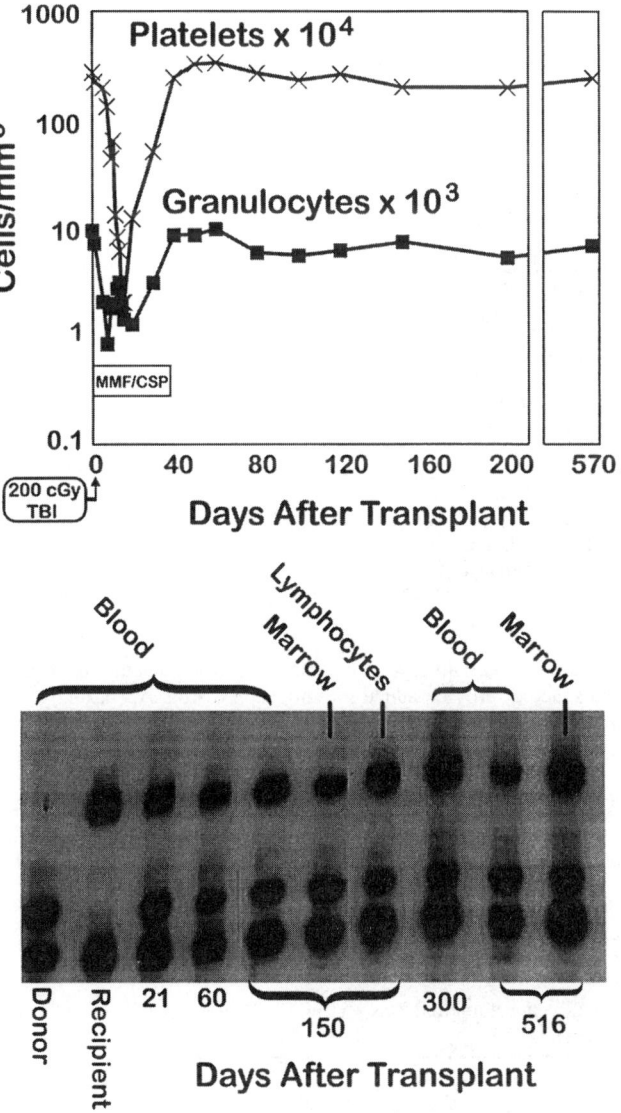

FIGURE 2. Granulocyte and platelet changes in a dog conditioned with a sublethal dose of 200 cGy TBI and given a marrow graft from a DLA-identical littermate on Day 0, followed by postgrafting immunosuppression with mycophenolate mofetil/cyclosporine (MMF/CSP) for no more than 35 days.[19] The bottom panel shows the results of testing for $(CA)_n$ dinucleotide repeats of donor and recipient cells before transplantation (lanes 1 and 2) and recipient cells after marrow transplantation (lanes 3 to 10). "Lymphocytes" includes lymphocytes and monocytes.

G-CSF–mobilized peripheral blood stem cells after 100 cGy TBI showed stable mixed chimerism in a majority of recipient dogs.

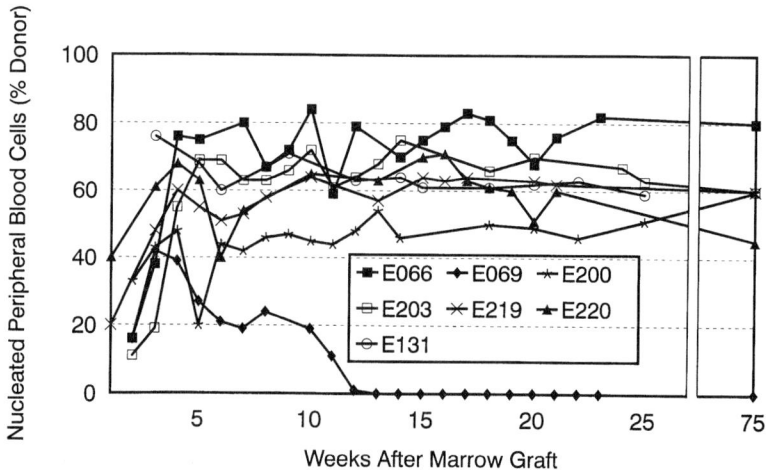

FIGURE 3. Percent donor nucleated peripheral blood cells after transplant in seven dogs given 200 cGy TBI and DLA-identical marrow grafts.[19] Two dogs received methotrexate/cyclosporine (E200, E203) and five were given mycophenolate mofetil/cyclosporine (E066, E069, E131, E219, E220) after transplant. Data were estimated by phosphorimage analysis of $(CA)_n$ dinucleotide repeat marker results.

An important question with regard to these studies was whether the role of TBI was to create marrow space or provide added immunosuppression. Accordingly, four dogs were given marrow grafts and postgrafting immunosuppression by MMF/CSP after either marrow irradiation (with sparing of lymphoid tissues) or lymphoid irradiation (with sparing of marrow) (unpublished observations). Although longer follow-up is needed, preliminary results suggested that lymphoid irradiation was effective in establishing mixed chimerism while marrow irradiation was not. Given these findings, it is possible that the small dose of TBI currently used for establishment of mixed chimerism can be replaced by other even less toxic means of T-cell suppression. Anasetti and coworkers from FHCRC have reported on successful second transplants in patients who had rejected their first transplants by using a conditioning regimen that combined a monoclonal antibody to CD3 (BC3) with

TABLE 8. Dogs Given a Sublethal Dose of TBI (200 cGy) and Marrow Grafts from DLA-Identical Littermates[19]

				% Donor Cells Estimated by Phosphorimage Analysis of $(CA)_n$ Dinucleotide Repeat Marker Results			
				Peripheral Blood			Popliteal Lymph Node
Dog Number	Postgrafting Immunosuppression[a]	Day of Test	Marrow	Buffy Coat Cells	Mononuclear Cells	Granulocytes	Lymphocytes (day posttransplant)
E200	MTX/CSP	135	85	86	54	91	55 (292 d)
E203		135	85	86	55	92	50 (292 d)
E131	MMF/CSP	180	44	55	49	54	50 (341 d)
E219		98	54	61	36	69	40 (255 d)
E220		98	53	60	35	68	35 (255 d)

[a]*Abbreviations:* CSP = cyclosporine; MMF = mycophenolate mofetil; MTX = methotrexate.

TABLE 9. Dogs Given Marrow Grafts from DLA-Identical Littermates, and MMF/CSP[a] after Transplant[19]

TBI Dose (cGy)	Number of Dogs with Rejection/ Number of Dogs Studied	Duration of Mixed Chimerism (Weeks)
100	6/6	3, 3, 10, 10, 10, 12
0	2/2	2, 2

[a]CSP = cyclosporine; MMF = mycophenolate mofetil; TBI = total body irradiation.

very high doses of corticosteroids.[21] The regimen was patterned after a second transplant program reported from Sloan Kettering, where investigators had combined high dose corticosteroids with antithymocyte globulin (ATG).[22] The relative contributions of steroids versus the anti-CD3 antibody in the establishment of successful second transplants are unknown. Early studies of the same dose and dose schedule of corticosteroids in dogs conditioned by 450 cGy TBI for DLA-identical marrow grafts showed that corticosteroids did not enhance engraftment, and all five dogs so treated rejected their allografts.[17] Conversely, preliminary studies in the same canine model using an anti-T-cell receptor $\alpha\beta$ antibody have shown sustained mixed hematopoietic chimerism in five of six dogs, suggesting that host T-cell suppression with a monoclonal antibody might one day be used as a substitute for or an adjunct to low-dose TBI (unpublished observations).

Much work on mixed allogeneic chimerism has been done in inbred strains of mice. Most investigators have used *in vivo* T-cell depletion whereby antibodies were combined with TBI at very high, but nevertheless sublethal doses. In other cases, TBI was given along with thymic irradiation and postgrafting CSP or high-dose CY. The first study was that reported by Cobbold and colleagues in 1986, in which pretransplant therapy with anti-CD4 and anti-CD8 monoclonal antibodies was combined with 600–850 cGy TBI delivered at the high dose rate of 35 cGy/min.[23] In another study, non-obese diabetic mice were given ≥750 cGy of TBI followed by very large doses of allogeneic marrow cells, on the order of ≥30 x 10^6 (≥1.5 x 10^9/kg).[24] In one report, mice were conditioned for allografts by 500 cGy TBI and then given 100 or 200 mg CY/kg after transplant.[25] In another report, anti-CD4 and CD8 monoclonal antibodies were combined with 3 Gy TBI and 7 Gy thymic irradiation to ensure engraftment.[26] That same group of investigators reported more recently that the need for thymic irradiation could be avoided by additional anti-CD4 and anti-CD8 monoclonal antibody therapy after transplant.[27,28] Persistent chimerism was obtained when murine recipients were given anti-CD4 and CD8 monoclonal antibodies along with 3 Gy of TBI administered at 100 cGy/min before transplant and antibody treatment against natural killer cells after transplant for at most 16 weeks.[29] Persistent long-term mixed chimerism in large random bred animal species achieved through the use of nonmyeloablative conditioning programs has not been reported outside of the present canine studies.

Taken together, the data in the preclinical animal models support the hypotheses 1–4 in TABLE 3 and show that allogeneic transplants can be accomplished safely and with little toxicity and result in stable mixed donor-host hematopoietic chimerism. Evidence in support for

TABLE 10. Sickle Cell Patient with Stroke before Transplant[30]

- 24 Months after HLA-Identical Sibling Transplant
- 10–20% Donor Chimerism
- 6.7% Hgb F, 30% Hgb S
- 100% Lansky Performance Score
- No Central Nervous System Symptoms
- No Transfusion Requirement

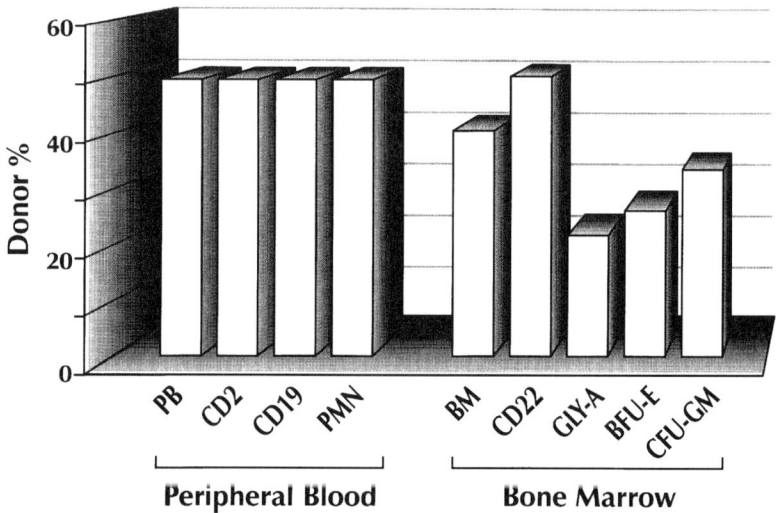

FIGURE 4. Percent donor chimerism in a thalassemia patient 4 years after transplantation of HLA-identical sibling marrow following a conditioning program of busulfan and cyclophosphamide.[31] Abbreviations: PB=peripheral blood; PMN=polymorphonuclear cells; BM=bone marrow; BFU-E=burst-forming unit erythrocytes; CFU-GM=colony forming units granulocytes/macrophages. (From Andrean's et al.[3] Reproduced with permission.)

hypothesis 5, namely that establishing mixed chimerism would be effective treatment in patients with genetic diseases, comes from at least two clinical publications in 1996 and one in 1997 that described observations after transplants for sickle cell disease and thalassemia major.[30–32] TABLE 10 shows 10–20% stable donor chimerism in a sickle cell disease patient who was transplanted from an HLA-identical sibling donor because of stroke and who is now more than two years after transplant without central nervous system or other sickle cell disease–related symptoms and not requiring transfusions. FIGURE 4 shows comparable data in a patient with thalassemia. Four years after transplantation, donor type chimerism ranged from 20–50% depending on the hematopoietic cell subset studied, and yet the patient did not require red blood cell transfusions. That report included data from at least two other patients showing a similar result.[31] Studies are ongoing in a canine model of severe hemolytic anemia due to pyruvate kinase deficiency to ask what degree of mixed chimerism is needed to accomplish cure. Previous studies had shown that complete replacement of hematopoiesis by donor cells was curative for this severe congenital canine disease.[33]

In conclusion, preclinical experiments combined with clinical observations have led to the development of a radically new concept in hematopoietic stem cell transplantation for genetic disorders in which the current highly toxic and myeloablative pretransplant conditioning regimens may be replaced with minimally toxic nonmyeloablative regimens focusing on intense temporary immunosuppression. Ultimately, host immunosuppression before transplantation may be accomplished by biological reagents, *e.g.* monoclonal antibodies to surface determinants on T cells, complemented by postgrafting immunosuppression directed at preventing both HVG and GVH reactions. We hypothesize that the resultant stable mixed donor-host hematopoietic chimerism will be sufficient to accomplish cure of clinical manifestations of genetic diseases including thalassemia major. This way, the efficiency of allografting as treatment for these diseases is exploited without exposing patients to the usual toxicities of this procedure.

REFERENCES

1. THOMAS, E. D., C. D. BUCKNER, J. E. SANDERS, T. PAPAYANNOPOULOU, C. BORGNA-PIGNATTI, P. DE STEFANO, K. M. SULLIVAN, R. A. CLIFT & R. STORB. 1982. Marrow transplantation for thalassaemia. Lancet ii: 227–229.
2. THOMAS, E. D., J. E. SANDERS, C. D. BUCKNER, T. PAPAYANNOPOULOU, C. BORGNA-PIGNATTI, P. DE STEFANO, K. M. SULLIVAN, H. J. DEEG, R. P. WITHERSPOON, F. R. APPELBAUM, R. A. CLIFT & R. STORB. 1985. Marrow transplantation for thalassemia. Ann. N.Y. Acad. Sci. **445**: 417–427.
3. LUCARELLI, G., M. GALIMBERTI, P. POLCHI, C. GIARDINI, P. POLITI, D. BARONCIANI, E. ANGELUCCI, F. MANENTI, C. DELFINI, G. AURELI & P. MORETTO. 1987. Marrow transplantation in patients with advanced thalassemia. N. Engl. J. Med. **316**: 1050–1055.
4. LUCARELLI, G., M. GALIMBERTI, P. POLCHI, E. ANGELUCCI, D. BARONCIANI, C. GIARDINI, P. POLITI, S. M. T. DURAZZI, P. MURETTO & F. ALBERTINI. 1990. Bone marrow transplantation in patients with thalassemia. N. Engl. J. Med. **322**: 417–421.
5. STORB, R., P. L. WEIDEN, T. C. GRAHAM, K. G. LERNER, N. NELSON & E. D. THOMAS. 1977. Hemopoietic grafts between DLA-identical canine littermates following dimethyl myleran. Evidence for resistance to grafts not associated with DLA and abrogated by antithymocyte serum. Transplantation **24**: 349–357.
6. SANTOS, G. W. & A. H. OWENS, JR. 1969. Allogeneic marrow transplants in cyclophosphamide treated mice. Transplant. Proc. **1**: 44–46.
7. STORB, R., R. B. EPSTEIN, R. H. RUDOLPH & E. D. THOMAS. 1969. Allogeneic canine bone marrow transplantation following cyclophosphamide. Transplantation **7**: 378–386.
8. STORB, R., C. D. BUCKNER, L. A. DILLINGHAM & E. D. THOMAS. 1970. Cyclophosphamide regimens in rhesus monkeys with and without marrow infusion. Cancer Res. **30**: 2195–2203.
9. STORB, R., E. D. THOMAS, C. D. BUCKNER, R. A. CLIFT, F. L. JOHNSON, A. FEFER, H. GLUCKSBERG, E. R. GIBLETT, K. G. LERNER & P. NEIMAN. 1974. Allogeneic marrow grafting for treatment of aplastic anemia. Blood **43**: 157–180.
10. DEEG, H. J., R. STORB, P. L. WEIDEN, R. F. RAFF, G. E. SALE, K. ATKINSON, T. C. GRAHAM & E. D. THOMAS. 1982. Cyclosporin A and methotrexate in canine marrow transplantation: Engraftment, graft-versus-host disease, and induction of tolerance. Transplantation **34**: 30–35.
11. STORB, R., H. J. DEEG, J. WHITEHEAD, F. APPELBAUM, P. BEATTY, W. BENSINGER, C. D. BUCKNER, R. CLIFT, K. DONEY, V. FAREWELL, J. HANSEN, R. HILL, L. LUM, P. MARTIN, R. MCGUFFIN, J. SANDERS, P. STEWART, K. SULLIVAN, R. WITHERSPOON, G. YEE & E. D. THOMAS. 1986. Methotrexate and cyclosporine compared with cyclosporine alone for prophylaxis of acute graft versus host disease after marrow transplantation for leukemia. N. Engl. J. Med. **314**: 729–735.
12. LUCARELLI, G., R. A. CLIFT, M. GALIMBERTI, P. POLCHI, E. ANGELUCCI, D. BARONCIANI, C. GIARDINI, M. ANDREANI, M. MANNA, S. NESCI, F. AGOSTINELLI, S. RAPA, M. RIPALTI & F. ALBERTINI. 1996. Marrow transplantation for patients with thalassemia. Results in class 3 patients. Blood **87**: 2082–2088.
13. GALIMBERTI, M., E. ANGELUCCI, D. BARONCIANI, C. GIARDINI, P. POLCHI, B. ERER, D. J. GAZIEV, C. PAZZAGLIA, A. CIARONI, M. BALDASSARRI, F. MARTINELLI & G. LUCARELLI. 1997. Bone marrow transplantation in thalassemia. The experience of Pesaro. Bone Marrow Transplantation **19**: 45–47.
14. STORB, R., R. F. RAFF, T. GRAHAM, F. R. APPELBAUM, H. J. DEEG, F. G. SCHUENING, H. SHULMAN & M. PEPE. 1993. Marrow toxicity of fractionated versus single dose total body irradiation is identical in a canine model. Int. J. Radiat. Oncol. Biol. Phys. **26**: 275–283.
15. STORB, R., R. F. RAFF, F. R. APPELBAUM, F. W. SCHUENING, B. M. SANDMAIER, T. C. GRAHAM & E. D. THOMAS. 1988. What radiation dose for DLA-identical canine marrow grafts? Blood **72**: 1300–1304.

16. STORB, R., R. F. RAFF, F. R. APPELBAUM, H. J. DEEG, T. C. GRAHAM, F. G. SCHUENING, H. SHULMAN, C. YU, E. BRYANT, R. BURNETT & K. SEIDEL. 1994. DLA-identical bone marrow grafts after low-dose total body irradiation: The effect of canine recombinant hematopoietic growth factors. Blood **84:** 3558–3566.
17. YU, C., R. STORB, B. MATHEY, H. J. DEEG, F. G. SCHUENING, T. C. GRAHAM, K. SEIDEL, R. BURNETT, J. L. WAGNER, H. SHULMAN & B. M. SANDMAIER. 1995. DLA-identical bone marrow grafts after low-dose total body irradiation: Effects of high-dose corticosteroids and cyclosporine on engraftment. Blood **86:** 4376–4381.
18. YU, C., E. OSTRANDER, E. BRYANT, R. BURNETT & R. STORB. 1994. Use of $(CA)_n$ polymorphisms to determine the origin of blood cells after allogeneic canine marrow grafting. Transplantation **58:** 701–706.
19. STORB, R., C. YU, J. L. WAGNER, H. J. DEEG, R. A. NASH, H.-P. KIEM, W. LEISENRING & H. SHULMAN. 1997. Stable mixed hematopoietic chimerism in DLA-identical littermate dogs given sublethal total body irradiation before and pharmacological immunosuppression after marrow transplantation. Blood **89:** 3048–3054.
20. YU, C., R. STORB, H. J. DEEG, F. G. SCHUENING, R. A. NASH & T. GRAHAM. 1995. Synergism between mycophenolate mofetil and cyclosporine in preventing graft-versus-host disease in lethally irradiated dogs given DLA-nonidentical unrelated marrow grafts [abstract]. Blood **86**(Supp. 1): 577a.
21. ANASETTI, C., P. J. MARTIN, R. STORB & J. A. HANSEN. 1994. Engraftment of allogeneic hematopoietic stem cells in patients conditioned only with anti-CD3 monoclonal antibody BC3 plus methylprednisolone [abstract]. Blood **84** (Supp. 1): 249a.
22. KERNAN, N. A., C. BORDIGNON, G. HELLER, I. CUNNINGHAM, H. CASTRO-MALASPINA, B. SHANK, N. FLOMENBERG, J. BURNS, S. Y. YANG, P. BLACK, N. H. COLLINS & R. J. O'REILLY. 1989. Graft failure after T-cell-depleted human leukocyte antigen identical marrow transplants for leukemia: I. Analysis of risk factors and results of secondary transplants. Blood **74:** 2227–2236.
23. COBBOLD, S. P., G. MARTIN, S. QIN & H. WALDMANN. 1986. Monoclonal antibodies to promote marrow engraftment and tissue graft tolerance. Nature **323:** 164–166.
24. LI, H., C. L. KAUFMAN, S. S. BOGGS, P. C. JOHNSON, K. D. PATRENE & S. T. ILDSTAD. 1996. Mixed allogeneic chimerism induced by a sublethal approach prevents autoimmune diabetes and reverses insulitis in nonobese diabetic (NOD) mice. J. Immunol. **156:** 380–388.
25. COLSON, Y. L., S. M. WREN, M. J. SCHUCHERT, K. D. PATRENE, P. C. JOHNSON, S. S. BOGGS & S. T. ILDSTAD. 1995. A nonlethal conditioning approach to achieve durable multilineage mixed chimerism and tolerance across major, minor, and hematopoietic histocompatibility barriers. J. Immunol. **155:** 4179–4188.
26. SHARABI, Y., V. S. ABRAHAM, M. SYKES & D. H. SACHS. 1992. Mixed allogeneic chimeras prepared by a non-myeloablative regimen: requirement for chimerism to maintain tolerance. Bone Marrow Transplantation **9:** 191–197.
27. TOMITA, Y., D. H. SACHS, A. KHAN & M. SYKES. 1996. Additional monoclonal antibody (mAB) injections can replace thymic irradiation to allow induction of mixed chimerism and tolerance in mice receiving bone marrow transplantation after conditioning with anti-T cell mABs and 3-Gy whole body irradiation. Transplantation **61:** 469–477.
28. TOMITA, Y., A. KHAN & M. SYKES. 1996. Mechanism by which additional monoclonal antibody (mAB) injections overcome the requirement for thymic irradiation to achieve mixed chimerism in mice receiving bone marrow transplantation after conditioning with anti-T cell mABs and 3-Gy whole body irradiation. Transplantation **61:** 477–485.
29. LEE, L. A., J. J. SERGIO & M. SYKES. 1996. Natural killer cells weakly resist engraftment of allogeneic, long-term, multilineage-repopulating hematopoietic stem cells. Transplantation **61:** 125–132.
30. WALTERS, M. C., M. PATIENCE, W. LEISENRING, J. R. ECKMAN, J. P. SCOTT, W. C. MENTZER, S. C. DAVIES, K. OHENE-FREMPONG, F. BERNAUDIN, D. C. MATTHEWS, R. STORB & K. M. SULLIVAN. 1996. Bone marrow transplantation for sickle cell disease. N. Engl. J. Med. **335:** 369–376.
31. ANDREANI, M., M. MANNA, G. LUCARELLI, P. TONUCCI, F. AGOSTINELLI, M. RIPALTI, S. RAPA, N. TALEVI, M. GALIMBERTI & S. NESCI. 1996. Persistence of mixed chimerism in patients transplanted for the treatment of thalassemia. Blood **87:** 3494–3499.

32. SULLIVAN, K. M., M. C. WALTERS, M. PATIENCE, W. LEISENRING, G. R. BUCHANAN, O. CASTRO, S. C. DAVIES, R. DICKERHOFF, J. R. ECKMAN, M. L. GRAHAM, K. OHENE-FREMPONG, D. POWARS, Z. R. ROGERS, J. P. SCOTT, L. STYLES, E. VICHINSKY, D. A. WALL, A. S. WAYNE, J. WILEY, J. WINGARD, N. BUNIN, B. CAMITTA, P. J. DARBYSHIRE, P. DINNDORF, T. KLINGEBIEL, L. MCMAHON, W. C. MENTZER, N. OLIVIERI, E. ORRINGER, R. PARKMAN, I. A. G. ROBERTS, J. E. SANDERS, F. O. SMITH & R. STORB. 1997. Collaborative study of marrow transplantation for sickle cell disease: aspects specific for transplantation of hemoglobin disorders. Bone Marrow Transplantation **19:** 102–105.
33. WEIDEN, P. L., R. STORB, T. C. GRAHAM & M. L. SCHROEDER. 1976. Severe hereditary haemolytic anaemia in dogs treated by marrow transplantation. Br. J. Haematol. **33:** 357–362.

Treatment of Iron Overload in the "Ex-Thalassemic"
Report from the Phlebotomy Program[a]

EMANUELE ANGELUCCI,[b,d] PIETRO MURETTO,[c] GUIDO LUCARELLI,[b] MARTA RIPALTI,[b] DONATELLA BARONCIANI,[b] BUKET ERER,[b] MARIA GALIMBERTI,[b] MAURO ANNIBALI,[b] CLAUDIO GIARDINI,[b] DJAVID GAZIEV,[b] SIMONA RAPA,[b] AND PAOLA POLCHI[b]

[b]*Divisione di Ematologia di Muraglia e Centro Trapianto Midollo Osseo,* [c]*Servizio Anatomia Patologica, Azienda Ospedale di Pesaro, Pesaro, Italy*

ABSTRACT: After successful marrow transplantation (BMT) iron overload remains an important cause of morbidity in Thalassemia. After BMT, patients have normal erythropoiesis capable of producing a hyperplastic response to phlebotomy so that this procedure can be contemplated as a method of mobilizing iron from overloaded tissues. Forty-one patients (mean age 16±2.9 years) with prolonged follow-up (range 2–7 years) after BMT were submitted to a moderate intensity phlebotomy program (6 ml/kg blood withdrawal at 14-day intervals) to reduce iron overload. Values are expressed as mean ± SD or as median with a range (25th–75th percentile). Serum ferritin decreased from 2,587 (2,129–4,817) to 280 (132–920) µg/l ($p < 0.0001$), total transferrin increased from 2.34±0.37 to 2.9±0.66 g/l ($p = 0.0001$), transferrin saturation decreased from 90%±14% to 39%±34% ($p < 0.0001$). Liver iron concentration evaluated on liver biopsy specimens decreased from 20.8 (15.5–28.1) to 3 (0.9–14.6) mg/g dry weight ($p < 0.0001$). Alanine amino-transaminase from 5.2±3.4 to 1.6±1.2 ($p < 0.0001$) times the upper level of normality. The histological grading for chronic hepatitis (Histology Activity Index) decreased from 4.2±2.4 to 2.3±1.8 ($p < 0.0001$). Phlebotomy is a safe, efficient, and widely applicable method to decrease iron overload in "ex-thalassemic."

Although marrow transplantation is a rational therapeutic approach for the cure of β-thalassemia major, there is no reason to expect that it will erase the damage resulting from years of thalassemia and its treatment. When transplantation is performed in patients with advanced disease, the correction of the congenital defect is not sufficient. Health and a normal life expectancy can only be achieved by curing the lesions that already existed at the time of transplant. Foremost among the complications of treated thalassemia are those that result from iron overload. After cure by BMT, patients still have disease processes acquired before transplantation as a consequence of thalassemia and its treatment. A spontaneous but slow drop in serum ferritin and liver iron and increases in serum total iron binding capacity as the years elapse after BMT has been observed.[1,2] For some patients

[a]Supported by Fondazione Berloni per la lotta contro la Talassemia, Pesaro, Italy
[d]Address for Correspondence: Doctor E. Angelucci, Divisione Ematologica e CentroTrapianto Midollo Osseo di Muraglia, Azienda Ospedale di Pesaro, 61100 Pesaro Italy. Telephone: 721 364077; Fax: 721 364057; E-mail, g.lucarelli@wnt.it

with mild iron overload, the rate of unloading was sufficient to reduce tissue iron levels to normal, but this was not achieved in patients who had severe iron overload at the time of transplant. After BMT, patients have normal erythropoiesis capable of producing a hyperplastic response to phlebotomy so that this procedure can be contemplated as a method of mobilizing iron from overloaded tissues. Here we report experience with this approach.

PATIENTS AND METHODS

From July 1991 to December 1992, 41 patients (19 males and 22 females) who had been regularly followed-up after transplantation in Pesaro for homozygous β-thalassemia were enrolled in a program of regular phlebotomy. Patients were eligible for this study if they had the following characteristics: (1) prognostic Class 2 or 3 before transplantation,[3] (2) the 2-year follow-up examinations revealed serum ferritin levels greater than 2,000 µg/l, and (3) the 2-year post-transplant liver biopsy revealed moderate or severe iron overload.[2] Patients with mixed chimerism[4] or active evidence of chronic graft-versus-host disease were excluded. Informed consent was obtained from all patients and parents after the procedure and risks have been explained in detail.

The post-transplant phlebotomy treatment was performed at several centers throughout Italy. The protocol consisted of phlebotomy of 6 ml/kg at 14-day intervals. Complete protocol and guidelines have been reported elsewhere.[5]

Annual follow-up in Pesaro included physical examination, complete blood count, serum ferritin (enzyme-linked immunosorbent assay, reference range 20–200 µg/l) total transferrin and unbound transferrin (expressed as g/l, normal values, respectively, 2.5–4 and 1.5–3.4), serum and alanine aminotransferase (ALT) (expressed as multiples of the upper limit of the reference range). A biopsy of the center of the right lobe of the liver with ultrasound guidance was performed annually. Liver biopsies were assessed by a coloration technique.[2,6] They were graded for inflammation according to the Histology Activity Index (HAI).[7] Hepatitis C virus (HCV) status was assessed with the latest- generation antibody-detection technique and with the polymerase chain reaction (PCR) using commercially available kits (Amplicor Hepatitis C virus test, Roche Diagnostic System Inc., Basel). Thirty-five patients (85%) were hepatitis C seropositive and 29 had HCV-RNA detectable in serum by PCR; no patient was hepatitis B surface antigen–positive. Two patients who received interferon therapy for HCV disease were evaluated for iron depletion but not for inflammatory lesions.

The liver iron concentration (LIC) was assayed by atomic absorption spectrophotometry[6,8] and expressed as mg/g dry weight (dw). Specimens with a total dry weight < 0.5 mg were not evaluated for iron content.

Treatment adherence was calculated as the ratio of phlebotomies performed to phlebotomies scheduled. Values were expressed as medians with a range (25th–75th percentile) or as means ± standard deviations. The paired Student's t test for means, was used to assess the significance of difference between comparison, and the Wilcoxon test was used for comparison of ordered values.

RESULTS

Before transplantation these 41 patients had received a mean number of 188±91 red cells transfusions. Only seven patients had received regular chelation; 20 were Class 2 and 21 Class 3. Before BMT, mean serum ferritin level was 4,127±1731 and mean liver iron concentration was 23.4±8.8 mg/g dw. All of them had received bone marrow from an HLA-identical sibling (thalassemia minor donor = 26, normal donor = 15). Mean time

TABLE 1. Adherence to Treatment and Iron Depletion

Characteristic	Mean ± S. D.
Months of therapy	38 ± 20
Phlebotomies (N)	54 ± 35
Adherence to treatment (%)	73 ± 24
Blood withdrawal (l)	15.1 ± 10
Iron removed (g)	6.3 ± 3.8

TABLE 2. Laboratory Measures of Iron Depletion

Parameter	before Phlebotomy	Last Follow-up	Two tailed p value
Serum ferritin (µg/l)	2,587 (2,129–4,817)	280 (132–920)	<0.0001[a]
Total transferrin (g/l)	2.34±0.37	2.9±0.66	<0.0001[b]
Unbound transferrin (g/l)	0.11(0.02–0.42)	1.84 (1–2.5)	<0.0001[a]
Transferrin saturation (%)	90±14	39±34	<0.0001[b]
Liver iron concentration (mg/g dw)	20.8 (15.5–28.1)	3 (0.9–14.6)	<0.0001[a]

Tests of significance were performed with paired Student's t test[b] for comparison of means ± SD and with the Wilcoxon test[a] for comparison of ordered values [median (25th–75th percentile)].

between the starting of the program and last follow-up was 3.5±0.6 years. The following parameters were registered before the beginning of the program and at last follow-up: age (years) 16±2.9 and 20±3; height (centimeters) 150±9 and 159±7; body weight (kilograms) 43±9 and 53±10, and hemoglobin (g/l) 126±15 and 127±16 (26 had received a thalassemia minor as marrow donor). Adherence to protocol (phlebotomies scheduled/done) was 72% ± 23 (range 18%–100%).

TABLE 1 describes the performance of the treatment program and estimates of iron removed by phlebotomy. TABLE 2 presents the laboratory assessments of iron removal as indicated by the levels of iron and transport proteins in serum and the iron concentrations in the liver before and after more than three years of follow-up. FIGURE 1 reports the behavior of serum ferritin in 15 patients who started the program 5 years after BMT. TABLE 3 reports inflammatory parameters in the 39 evaluable patients before and after the course

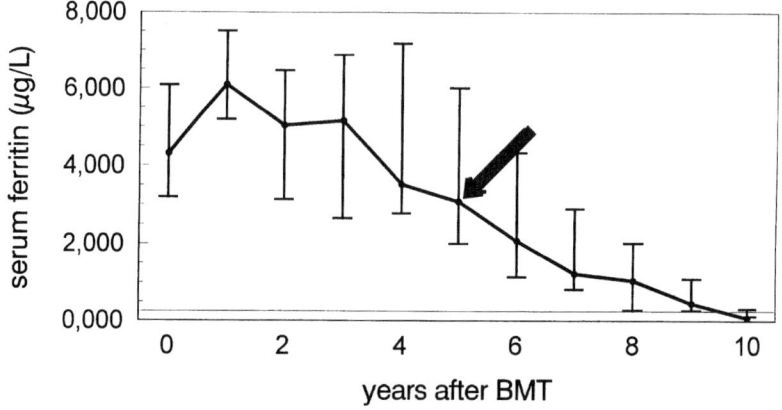

FIGURE 1. Serum ferritin (µg/l) behavior in 15 patients who started the program 5 years after BMT. The line indicates the normal range. Values are expressed as medians with a range (25th to 75th percentile)

TABLE 3. Inflammatory Lesions and Liver Fibrosis[a]

Parameter	Before Phlebotomy	Last Follow-up	Two tailed p value
ALT (times upper level)	5.2±3.4	1 7±1.2	<0.0001[b]
Histology activity index[7]	4.2±2.4	2.3±1.8	<0.0001[b]
Fibrosis[7]	3 (3–3)	3 (1–3)	NS[c]

[a]Data were available for 39 patients.
Tests of significance were performed with paired Student's t test[b] for comparison of means ± SD and with the Wilcoxon test[c] for comparison of ordered values [median (25th–75th percentile)]. Thirty-three patients were anti-HCV seropositive and 27 had HCV viremia as detected by PCR. Histology activity index include piecemeal necrosis, intralobular degeneration, and portal inflammation.[18]

of phlebotomy. The grading[9] of chronic hepatitis (periportal necrosis + intralobular degeneration + portal inflammation)[7] and transaminase values showed a trend towards a uniform decrease in parallel with liver iron content, but this was not the case for the fibrosis score (staging of chronic hepatitis[9]). FIGURE 2 reports the behavior of ALT in the 15 patients who started the program 5 years after BMT.

By May 1997, 16 patients achieved a normal liver iron content: 0.9±0.4 (range 0.28–1.58) mg/g dw compared with pre-treatment values of 16.5±8 (range 3.3–29.3). All the others patients are continuing regular treatment.

DISCUSSION

Bone marrow transplantation is the only present accessible curative treatment for homozygous, β-thalassemia.[3] Because of the normal erythropoiesis achieved and the very limited excretion of excess iron, phlebotomy appeared to be appropriate to remove excess transfusional iron acquired before BMT. Patients were enrolled on this program on the basis of an indirect or semiquantitative estimate of iron overload using the serum ferritin.[6,10,11] Thus patients had very different levels of iron stores at enrollment: liver iron

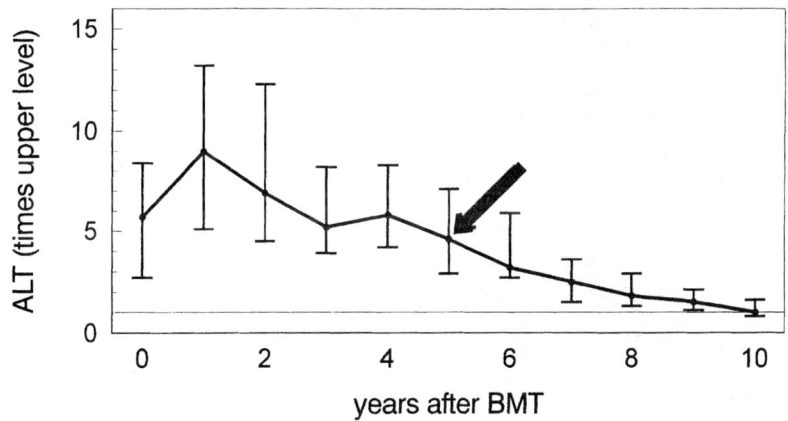

FIGURE 2. ALT (times upper level of normal range) behavior in 15 patients who started the program 5 years after BMT. The line indicates the normal range. Values are expressed as medians with a range (25th to 75th percentile)

concentration ranged from 3.3 to 57.18 mg/g dw. Some patients achieved normal liver iron concentrations in a few months while others still have severe iron overload after more than 3 years of therapy.

Adherence to protocol in the 41 treated patients was only 72%±24, despite treatment being designed to maintain an almost completely normal life. Psychological rather than medical difficulties were encountered. No cases of graft failure, prolonged anemia, or protein depletion were seen, while it was possible to achieve normal liver iron concentrations. This study clearly demonstrates that a moderately intensive phlebotomy program is safe for thalassemic patients after BMT and this form of therapy is likely to be much safer, cheaper, and more widely applicable than alternative iron chelation therapy.[12] During the treatment there was a significant decrease in transaminase levels, confirmed by significant improvement of histologic grading of chronic hepatitis. There is much debate about the severity and likelihood of progression of HCV disease,[13-15] and on the possible effect of iron on virus virulence and response to interferon therapy.[16,17] The role of cofactor in HCV disease progression has been emphasized[15] and our experience suggests that iron, at least at the level reported here, could be one of these cofactors for patients with a history of thalassemia. In the present series on 35 anti–HCV positive patients 20 (57%) presented the criteria for interferon therapy[18] before phlebotomy and only 10 (28%) at the last follow-up. These data clearly indicate that anti–HCV positive ex-thalassemic patients should be iron depleted before evaluation for interferon therapy. Further follow-up is necessary to evaluate a possible effect of iron depletion on liver fibrosis.

REFERENCES

1. LUCARELLI, G., E. ANGELUCCI, C. GIARDINI, D. BARONCIANI, M. GALIMBERTI, P. POLCHI et al. 1993. Fate of iron stores in thalassemia after bone marrow transplantation. Lancet **342:** 1388–1391.
2. MURETTO, P., S. DEL FIASCO, E. ANGELUCCI & G. LUCARELLI. 1994. Bone marrow transplantation in thalassemia: Modification of hepatic iron overload and related pathologies after long-term engrafting. Liver **14:** 14–24.
3. LUCARELLI, G., M. GALIMBERTI, P. POLCHI, E. ANGELUCCI, D. BARONCIANI & C. GIARDINI et al. 1990. Bone marrow transplantation in patients with thalassemia. N. Engl. J. Med. **322:** 417–421.
4. ANDREANI, M., M. MANNA, G. LUCARELLI, P. TONUCCI, F. AGOSTINELLI, M. RIPALTI et al. 1996. Persistence of mixed chimerism in patients transplanted for the treatment of thalassemia. Blood **87:** 3494–3499.
5. ANGELUCCI, E., P. MURETTO, G. LUCARELLI, M. RIPALTI, D. BARONCIANI, B. ERER et al. 1997. Phlebotomy to reduce iron overload in patients cured of thalassemia by bone marrow transplantation. Blood **90:** 994–998.
6. ANGELUCCI, E., D. BARONCIANI, G. LUCARELLI, M. BALDASSARI, M. GALIMBERTI, C. GIARDINI et al. 1995. Needle liver biopsy in thalassaemia: Analyses of diagnostic accuracy and safety in 1184 consecutive biopsies. Br. J. Haematol. **89:** 757–761.
7. KNODELL, R. G., K. G. ISHAK, W. C. BLACK, T. S. CHEN, R. CRAIG, N. KAPLOWITZ et al. 1981. Formulation and application of a numerical scoring system for assessing histological activity in asymptomatic chronic active hepatitis. Hepatology **1:** 431–435.
8. SORIANO-CUBELLS, M. J. & L. APARISI-QUERADA.1984. Rapid determination of copper, iron and zinc in liver biopsies. Atomic Spectroscopy **5:** 217–222.
9. DESMET, V. J., M. GERBER, J. H. HOOFNAGLE, M. MANNS & P. J. SCHEUER. 1994. Classification of chronic hepatitis. Diagnosis, grading and staging. Hepatology **19:** 1513–1520.
10. FINCH, C. A., B. BELLOTTI, S. STRAY, D. A. LIPSCHITZ, J. D. COOK, M. J. PIPPARD et al. 1986. Plasma ferritin determination as a diagnostic tool. West J. Med. **145:** 657–663.
11. BRITTENHAM, G. M., A. R. COHEN, C. MCLAREN, M. B. MARTIN, P. M. GRIFFITH, A. W. NIENHUIS et al. 1993. Hepatic iron stores and plasma ferritin concentration in patients with sickle cell anemia and thalassemia major. Am. J. Hematol. **42:** 81–85.

12. KONTOGHIORGHES, G. J. 1995. Comparative efficacy and toxicity of desferrioxamine, deferiprone and other iron and aluminium chelating drugs. Toxicol. Lett. **80:** 1–18.
13. TONG, M. Y., N. S. EL-FARRA, A. R. REIKES & R. L. CO. 1995. Clinical outcomes after transfusion-associated hepatitis C. N. Engl. J. Med. **332:** 1463–1466.
14. TERRAULT, N. & T. WRIGHT. 1995. Interferon and hepatitis C. N. Engl. J. Med. **332:** 1509–1511.
15. ALTER, H. J. 1995. To C or not to C: these are the questions. Blood **85:** 1681–1695.
16. OLYNYK, J. K., K. R. REDDY, A. M. DI BISCEGLIE, L. J. JEFFER, T. I. PARKER, J. L. RADIK *et al.* 1995. Hepatic iron concentration as a predictor of response to interferon alfa therapy in chronic hepatitis. Gastroenterology **108:** 1104–1109.
17. BARTON, A. N., B. F. BANNER, E. E. CABLE & H. L. BANKOVSKY. 1995. Distribution of iron in the liver predicts the response of chronic hepatitis C infection to interferon therapy. Am. J. Clin. Pathol. **103:** 419–424.
18. HOOFNAGLE, J. H. & A. M. DI BISCEGLIE. 1997. The treatment of chronic viral hepatitis. N. Engl. J. Med. **336:** 347–356.

Late Effects of Bone Marrow Transplantation for Thalassemia[a]

ANTONIO PIGA,[b,d] FILOMENA LONGO,[b] VINCENZO VOI,[b] SILVIA FACELLO,[b] ROBERTO MINIERO,[b] AND BERND DRESOW[c]

[b]*Department of Pediatrics, Hematology, Oncology Division, University of Torino, Italy*
[c]*Medizinische Biochemie, University of Hamburg, Germany*

> ABSTRACT: Long term effects of BMT in thalassemia were monitored in 33 patients transplanted between 1987 and 1995 and compared with 155 patients matched for age and treated during the same period with conventional therapy (CT). The incidence of fulminant sepsis and growth impairment was significantly higher in transplanted patients, whereas the occurrence of hypothyroidism, hypogonadism, and cardiopathy was higher in CT patients. For diabetes, liver disease, and severe infections, the differences were not statistically significant. After BMT we performed monthly erythrocytaferesis for iron removal in 23 (70%) patients, obtaining a complete normalization of iron stores in 91% of cases; among untreated patients, 60% had evidence of iron up to 8-3 years after BMT. Protection against poliovirus, tetanus, diphtheria, and hepatitis B has been lost in 74%, 47%, 78%, and 44%, respectively. After BMT a careful follow-up is needed to monitor and treat late transplant-related and thalassemia-related complications.

Most of the papers on bone marrow transplantation (BMT) for thalassemia focused on survival patterns,[1–4] whereas little data on late effects are available.[5,6]

Yet long-term complications of thalassemic patients treated with conventional therapy (CT) (transfusion and iron chelation)[7–12] or long-term sequelae of BMT for other diseases are well known.

We analyzed late effects of BMT in a homogeneous group of thalassemic patients and compared them to a matched group of subjects treated with conventional therapy.

PATIENTS

Transplanted Subjects

From our series of 257 consecutive subjects with transfusion-dependent homozygous β-thalassemia, we considered for this study 33 patients that had been successfully transplanted between 1987 and 1995. All donors were HLA-identical siblings. Conditioning regimen included busulfan (14–16 mg/kg) and cyclophosphamide (200 mg/kg), GVHD prophylaxis was done with cyclosporine A and a short course of methotrexate. We did not consider the first 12 months after BMT.

Erythrocytapheresis was performed monthly utilizing a Baxter CS3000 blood cell separator and removing 10% of blood volume on the average. No patient received any treatment for iron overload during the first two years post-BMT.[13] All patients and donors had been fully vaccinated against polio, tetanus, and diphtheria after birth according to the

---

[a]This work was supported by grants from Italian MURST (40% and 60%).
[d]Address for correspondence: Dr. Antonio Piga, Piazza Polonia 94, 10126 Torino, Italy. Tel: +39 11 3135291; Fax: +39 11 3135309; and E-mail: piga@pediatria.unito.it

Italian schedule (tetanus-diphtheria-polio, one administration at months 3, 4, and 13 months, polio repeated during the third year, tetanus-diphtheria in the sixth year, and then tetanus once every tenth year). For hepatitis B, 28 patients had been vaccinated 2.4–6.7 years (average = 3.8) before the BMT with a full cycle of a purified immunizing HBsAg preparation (HeVacB) obtained from donor sera, whereas five patients had been found immune. We checked the antibody levels to tetanus, diphtheria, poliomyelitis, and hepatitis B, and we performed a booster in the patients that had lost the coverage.[14]

Conventionally Treated Subjects

From the remaining 224 consecutive patients we included in the analysis all the 155 subjects matched for age with transplanted ones. All were regularly transfused to maintain a mean hemoglobin of 12–13 g%. Pretransfusional Hb ranged from 9.5 to 12. Chelation had been prescribed as a daily intramuscular injection of 20 mg/kg/d of desferrioxamine from 1970 to 1977, then as an 8–12 hours subcutaneous infusion of 30–60 mg/kg/day.

We divided these patients in two groups: high and low chelation (HC group and LC group), based on whether the mean number of desferal infusions per year had been more or less than 225, respectively. For patients who started chelation therapy before 1978, *i.e.*, before slow subcutaneous infusion had been set up, intramuscular-injection frequency has been calculated in the same way.

METHODS

Survival and disease-free cumulative frequencies for major complications were calculated by the Kaplan-Meier method, and the extension of Gehan's generalized Wilcoxon test was used to test for differences between the groups. The software Statistica for Windows® (release 5.0(1995), StatSoft, inc., Tulsa, OK, USA) has been utilized. Endpoints for censoring have been considered respectively: survival: death; heart disease: heart failure and/or symptomatic cardiopathy affecting quality of life and/or echocardiographic or ECG Holter abnormalities requiring medication; diabetes: insulin-dependent diabetes or severe glucose tolerance alteration requiring medication; liver disease: cirrhosis or active chronic hepatitis or severe fibrosis on biopsy, and/or mean ALT levels > 100 mU/ml; hypothyroidism: date of starting thyroxin medication; hypogonadism: date of starting medication; height growth failure: loss of two centiles or height < 3° centile corrected for genetic target; infections: septicemia and/or severe infections requiring hospitalization; fatal sepsis: fulminant sepsis as first cause of death.

Magnetic biosusceptometry (SQUID) or chemical analysis on biopsy sample have been utilized to measure the liver iron concentration (LIC), as reference marker of iron overload: an upper limit of 0.7 mg/g wet weight has been considered for normal iron stores.

RESULTS

The median age of the three groups (BMT, high and low chelation) was 18.6, 18.9 and 19 years, respectively (p = ns). Of 14 deaths observed, five have been a fatal sepsis, three occurring in BMT group, one in LC group, and one in a 6-year-old girl HC; only this last one had her spleen (TABLE 1).

All seven heart failures and the 2 leukemias occurred in LC patients. Survival patterns are shown in FIGURE 1, there was a significant difference between LC group and the other two. The probability of overall survival and disease-free survival at 25 years of life for the three groups are shown in TABLE 1. The risk of hypothyroidism and hypogonadism was significantly higher with conventional treatment ($p = 0.02$). HC and BMT group did not show any significant differences in survival and complication-free patterns, whereas LC group had a worst pattern in all the situations except growth failure and sepsis.

Twenty-three (70%) of 33 transplanted patients underwent an erythrocytapheresis program: on the average each patient had 16.8 sessions in 1.9 years, removing 282 ± 73 mg of iron (range 90–416) every time; 21 out of 23 obtained a complete normalization of iron stores. Among 10 untreated patients, 6 had evidence of iron overload (liver iron concentration at SQUID or biopsy > 0.7 mg/g w.w.) up to 8.3 years after BMT.

Protection against polio, tetanus, diphtheria, and hepatitis B has been lost in 74%, 47%, 78%, and 44%, respectively. After a booster, a protective Ab level has been reached only for tetanus and polio.

DISCUSSION

Many results of BMT[1,6] or conventional treatment[7,9,15] for thalassemia are published, but a true comparison of these two approaches is lacking for several reasons: it is difficult to obtain homogeneous groups in chronic diseases; subcutaneous chelation therapy is prescribed from 20 years and a high compliance is hard to maintain; in the past BMT has been offered mainly to younger patients; furthermore it may be difficult to understand if a post-transplant event is more linked to the BMT or to the thalassemia, i.e., early damage from iron overload. We managed to match our transplanted patients for age in a 1:5 ratio with

TABLE 1. Characteristics and Probability of Survival

	Bone Marrow Transplantation	Conventional Treatment			X^2	p
		all	high chelation	low chelation		
Patients (N)	32	115	111	44		
Age (mean)	18.6	18.9	18.9	19.0		
Deaths (N)	3	11	1	10		
Causes of Death						
Sepsis	3	2	1	1		
Heart Failure	—	7	—	7		
Leukemia	—	2	—	2		
Survival						
Disease-free Survival for:	82%	89%	99%	70%	18.99	<0.0001
Heart Disease	88%	77%	95%	33%	34.37	<0.0001
Hypothyroidism	92%	68%	75%	52%	17.38	<0.0001
Growth Failure	67%	83%	81%	85%	3.04	ns
Diabetes	95%	90%	95%	78%	11.73	<0.01
Liver Disease	86%	78%	89%	54%	13.07	<0.001
Serious Infections	78%	75%	77%	68%	2.94	ns
Fatal Sepsis	82%	98%	99%	96%	1.98	ns
Tumors	100%	100%	100%	98%	—	—
All Complications	78%	64%	70%	50%	12.56	<0.01

*a*Characteristics and probability of survival and disease-free survival at 25 years of age in 187 thalassemic patients, who underwent bone marrow transplantation ($N = 32$), or were conventionally treated ($N = 155$) with transfusion and chelation with high ($N = 111$) or low ($N = 44$) compliance χ^2 and p refer to the comparison among the three groups. (ns = not significant.)

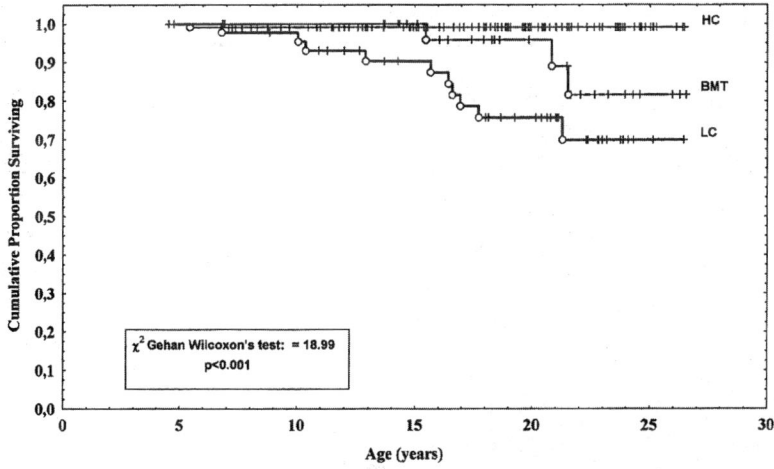

FIGURE 1. Overall survival in 187 thalassemic patients: 32 transplanted patients (BMT), compared to 155 conventionally treated patients, 111 of them with high chelation (HC) and 44 with low chelation (LC).

conventionally treated patients, as we take care of a large series of thalassemic patients whose data on transfusion and chelation have been accurately stored in a computerized clinical record.[16]

As is well known, heart failure resulted as the main cause of death in the LC group, conditioning the significantly lower survival pattern of these patients.[7,17] Today it is not possible to know if BMT or HC effectively prevents the progression of cardiac disease or simply delays its appearance. A longer follow-up will probably answer this question.

Interestingly, fatal sepsis has been the second cause of death (36%). Even if the numbers are too small to verify a difference in the three groups, BMT patients seem more prone to this complication. A transplanted-related immune defect is unlikely: all three subjects were well being, off therapy, and more than one year after BMT (1.2, 3.8, and 6 years, respectively). We suppose a lower level of attention to prevent overwhelming infections in splenectomized transplanted patients in comparison with conventionally treated ones. In these patients, in fact, the need of prevention is reinforced monthly at transfusion, whereas the transplanted patients after the first year of intensive post-transplant follow-up, tend to consider themselves "cured."

Bone marrow transplantation and conventional treatment with high chelation level seem to offer similar results. Transplanted patients and well chelated patients showed a similar pattern on Kaplan-Meier curves. A possible explanation is that a seven-year follow-up could be too short for the appearance of certain clinical complications such as cirrhosis or tumors.[18–20] Even if none of the differences is significant, BMT tends to protect more than high chelation from hypothyroidism and hypogonadism. This could mean that regular chelation does not protect completely from iron oxidative damage on certain tissues. Growth failure is the only complication where low chelation seems to protect better than high chelation and BMT.[21–23] This could be due to the toxic effect of desferrioxamine on one side and of conditioning regimen on the other.

Phlebotomy has been demonstrated to be effective in reducing iron stores[24] in transplanted patients. We utilized erythrocytapheresis as a larger amount of iron can be removed in each session, saving plasma and mononucleated cells.[13] This approach resulted in safe and effective normalizing of iron stores. Even if we did not observe any complications of iron overload after BMT, a longer follow-up will clarify if a real prevention of these complications has been achieved. Still, the spontaneous decline of iron stores in untreated patients is very slow and stresses the utility of intervention.

After BMT, a careful follow-up is needed to monitor and treat late transplant-related and thalassemia-related complications.

REFERENCES

1. LUCARELLI, G. et al. 1995. Bone marrow transplantation in thalassemia. Sem. Hematol. **32**(4): 297–303.
2. APPERLEY, J. F. 1993. Bone marrow transplant for the haemoglobinopathies: Past, present and future. Baillieres Clin. Haematol. **6**(1): 299–325.
3. LUCARELLI, G. et al. 1996. Marrow transplantation for patients with thalassemia: Results in class 3 patients. Blood **87**(5): 2082–2088.
4. LUCARELLI, G. et al. 1990. Bone marrow transplantation in patients with thalassemia. N. Engl. J. Med. **322**: 417–421.
5. LUCARELLI, G. 1997. Bone marrow transplantation for thalassaemia. J. Int. Med. (Suppl.) **740**: 49–52.
6. GALIMBERTI, M. et al. 1997. Bone marrow transplantation in thalassemia. The experience of Pesaro. Bone Marrow Transplantation **19**: 45–47.
7. OLIVIERI, N. F. et al. 1994. Survival in medically treated patients with homozygous β thalassemia. N. Engl. J. Med. **331** (9): 574–578.
8. PIGA, A. et al. 1997. Mortality and morbidity in thalassemia with conventional treatment. Bone Marrow Transplantation **19**: 11–13.
9. GABUTTI, V. & A. PIGA. 1996. Results of long-term iron-chelating therapy. Acta Haematol. **95**: 26–36.
10. LOCASCIULLI, A. et al. 1997. Morbidity and mortality due to liver disease in children undergoing allogenic bone marrow transplantation: a 10-year prospective study. Blood **9**: 3799–3805.
11. LOCATELLI, F. et al. 1993. Late effects in children after bone marrow transplantation: a review. Haematologica **78**: 319–328.
12. DUELL, T. et al. 1997. Health and functional status of long-term survivors of bone marrow transplantation. EBMT Working Party on Late Effects and EULEP Study Group on Late Effects. European Group for Blood and Marrow Transplantation. Ann. Intern. Med. **126**(3). 184–192.
13. PIGA, A. et al. 1995. Iron overload after bone marrow transplantation in thalassemia. Blood **86** (10) (Suppl 1): 401a.
14. GAROFALO, F. et al. 1997. Antibody levels and response to vaccinations 4–6 years after BMT in thalassemia. Bone Marrow Transplantation **19**: 145–146.
15. OLIVIERI, N. F. & G. M. BRITTENHAM. 1997. Iron-chelating therapy and the treatment of thalassemia. Blood **89**: 739–776.
16. GABUTTI, V. et al. 1993. Computhal: A computerized clinical record for thalassemia. Ciba-Geigy.
17. BRITTENHAM, G. M. et al. 1994. Efficacy of deferoxamine in preventing complications of iron overload in patients with thalassemia major. N. Engl. J. Med. **331** (9): 567–573.
18. WHITERSPOON, R. P. et al. 1989. Secondary cancers after bone marrow transplantation for leukaemia or aplastic anaemia. N. Engl. J. Med. **321**: 784–789.
19. RUSSO, A. & G. SCHILIRO. 1987. Thalassemia major and malignancies. Am. J. Hematol. **24**: 11–112.
20. MINIERO, R. & P. SARACCO. 1988. Cancer in thalassemia and other hemoglobinopathies. Am. J. Hematol. **27**: 74.
21. SANDERS, J. E. 1991. The impact of marrow transplant preparative regimens on subsequent growth and development. Sem. Hematol. **28**: 244–249.
22. COHEN, A. et al. 1995. Growth in patients after allogeneic bone marrow transplant for hematological diseases in childhood. Bone Marrow Transplantation **15**(3): 343 348.

23. DE SIMONE, M. *et al.* 1995. Growth and endocrine function following bone marrow transplantation for thalassemia. Bone Marrow Transplantation **15**(2): 227–233.
24. ANGELUCCI, E. *et al.* 1997. Phlebotomy to reduce iron overload in patients cured of thalassemia by bone marrow transplantation. Italian Cooperative Group for Phlebotomy Treatment of Transplanted Thalassemia Patients. Blood **90:** 994–998.

In Utero Transplantation for Thalassemia

ALAN W. FLAKE[a] AND ESMAIL D. ZANJANI[b]

[a]*Children's Institute of Surgical Science, Children's Hospital of Philadelphia, Philadelphia, Pennsylvania 19104, USA*

[b]*Department of Medicine, University of Nevada, Veterans Administration Medical Center, Reno, Nevada 89520, USA*

ABSTRACT: In utero hematopoietic stem cell transplantation is a promising approach for the treatment of a variety of congenital hematologic diseases. Although the approach has been successful for immunodeficiency syndromes, attempts thus far to treat the hemoglobinopathies have failed. In most of these cases the late gestational age at transplantation, source of donor cells, or procedure-related complications, provide an explanation for failure. Nevertheless the biology of thalassemia, in the context of prenatal transplantation, requires examination. In contrast to postnatal bone marrow transplant regimens, engraftment after in utero transplantation requires donor cells to effectively compete for developing receptive sites in the recipient hematopoietic microenvironment. Effective prenatal treatment of thalassemia will depend on the ability of normal cells to engraft and compete in the thalassemic microenvironment. Clinical observations after bone marrow transplantation of amelioration of anemia in β-thalassemia by relatively low degrees of mixed chimerism, and the apparent selective advantage observed for donor erythropoiesis, suggest prenatal transplantation could succeed. Prenatal strategies involving multiple transplants, donor-specific tolerance induction, and postnatal same-donor transplants should be considered.

In utero hematopoietic stem cell (HSC) transplantation is a therapeutic approach that can potentially treat a variety of congenital hematologic diseases. There is theoretical, experimental, and limited clinical support for its application to the thalassemia disorders. The only current curative therapy for thalassemia is postnatal bone marrow transplantation (BMT). Despite excellent results with HLA-identical BMT, concerns related to the toxicity of BMT prevent its widespread application. Thus, approaches to transplantation that could reduce treatment-related morbidity and mortality are needed. Theoretically, prenatal transplantation could avoid much of the risk of postnatal BMT. The purpose of this report is to review the current status of *in utero* HSC transplantation in the specific context of the prenatal treatment of the thalassemia disorders.

THEORETICAL BASIS FOR *IN UTERO* HEMATOPOIETIC STEM CELL TRANSPLANTATION

The early gestational fetal environment is unique and may offer advantages for the transplantation and engraftment of foreign HSC. These potential advantages are based on events of normal hematopoietic and immunologic ontogeny (FIG. 1). During development,

---

[a]Address for correspondence: Alan W. Flake, M.D., Director, Children's Institute of Surgical Science, Children's Hospital of Philadelphia, 34th Street and Civic Center Blvd., Philadelphia, Pennslylvania 19104. Tel: 215/590-3188; Fax: 215/590-3324; E-mail: flake@email.chop.edu

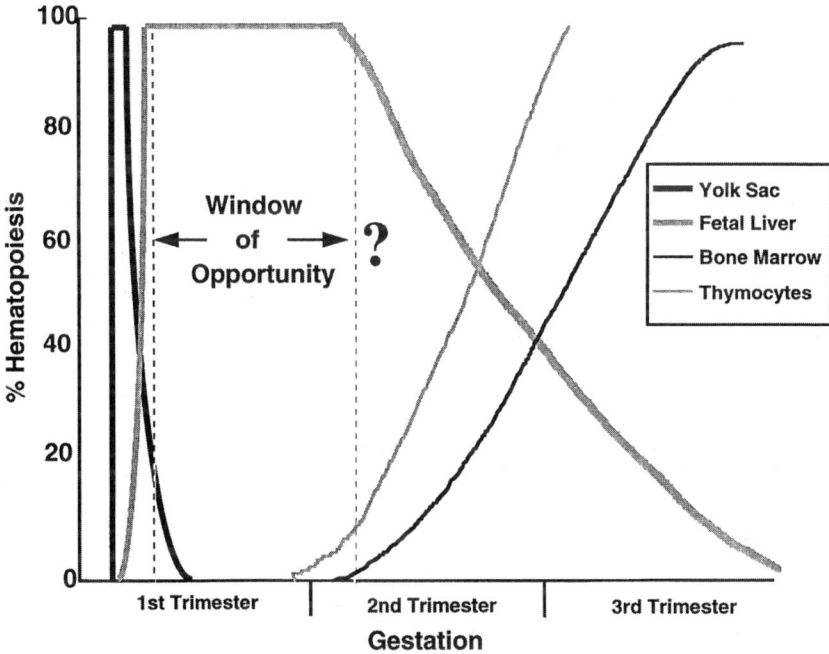

FIGURE 1. Schematic of normal hematopoietic and immunologic ontogeny. The window of opportunity is the optimal theoretical period for engraftment of donor cells. The limits of this window in humans are poorly defined and the late limit may be extended indefinitely in circumstances of genetic T-cell deficiency (SCID).

hematopoiesis goes through a sequence of migrational events, from the yolk sac and/or periaortic splanchnopleure, to the fetal liver, and finally to the bone marrow.[1,2] The transition of hematopoiesis from the fetal liver to the bone marrow is particularly interesting from a potential therapeutic perspective. The fetal liver becomes a hematopoietic organ precipitously at 5–7 weeks gestation. There is then a prolonged period of transition from the time that hematopoiesis is first observed in the bone marrow (around 12 weeks gestation) to the point at which it becomes the dominant source of hematopoiesis (after 34 weeks gestation). During this time the bone marrow compartment is exponentially expanding in both size and cellularity, suggesting that new sites for hematopoiesis are constantly forming and being occupied by migrating HSC. Thus engraftment of donor HSC should be possible on a competitive basis. This concept of competitive population of forming hematopoietic niches is fundamental to *in utero* HSC transplantation and is one of the conceptual differences that separate prenatal from postnatal BMT. In postnatal transplantation, myeloablation is generally used with the ultimate aim of replacement of host hematopoiesis. In prenatal transplantation, engraftment occurs by competitive population of available sites. The goal is an adequate level of mixed chimerism to clinically ameliorate a disease.

The second major advantage provided by normal ontogeny is immunologic tolerance. Fetal immunologic tolerance was first experimentally tested by the classic experiments of Billingham and Medawar characterizing the phenomenon of "acquired immunologic tolerance."[3] There is now a large body of experimental evidence for the central role of the fetal thymus in self recognition and tolerance for foreign antigens.[4,5] The details of thymic processing are still being elucidated but the critical events have now been defined. Thymocytes are positively selected for recognition of self Class I or Class II MHC antigens which are presented by thymic epithelial cells of thymic stromal origin. Lack of MHC recognition results in programmed cell death. Thymocytes that recognize self MHC are then negatively selected by high affinity recognition of "self" antigen in association with self MHC. Self-antigen presentation is directed by thymic dendritic cells which are derived from HSCs. The end result is a repertoire of single positive (CD4+ or CD8+) functionally competent lymphocytes that recognize foreign antigen in association with self MHC. Single positive (post thymic) lymphocytes are first seen in the peripheral circulation of the fetus at around 12–14 weeks gestation.[6] Theoretically, transplantation of foreign cells prior to completion of the thymic negative selection process would result in processing of foreign antigen as "self" with secondary specific tolerance on the basis of clonal deletion. The combined advantages of receptivity for engraftment and specific tolerance induction could avoid most of the current problems related to postnatal bone marrow transplantation. In addition, treatment of the disease prior to its clinical manifestations would avoid many of the quality of life issues currently existent with postnatal therapies (TABLE 1).

EXPERIMENTAL SUPPORT FOR *IN UTERO* HSC TRANSPLANTATION

The most convincing support for the feasibility of *in utero* HSC transplantation are the observations of natural chimerism arising from shared placental circulation in dizygotic cattle twins.[7] The original observation of chimerism in bovine twins has now been extended to a number of other species, most notably primates[8] and humans.[9] Chimeric individuals share their siblings blood elements and are specifically tolerant for skin or organ grafts from their donor siblings.[10,11] The degree of chimerism can range from microchimerism to near complete replacement by donor cells and appears to be permanent in the animals studied. This demonstrates that, at least under certain circumstances, in an otherwise normal hematopoietic microenvironment, allogeneic cells can effectively compete with recipient cells and achieve high levels of sustained donor cell expression.

Experimental studies on *in utero* HSC transplantation have been performed in a number of animal models. The early studies by Fleischman and Mintz[12] demonstrating correction of genetic anemia in the W/W^v mouse by transplacental injection of normal donor cells, confirmed the ability to reconstitute a hematopoietic microenvironment with a primary stem cell deficiency by *in utero* transplantation. Subsequently, in a mouse severe combined immunodeficiency disease (SCID) model in which there is a selective lineage advantage for normal lymphocytes, Blazer and colleagues[13] achieved full lymphocyte reconstitution after intraperitoneal transplantation of normal bone marrow. The levels of bone marrow engraftment were low. This experimentally confirms the concept that a selective lineage advantage

TABLE 1. Advantages of *in Utero* HSC Transplantation

Advantage	Effect
Immunologic Tolerance	No HLA-Restriction/Immunosuppression
BM Space Available	No Myeloblation
Sterile "Isolation"	No Post-transplant Isolation
Proliferative Environment	Potential Competitive Advantage-Normal Cells
Preempts Clinical Disease	Avoids Complicating Morbidity/Suffering

results in peripheral amplification of donor cell engraftment for that lineage, a concept that may be important in a number of human diseases, including the thalassemias.

In large animal studies, the sheep has been most informative. Transplantation of allogeneic fetal liver-derived HSC into early gestational fetal lamb recipients results in multilineage chimerism with levels of sustained donor cell engraftment of 10–20% without myeloablation, or immunosuppression.[14] Studies utilizing differences at the β-hemoglobin locus in sheep have confirmed sustained donor hemoglobin levels as high as 20–30% after a single intrauterine transplant.[15] It is important to note that these are hematopoietically normal sheep, proving that at least in the sheep, normal hematopoiesis is not prohibitive to competitive population by donor cells. Other studies in this model have confirmed the concept of an immunologic "window of opportunity." Transplantation of cells after approximately 80 days gestation resulted in failure of engraftment, presumably on an immunologic basis. In addition, dose/engraftment curves suggest saturation kinetics, *i.e.* engraftment plateaus with increasing doses of donor cells suggesting saturation of available recipient receptive sites.[16] This has been supported by the observation that improved engraftment occurs when a given donor cell dose is divided into three aliquots and transplanted at intervals of 1 week. This presumably allows time for renewal of available recipient niches for the engraftment of HSC. Homing studies in the allogeneic sheep model suggest that engraftment recapitulates ontogeny.[17] When transplants are performed prior to bone marrow hematopoiesis, donor cells engraft primarily in the fetal liver. Following initiation of bone marrow hematopoiesis, cells preferentially home and engraft in the bone marrow. Finally, studies in the allogeneic sheep model have defined the sensitivity of the fetus to graft versus host disease (GVHD).[18] The occurrence of GVHD is related purely to T-cell dose and complete T-cell depletion increases the rate of failure of engraftment. Allogeneic engraftment has also been demonstrated in the normal fetal primate,[19] goat,[20] and mouse[21] following *in utero* transplantation.

One remarkable aspect of fetal tolerance is that it extends across even widely disparate species barriers. Xenogeneic chimerism after *in utero* HSC transplantation has now been documented in the human-sheep,[22] human-baboon,[23] human-mouse,[24] pig-sheep,[25] and rat-mouse[26] species combinations. The human-sheep model has been the most studied and most informative with respect to clinical transplantation. This model allows unequivocal detection of donor cells as well as phenotypic characterization of engraftment using the large number of defined human differentiation antigens. In this model, transplantation of preimmune fetal lambs (48–54 days gestation) by intraperitoneal injection of human fetal liver–derived hematopoietic cells (2×10^9–1×10^{10} cells/kg estimated fetal body wt.) results in stable, multilineage, human cell engraftment in a subset of the transplanted animals. The human-sheep chimerism created in the original experiments has now persisted for over 4 years.

A major question raised by the early studies in the allogeneic model was whether true pluripotent HSC were engrafted after *in utero* transplantation? This question has fundamental implications for the longevity of engraftment and the ability to permanently cure a patient by the prenatal approach. To address this question we separated human cells from sheep bone marrow harvested from 3-year-old human-sheep chimeras using the human CD45 antigen for positive selection.[27] The pooled human cells were then retransplanted into second-generation fetal lamb recipients. The documentation of long-term multilineage human chimerism in the second-generation recipients represents definitive evidence that chimerism after *in utero* transplantation is secondary to engraftment of true HSC and that it can, at least potentially, persist for the lifetime of the recipient.

The human-sheep model has also been extremely useful as an assay system for the repopulating potential and safety of human donor cell populations for clinical *in utero* transplantation. The model can be used as a rapid and specific assay for the presence of long-term repopulating cells in any human cell population.[28,29] In addition, xenogeneic

GVHD is easily induced and appears to be equal in its manifestations and severity to allogeneic GVHD. Using this model we have confirmed that all unprocessed postnatal sources of donor cells, including human cord blood, uniformly cause lethal GVHD.[30] In contrast, adult BM enriched for CD34, or more highly enriched populations, have the ability to engraft the fetus without causing GVHD.[28,29,31–33]

CLINICAL EXPERIENCE WITH *IN UTERO* TRANSPLANTATION

Theoretically, any disease that can be prenatally diagnosed and is treatable by BMT after birth could be treated by *in utero* transplantation. In reality however, the biology of each disease is different, and some diseases are much more biologically favorable than others.[34] The most favorable diseases have a selective advantage for donor cells or require only a very low level of engraftment and donor cell expression to clinically ameliorate the disease. Other diseases that require near-complete replacement of defective cells or require population of the CNS with normal cells are, at the present time, much less likely to be effectively treated by *in utero* transplantation.

We are aware of a total of 24 *in utero* HSC transplants reported or discussed in the literature including the initial report by Linch[35] in 1986. They have been performed for a variety of diseases, at various gestational ages, using different donor cell preparations, and modes of transplantation, and are reviewed elsewhere.[34] Clinical success has thus far been confined to the immunodeficiency disorders. Touraine[36,37] has reported two successful cases: one patient with "bare lymphocyte syndrome" and the other patient a female with presumed autosomal SCID. In both cases fetal liver- and thymus-derived donor cells were used and analysis is complicated by multiple transplants from different donors including postnatal transplants in the SCID patient. There has been minimal engraftment data published on these patients, particularly beyond one year of age, but they are reported to be healthy.[38] Two cases of successfully treated X-linked SCID have recently been reported. One of these is very preliminary (3.5 months of age) and contains very little data on immunologic function.[39] The other has documented evidence of donor progenitor cells in the bone marrow, with complete T-lymphocyte reconstitution, and remains healthy at 22 months of age.[40] In both cases, CD34-enriched paternal bone marrow cells were transplanted into the peritoneal cavity.

In the majority of failures, no donor cell engraftment or expression has been documented. In a significant number of these cases an explanation for failure is apparent. In eight attempts, fetuses without an inherent defect in cellular immunity were transplanted at a gestational age when rejection would be anticipated (after 16 weeks gestation). Four fetuses either had procedure-related deaths or were electively terminated after umbilical blood sampling suggested no engraftment (see below). In other cases, donor cell preparations were used that, in retrospect, were suboptimal. For instance, we have had difficulty engrafting T-cell depleted adult marrow without enrichment in the sheep model and cryopreserved fetal liver may not be a viable source of stem cells for fetal engraftment. The failures in patients with thalassemia disorders will be discussed in more detail below.

THALASSEMIAS AND *IN UTERO* BONE MARROW TRANSPLANTATION

There have been nine reported attempts to treat hemoglobinopathies by *in utero* transplantation (TABLE 2). Five have been for β-thalassemia major, three for α-thalassemia-1, and one for sickle cell disease. Of the five cases of β-thalassemia major, two died from procedure-related complications that, in retrospect, were preventable. Two of the remaining three were transplanted at 18 and 19 weeks gestation which would be expected to fail on an immunologic basis. The remaining case was transplanted at 12 weeks gestation with fetal liver–derived cells and was initially reported as engrafted by Touraine on the basis of

TABLE 2. Clinical Experience with *in Utero* HSC Transplantation for Hemoglobinopathies

Donor Cell Source	Gestational Age (weeks)	Disease Treated	Postnatal Outcome	Reference
Fetal liver	12	β-Thalassemia major	Alive, not engrafted	38
Fetal liver	19	β-Thalassemia major	Intrauterine death	
Sibling TCD BM	25	β-Thalassemia	No engraftment, clinical status c/w primary disease	56
Maternal TCD BM	18	α-Thalassemia 1	Terminated at 24 wks, + donor cells in extramedullary hematopoiesis	41
Fetal Liver	14	β-Thalassemia major	Septic abortion	41
Cryopreserved Fetal Liver	15	α-Thalassemia-1	No detectable engraftment	42
	18	β-Thalassemia major		
	13	Sickle Cell Disease		
Paternal CD34 Enriched	13	α-Thalassemia-1	PCR detectable α-gene, ? Tolerance	45

detectable Y-chromosome by PCR and 0.9% HbA at birth. This increased to 30% HbA at one year of age but no follow-up engraftment data have been provided.[38] The child has since been stated to have lost the engraftment and remains transfusion dependent. It is, in our opinion, somewhat doubtful that this patient was ever engrafted by donor HSCs because of the transient presence of PCR-detectable donor cells and the normal variability of HbA levels in β-thalassemia patients.

The three patients treated for α-thalassemia are of interest. The first case was transplanted at 18 weeks gestation with T-cell depleted maternal marrow. There was no evidence of engraftment at 24 weeks by percutaneous umbilical blood sampling and the pregnancy was terminated.[41] Analysis at autopsy revealed marked extramedullary hematopoiesis with donor cells identified in extramedullary sites. This case is important in that it confirms the sheep data in which donor cells are not peripherally expressed until later in gestation. We feel strongly that peripheral blood sampling should not be used as an indicator of engraftment. A second case was transplanted at 15 weeks gestation by a single injection of cryopreserved fetal liver–derived cells.[42] There is data to suggest that cryopreservation may damage the ability of fetal liver HSC to engraft in the human. Postnatal treatment of SCID patients failed when cryopreserved fetal liver was used but was successful when similar doses of fresh fetal liver cells were used.[43,44] In addition, as discussed below, there may be biological disadvantages in α-thalassemia for donor cell competition and engraftment. The final case of α-thalassemia was transplanted by a series of three transplants of CD34-enriched paternal marrow, at 13, 18, and 23 weeks gestation.[45] The fetus required repeated intrauterine transfusions to survive to term and by report has a trace positive PCR signal for α-globin gene in cord blood and bone marrow and evidence of donor-specific tolerance by mixed lymphocyte reaction. The child remains healthy but transfusion dependent at 1 year of age. These observations have not yet been published.

In summary, there is not yet convincing evidence for the efficacy of *in utero* transplantation in the treatment of the thalassemia disorders, but it does not appear to have been adequately tested. There have been very few cases attempted and with the exception of the final case of α-thalassemia, none of the transplants were performed in what we would currently consider to be an optimal manner. We discuss below why we remain optimistic about the potential for this approach and what we would currently use as a transplantation strategy for the appropriate thalassemia candidate.

BIOLOGIC CONSIDERATIONS FOR THE PRENATAL TREATMENT OF THALASSEMIA

The prenatal hematopoietic biology of the α- and β-thalassemias in the context of *in utero* transplantation are different and should be considered separately. In the case of α-thalassemia-1, α-globin–dependent hemoglobin production (Hb F) begins at 8 weeks gestation.[46] By 10 weeks physiologic evidence of fetal anemia can be observed sonographically as placentomegaly. By 12–14 weeks fetal hydrops (high output cardiac failure) may be observed.[47] During this time the fetus develops ineffective erythropoiesis in the fetal liver and abnormal sites of extramedullary hematopoiesis. The fetal hematopoietic microenvironment is hypercellular and may not be optimal in terms of available receptive sites or donor cell competition. We are therefore relatively pessimistic about the possibility of achieving significant levels of engraftment in this disease. As suggested by one of the cases discussed above however, it may be possible to induce tolerance for postnatal transplantation from the same donor. In contrast, β-globin–dependent hemoglobin production does not occur until after birth. Production of Hb F is normal in β-thalassemia major and therefore the fetal microenvironment is relatively normal. Ineffective erythropoiesis begins with the switch to adult hemoglobin after birth and may provide a postnatal selective advantage for donor-derived erythropoiesis.

Two fundamental questions regarding *in utero* transplantation for β-thalassemia are appropriate. Can donor cells engraft in a hematopoietically normal host and if so, will the level of engraftment be adequate for clinical effect? The question of engraftment can only be answered indirectly from the experimental data presented above. In natural and experimental models of prenatally induced chimerism, either allogeneic or xenogeneic chimerism can be induced in recipients with normal hematopoiesis. Depending upon the animal species and experimental conditions, the level of chimerism ranges from minimal to adequate for correction of thalassemia. We have also documented the presence of significant levels (approximately 20%) of donor-derived primitive progenitors (CD34+/CD38-) in the bone marrow of our successfully treated patient with X-linked SCID.[40] It is therefore reasonable to expect that with an appropriately performed transplant, at least some level of donor cell engraftment could be achieved in thalassemia.

There is both experimental and clinical data available that supports the concept of treatment of thalassemia by the creation of mixed chimerism. Rubin and colleagues[48] demonstrated in neonatal homozygous $Hbb^{th}/IIbb^{th}$ mice that intraperitoneal injection of syngeneic fetal liver cells could result in increasing erythroid chimerism over time and that there was a selective amplification of donor erythropoiesis with levels of erythrocyte chimerism in the peripheral circulation of as high as 30% at the same time that less than 1% of peripheral blood mononuclear cells were of donor origin. Similarly, van den Bos and colleagues[49] in a heterozygous ($Hba^{th}/+$) α-thalassemia mouse model showed correction of anemia by mixed chimerism by transplantation of normal syngeneic BM after sublethal irradiation. Once again, there was evidence of selective donor erythroid expression with levels of donor-derived clonogenic progenitors at 20–30% and levels of erythroid chimerism much greater than 50%. Possible explanations for the selective advantage of donor erythropoiesis in these models include an advantage for erythroid-committed progenitors due to host ineffective erythropoiesis and/or the relative half lives of mature donor and recipient red cells. At least in the α-thalassemia model, the difference in red cell survival cannot fully explain the degree of peripheral donor erythroid expression suggesting a true lineage selective advantage at the progenitor level.

Even more compelling are observations on mixed chimerism after postnatal BMT. The experience from Lucarelli and colleagues is most informative.[50] In their subset of patients with stable mixed chimerism after BMT, β-globin synthesis exceeds engraftment. With levels of BM donor cell engraftment of 25–75%, peripheral normal Hb levels are 10–13.5

g/dL. Patients with 20% donor-derived BM engraftment have complete clinical amelioration of their disease. In addition, there are anecdotal reports of patients with as little as 5% donor cells in the BM with minimal transfusion requirement, essentially converting a β-thalassemia major phenotype to an intermedia phenotype.[51] These levels of donor cell engraftment have been consistently achieved after *in utero* transplantation in the sheep model and can potentially be accomplished clinically.

At the very least one could expect microchimerism, or very low, non therapeutic levels of donor cell chimerism after *in utero* transplantation. There is abundant evidence that the presence of even low levels of chimerism correlate with the presence of donor-specific tolerance.[52,53] A strategy of prenatal transplantation to achieve postnatal tolerance for same donor BMT would potentially allow postnatal treatment with a minimal myelopreparative regimen and therefore mimimal toxicity. There is a relevant case report from Or and colleagues[54] of a patient with stable 4–7% mixed chimerism for 5 years after BMT at 18 months of age. The patient had an intermedia phenotype requiring only 8 transfusions over 4 years. He then underwent a same donor second transplant using mobilized peripheral blood stem cells and a non-myeloablative conditioning regimen with no post transplant immunosuppression. At 18 months after the second transplant the patient has 100% donor engraftment and normal Hb levels. This single case suggests that the presence of low level chimerism allows second same donor transplants with minimal toxicity and that the second transplant can dramatically improve engraftment. It lends direct support to the feasibility of the strategy outlined above.

THE "OPTIMAL" STRATEGY FOR *IN UTERO* TRANSPLANTATION FOR THALASSEMIA

The clinical approach to *in utero* transplantation is evolving as information from experimental and clinical experience accumulates. Therefore, any "optimal" strategy outlined today may become rapidly outmoded. Nevertheless, the algorithm which we would currently follow is shown in FIGURE 2. This algorithm presumes the appropriate expertise and

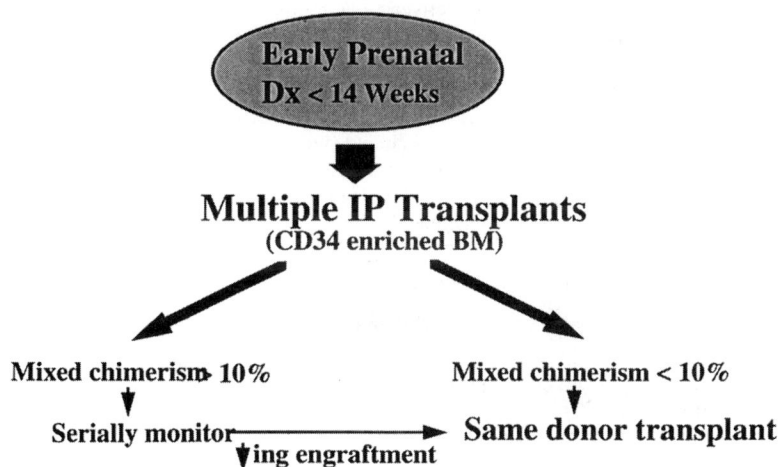

FIGURE 2. Algorithm for a potential strategy for application of *in utero* HSC transplantation to the thalassemia syndromes. The rationale is explained in the text.

TABLE 3. Considerations for Donor Cell Source

	Pros	Cons
Fetal Liver	Proliferation/Homing? No GVHD	Safety Ethics? Non-renewable
Adult BM	Safe Renewable	GVHD Proliferation/Homing?
Enriched BM	Safe Renewable No GVHD	Proliferation/Homing?

commitment of the center performing the transplant, as well as the performance of appropriate prenatal counseling and informed consent of the parents. The ethical framework for experimental fetal therapy is beyond the scope of this chapter but is well developed and has been outlined, for fetal intervention in general,[55] and *in utero* transplantation specifically,[34] elsewhere. The prenatal diagnosis must be made early so that there is adequate time to perform the initial transplant prior to 14 weeks gestation. At the present time the overiding considerations regarding the source of donor cells are maternal and fetal safety and renewability for postnatal same donor transplants (TABLE 3). These considerations exclude the use of fetal liver–derived cells and cord blood, and favor the use of enriched adult donor cell sources. There is little or no evidence favoring one form of enrichment over another. The important considerations are sterility and quality, and exhaustive T-cell depletion to avoid GVHD. We currently use a process based on positive selection of $CD34^+$ cells and negative selection of $CD3^+$ cells. We would recommend a series of at least three ultrasound-guided, intraperitoneal transplants spaced 1 week apart. The technical skill required to perform these transplants safely should not be underestimated and extensive experience with fetal injection procedures at early gestational age is required. Extrapolation of experience with late gestational procedures is not adequate. Following the transplants, no special monitoring is required until after the age of fetal viability, at which time the fetus should be followed by serial ultrasounds to assess growth and look for evidence of possible GVHD. Following delivery, the ability to assess engraftment by sensitive detection methodology is a prerequisite for the institution performing the transplant. Low levels of engraftment (< 10%) should be retransplanted early using minimal preparative regimens prior to the requirement for multiple transfusions. We would favor the philosophy that multiple postnatal transplants can be performed, if necessary, using minimally toxic preparative regimens, to achieve stepwise improvements of engraftment rather than attempt to achieve high levels of engraftment with a single postnatal transplant at the expense of preparative regimen toxicity. If higher levels of engraftment are present (> 10%) the patients engraftment dynamics can be followed serially over time to assess the need for further transplants.

SUMMARY

In utero HSC transplantation differs from postnatal BMT because engraftment depends upon competitive population of receptive sites in the recipient BM. There is ample evidence from experimental and natural models of *S* transplantation that donor cells can effectively compete in the fetal microenvironment to permanently engraft HSC. This engraftment is favored by diseases in which there is a selective advantage for donor cells but can clearly be achieved in the normal recipient microenvironment. Although clinical success thus far is limited to the immunodeficiency disorders, the approach has not been adequately tested as yet for the thalassemias. The establishment of mixed chimerism in thalassemia results in selective amplification of donor erythroid expression in the periphery, providing therapeutic benefit for even low levels of donor cell chimerism. In addition, the presence of mixed chimerism at any level should be associated with donor specific tolerance providing the opportunity of same donor transplants after birth with minimal toxicity. Therefore, there is reason to be optimistic that in the future, *in utero* transplantation may play a role in selected fetuses affected with the thalassemia disorders.

REFERENCES

1. METCALF, D. & M. A. S. MOORE. 1971. In Embryonic Aspects of Haemopoiesis. A. Neuberger & E. L. Tatum, Eds: Chapter 4. North-Holland Publishing Co. Amsterdam.
2. TAVIAN, M., L. COULOMBEL, D. LUTON, H. SAN CLEMENTE, F. DIETERLEN-LIEVRE & B. PEAULT. 1996. Aorta-associated CD34+ hematopoietic cells in the early human embryo. Blood **87:** 67–72.
3. BILLINGHAM, R., L. BRENT & P. B. MEDAWAR. 1953. Actively acquired tolerance of foreign cells. Nature **172:** 603–607.
4. SPRENT, J. 1995. Central tolerance of T cells. Int. Rev. Immunol. **13:** 95–105.
5. ANDERSON, G., N. MOORE, J. OWEN & E. JENKINSON. 1996. Cellular interactions in thymocyte development. Annu. Rev. Immunol. **14:** 73–99.
6. STROMINGER, J. L. 1989. Developmental biology of T cell receptors. Science **244:** 943–949.
7. OWEN, R. D. 1945. Immunogenetic consequences of vascular anastomoses between bovine cattle twins. Science **102:** 400–401.
8. PICUS, J., W. ALDRICH & N. LETVIN. 1985. A naturally occurring bone-marrow chimeric primate. Transplantation **39:** 297–303.
9. VAN DIJK, B., D. BOMMSMA & A. DE MAN. 1996. Blood group chimerism in human multiple births is not rare. Am. J. Med. Genet. **61:** 264–268.
10. ANDERSON, D., R. BILLINGHAM, G. LAMPKIN & P. MEDAWAR. 1951. The use of skin grafting to distinguish between monozygotic and dizygotic twins in cattle. Heredity **5:** 379–397.
11. SIMONSEN, M. 1955. The acquired immunity concept in kidney homotransplantation. Ann. N.Y. Acad. Sci. **59:** 448–452.
12. FLEISCHMAN, R. & B. MINTZ. 1979. Prevention of genetic anemias in mice by microinjection of normal hematopoietic cells into the fetal placenta. Proc. Natl. Acad. Sci. USA **76:** 5736–5740.
13. BLAZER, B., P. TAYLOR & D. VALLERA. 1995. In utero transfer of adult bone marrow cells into recipients with severe combined immunodeficiency disorder yields lymphoid progeny with T- and B-cell functional capabilities. Blood **86:** 4353–4366.
14. ZANJANI, E. D., J. L. ASCENSAO, A. W. FLAKE, M. R. HARRISON & M. TAVASSOLI. 1992. The fetus as an optimal donor and recipient of hemopoietic stem cells. Bone Marrow Transplant. **10:** 107–114.
15. FLAKE, A. W., M. R. HARRISON, N. S. ADZICK & E. D. ZANJANI. 1986. Transplantation of fetal hematopoietic stem cells in utero: the creation of hematopoietic chimeras. Science **233:** 776–778.
16. FLAKE, A. & E. ZANJANI. 1997. Cellular therapy. New trends and controversies in fetal diagnosis and therapy. Obstet. Gynecol. Clin. N. Am. **24:** 159–177.
17. ZANJANI, E. D., J. L. ASCENSAO & M. TAVASSOLI. 1992. Homing of liver-derived hemopoietic stem cells to fetal bone marrow. Trans. Assoc. Am. Physicians. **105:** 7–14.
18. CROMBLEHOLME, T. M., M. R. HARRISON & E. D. ZANJANI. 1990. In utero transplantation of hematopoietic stem cells in sheep: the role of T cells in engraftment and graft-versus-host disease. J. Pediatr. Surg. **25:** 885–892.
19. HARRISON, M. R., R. N. SLOTNICK, T. M. CROMBLEHOLME, M. S. GOLBUS *et al*. 1989. In-utero transplantation of fetal liver haemopoietic stem cells in monkeys. Lancet **2:** 1425–1427.
20. PEARCE, R., D. KIEHM, D. ARMSTRONG, P. LITTLE *et al*. 1989. Induction of hematopoietic chimerism in the caprine fetus by intraperitoneal injection of fetal liver cells. Experientia **45:** 307–308.

21. CARRIER, E., T. LEE, M. BUSCH & M. COWAN. 1995. Induction of tolerance in nondefective mice after in utero transplantation of major histocompatibility complex-mismatched fetal hematopoietic stem cells. Blood. **86:** 4681–4690.
22. ZANJANI, E. D., M. G. PALLAVICINI, J. L. ASCENSAO, A. W. FLAKE *et al.* 1992. Engraftment and long-term expression of human fetal hemopoietic stem cells in sheep following transplantation in utero. J. Clin. Invest. **89:** 1178–1188.
23. SHIELDS, L., E. BRYANT, T. EASTERLING & R. ANDREWS. 1995. Fetal liver cell transplantation for the creation of lymphhematopoietic chimerism in the fetal baboon. Am. J. Obstet. Gynecol. **173:** 1157–1160.
24. PALLAVICINI, M. G., A. W. FLAKE, D. MADDEN, C. BETHEL *et al.* 1992. Hemopoietic chimerism in rodents transplanted in utero with fetal human hemopoietic cells. Transplant. Proc. **24:** 542–543.
25. HEDRICK, M. H., H. E. RICE, D. H. SACHS, E. D. ZANJANI & A. W. FLAKE. 1993. Creation of pig-sheep xenogeneic hematopoietic chimerism by the in utero transplantation of hematopoietic stem cells. Transplant. Sci. **3:** 23–26.
26. RICE, H. E., M. H. HEDRICK & A. W. FLAKE. 1994. In utero transplantation of rat hematopoietic stem cells induces xenogeneic chimerism in mice. Transplant. Proc. **26:** 126–128.
27. ZANJANI, E. D., A. W. FLAKE, H. RICE, M. HEDRICK & M. TAVASSOLI. 1994. Long-term repopulating ability of xenogeneic transplanted human fetal liver hematopoietic stem cells in sheep. J. Clin. Invest. **93:** 1051–1055.
28. KAWASHIMA, I., E. D. ZANJANI, G. ALMAIDA PORADA, A. W. FLAKE *et al.* 1996. CD34+ human marrow cells that express low levels of Kit protein are enriched for long-term marrow-engrafting cells. Blood **87:** 4136–4142.
29. CIVIN, C., G. ALMEIDA-PORADA, M.-J. LEE, J. OLWEUS *et al.* 1996. Sustained, retransplantable, multilineage engraftment of highly purified adult human bone marrow stem cells in vivo. Blood **88:** 4102–4109.
30. ZANJANI, E. D., A. W. FLAKE, H. E. RICE, M. H. HEDRICK & M. TAVASSOLI. 1993. An in vivo comparison of potential human donor hematopoietic stem cell sources for bone marrow transplantation using the human/sheep xenograft model. Blood **82 (Suppl. 1):** 655a (Abstract 2605).
31. SROUR, E. F., E. D. ZANJANI, K. CORNETTA, C. M. TRAYCOFF *et al.* 1993. Persistence of human multilineage, self-renewing lymphohematopoietic stem cells in chimeric sheep. Blood **82:** 3333–3342.
32. TRAYCOFF, C. M., R. HOFFMAN, E. D. ZANJANI, K. CORNETTA *et al.* 1994. Measurement of marrow repopulating potential of human hematopoietic progenitor and stem cells using a fetal sheep model. Prog. Clin. Biol. Res. **389:** 281–291.
33. UCHIDA, N., J. COMBS, S. CHEN, E. ZANJANI *et al.* 1996. Primitive human hematopoietic cells displaying differential efflux of the rhodamine 123 dye have distinct biological activities. Blood **88:** 1297–1305.
34. FLAKE, A. & E. ZANJANI. 1998. In utero hematopoietic stem cell transplantation: A status report. J. Am. Med. Assoc. **278:** 932–937.
35. LINCH, D., C. RODECK & K. NICOLAIDES. 1986. Attempted bone marrow transplantation in a 17 week fetus. Lancet **1:** 1382.
36. TOURAINE, J. L. 1991. Stem cell transplantation in primary immunodeficiency, with special reference to the first prenatal, in utero, transplants. Allergol. Immunopathol. (Madr) **19:** 49–51.
37. TOURAINE, J. L., D. RAUDRANT, C. ROYO, A. REBAUD *et al.* 1989. In-utero transplantation of stem cells in bare lymphocyte syndrome. Lancet **1:** 1382.
38. TOURAINE, J. 1996. Treatment of human fetuses and induction of immunological tolerance in humans by in utero transplantation of stem cells into fetal recipients. Acta Haematol. **96:** 115–119.
39. WENGLER, G., A. LANFRANCHI, T. FRUSCA, R. VERARDI *et al.* 1996. In-utero transplantation of parental CD34 haematopoietic progenitor cells in a patient with X-linked severe combined immunodeficiency (SCIDX1). Lancet **348:** 1484–1487.
40. FLAKE, A., M.-G. RONCAROLO, J. PUCK, G. ALMEIDA-PORADA *et al.* 1996. Treatment of X-linked severe combined immunodeficiency by in utero transplantation of paternal bone marrow. N. Engl. J. Med. **335:** 1806–1810.
41. COWAN, M. & M. GOLBUS. 1994. In utero hematopoietic stem cell transplants for inherited disease. Am. J. Pediatr. Hemat./Oncol. **16:** 35–42.

42. WESTGREN, M., O. RINGDEN, E.-N. STURLA, E. SVERKER et al. 1996. Lack of evidence of permanent engraftment after in utero fetal stem cell transplantation in congenital hemoglobinopathies. Transplantation **61:** 1176–1179.
43. GUPTA, S., R. PAHWA, R. O'REILLY, R. GOOD & F. SIEGEL. 1976. Ontogeny of lymphocyte subpopulations in human fetal liver. Proc. Natl. Acad. Sci. USA **73:** 919–922.
44. PAHWA, R., S. PAHWA, R. GOOD, G. INCEFY & R. O'REILLY. 1977. Rationale for combined use of fetal liver and thymic for immunological reconstitution in patients with severe combined immunodeficiency. Proc. Natl. Acad. Sci. USA **74:** 3002–3005.
45. HAYWARD, A., J. HOBBINS, R. QUINONES, R. GILLER et al. 1996. Microchimerism and tolerance following intrauterine transplantation and transfusion for a-thalassemia-1. Presented at the In Utero Stem Cell Transplantation and Gene Therapy Conference. Reno, NV, 1996.
46. BUNN, H. & B. FORGET. 1986. In Hemoglobin Structure. Chapter 2: 13–35. W. B. Saunders. Philadelphia.
47. LAM, Y., A. GHOSH, M. TANG, C. LEE & S. SIN. 1997. Second-trimester hydrops fetalis in pregnancies affected by homozygous α thalassemia-1. Prenat. Diagn. **17:** 267–269.
48. BETHEL, C., D. MURUGESH, M. HARRISON, N. MOHANDAS & E. RUBIN. 1993. Selective erythroid replacement in murine b-thalassemia using fetal hematopoietic stem cells. Proc. Natl. Acad. Sci. USA **90:** 10120–10124.
49. VAN DEN BOS, C., D. KIEBOOM, J. VAN DER SLUIJS, M. BAERT et al. 1994. Selective advantage of normal erythrocyte production after bone marrow transplantation of a-thalassemic mice. Exp. Hematol. **22:** 441–446.
50. ANDREANI, M., M. MANNA, G. LUCARELLI, P. TONUCCI et al. 1996. Persistence of mixed chimerism in patients transplanted for the treatment of thalassemia. Blood **87:** 3494–3499.
51. KAPELUSHNIK, J., R. OR, D. FILON, A. NAGLER et al. 1995. Analysis of β-globin mutations shows stable mixed chimerism in patients with thalassemia after bone marrow transplantation. Blood **86:** 3241–3246.
52. KAUFMAN, C. L. & S. T. ILDSTAD. 1994. Induction of donor-specific tolerance by transplantation of bone marrow. Therap. Immunol. **1:** 101–111.
53. SYKES, M. 1996. Immunobiology of transplantation. FASEB J. **10:** 721–730.
54. OR, R., J. KAPELUSHNIK, E. NAPARSTEK, A. NAGLER et al. 1996. Second transplantation using allogeneic peripheral blood stem cells in a β-thalassaemia major patient featuring stable mixed chimaerism. Br. J. Haematol. **94:** 285–287.
55. FLETCHER, J. C. 1992. Fetal therapy, ethics and public policies. Fetal Diagn Ther. **7:** 158–168.
56. SLAVIN, S., E. NAPARSTEK & M. ZIEGLER. 1992. Clinical application of intrauterine bone marrow transplantation for treatment of genetic disease—feasibility studies. Bone Marrow Transplant. **1:** 189–190.

Unrelated and HLA-Nonidentical Related Donor Marrow Transplantation for Thalassemia and Leukemia

A Combined Report from the Seattle Marrow Transplant Team and the International Bone Marrow Transplant Registry[a]

K. M. SULLIVAN,[b-d] C. ANASETTI,[c,d] M. HOROWITZ,[e] P. A. ROWLINGS,[e] E. W. PETERSDORF,[c,d] P. J. MARTIN,[c,d] R. A. CLIFT,[c] M. C. WALTERS,[c,d] T. GOOLEY,[c] J. SIERRA,[c] J. E. ANDERSON,[c,d] J. BJERKE,[c] M. SIADAK,[c] M. E. D. FLOWERS,[c] R. A. NASH,[c,d] J. E. SANDERS,[c,d] F. R. APPELBAUM,[c,d] R. STORB,[c,d] AND J. A. HANSEN[c,d]

[c]*Fred Hutchinson Cancer Research Center, the [d]University of Washington School of Medicine, Seattle, Washington, USA*

[e]*International Bone Marrow Transplant Registry and the Medical College of Wisconsin, Milwaukee, Wisconsin, USA*

ABSTRACT: Allogeneic marrow transplantation is curative therapy for thalassemia, but fewer than 30% of patients have an HLA-identical sibling marrow donor. Selection of alternative donors of hematopoietic stem cells (unrelated individuals or HLA-nonidentical family members) has been aided by establishment of world-wide donor registries now exceeding 3.6 million volunteers and by DNA-based HLA typing to more closely match potential donors. Coupled with improved methods to control graft-versus-host disease and prevent fungal and cytomegalovirus infection, remarkable progress has been made in alternative donor transplantation. For patients 50 years of age or younger, with recently diagnosed chronic myelogenous leukemia (CML) in chronic phase, 1- and 5-year survivals after HLA-A, B, DRB1 identical unrelated marrow transplantation in Seattle are 82% and 74%, respectively. These results are essentially identical to outcome in similar patients given HLA-matched sibling allografts. However, the world-wide number of alternative donor transplants for thalassemia remains limited to date: 4 unrelated and 60 HLA-nonidentical related transplants have been reported to the IBMTR since 1969 with actuarial overall survival of 75%. Using the paradigm of CML, it is likely that access to curative therapy of thalassemia will improve with optimal HLA typing and donor selection early in the course of disease.

---

[a]This work supported by Grants AI 2958, AI 33484, AR 39153, CA 18029, CA 18221, CA 40053 and HL 36444 from the National Institutes of Health, Department of Health and Human Services. Additional sponsors of the International Bone Marrow Transplant Registry are listed in the appendix.

[b]Address for correspondence: Keith M. Sullivan, M.D., Fred Hutchinson Cancer Research Center, 1100 Fairview Ave. N., D5-360, P.O. Box 19024, Seattle, WA 98109-1024. Tel: 206/667-4416; Fax: 206/667-2147; E-mail: ksulliva@fhcrc.org

Marrow transplantation from HLA-identical sibling donors is an increasingly employed treatment for a number of malignant and non-malignant disorders. With disease-free survival of 80–90% after HLA-matched sibling transplantation for early stage thalassemia, chronic phase leukemia, and severe aplastic anemia, marrow grafting is now being applied in other conditions for the prevention of long-term morbidity and mortality.[1-6] Unfortunately, fewer than 30% of individuals in an average size family have an HLA-identical sibling, which has led to considerable interest in stem cell transplantation from alternative donors, such as HLA-nonidentical family members and unrelated volunteers. While initial reports affirmed the feasibility of this approach, rates of graft failure and graft-versus-host disease (GVHD) were more frequent than seen with matched sibling allografts.[7-12] However, recent advances in molecular techniques for high-resolution HLA typing to select closely matched unrelated donors and supportive care regimens to control GVHD and prevent cytomegalovirus infections have improved the outcome of transplantation from alternative donors.[13-21]

Due to the currently limited number of unrelated transplants for thalassemia, we will use the paradigm of chronic myelogenous leukemia (CML) for consideration in thalassemia. The following reviews the current status of alternative donor transplants for leukemia at the Fred Hutchinson Cancer Research Center (FHCRC) and the worldwide experience with mismatched related and unrelated transplants for thalassemia reported to the International Bone Marrow Transplant Registry (IBMTR).

DONOR REGISTRIES

Established in 1986, the National Marrow Donor Program (NMDP) is a network funded by the U.S. Congress to coordinate searches for unrelated donors.[22] With more than 2.5 million Americans joining the NMDP, the probability among Caucasians of finding a matched unrelated donor exceeds 70%. However, due to fewer individuals of minority ethnic groups in the registry and their greater potential for HLA polymorphisms, the likelihoods of matching for Hispanic, Asian/Pacific, and black individuals are, respectively, 62%, 45%, and 24%.[23] As efforts proceed with minority recruitment, these donor-matching rates will continue to improve. Meanwhile, world-wide efforts to coordinate computer searches continue. Located in the Netherlands, the Eurodonor Foundation compiles a directory of 30 registries in 26 countries. This database includes 3.6 million donors typed for HLA-A and B with more than 1.0 million donors also typed for HLA-DR.[23]

HLA TYPING TECHNIQUES AND TERMINOLOGY

Human leukocyte antigens (HLA) identify regions on cell surfaces of transplantation importance.[24] Increasing degrees of HLA disparity between donor and recipient increase the likelihood of graft failure or GVHD. Aided by DNA technology, over 200 antigens/alleles are currently defined at the HLA-A, B, and DR loci. This compares to 105 A, B, and DR antigens serologically defined in 1990. Current techniques use DNA-based technology (PCR amplification and sequence-specific oligonucleotide probes) for typing of class II HLA-DR and DQ genes. Additional class I alleles are likely to be defined in the future with use of these new techniques.

Protocols for unrelated donor transplants at FHCRC are based on patient age: individuals 36–55 years old require an HLA-A, B, DRB1 identical donor. Those less than 36 years old may have an unrelated donor with a one locus minor HLA-mismatch.

Class I mismatch: HLA-A or B antigens or alleles belonging to the same crossreactive (CREG) group.[25,26] Three of four A and B antigens match as do both DRB1 alleles. *Class II mismatch:* Pairs of disparate DRB1 alleles belong to the same serologically defined DR group. Four of four A and B antigens match while one of two DRB1 alleles match.

A genotypic mismatch exists within the family when there is HLA identity for one haplotype (confirmed by family segregation studies) and differences on the unshared haplotype. *Zero antigen mismatch:* Donor and patient are phenotypically matched on the nonshared haplotype for HLA-A, B, C, DRB1, and DQB1. *One antigen mismatch:* The donor is nonidentical for one HLA-A, B, C, DRB1, or DQB1 antigen/allele. HLA-C and/or DQ disparity is not considered a second/third mismatch when either A, B, or DRB1 is disparate. *Two/three antigen mismatch:* The donor and patient are mismatched for two or three HLA-A, B, or DRB1 antigens/alleles. Because of the severity of complications, such mismatched pairs are not routinely considered for transplantation.

COMPLICATIONS OF ALLOGENEIC TRANSPLANTATION

TABLE 1 summarizes published data from Seattle for patients with unmodified HLA-identical marrow grafts from siblings and unrelated donors. All patients had hematologic malignancies and received GVHD prophylaxis with a regimen of four doses of methotrexate (MTX) and 180 days of daily cyclosporine (CSP) posttransplant.[16] Graft failure was exceedingly rare in matched sibling allografts but ranged from 1% (acute leukemia) to 6% (CML) in unrelated marrow recipients.[8,9,27,28] Grade II–IV (moderate-life threatening) acute GVHD was increased in unrelated transplant recipients as was grade III–IV GVHD.[29,30] Clinical extensive chronic GVHD also increased in frequency.[31,32] FIGURE 1 depicts the probability of developing chronic GVHD among patients with hematologic malignancies surviving beyond Day 150 posttransplant.[32] Chronic GVHD had an earlier onset among

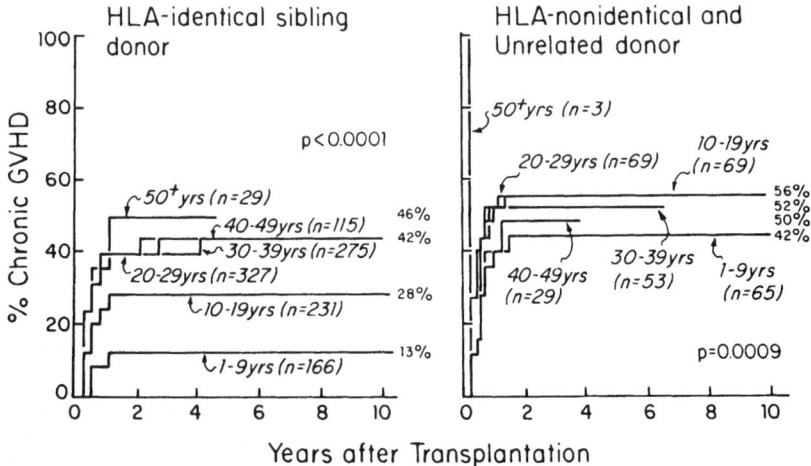

FIGURE 1. Probability of developing clinical extensive chronic graft-versus-host disease (GVHD) in relation to age of recipients of HLA-identical sibling (*left*) or HLA-nonidentical or unrelated (*right*) marrow transplants. (From Sullivan *et al.*[32] Reproduced by permission.)

TABLE 1. Complications of Allogeneic Transplantation (MTX/CSP)

Events in Patients with Hematologic Malignancy	HLA-Identical Marrow Donor	
	Sibling	Unrelated
Graft failure	<1%	1–6%
Acute GVHD (grade II-IV)	35%	78%
Acute GVHD (grade III-IV)	14%	37%
Chronic GVHD (extensive)	33%	64%

mismatched and unrelated transplant patients, and in contrast to the matched sibling recipients, children and young adults did not exhibit a lower risk of developing chronic GVHD. Of note, many patients do not develop chronic GVHD after allogeneic transplantation, and immunosuppression can be successfully discontinued 180 days after transplant with self-sustained graft-host tolerance.

COMPLICATIONS OF UNRELATED TRANSPLANTATION

TABLE 2 compares results in patients less than 36 years old receiving marrow from HLA-identical unrelated donors with individuals receiving one antigen minor mismatched unrelated marrow.[33] Subsequent analysis showed that HLA-C mismatching was an independent factor associated with graft failure, thereby demonstrating that these gene products have transplantation importance.[28] The increase in clinically severe acute GVHD, however, was mainly due to DRB1 mismatching.[34] An increase in the cumulative incidence of chronic GVHD was also observed.[33] FIGURE 2 depicts this increase among children given HLA matched and mismatched unrelated marrow grafts.[35] All surviving patients had chronic GVHD resolve and immunosuppressive treatment was discontinued between the second and third year posttransplant.

Unrelated Transplantation for Acute Leukemia

TABLE 3 details results of unrelated donor transplants performed in Seattle for acute leukemia between September 1979 and June 1994.[36] Most patients were transplanted in relapse or beyond first complete remission (CR). Kaplan-Meier (KM) estimates of relapse and disease-free survival were remarkably similar to results obtained with matched sibling donors.[37,38]

TABLE 2. Complications of Unrelated Transplantation (MTX/CSP)

Events in Patients (< 36 years old) with Hematologic Malignancy	Unrelated Bone Marrow Donor	
	Matched at A, B and DRBI	One Ag Mismatch at A, B or DRBI[a]
Graft failure	3%	5%
Acute GVHD (grade II-IV)	78%	94%
Acute GVHD (grade Ill-IV)	36%	51%[b]
Chronic GVHD (extensive)	61%	74%

[a] Class I mismatch within a cross reactive group (CREG); Class II mismatch was DR identical but DRBI nonidentical.
[b] 34% GVHD for CREG mismatch but 61% GVHD for DRBI mismatch.

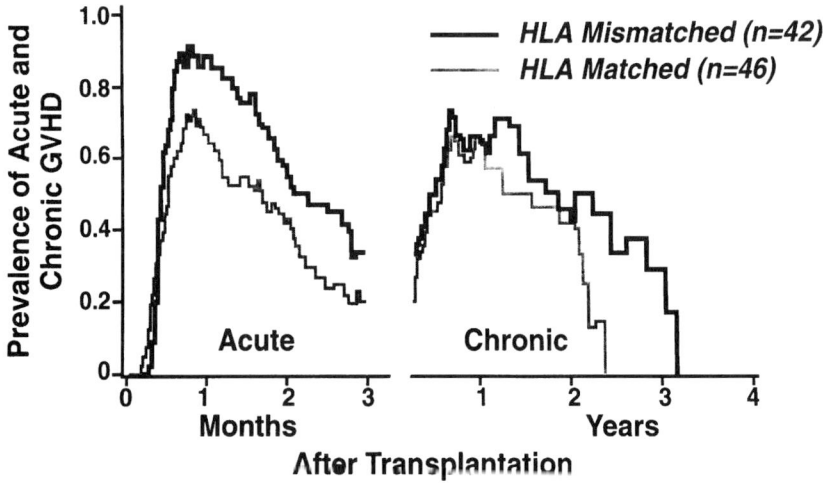

FIGURE 2. Prevalence of grade II-IV acute and clinical extensive chronic graft-versus-host disease (GVHD) requiring treatment among children given HLA-matched and mismatched unrelated marrow transplants. Chronic GVHD resolved and all immunosuppressive therapy was discontinued 2.4 years (HLA-matched) and 3.2 years (HLA-mismatched) posttransplant. (From Balduzzi et al.[35] Reproduced by permission.)

Unrelated Transplantation for CML

TABLE 4 presents the probability of relapse and survival after unrelated marrow transplantation in Seattle for CML.[21,39] Again, relapse and mortality increased in patients with advanced disease who were transplanted in accelerated phase (AP) or blast crisis (BC). Among the 152 patients in chronic phase transplanted from an HLA-A, B, DRB1 identical unrelated donor, survival was similar for all age groupings through 50 years of age, thereafter, survival was substantially reduced (FIG. 3).

TABLE 5 restricts the analysis to patients 50 years of age or younger with CML in chronic phase.[21] As shown in TABLE 5 and FIGURE 4, time from diagnosis of CML to transplant was inversely correlated with overall survival. This relationship had been previously observed among chronic phase CML patients given matched sibling transplants.[4] As shown in TABLE 5, survival in newly diagnosed patients was remarkably similar for HLA-identical unrelated and matched sibling marrow recipients.[4,21]

TABLE 3. Unrelated Transplantation for Acute Leukemia (1979–1994)

Disease Status at Transplant	Number Patients	Three Year KM Estimates	
		Leukemia Relapse	Disease-free Survival
CR-1	11	20%	55%
CR-2	35	41%	31%
CR-3+	20	35%	26%
Relapse	94	76%	12%

TABLE 4. Unrelated Transplants for CML

Outcome of Transplant	CML Status at Marrow Transplantation			
	Chronic (N = 204)	Accelerated (N = 79)	Blast Crisis rem (N = 18)	Blast Crisis (N = 32)
Relapse	7%	14%	17%	56%
1 year Survival	67%	54%	44%	28%
5 year Survival	55%	39%	32%	0

Unrelated and HLA-Nonidentical Related Transplantation for Thalassemia

The largest single center experience of marrow transplantation for thalassemia is from the team in Pesaro. Through June 1996, that group performed 805 transplants for thalassemia: 780 from HLA-identical related donors, 24 from WA-nonidentical related, and one from an unrelated donor.[40] This small number of alternative donor transplants was also seen in reports from the United States where only four alternative donor allografts were reported.[41,42] Similarly, few other unrelated transplants have been reported.[43]

Accordingly, we obtained approval from the Statistical Center of the IBMTR to review data of alternative donor transplants for thalassemia reported from 22 teams worldwide between 1969 and 1996. The analysis was not reviewed by the IBMTR Advisory Committee. TABLES 6 and 7 display patient characteristics and outcome of the 64 patients. As with the published United States experience, many patients did not have a pretransplant liver biopsy and further Pesaro classification of the thalassemia was not recorded.[41] Nonetheless, it is likely that most were class 2 or class 3 patients with hepatomegaly and irregular iron chelation histories. Forty-eight of the 64 patients survived, with 18 of the survivors experiencing recurrence of thalassemia. Of the 60 patients with genotypically HLA-nonidentical related donors, 39 have information provided concerning the degree of HLA mismatching: 24 had phenotypically matched parental donors, 11 had one-antigen, and 4 had two-antigen mismatched related donors. The number of surviving patients in the three

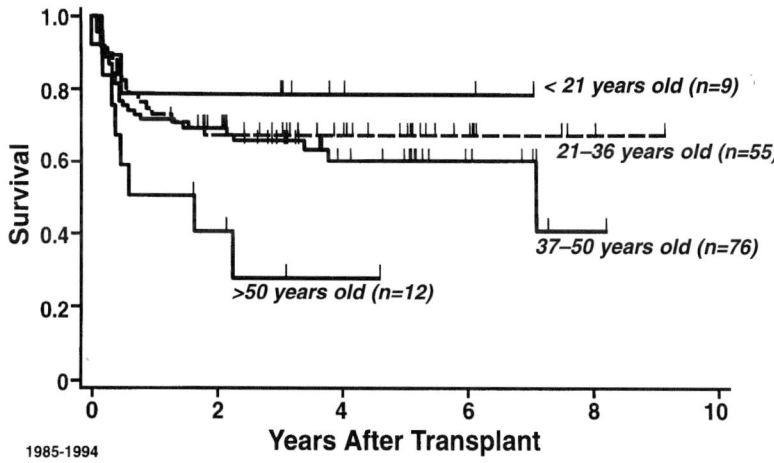

FIGURE 3. Probability of survival in relation to age at transplant of patients with chronic myelogenous leukemia in chronic phase given HLA-A, B, DRB1-identical unrelated marrow grafts in Seattle. (From Hansen et al.[21] Reproduced by permission.)

TABLE 5. Survival of Patients with CML in Chronic Phase (HLA-Identical Donors)[a]

Overall Survival after BMT	Time from Diagnosis to Marrow Transplantation			
	> 3 years Unrelated Donor ($N = 38$)	1–3 years Unrelated Donor ($N = 55$)	< 1 Year Unrelated Donor ($N = 51$)	< 1 year Sibling ($N = 218$)
1 year	57%	75%	82%	86%
3 years	57%	66%	74%	80%
5 years	50%	62%	74%	77%

[a]Patients < 50 years old transplanted in Seattle.

groups is 19 (79%), 7 (64%), and 2 (50%), respectively. FIGURE 5 depicts actuarial overall survival in patients given HLA-mismatched related marrow grafts.

DISCUSSION AND FUTURE DIRECTIONS

The world experience with alternative donor transplantation for thalassemia remains very limited. Moreover, the small number of cases span nearly three decades and only 11 (17%) of the 64 patients have been transplanted since January 1993. Thus, most were unlikely to have benefited from improved supportive care techniques and DNA typing technologies.[13,15,18,19,44] Using the paradigm of improved outcome in recent years for patients with newly diagnosed CML described above, it is likely that results of alternative donor transplantation for thalassemia will improve with enhanced supportive care, optimal techniques of HLA matching, and donor selection early in the disease. Current results in children undergoing marrow transplantation for leukemia clearly support this hypothesis.[35]

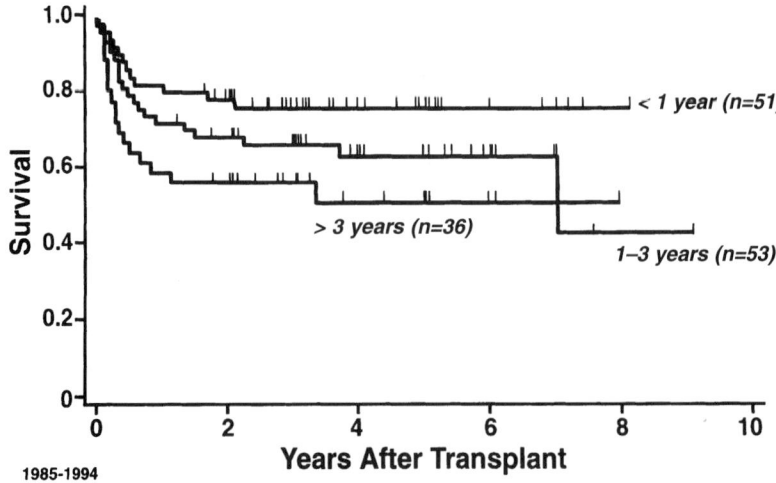

FIGURE 4. Probability of survival in patients with chronic myelogenous leukemia in chronic phase who were 50 years of age or younger at the time of transplant in Seattle from HLA-A, B, DRB1 identical unrelated donors. Outcome is displayed in relation to time from diagnosis of leukemia to marrow transplantation. (From Hansen *et al.*[21] Reproduced by permission.)

TABLE 6. Mismatch Related BMT for Thalassemia (IBMTR)[a]

Number of patients	60
Median age (range)	6 (1–19) years
Conditioning	Busulfan + cyclophosphamide + other ($N = 54$)
GVHD prophylaxis	Methotrexate/cyclosporine ($N = 27$)
	Tcell depletion ($N = 8$)
Transplant outcome	28 Alive and engrafted
	17 Alive with recurrence
	15 Died

[a]22 transplant teams (1969–1996).

Thus it is incumbent upon the physician to identify patients for HLA typing early in the course of the disease. This appears especially important in thalassemia early at the onset of noncompliance or cessation of chelation therapy. This lesson of improved results with early patient identification has been well demonstrated in CML, acute leukemia, and more recently, sickle cell disease.[5,45] Explaining the details of treatment options, results to date and areas of incomplete information are key to the patient education and consent process.[46] Only with suffcient recent experience will we be able to accurately judge the late effects and quality of life after alternative donor transplantation for thalassemia.[47]

Will alternative donor transplants early in the course of thalassemia be met with an increased rate of graft failure? The experience with chronic phase CML could suggest such an increase. Frequent monitoring for mixed donor-host hematopoietic chimerism may presage recurrence of thalassemia, although some patients with thalassemia and sickle cell disease exhibit stable mixed hematopoietic chimerism for many years and remain free of disease.[5,48–50] Hence, even a small fraction of donor-derived cells may ameliorate disease symptoms. Recent preclinical approaches of pharmacological immunosuppression to stabilize mixed chimerism may be of future clinical benefit in promoting corrective levels of hemoglobin synthesis.[51]

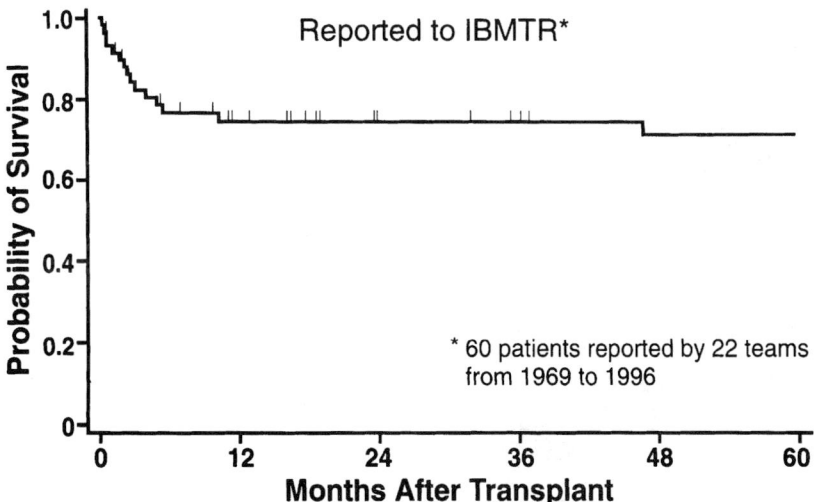

FIGURE 5. Probability of survival in 60 patients with thalassemia given marrow allografts from genotypically HLA-nonidentical family members reported to the International Bone Marrow Transplant Registry (IBMTR).

TABLE 7. Unrelated BMT for Thalassemia (IBMTR)[a]

Number patients (age)	4 (1, 2, 11, 16 years old)
Conditioning	Busulfan + cyclophosphamide + other ($N = 3$)
GVHD Prophylaxis	Methotrexate/cyclosporine ($N = 3$) Tcell depletion ($N = 1$)
Transplant Outcome	2 Alive and engrafted 1 Alive with recurrence 1 Died

[a]1989–1996.

ACKNOWLEDGMENTS

We wish to thank Melissa Regan for editorial assistance and Melodee Nugent for statistical assistance.

APPENDIX: Additional support for the IBMTR is provided by grants from Alpha Therapeutic Corporation; Amgen, Inc; Anonymous; Astra Pharmaceutical; Baxter Healthcare Corporation; Bayer Corporation; Biogen; Blue Cross and Blue Shield Association; Lynde and Harry Bradley Foundation; Bristol-Myers Squibb Company; Frank G. Brotz Family Foundation; CellPro, Inc; Centeon; Center for Advanced Studies in Leukemia; Chimeric Therapies; Chiron Therapeutics; Charles E. Culpeper Foundation; Eleanor Naylor Charitable Trust; Eppley Foundation for Research; Genetech, Inc; Glaxo Wellcome Company; Hoechst Marion Roussel, Inc; Immunex Corporation; Janssen Pharmaceutica; Kettering Family Foundation; Kirin Brewery Company; Robert J. Kleberg, Jr. and Helen C. Kleberg Foundation; Herbert H. Kohl Charities, Inc., Eli Lilly Company Foundation; Nada and Herbert P. Mahler Charities; Milstein Family Foundation; Milwaukee Foundation/Elsa Schoeneich Research Fund; Samuel Roberts Noble Foundation; Novartis Pharmaceuticals; Ortho Biotech Corporation; John Oster Family Foundation; Elsa U. Pardee Foundation; Jane and Lloyd Pettit Foundation; Alirio Pfiffer Bone Marrow Transplant Support Association; Pfizer, Inc.; Pharmacia and Upjohn; RGK Foundation; Schering-Plough International; Walter Schroeder Foundation; Searle; Stackner Family Foundation; Starr Foundation; Joan and Jack Stein Charities; and Wyeth-Ayerst Laboratories.

REFERENCES

1. THOMAS, E. D., C. D. BUCKNER, J. E. SANDERS, T. PAPAYANNOPOULOU, C. BORGNA-PIGNATTI, P. DE STEFANO, K. M. SULLIVAN, R. A. CLIFT & R. STORB. 1982. Marrow transplantation for thalassaemia. Lancet **2:** 227–229.
2. LUCARELLI, G., M. GALIMBERTI, P. POLCHI, E. ANGELUCCI, D. BARONCIANI, C. GIARDINI, M. ANDREANI, F. AGOSTINELLI, F. ALBERTINI, R. A. CLIFT. 1993. Marrow transplantation in patients with thalassemia responsive to iron chelation therapy. N. Engl. J. Med. **329:** 840–844.
3. STORB, R., R. ETZIONI, C. ANASETTI, F. R. APPELBAUM, C. D. BUCKNER, W. BENSINGER, E. BRYANT, R. CLIFT, H. J. DEEG, K. DONEY, M. FLOWERS, J. HANSEN, P. MARTIN, M. PEPE, G. SALE, J. SANDERS, J. SINGER, K. M. SULLIVAN, E. D. THOMAS & R. P. WITHERSPOON. 1994. Cyclophosphamide combined with antithymocyte globulin in preparation for allogeneic marrow transplants in patients with aplastic anemia. Blood **84:** 941–949.

4. CLIFT, R. A., C. D. BUCKNER, E. D. THOMAS, W. I. BENSINGER, R. BOWDEN, E. BRYANT, H. J. DEEG, K. C. DONEY, L. D. FISHER, J. A. HANSEN, P. MARTIN, G. B. MCDONALD, J. E. SANDERS, G. SCHOCH, J. SINGER, R. STORB, K. M. SULLIVAN, R. P. WITHERSPOON & F. R. APPELBAUM. 1994. Marrow transplantation for chronic myeloid leukemia: A randomized study comparing cyclophosphamide and total body irradiation with busulfan and cyclophosphamide. Blood **84:** 2036–2043.
5. WALTERS, M. C., M. PATIENCE, W. LEISENRING, J. R. ECKMAN, J. P. SCOTT, W. C. MENTZER, S. C. DAVIES, K. OHENE-FREMPONG, F. BERNAUDIN, D. C. MATTHEWS, R. STORB & K. M. SULLIVAN. 1996. Bone marrow transplantation for sickle cell disease. N. Engl. J. Med. **335:** 369–376.
6. SULLIVAN, K. M. & D. E. FURST. 1997. The evolving role of blood and marrow transplantation for the treatment of autoimmune diseases. J. Rheumatol. **24**(suppl 48): 1–4.
7. HANSEN, J. A., R. A. CLIFT, E. D. THOMAS, C. D. BUCKNER, R. STORB & E. R. GIBLETT. 1980. Transplantation of marrow from an unrelated donor to a patient with acute leukemia. N. Engl. J. Med. **303:** 565–567.
8. BEATTY, P. G., R. A. CLIFT, E. M. MICKELSON, B. NISPEROS, N. FLOURNOY, P. J. MARTIN, J. E. SANDERS, P. STEWART, C. D. BUCKNER, R. STORB, E. D. THOMAS & J. A. HANSEN. 1985. Marrow transplantation from related donors other than HLA-identical siblings. N. Engl. J. Med. **313:** 765–771.
9. ANASETTI, C., P. G. BEATTY, R. STORB, P. J. MARTIN, M. MORI, J. E. SANDERS, E. D. THOMAS & J. A. HANSEN. 1990. Effect of HLA incompatibility on graft-versus-host disease, relapse, and survival after marrow transplantation for patients with leukemia or lymphoma. Hum. Immunol. **29:** 79–91.
10. MCGLAVE, P., G. BARTSCH, C. ANASETTI, R. ASH, P. BEATTY, J. GAJEWSKI & N. A. KERNAN. 1993. Unrelated donor marrow transplantation therapy for chronic myelogenous leukemia: initial experience of the National Marrow Donor Program. Blood **81:** 543–550.
11. KERNAN, N. A., G. BARTSCH, R. C. ASH, P. G. BEATTY, R. CHAMPLIN, A. FILIPOVICH, J. GAJEWSKI, J. A. HANSEN, J. HENSLEE-DOWNEY, J. M. MCCULLOUGH, P. MCGLAVE, H. A. PERKINS, G. L. PHILLIPS, J. SANDERS, D. STRONCEK, E. D. THOMAS & K. G. BLUME. 1993. Retrospective analysis of 462 unrelated marrow transplants facilitated by the National Marrow Donor Program (NMDP) for treatment of acquired and congenital disorders of the lymphohematopoietic system and congenital metabolic disorders. N. Engl. J. Med. **328:** 593–602.
12. BEARMAN, S. I., M. MORI, P. G. BEATTY, W. G. MEYER, C. D. BUCKNER, F. B. PETERSEN, J. E. SANDERS, C. ANASETTI, P. MARTIN, F. R. APPELBAUM & J. A. HANSEN. 1994. Comparison of morbidity and mortality after marrow transplantation from HLA-genotypically identical siblings and HLA-phenotypically identical unrelated donors. Bone Marrow Transplant. **13:** 31–35.
13. CHOO, S. Y., G. C. STARLING, C. ANASETTI & J. A. HANSEN. 1993. Selection of an unrelated donor for marrow transplantation facilitated by the molecular characterization of a novel HLA-A allele. Hum. Immunol. **36:** 20–26.
14. PETERSDORF, E. W., A. G. SMITH, E. M. MICKELSON, G. M. LONGTON, C. ANASETTI, S. Y. CHOO, P. J. MARTIN & J. A. HANSEN. 1993. The role of HLA-DPB1 disparity in the development of acute graft-versus-host disease following unrelated donor marrow transplantation. Blood **81:** 1923–1932
15. PETERSDORF, E. W., J. F. STANLEY, P. J. MARTIN & J. A. HANSEN. 1994 Molecular diversity of the HLA-C locus in unrelated marrow transplantation. Tissue Antigens **44:** 93–99.
16. STORB, R., M. PEPE, H. J. DEEG, C. ANASETTI, F. R. APPELBAUM, W. BENSINGER, C D. BUCKNER, R. A. CLIFT, K. DONEY, J. HANSEN, P. MARTIN, M. PETTINGER, J. E. SANDERS, J. SINGER, P. STEWART, K. M. SULLIVAN, E. D. THOMAS & R. P. WITHERSPOON. 1992. Long-term follow-up of a controlled trial comparing a combination of methotrexate plus cyclosporine with cyclosporine alone for prophylaxis of graft-versus-host disease in patients administered HLA-identical marrow grafts for leukemia. (Letter to the Editor). Blood **80**: 560–561.
17. NASH, R. A., L. A. PINEIRO, R. STORB, H. J. DEEG, W. E. FITZSIMMONS, T. FURLONG, J. A. HANSEN, T. GOOLEY, R. M. MAHER, P. MARTIN, P. A. MCSWEENEY, K. M. SULLIVAN, C. ANASETTI & J. W. FAY. 1996. FK506 in combination with methotrexate for the prevention of graft-versus-host disease after marrow transplantation from matched unrelated donors. Blood **88:** 3634–3641.

18. GOODRICH, J. M., R. A., BOWDEN, L. FISHER, C. KELLER, G. SCHOCH & J. D. MEYERS. 1993. Ganciclovir prophylaxis to prevent cytomegalovirus disease after allogeneic marrow transplant. Ann. Intern. Med. **118:** 173–178.
19. LANINO, E., C. ANASETTI, G. LONGTON, R. ETZIONI, R. BOWDEN & J. A. HANSEN. 1993. Prevention of cytomegalovirus disease with ganciclovir in recipients of marrow transplants from unrelated donors [abstract]. Blood **82:** 1359a.
20. ANASETTI, C. & J. HANSEN. 1993. Bone marrow transplantation from HLA-partially matched related donors and unrelated volunteer donors. *In* Bone Marrow Transplantation. S. J. Forman, K. G. Blume & E. D. Thomas, Eds.: 665–679. Blackwell Scientific Publications. Cambridge, MA.
21. HANSEN, J. A., T. A. GOOLEY, P. J. MARTIN, F. APPELBAUM, T. R. CHAUNCEY, R. A. CLIFT, E. W. PETERSDORF, J. RADICH, J. E. SANDERS, R. F. STORB, K. M. SULLIVAN & A. ANASETTI. 1998. Bone marrow transplants from unrelated donors for patients with chronic myeloid leukemia. N. Engl. J. Med. **338:** 962–968.
22. MCCULLOUGH, J., J. HANSEN, H. PERKINS, D. STRONCEK & G. BARTSCH. 1989. The National Marrow Donor Program: How it works, accomplishments to date. Oncology **3:** 63–72.
23. ANASETTI, C. 1997. Marrow transplantation from unrelated volunteer donors. Bone Marrow Transplant. **19**(suppl 2): 57–59.
24. HANSEN, J. A., S. Y. CHOO, D. E. GERAGHTY & E. MICKELSON. 1990. The HLA system in clinical marrow transplantation. Hematol. Oncol. Clin. N. Am. S. J. Forman, Ed.: 507–515. W. B. Saunders Co. Philadelphia, PA.
25. RODEY, G. E. & T. C. FULLER. 1987. Public epitopes and the antigen structure of the HLA molecules. Crit. Rev. Immunol. **7:** 3–229.
26. National Marrow Donor Center Manual of Operations. 1992 edition. Minnneapolis, MN
27. ANASETTI, C., D. AMOS, P. G. BEATTY, F. R. APPELBAUM, W. BENSINGER, C. D. BUCKNER, R. CLIFT, K. DONEY, P. J. MARTIN, E. MICKELSON, B. NISPEROS, J. O'QUIGLEY, R. RAMBERG, J. E. SANDERS, P. STEWART, R. STORB, K. M. SULLIVAN, R. P. WITHERSPOON, E. D. THOMAS & J. A. HANSEN. 1989. Effect of HLA compatibility on engraftment of bone marrow transplants in patients with leukemia or lymphoma. N. Engl. J. Med. **320:** 197–204.
28. PETERSDORF, E. W., G. M. LONGTON, C. ANASETTI, E. M. MICKELSON, S. K. MCKINNEY, A. G. SMITH, P. J. MARTIN & J. A. HANSEN. 1997. Association of HLA-C disparity with graft failure after marrow transplantation from unrelated donors. Blood **89:** 1818–1832.
29. GLUCKSBERG, H., R. STORB, A. FEFER, C. D. BUCKNER, P. E. NEIMAN, R. A. CLIFT, K. G. LERNER & E. D. THOMAS. 1974. Clinical manifestations of graft-versus-host disease in human recipients of marrow from HL-A-matched sibling donors. Transplantation **18:** 295–304.
30. BEATTY, P. G., J. A. HANSEN, G. M. LONGTON, E. D. THOMAS, J. E. SANDERS, P. J. MARTIN, S. I. BEARMAN, C. ANASETTI, E. W. PETERSDORF, E. M. MICKELSON, M. S. PEPE, F. R. APPELBAUM, C. D. BUCKNER, R. A. CLIFT, F. B. PETERSEN, P. S. STEWART, R. F. STORB, K. M. SULLIVAN, M. C. TESLER & R. P. WITHERSPOON. 1991. Marrow transplantation from HLA-matched unrelated donors for treatment of hematologic malignancies. Transplantation **51:** 443–447.
31. SULLIVAN, K. M., H. M. SHULMAN, R. STORB, P. L. WEIDEN, R. P. WITHERSPOON, G. B. MCDONALD, M. M. SCHUBERT, K. ATKINSON & E. D. THOMAS. 1981. Chronic graft-versus-host disease in 52 patients: adverse natural course and successful treatment with combination immunosuppression. Blood **57:** 267–276.
32. SULLIVAN, K. M., E. AGURA, C. ANASETTI, F. R. APPELBAUM, C. BADGER, S. BEARMAN, K. ERICKSON, M. FLOWERS, J. A. HANSEN, T. LOUGHRAN, P. MARTIN, D. MATTHEWS, E. PETERSDORF, J. RADICH, S. RIDDELL, D. ROVIRA, J. SANDERS, F. SCHUENING, M. SIADAK, R. STORB & R. P. WITHERSPOON. 1991. Chronic graft-versus-host disease and other late complications of bone marrow transplantation. Sem. Hematol. **28:** 250–259.
33. BEATTY, P. G., C. ANASETTI, J. A. HANSEN, G. M. LONGTON, J. E. SANDERS, P. J. MARTIN, E. M. MICKELSON, S. Y. CHOO, E. W. PETERSDORF, M. S. PEPE, F. R. APPELBAUM, S. I. BEARMAN, C. D. BUCKNER, R. A. CLIFT, F. B. PETERSEN, J. SINGER, P. S. STEWART, R. F. STORB, K. M. SULLIVAN, M. C. TESLER, R. P. WITHERSPOON & E. D. THOMAS. 1993. Marrow transplantation from unrelated donors for treatment of hematologic malignancies: Effect of mismatching for one HLA locus. Blood **81:** 249–253.

34. PETERSDORF, E. W., G. M. LONGTON, C. ANASETTI, P. J. MARTIN, E. M. MICKELSON, A. G. SMITH & J. A. HANSEN. 1995. The significance of HLA-DRB1 matching on clinical outcome after HLA-A, B, DR identical unrelated donor marrow transplantation. Blood **86:** 1606–1613.
35. BALDUZZI, A., T. GOOLEY, C. ANASETTI, J. E. SANDERS, P. J. MARTIN, E. W. PETERSDORF, F. R. APPELBAUM, C. D. BUCKNER, D. MATTHEWS, R. STORB, K. M. SULLIVAN & J. A. HANSEN. 1995. Unrelated donor marrow transplantation in children. Blood **86:** 3247–3256.
36. SIERRA, J., B. STORER, J. A. HANSEN, J. W. BJERKE, P. J. MARTIN, E. W. PETERSDORF, F. R. APPELBAUM, E. BRYANT, T. R. CHAUNCEY, G. SALE, J. E. SANDERS, R. STORB, K. M. SULLIVAN & C. ANASETTI. 1997. Transplantation of marrow cells from unrelated donors for treatment of high-risk acute leukemia: The effect of leukemic burden, donor HLA-matching, and marrow cell dose. Blood **89:** 4226–4235.
37. APPELBAUM, F. R., L. D. FISHER & E. D. THOMAS AND THE SEATTLE MARROW TRANSPLANT TEAM. 1988. Chemotherapy v marrow transplantation for adults with acute nonlymphocytic leukemia: A five-year follow-up. Blood **72:** 179–184.
38. SULLIVAN, K. M., P. L. WEIDEN, R. STORB, R. P. WITHERSPOON, A. FEFER, L. FISHER, C. D. BUCKNER, C. ANASETTI, F. R. APPELBAUM, C. BADGER, P. BEATTY, W. BENSINGER, R. BERENSON, C. BIGELOW, M. A. CHEEVER, R. CLIFT, H. J. DEEG, K. DONEY, P. GREENBERG, J. A. HANSEN, R. HILL, T. LOUGHRAN, P. MARTIN, P. NEIMAN, F. B. PETERSEN, J. SANDERS, J. SINGER, P. STEWART & E. D. THOMAS. 1989. Influence of acute and chronic graft-versus-host disease on relapse and survival after bone marrow transplantation from HLA-identical siblings as treatment of acute and chronic leukemia. Blood **73:** 1720–1728.
39. HANSEN, J. A., E. W. PETERSDORF, S. Y. CHOO, P. J. MARTIN & C. ANASETTI. 1995. Marrow transplantation from HLA partially matched relatives and unrelated donors. Bone Marrow Transplant. **15:** S128–S139.
40. GALIMABERTI, M., E. ANGELUCCI, D. BARONCIANI, G. GIARDINI, P. POLCHI, B. ERER, D. J. GAZIEV, C. PAZZAGLIA, A. CIARONI, M. BALDASSARRI, F. MARTINELLI & G. LUCARELLI. 1997. Bone Marrow Transplantation in Thalassemia: The experience of Pesaro. Bone Marrow Transplant. **19**(suppl 2): 45–47.
41. WALTERS, M. C., K. M. SULLIVAN, R. J. O'REILLY, F. BOULAD, J. BROCHSTEIN, K. BLUME, M. AMYLON, F. L. JOHNSON, M. KLEMPERER, J. GRAHAM-POLE, F. R. APPELBAUM, J. A. HANSEN, J. E. SANDERS, R. STORB & E. D. THOMAS. 1994. Bone marrow transplantation for thalassemia: The USA experience. Am. J. Ped. Hematol. Oncol. **16:** 11–17.
42. CLIFT, R. A. & F. L. JOHNSON. 1997. Marrow transplants for thalassemia: the USA experience. Bone Marrow Transplant **19**(suppl 2):57–59.
43. CONTU, L., G. LA NASA & M. ARRAS. 1994. Bone marrow transplantation in beta-thalassemia. Bone Marrow Transplant. **13:** 329–331.
44. SANTAMARIA, P., N. L. REINSMOEN, A. L. LINDSTROM et al. 1994. Frequent HLA class I and DP sequence mismatches in serologically (HLA-A, HLA-B, HLA-DR) and molecularly (HLA-DRB1, HLA-DQAI, HLA-DQBI) HLA-identical unrelated marrow transplant pairs. Blood. **83:** 280–287.
45. SULLIVAN, K. M., M. C. WALTERS, M. PATIENCE, W. LEISENRING, G. R. BUCHANAN, O. CASTRO, S. C. DAVIES, R. DICKERHOFF, J. R. ECKMAN, M. L. GRAHAM, K. OHENE-FREMPONG, D. POWARS, Z. R. ROGERS, J. P. SCOTT, L. STYLES, E. VICHINSKY, D. A. WALL, A. S. WAYNE, J. WILEY, J. WINGARD, N. BUNIN, B. CAMITTA, P. J. DARBYSHIRE, P. DINNDORF, T. KLINGEBIEL, L. MCMAHON, W. C. MENTZER, N. OLIVIERI, E. ORRINGER, R. PARKMAN, I. A. G. ROBERTS, J. E. SANDERS, F. O. SMITH & R. STORB. 1997. Collaborative study of marrow transplantation for sickle cell disease: aspects specific for transplantation of hemoglobin disorders. Bone Marrow Transplant. **19**(suppl 2) 102–105.
46. DOVER, G. L. & D. VALLE. 1994. Therapy for beta-thalassemia—a paradigm for the treatment of genetic disorders [editorial]. N. Engl. J. Med. **331:** 609–610.
47. SULLIVAN, K. M. 1997. Long-term follow-up and quality of life after hematopoietic stem cell transplantation. J. Rheumatol. **24**(suppl 48) 46–52.
48. ANDREANI, M., M. MANNA, G. LUCARELLI, P. TONUCCI, F. AGOSTINELLI, M. RIPALTI, S. RAPA, N. TALEVI, M. GALIMBERTI & S. NESCI. 1996. Persistence of mixed chimerism in patients transplanted for the treatment of thalassemia. Blood **87:** 3494–3499.

49. MANNA, M., S. NESCI, G. LUCARELLI, P. TONUCCI, M. RIPALTI, S. RAPA, F. AGOSTINELLI & M. ANDREANI. 1997. Mixed chimerism after bone marrow transplantation in Thalassemia. Bone Marrow Transplant. **19**(suppl. 2):87–88.
50. WALTERS, M. C., M. PATIENC, W. LEISENRING, Z. R. ROGERS, P. DINNDORF, S. C. DAVIES, I. A. G. ROBERT, A. YEAGER, J. KURTZBERG, N. BUNIN, J. P. SCOTT, D. A. WALL, A. S. WAYNE, J. WILEY, P. J. DARBYSHIRE, W. C. MENTZEN, F. O. SMITH & K. M. SULLIVAN. 1997. Collaborative multicenter investigation of marrow transplantation for sickle cell disease: Current results and future directions. Biol. Blood Marrow Transplantation **3**: 310–315.
51. STORB, R., C. YU, J. L. WAGNER, H. J. DEEG, R. A. NASH, H.-P. KIEM, W. LEISENRING & H. SHULMAN. 1997. Stable mixed hematopoietic chimerism in DLA-identical littermate dogs given sublethal total body irradiation before and pharmacological immunosuppression after marrow transplantation. Blood **89**: 3048–3054.

Relationship between Genotype and Phenotype

Thalassemia Intermedia[a]

RENZO GALANELLO[b] AND ANTONIO CAO

Istituto di Clinica e Biologia dell'Età Evolutiva, Ospedale Regionale per le Microcitemie Azienda A.S.L., 8 Cagliari, Italy

ABSTRACT: Thalassemia intermedia encompasses a number of clinical conditions ranging in severity from β-thalassemia carrier state to transfusion-dependent thalassemia major. The molecular bases of thalassemia intermedia, only partially defined, are very heterogeneous, but in general any factor able to reduce the globin-chain imbalance results in a milder form of thalassemia. These factors are the presence of a silent or mild β-thalassemia allele, associated with a high residual β-globin production, and the coinheritance of α-thalassemia or of genetic determinants that increase the γ-chain production. Less frequent mechanisms are double heterozygosity for β-thalassemia and triplicated α genes, and the presence of a hyperunstable hemoglobin variant. However, for a consistent number of β^0-thalassemia homozygotes with a thalassemia intermedia phenotype the modifying factor has not been defined yet. In contrast, there are simple β-thalassemia carriers who, for unknown reasons, have an unusually severe clinical phenotype.

The progress in molecular biology and the wide availability of methods for DNA analysis have allowed the definition of globin gene defects in thalassemia syndromes and partially elucidated the relationship between genotype and phenotype. This knowledge has been helpful in clinical practice for the prediction of the phenotype in genetic counseling and prenatal diagnosis, and for planning the appropriate treatment in homozygous β-thalassemia patients. These patients most commonly present a severe transfusion-dependent anemia from the first year of life, a condition known as thalassemia major. However, a minority of patients show a mild clinical picture of survival without a regular transfusion requirement. This condition, defined as thalassemia intermedia, is extremely heterogeneous and encompasses a wide spectrum of phenotypes ranging in severity from a severe anemia, with hepato-splenomegaly and marked thalassemia-like bone modifications, to a moderate microcytic hypochromic anemia with barely enlarged spleen and almost absent facial bone alterations.

Thalassemia intermedia is equally very heterogeneous at the genotype level. These patients are most commonly homozygotes or compound heterozygotes for β-thalassemia, having both β-globin loci affected. Less frequently only a single β-globin locus is mutated,

---

[a]This work supported by CNR-Progetto Strategico nel Mezzogiorno N. 95.0467153st 75; MPI 60% Theleton Prog. no. E 502 and Legge Regionale 30.04.1990 n.11 Regione Sardegna.

[b]Address for correspondence: Renzo Galanello, Ospedale Regionale per le Microcitemie, Via Jenner s.n., 09121 Cagliari, Phone: + 39 70 6095508; Fax: + 39 70 6095509; e-mail: renzo.galanell@mcweb.unica.it

the other being completely normal (TABLE 1). In this paper the relationship between molecular mechanisms and clinical aspects of this disorder will be discussed.

THALASSEMIA INTERMEDIA ASSOCIATED WITH HOMOZYGOUS OR COMPOUND HETEROZYGOUS β-THALASSEMIA

The degree of globin-chain imbalance is the main determinant of the severity of thalassemia syndromes. The absent or reduced production of β-globin leads to a relative excess of α-chains, which are highly unstable and precipitate in the bone marrow erythroid precursors causing membrane damage and cell death.

This ineffective erythropoiesis is the principal determinant of anemia, while peripheral hemolysis of mature red cells containing α-chain inclusions and the overall reduction in hemoglobin synthesis per cell are secondary mechanisms. In homozygous β-thalassemia patients any inherited or acquired factor able to reduce the degree of globin imbalance may thus produce milder clinical forms.

Three main factors have been so far identified: (1) presence of mild or silent β-thalassemia alleles; (2) coinheritance of α-thalassemia; and (3) coinheritance of determinants associated with increased γ-chain production.

Presence of Mild or Silent β-Thalassemia Alleles

Mild β-thalassemia mutations (TABLE 2) are characterized by a residual high β-chain production (Baysal & Carver[1] present detailed references to individual mutations). This group of molecular defects includes transcriptional mutants in the proximal CACCC box and in the TATA box, consensus sequence, and polyadenylation mutants. Homozygotes or compound heterozygotes for these mild mutations usually have thalassemia intermedia, while compound heterozygosity for a mild and severe mutation may produce either thalassemia intermedia or thalassemia major. Some of these mutations are ethnic specific: -87 C→T and IVS 1-6 T→C are common in Mediterraneans, -29 A→G and -88 C→T are frequently found in blacks.

It is interesting to note that among promoter mutations, different substitutions at the same position may produce different phenotypes. In fact, the common Mediterranean -87 C→G mutation in interaction with a severe β-thalassemia defect usually results in tha-

TABLE 1. Molecular Mechanisms for β-Thalassemia Intermedia

Homozygotes
Reduction of globin chain imbalance
Silent and mild β-thalassemia mutations
homozygosity
compound heterozygosity with severe mutation
Coinheritance of α-thalassemia
Coinheritance of genetic determinants increasing HbF
Heterozygotes:
Worsening of globin chain imbalance
coinheritance of triplicated α-globin locus
compound heterozygosity with pancellular HPFH
hyperunstable globins
unknown mechanism
Associated globin variant
compound heterozygosity with some β-globin variants

lassemia intermedia, while the C→T substitution at the same position is associated with thalassemia major.

Another group of mild β-thalassemia mutations in the first exon (cod 19, 26, and 27) is associated with nucleotide substitutions, which modify the DNA sequence of this region making it more similar to a splicing donor site. The consequence is an aberrant splicing of precursor mRNA through these activated sites, with a consequent decrease in normal splicing. These mutations, being in exon 1, result also in abnormal hemoglobin production. Hb E (cd 26 G→A) is very common in Southeast Asians and Hb Knossos (cd 27 G→T) has been described in Mediterraneans. Homozygotes for both Hb E and Hb Knossos have a mild thalassemia intermedia. Compound heterozygosity for Hb Knossos and severe β-thalassemia result in the typical thalassemia intermedia, while compound heterozygosity for HbE and β^0 or β^+ thalassemia results in severe thalassemia major. The IVS1-6 T→C substitution, referred to as the Portuguese form of β-thalassemia,[2] accounts for the majority of the β^+ thalassemia intermedia in the Mediterranean area, both in the homozygous state and in combination with severe β-gene defect. However, the same mutation has been reported in a severe form in Spain and Lebanon.[3,4]

Silent β-thalassemia (TABLE 2) belongs to a peculiar group of thalassemic defects characterized in the heterozygous state by normal MCV and MCH, normal or more frequently borderline HbA_2, and normal HbF. Globin chain synthesis ratio is only slightly imbalanced, and sometimes even normal. This phenotype may escape detection by the usual screening methods, but a careful evaluation of HbA_2 may lead to correct identification by DNA analysis. The most common silent β-thalassemia mutation is -101 C→T within the distal CACCC box, present mainly in Mediterranean population.[5] Compound heterozygosity of -101 mutation with a severe mutation always produces a very mild thalassemia intermedia. Frequently the diagnosis is made in adulthood or even in the elderly.

A peculiar mutation of this group is the IVS2 844 C→G substitution within the consensus sequence of the IVS2 acceptor splice site.[6] Carriers of this mutation are hematologically silent or with very mild modifications; homozygotes have the typical manifestations of heterozygotes for β-thalassemia, while compound heterozygotes for this and a severe mutation may have the phenotype of thalassemia intermedia or of transfusion-dependent thalassemia major. The phenotype associated with IVS2-844 mutation in combination with severe β-thalassemia is therefore unpredictable.

TABLE 2. Mild and Silent β-Thalassemia Mutations

MILD
    Transcription
        -88 C→T, -87 C→G, -86 C→A, -31 A→G, -30 T→A, -29 A→G
    Splice site activation
        cd 19 A→G (Hb Malay), cd 26 G→A (HbE), cd 27 G→T (Hb Knossos)
    Consensus sequence
        IVS 1-6 T→C
    Polyadenmilation
        AATAAA→AACAAA
        AATGAA→AATAGA
            →A(-AATAA)
SILENT
    Transcription
        promoter -101 C→ , -92 C→T
            -5' UTR + 1 A→C, +10-T, +33 C→G
            -3' UTR + C→G
        Consensus sequence: IVS2-844 C→G
        Polyadenylation: AATAA<u>A</u>→AATAAG

Coinheritance of α-Thalassemia

Coinheritance with homozygous β-thalassemia of α-thalassemia leads to a reduction in the excess of α-chain pool and inclusion-body formation in erythroid precursors. Extensive studies in Mediterranean and Southeast Asian patients have shown a significant difference in the frequency of α-thalassemia between thalassemia intermedia and thalassemia major.[7-9] However, the ameliorating effect depends both on the type of coinherited α-thalassemia and on the severity of β-thalassemia mutation. In homozygotes for β$^+$-thalassemia, who have some residual β-globin chain output, even a single α-globin gene deletion (-α/αα) is able to ameliorate the clinical picture. Homozygotes for β^0-thalassemia may have a beneficial effect by the coinheritance of two α-globin genes deletion (-α/-α) or of a non-deletion defect in the α2 gene.

However since each genetic combination is associated with a wide range of clinical outcomes, the definition of the α-globin genotype in any single patient may not have an absolute value in the prediction of the clinical phenotype.

Coinheritance of Determinants Associated with Increased γ-Chain Production

The increase in γ-chain production has an ameliorating effect on the clinical picture of homozygous β-thalassemia, not only by reducing the overall α/non α-globin–chain imbalance but also by producing a net increase in total hemoglobin synthesis. Several genetic determinants able to enhance γ-globin chains in β-thalassemia homozygotes have been identified (TABLE 3).

The first group includes those β-thalassemia defects with an intrinsic propensity to increase γ-chain output. This is clearly shown by the variable increase in HbF levels in heterozygotes for these defects. Deletion δβ-thalassemia refers to a group of complex β-thalassemia defects resulting from deletions of variable extent of the β-globin gene cluster, which remove δ and β gene.[10] These mutations are characterized by absent δ- and β-globin chain and increased γ-chain production. Homozygotes for δβ-thalassemia, and less consistently, compound heterozygotes with β-thalassemia, have the clinical phenotype of thalassemia intermedia.

Hb Lepore is a δβ fusion chain resulting from non-homologous crossing over between δ- and β-globin genes.[11] This determinant is usually associated with slightly increased HbF levels. Homozygotes for Hb Lepore and compound heterozygotes for this mutation and severe β-thalassemia show a heterogeneous clinical picture ranging from thalassemia major to thalassemia intermedia.

TABLE 3. Genetic Determinants Increasing HbF in Homozygotes for β-Thalassemia

Intrinsic to the β-thalassemia mutation
Deletion δβ thalassemia
5' β promoter deletion
Hb Lepore
Associated Gγ or Aγ promoter mutation
196 C→T Aγ linked to β^{0}39 C→T
158 C→T Gγ linked to FS cd 6 - A
FS cd 8 - AA
IVS2-1 G→A
β^{0}39 C→T
Related to coinherited heterocellular HPFH

The 5′ β promoter deletions, even if widely different in size, have in common the loss of the region from position -125 to +78 (relative to the Cap site) which includes the CACCC, CAAT, and TATA boxes.[12–15] Interestingly homozygotes for three common β promoter mutations, namely -88 C→T, -87 C→G, and -29 A→G, also show very high levels of HbF (average values: 64.5%, 32.5%, and 60.6% respectively). It is possible that when the β promoter region is involved there is a reduced interaction with transcription factors and LCR in favor of γ promoter interaction. Another group of determinants able to increase HbF production are mutations in the Gγ or Aγ promoter region associated with β-thalassemia mutations.

The most common is -158 C→T Gγ promoter substitution, which is in linkage disequilibrium with frameshift cd 6 (-A), frameshift cd 8 (-AA), and IVS2-1 G→A β-thalassemia.[16] This mutation leads to enhanced γ chain production, mainly Gγ chains, under conditions of erythropoietic stress, partially compensating for absent β chain synthesis in homozygotes for the previous reported β-thalassemia mutations, with consequent amelioration of globin chain imbalance and of the clinical phenotype. The -158 C→T Gγ promoter substitution has been found occasionally in subjects with the mild β$^+$IVS1-6 T→C and with the severe β^{0}39 C→T mutation associated with haplotype IV and IX respectively[17] (Galanello et al., unpublished observations). The usual severe clinical picture of homozygous β^{0}39 is ameliorated by the presence of -158 C→T substitution, resulting in thalassemia intermedia.

The non-deletion HPFH mutation C→T at position -196 in the Aγ promoter, when linked "in cis" to the β^{0}39 mutation, results in the so-called Sardinian non-deletion δβ-thalassemia, characterized in the heterozygous state by high HbF levels in the order of 12 to 17%, normal HbA2, and moderate red blood cell indices modifications, and in the compound heterozygous state with β^{0}39 mutation by the typical clinical features of thalassemia intermedia.[18]

Molecular analysis of 91 β^0 thalassemia intermedia Sardinian patients showed that there are two genetic determinants able to increase γ chain production, i.e., 196 Aγ C→T mutation associated with β^{0}39 nonsense mutation and -158 Gg C→T mutation, which is associated in 100% of the cases with frameshift mutation (-A) at codon 6 and less frequently with β^{0}39 nonsense mutation (TABLE 4).[9] These genetic determinants have been found in 33 out of 91 patients accounting for 36% of the cases of β^0 thalassemia intermedia in our population (Galanello et al. unpublished observations).

Heterocellular HPFH is defined as an increase in HbF levels of > 1.0%, distributed among 15 to 20% of red cells, referred to as F cells. Normal subjects have HbF levels of < 1.0% and F cells < 4.0%. In two large families of Sardinian and Asian origin it has been shown that the coinheritance of heterocellular HPFH, demonstrated by the presence of increased F levels in normal members of these families, is able to ameliorate the clinical picture in homozygotes for β^0-thalassemia with Hb levels of 10–12 g/dl.[19,20]

This type of HPFH is unlinked to β-globin cluster and its genetics is quite heterogeneous. The identification of genes involved in γ-globin chain production control is under active investigation and candidate regions have been defined in chromosome 6q 22.3-23.1 and Xp 22.2-22.3.[21,22]

The coinheritance of such types of HPFH may account for the mild clinical picture of thalassemia intermedia present in a minority of homozygotes or compound heterozygotes

TABLE 4. Genetic Determinants Associated with Increased γ Chain Production in Sardinian β^0-Thalassemia Intermedia

γ Gene Promoter Mutation	β Gene Mutation	N of Patients
-196 Aγ C→T	β^{0}39 C→T	6
-158 Gγ C→T	β^{0}39 C→T	6
-158 Gγ C→T	β^{0}6 - A	21

for β^0-thalassemia or severe β^+ thalassemia, who show at molecular level no evident modifying factors.

THALASSEMIA INTERMEDIA IN HETEROZYGOTES FOR β-THALASSEMIA

Several patients with thalassemia intermedia have only a single β-globin gene affected and therefore are considered heterozygotes for β-thalassemia. The worsening of globin-chain imbalance in the majority of cases results from the coinheritance with heterozygous β-thalassemia of one or two extra α-globin genes, due to heterozygous or homozygous state for triplicated α-gene complex ($\alpha\alpha\alpha/\alpha\alpha$ or $\alpha\alpha\alpha/\alpha\alpha\alpha$). The clinical phenotype of β-thalassemia heterozygotes with interacting homozygosity for α-globin gene triplication is a moderate to relatively severe thalassemia intermedia, occasionally requiring transfusion therapy.[23–25] Heterozygotes for severe β-thalassemia mutations with one extra α-globin gene ($\alpha\alpha\alpha/\alpha\alpha$) show more heterogeneous clinical features. Most of the cases present a severe carrier phenotype with raised HbF levels and increased reticulocyte count, but sometimes this genetic interaction results in typical thalassemia intermedia.

The compound heterozygosity for severe β-thalassemia with both deletion and non deletion pancellular HPFH results in a mild thalassemia intermedia phenotype.

Hyperunstable hemoglobins are a group of hemoglobin variants able to produce the clinical picture of thalassemia intermedia of variable severity when present in heterozygous state.[26] For this reason, they are also referred to as dominant β-thalassemias. Short-time incubation and pulse-chase globin-chain synthesis experiments have clearly shown that these β variants undergo rapid aggregation and precipitation in bone marrow erythroid precursors. The continuous degradation of these β variants exhausts the cell proteolytic capacity, leading to accumulation of excess free α chains in a greater amount than that observed in β-thalassemia heterozygotes. Both α and β variant globins precipitate, leading to inclusion-body formation and cell damage. Due to the inability to form tetramers with α chains and to the early degradation, these variants are usually not detectable in peripheral blood by common detection methods. At the molecular level, four distinct groups have been defined: single base substitutions, deletion of intact codons, premature termination resulting in truncated β-globin chains, and frameshift mutations producing elongated β-globin chains. The clinical phenotype of carriers of these hyperunstable variants is markedly heterogeneous, varying from a severe carrier state to a serious transfusion-dependent anemia. Besides ineffective erythropoiesis, there is also a consistent hemolytic component. Sometimes splenectomy may eliminate transfusion dependency. These disorders are rare and have been described in many ethnic groups. The presence of hyperunstable hemoglobins should be suspected in any patient with thalassemia intermedia phenotype when both parents are hematologically normal.

Recently several patients with the typical thalassemia intermedia clinical picture have been reported, in whom only a single β gene is affected by a β-thalassemia mutation. In three families studied in our hospital the phenotype of six patients is characterized by moderate to severe microcytic and hypochromic anemia, splenomegaly, mild jaundice, marked α/non α imbalance, slight to moderate HbF increase, and nucleated red cells in peripheral blood. Sequence analysis of the β-globin gene from these patients revealed only heterozygosity for the codon 39 nonsense mutation (FIG. 1). Extensive analysis of β-globin gene cluster, LCR and α-globin genes in these families failed to identify any other associated molecular defect. One of the parents was heterozygous for codon 39 nonsense mutation with a typical carrier phenotype, the other was hematologically normal and had normal β-globin gene sequence. We postulated the presence of an atypical β-thalassemia

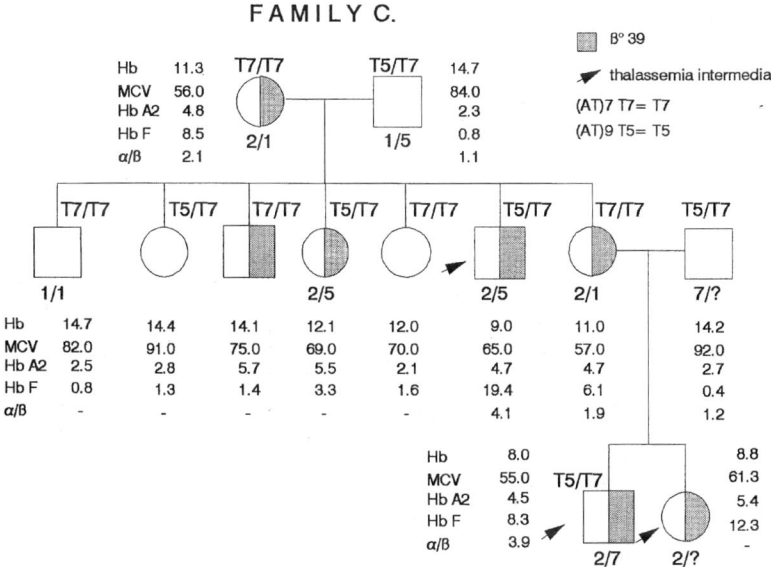

FIGURE 1. Pedigree of a family with heterozygous β–thalassemia and thalassemia intermedia phenotype.

determinant not linked to the β-globin cluster, which can worsen the α/non-α imbalance, leading to ineffective erythropoiesis.

Finally, compound heterozygosity for β-thalassemia and some structural β-chain variants may result in clinical and hematological features of β-thalassemia intermedia. The most common interacting variants are HbD Los Angeles (β121 glu→gen), HbC (β6 glu→lys), HbO-Arab (β121 glu→lys), and some electrophoretically silent variants such as Hb City of Hope (β69 gly→ser). The globin-chain imbalance in combination with the modified structural and functional characteristics of the Hb variant may produce a more severe phenotype compared to that observed in simple heterozygotes and even homozygotes for these variants.[27,28]

CONCLUSIONS

The knowledge of the relationship between genotype and phenotype has important implications for the screening of β-thalassemia carriers, genetic counselling, and prenatal diagnosis and for planning appropriate treatment of the patients.

When the presence of a mild to silent β-thalassemia mutation is suspected, accurate methods for identification should be used. The definition of β-thalassemia mutation and appropriate analysis of the α- and γ-globin genes in prospective parents may be useful in genetic counselling, allowing prediction of the clinical phenotype. The differentiation at presentation between thalassemia major and thalassemia intermedia is essential to design an appropriate treatment. In fact, the precise prediction of a mild phenotype may avoid needless transfusions and their complications, while the diagnosis of thalassemia major will allow an early start of the transfusion program, thus preventing hypersplenism and red cell antigen sensitization. Unfortunately, the accurate identification of these two phenotypes at the onset is sometimes difficult. Nevertheless, a careful analysis of clinical, hematologic, genetic, and molecular data may allow a reasonable aptitude for treatment

The contrasting clinical phenotypes (severe and mild) observed in patients with the same β-thalassemia mutation may be related to undefined determinants able to modify the globin-chain imbalance. For example, there is little information on the proteolytic mechanism in the erythroid precursors and the control of γ-globin chain production has been only partly clarified. Moreover, the tendency of some physicians to regularly transfuse thalassemic patients when the hemoglobin falls below 7.5 g/dl may be the cause for some phenotypic differences.

In conclusion, although a large body of information has been achieved on molecular mechanisms of thalassemia and this resulted in a better understanding of the clinical heterogeneity of thalassemic syndromes, the reason for the mild clinical expression in a consistent number of patients with thalassemia intermedia still remains to be elucidated.

ACKNOWLEDGMENTS

We thank Valeria Siccardo for editorial assistance.

REFERENCES

1. BAYSAL, E. & M. F. H. CARVER. 1995. The β and δ-thalassemia repository. Hemoglobin **19**: 213–236.
2. TAMAGNINI, G. P. et al. 1983. β$^+$-thalassemia-Portuguese type: clinical, hematological and molecular studies of a newly defined form of β thalassemia. Br. J. Haematol. **54**: 189–200.
3. CHEHAB, F. F. et al. 1987. The molecular basis of β-thalassemia in Lebanon: Application to prenatal diagnosis. Blood **69**: 1141–1145.
4. AMSELEM, S. et al. 1988. Determination of the spectrum of β-thalassemia genes in Spain by use of dot-blot analysis of amplified β-globin DNA. Am. J. Hum. Genet. **43**: 95–100.
5. GONZALEZ-REDONDO, J. M. et al. 1989. A C→T substitution nt-101 in a conserved DNA sequence of the promoter region of the β-globin gene is associated with "silent" β-thalassemia. Blood **73**: 1705–1711.
6. MURRU, S. et al. 1991. Molecular characterization of β-thalassemia intermedia in patients of Italian descent and identification of three novel β-thalassemia mutations. Blood **77**: 1342–1347.
7. WAINSCOAT, J. S. et al. 1983. Thalassemia intermedia—the interaction of α and β-thalassemia. Br J Haematol **53**: 411–416.
8. THEIN, S. L. et al. 1988. The molecular basis of thalassemia major and thalassemia intermedia in Asian Indians: application to prenatal diagnosis. Br. J. Haematol. **70**: 225–231.
9. GALANELLO, R. et al. 1989. Molecular analysis of β^0-thalassemia intermedia in Sardinia. Blood **74**: 823–827.
10. WOOD, W. G. 1993: Increased HbF in adult life. Bailliere's Clin. Hematol. **6**: 177–213.
11. BAIRD, M. et al. 1981. Localization of the site of recombination in formation of the Lepore Boston globin gene. J. Clin. Invest **68**: 560.
12. PADANILAM, B. J. et al. 1984. Partial deletion of the 5'β-globin gene region causes β^0-thalassemia in members of an American black family. Blood **64**: 941–944.
13. POPOVITCH, B. W. et al. 1986. Molecular characterization of an atypical β-thalassemia caused by a large deletion in the 5'β-globin gene region. Am. J. Hum. Genet. **39**: 797–810.
14. DIAZ-CHICO, J. C. et al. 1987. An ~300 bp deletion involving part of the 5'β-globin gene region is observed in members of a Turkish family with β-thalassemia. Blood **70**: 583–586.
15. GILMAN, J. G. 1987. The 12.6 kilobase deletion in Dutch β^0-thalassemia. Br. J. Haematol. **67**: 369–372.
16. GILMAN, J. G. & T. H. J. HUISMAN. 1985. DNA sequence variation associated with elevated fetal ^{G}γ globin production. Blood **66**: 783–787.

17. EFREMOV, D. G. et al. 1994. Possible factors influencing the haemoglobin and fetal haemoglobin levels in patients with beta-thalassemia due to a homozygosity for the IVS 1–6 (T→C) mutation. Br. J. Haematol.
18. PIRASTU, M. et al. 1984. Multiple mutations produce $\delta\beta^0$-thalassemia in Sardinia. Science **223**: 924–930.
19. CAPPELLINI, M. D., G. FIORELLI & L. F. BERNINI. 1981. Interaction between homozygous β^0-thalassaemia and the Swiss type of hereditary persistence of fetal haemoglobin. Br. J. Haematol. **48**: 561–572.
20. THEIN, S. L. & D. J. WEATHERALL. 1989. A non-deletion hereditary persistence of fetal hemoglobin (HPFH) determinant not linked to the β-globin gene complex. *In* Hemoglobin Switching. Part B: Cellular and Molecular Mechanisms. G. Stamatoyannopoulos & A. W. Nienhuis Eds.: 97–111. Alan R Liss. New York.
21. CRAIG, J. E. et al. 1996. Dissecting the loci controlling fetal haemoglobin production on chromosomes 11p and 6q by the regressive approach. Nature Genetics **12**: 58–64.
22. DOVER, G. J. et al. 1992. Fetal hemoglobin levels in sickle cell disease and normal individuals are partially controlled by an X-linked gene located at Xp22.2. Blood **80**: 816–824.
23. GALANELLO, R. et al. 1983. A family with segregating triplicated α-globin locus and β-thalassemia. Blood **62**: 1035–1040.
24. CAMASCHELLA, C. et al. 1987. A benign form of thalassemia intermedia may be determined by the interaction of triplicated α locus and heterozygous β-thalassemia. Br. J. Haematol. **66**: 103–107.
25. TRAEGER-SYNODINOS, J. et al. 1996. The triplicated α-globin gene locus in β-thalassemia heterozygotes: clinical, haematological, biosynthetic and molecular studies. Br. J. Haematol. **95**: 467–471.
26. THEIN, S. L. et al. 1990. Molecular basis of dominantly inherited inclusion body β-thalassemia. Proc. Natl. Acad. Sci. USA **87**: 3924–3928.
27. HUISMAN, T. H. J. 1990. Silent β-thalassemia and thalassemia intermedia. Haematologica **75**: 1–8.
28. KUTLAR, A. et al. 1989. β-thalassemia intermedia in two Turkish families is caused by the interaction of Hb Knossos [β27(B9)Ala→Ser] and of Hb City of Hope [β69(E13)Gly→Ser] with β^0-thalassemia. Hemoglobin **13**: 7–16.

The Hemoglobin E Syndromes

D. C. REES,[a,c] L. STYLES,[b] E. P. VICHINSKY,[b] J. B. CLEGG,[a] AND D. J. WEATHERALL[a]

[a]MRC Molecular Haematology Unit, Institute of Molecular Medicine, The John Radcliffe, Headley Way, Headington, Oxford, OX3 9DS, United Kingdom

[b]Department of Hematology, Children's Hospital, Oakland, California, USA

ABSTRACT: Heterozygotes and homozygotes for HbE (β26, GAG-AAG, Glu-Lys) are microcytic, minimally anemic, and asymptomatic. The microcytosis is attributed to the β thalassemic nature of the β^E gene, whereas the *in vitro* instability of HbE does not contribute to the phenotype. However, the compound heterozygote state HbE/β thalassemia results in a variable, and often severe anemia, with the phenotype ranging from transfusion dependence to a complete lack of symptoms. This has been well documented in Thailand, but the basis of the interaction and the cause of the variability remains unexplained. We have studied 50 HbE/β thalassemics from the UK and 16 from Oakland, CA and assessed the role of HbE instability. Time-course globin chain synthesis experiments have shown that instability is not an important factor in the steady state, but that at 41°C newly synthesized Hb molecules are unstable. We have identified one family in which HbE interacts with pyrimidine 5′ nucleotidase deficiency to cause severe anemia with Hb instability. The UK individuals, mostly of Bengali origin, have Hb's from 4.5-11 g/dl. The β thalassemia mutation, α thalassemia and the Xmn 1 Gγ polymorphism do not explain this variability, but the relative and absolute amounts of HbF correlate significantly with total Hb. The Oakland individuals, mostly from Southeast Asia, show similar variation in Hb, which again is largely unexplained.

Hemoglobin E (HbE), the fourth abnormal hemoglobin to be discovered, was identified in 1954, and it is of interest that the propositus with HbE/β-thalassemia, was of Hindu/Guatemalan/Spanish and Italian ancestry, a combination which has not been reported since.[1] Following this, intermittent progress has been made in understanding the pathophysiology and natural history of the HbE syndromes, particularly HbE/β-thalassemia, much of the work being done in Thailand (TABLE 1). HbE is most prevalent in and around Thailand, with large numbers affected further south into Indonesia and east to Bangladesh and Northeast India. Significant numbers are also found in Sri Lanka, with approximately half the cases of thalassemia involving HbE.[2] HbE is also increasingly common in Europe and North America, with the increasing size and importance of Southeast Asian and Bengali immigrant communities.

HbE trait and homozygous HbE result in hypochromic microcytosis and minimal anemia, but HbE/β-thalassemia causes a surprisingly severe and variable anemia.[3,4] The interaction between HbE and β-thalassemia is partly explained by the thalassemic nature of the β^E gene,[5,6] but the frequent occurrence of transfusion dependence is unexpected, particu-

[c]Address for correspondence: D. C. Rees, MRC Molecular Haematology Unit, Institute of Molecular Medicine, The John Radcliffe, Headley Way, Headington, Oxford, OX3 9DS, UK. Telephone: +44 1865 222377; fax: +44 1865 222500; e-mail: drees@hammer.imm.ox.ac.uk

TABLE 1. Major Advances in the Understanding of HbE Syndromes

Year	Discovery	Reference
1954	Electrophoretic variant HbE identified	1
1955	First description of HbE/β-thalassemia	14
1956	Detailed study of HbE/β-thalassemia, HbE trait, and HbE homozygotes	3
1957	First description of HbE/HbS double heterozygote	15
1961	Identification of β26 glu-lys change	16
1961	Ferrokinetics demonstrate ineffective erythropoiesis	17
1972	Normal oxygen affinity shown	18
1974	Oxidative instability demonstrated	19
1980	Reduced levels of $β^E$ mRNA shown	6
1982	$β^E$ mutation, GAG-AAG, activates cryptic splice site	5
1985	Co-inheritance of α-thalassemia increases Hb in HbE/β-thalassemia	20
1988	Variable phenotype of HbE/β-thalassemia established	4
1993	Xmn1 Gγ promoter ameliorates anemia in HbE/β-thalassemia	21

larly when the homozygous state for HbE is so mild. Equally, the wide range of steady-state hemoglobins, between 3 and 11g/dl in Thailand, is not easily explained, even when α-thalassemia, the nature of the β-thalassemia mutation, and cis-acting determinants of HbF are included in the analysis. Although other well-defined thalassemic genotypes, such as IVS 1-6 homozygosity[7] show marked variability in phenotype, the differences in hemoglobin in HbE/β thalassemics are particularly marked.

HbE is known to be unstable *in vitro* and it is possible that this may contribute to the severity and variability in HbE/β-thalassemia. The oxidative stress resulting from free α chains within the HbE/β-thalassemic red cell might result in the precipitation of HbE molecules, stressing the proteolytic capacity of the cell and further damaging its membrane. Small variations in oxidative stress and proteolytic capacity might provoke catastrophic precipitation of HbE and severe anemia.

In this study, we have investigated the possible clinical importance of HbE instability in the HbE syndromes, and also characterized a group of HbE/β-thalassemics living in the United Kingdom and North America, to try and identify determinants of severity.

CLINICAL MANIFESTATIONS OF HbE INSTABILITY

There are few published studies suggesting that the instability of HbE can be clinically important. Dapsone-associated Heinz body hemolytic anemia has been described in a Cambodian woman with HbE trait,[8] although it was not possible to confirm the absence of enzymopathies and membranopathies in the steady state; it also seems unlikely that such a reaction occurs frequently, given that many millions of people with HbE must have been exposed to dapsone. A study in Thailand also observed that whereas HbE homozygotes and heterozygotes do not have protection against malaria, HbE carriers who had recently eaten fava beans are significantly protected[9]; this surprising observation is unexplained, but a possible interaction between fava beans and HbE instability is possible.

HbE SYNTHESIS *IN VITRO*

We have studied the stability of hemoglobin E in a number of conditions, using time-course globin-chain synthesis analysis with [^{3}H]leucine for periods up to two hours at 37°C. Specific activity of the globin chains, i.e. the ratio of newly synthesized, tritiated globin chains to old, unlabeled chains, should increase linearly with time if the hemoglobin is stable; if newly synthesized hemoglobin molecules are unstable, the radioactive incorporation will plateau as the hemoglobin molecules containing new chains are precipitated and proteolysed.[10] This approach has the advantage of assessing the stability of newly synthesized globin chains within the physiological environment of the red cell.

We have recently studied a Bangladeshi family in which the genes for both HbE and pyrimidine 5' nucleotidase (P5'N) deficiency are segregating. The individual homozygous for both HbE and P5'N deficiency had severe anemia with a hemoglobin level of 2.8g/dl, MCV 60fl, and 7% reticulocytes.[11] Using time-course globin-chain synthesis experiments, linear incorporation of radioactivity was shown in P5'N and HbE homozygotes, but a marked plateau occurred in the P5'N-deficient HbE homozygote (FIG. 1), thus showing that this interaction causes instability of HbE, possibly because of the increased intracellular oxidative stress resulting from the enzymopathy. Although this interaction is unlikely to be a common cause of phenotypic variability in thalassemia, and may well be unique, it demonstrates that HbE's instability can be of pathological importance.

We have carried out similar time-course incubations using blood from untransfused HbE/β-thalassemics (FIG. 2). The rates of synthesis of the three globin chains are linear over the two-hour incubation, suggesting that significant instability does not occur in the steady state; the slight plateau occurring during α-globin synthesis probably reflects the inevitable loss of excess α chains. A similar result was found with HbE/β-thalassemia bone marrow. Most of these experiments are carried out on washed blood, with the white cells removed, to maximize incorporation and avoid synthesis of non-globin proteins. To ensure that washing does not remove small molecules from the cell that might potentiate instability and proteolysis, similar experiments have been performed by directly incubating whole blood with [³H]leucine: again radioactivity increases linearly, with no suggestion of instability.

These results have been corroborated by Percoll(Pharmacia, UK)/meglamine density gradient centrifugation using blood from an untransfused, HbE/β⁺-thalassemia (IVS 1-5) compound heterozygote, separating the red cells into very dense (old cells), intermediate, and less dense (new cells) fractions.[12] There is the expected, relative increase in HbF as the cells age, but no effective change in the ratio of HbE to HbA. Significant instability of HbE would be expected to lead to it decreasing relative to HbA as the cells age (FIG. 3).

We have performed a further series of experiments with incubations performed at 41°C, to simulate the core temperature that might occur during a febrile illness; this leads to a marked plateau in the rate of globin synthesis, suggestive of hemoglobin instability. A similar effect was not seen in control experiments using blood from an untransfused thalassemia intermedia patient without HbE (FIG. 4). However, homozygous HbE blood also showed this temperature-dependent plateau. A similar effect was achieved with HbE/β-thalassemia cells when an incubation temperature of 39°C was used. These data suggest that relatively low grade fevers, as commonly occur in tropical areas, can cause significant instability of HbE, which might be predicted to cause a marked fall in hemoglobin. We are not aware of any controlled clinical studies that sought hemolysis during febrile illnesses in HbE/β-thalassemics, although anecdotally sudden drops in Hb do occur coincident with such fevers. This phenomenon may explain some of the observed variability in Hb levels in genotypically similar HbE/β-thalassemics.

HbE/β THALASSEMIA IN THE UNITED KINGDOM AND NORTH AMERICA

We have analyzed the clinical, phenotypic, and genotypic details of 50 individuals resident in the United Kingdom and of 16 from Oakland, California. The British sample includes at least 90% of those with HbE/β-thalassemia resident in the United Kingdom, attending more than 15 different hospitals. The ages range from 1 year to 60 years, with

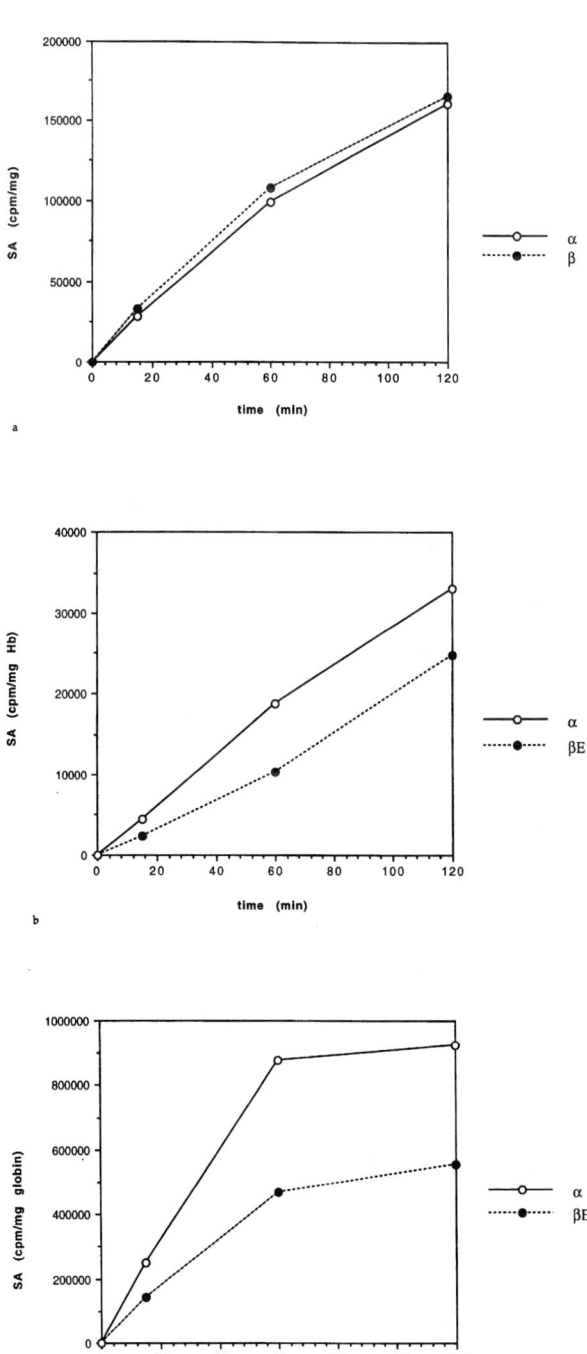

FIGURE 1. Time-course specific activity graphs for (**a**) pyrimidine 5′ nucleotidase deficiency, (**b**) homozygous HbE, and (**c**) homozygous HbE and pyrimidine 5′ nucleotidase deficiency.

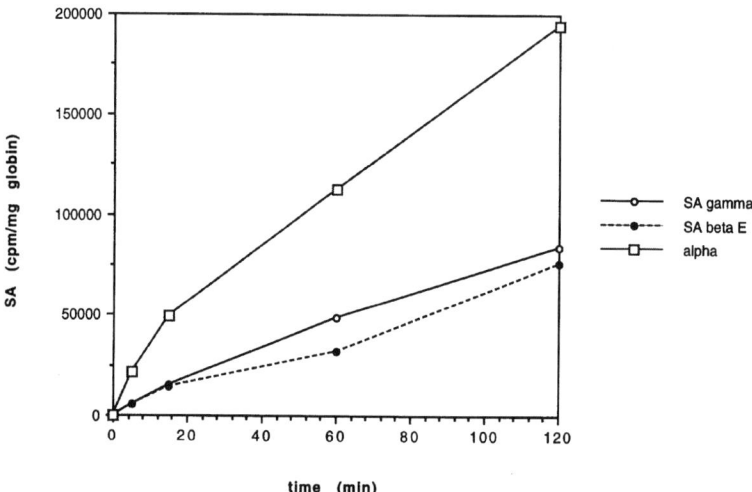

FIGURE 2. Time-course specific activity graph for HbE/β-thalassemia at 37°C.

40% being under the age of 10. Fifty percent are from Bangladesh and 26% from Pakistan and India; the remainder are from Southeast Asia. Fifty-six percent of the β-thalassemia alleles are due to the IVS 1-5 G-C severe β$^+$ mutation. The remainder are all β^0 thalassemia mutations. 78% of the individuals are heterozygous +/− at the *Xmn1* cleavage site at

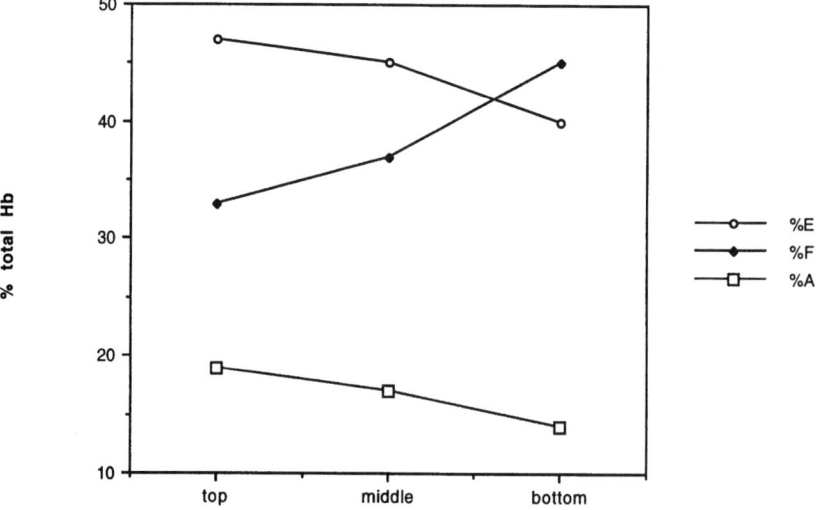

FIGURE 3. % HbE, HbF and HbA in a patient with HbE/ β$^+$-thalassemia in the top (young), middle, and bottom (old) fractions of red cells following density gradient centrifugation.

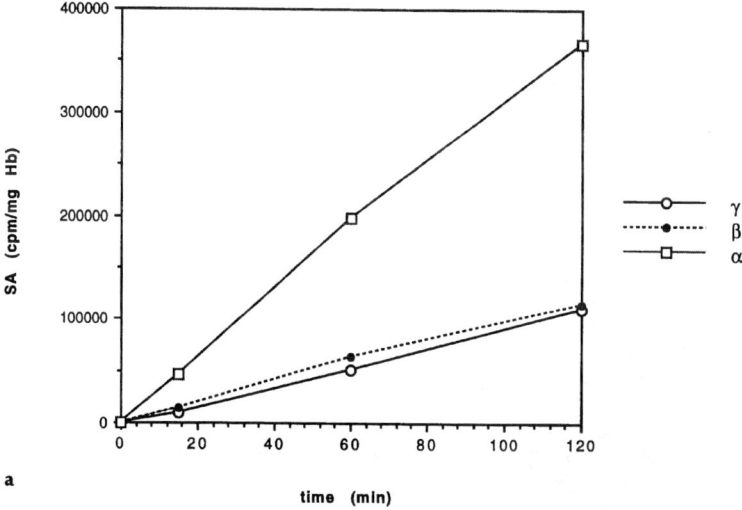

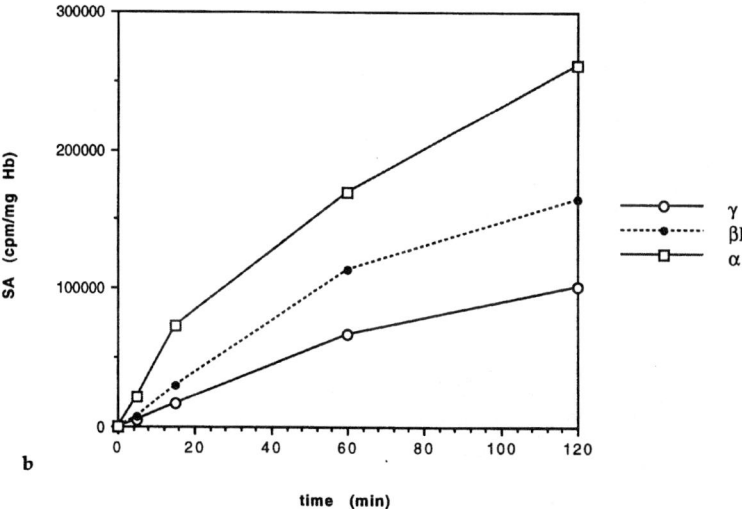

FIGURE 4. Time-course specific activity graph for thalassemia intermedia (**a**) and HbE/β thalassemia (**b**) both at 41°C.

position -158 of the Gγ gene, 17% -/- and 5% +/+. Only one individual was found with deletional α^+ thalassemia and there were no triplicated α genes. Fifty percent of the patients were treated with regular, frequent blood transfusions (mean age at starting 8.8, range 0.5–33), and 44% had been splenectomized (mean age 13.1, range 3.5–33). 32% were both splenectomized and transfusion dependent (31% splenectomized first, 63% splenectomized when transfusion dependent, 6% splenectomy and transfusions started together). Three patients have undergone bone marrow transplantation successfully.

Transfusion dependence was not predicted by the β^+/β^0-thalassemia nor the *Xmn1* status of the individuals. The most significant factor associated with early transfusion dependence was being born in the UK, as opposed to being born overseas (FIG. 5). Reliable pre-transfusion, hematological data were not available.

In the untransfused patients, the mean Hb was 7.6 g/dl (range 4.6–10.5), and again the variance not explained by splenectomy, sex, α-thalassemia, β^+/β^0-thalassemia, nor the *Xmn1* polymorphism. Multiple regression analysis of Hb versus α/non-α globin chain synthesis ratios, age, % reticulocytes Gγ/Aγ ratios, and %HbF explains 66% of the variance in hemoglobin ($p = 0.03$), with %F having the only significant regression coefficient (0.09, $p = 0.021$). Whereas %HbF (and absolute HbF) correlates positively with total hemoglobin ($R = 0.59, p = 0.0025$), %HbE shows a similarly significant negative correlation ($R = -0.52, p = 0.009$) (FIG. 6). The %HbF did not vary significantly with sex, splenectomy, and *Xmn1*. Multiple regression analysis of %HbF versus age, α/γ total counts ratio, % reticulocytes, and Gγ/Aγ ratio explain 83% of the variability. Age (-0.77, $p = 0.001$) and α/γ total counts ratio (-1.38, $p = 0.002$) had significant regression coefficients.

The Oakland patients differ from the United Kingdom sample in that they are nearly all from Southeast Asia, all have β^0-thalassemia mutations and attend a single center. The average age is 10.4 years (0.5–21), 44% are transfusion dependent, and 38% have been

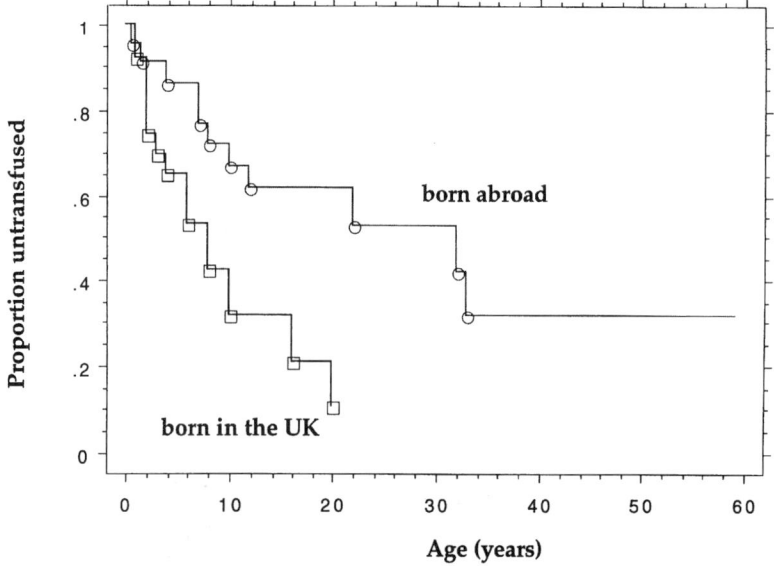

FIGURE 5. Kaplan-Meier plot comparing transfusion dependence in HbE/β-thalassemics born in the United Kingdom and born overseas.

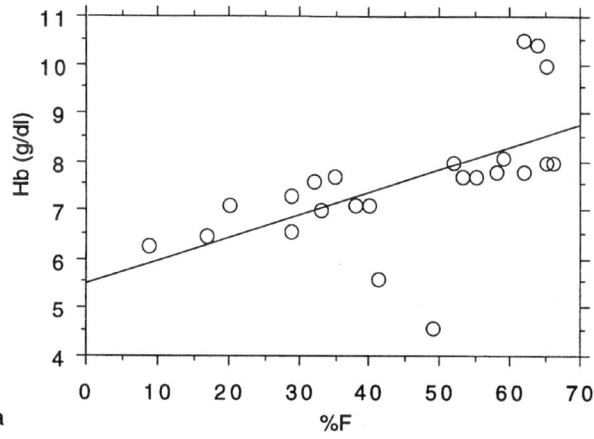

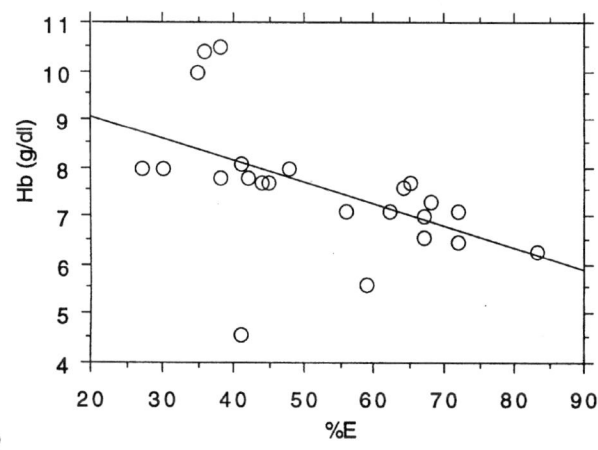

FIGURE 6. Regression plots of total hemoglobin versus %HbF (**a**) and %HbE (**b**).

splenectomized, similar to the United Kingdom. Three of sixteen patients have deletional α-thalassemia (all siblings). The general findings of the United Kingdom study are also true in this group, although statistical analysis is limited by the relatively small numbers. Analysis of the combined United Kingdom and Oakland patients does not differ from that of the United Kingdom group alone.

DISCUSSION

Hemoglobin instability does not seem important in steady-state HbE/β-thalassemia, but there is *in vitro* evidence that under conditions of fever and oxidative stress, instability may contribute to a fall in hemoglobin to an extent that does not occur in other forms of thalassemia. HbE/β-thalassemia shows the same clinical variability in the United States of America and United Kingdom as has previously been documented in Thailand; genotypic analysis does not adequately explain this variation. The only significant determinant of total hemoglobin was %HbF. Some of the variation in HbF production is determined by age, but differences in the α/γ total counts ratio is also a highly significant determinant; the α/γ synthesis ratio is determined by a number of largely unidentified *cis*- and *trans*-acting factors.

The current clinical management of these patients is varied, involving regular blood transfusions, splenectomy, and bone marrow transplantation in various combinations. There is no reliable way of predicting severity, with genotypic information being of limited value. Similarly, the clinical indications for regular transfusions and splenectomy are not well defined, with inconsistent practice in the United Kingdom, and presumably much of the rest of the world. The role of hydroxyurea and butyrate analogues is not established, although one Oakland patient has responded well to hydroxyurea and a study of 13 HbE/β-thalassemics in Thailand showed a 10% Hb increase in hemoglobin.[13]

HbE/β-thalassemia is the commonest form of severe thalassemia in the world and is most prevalent in the rapidly expanding and increasingly influential countries of Southeast Asia. It is also of growing importance in Europe, North America, and Australia, where the emphasis has traditionally been on Southern Europeans. Studies are needed to define the optimum clinical management, with particular consideration of HbF augmentation, which may be particularly beneficial in this disease, in which patients often hover on the brink of transfusion dependence.

REFERENCES

1. ITANO, H. A., W. R. BERGREN & P. STURGEON. 1954. Identification of a fourth abnormal human hemoglobin. J. Am. Chem. Soc. **76**: 2278.
2. WEATHERALL, D. J. & J. B. CLEGG. 1981. The Thalassaemia Syndromes. 3rd edit. Blackwell. Oxford. U.K.
3. CHERNOFF, A. I., V. MINNICH, S. NA-NAKORN, S. TUCHINDA, C. KASHEMSANT & R. R. CHRENOFF. 1956. Studies on hemoglobin E I. The clinical, hematologic, and genetic characteristics of the hemoglobin E syndromes. J. Lab. Clin. Med. **47(3)**: 455–489.
4. FUCHAROEN, S., P. WINICHAGOON, P. POOTRAKUL, A. PIANKIJAGUM & P. WASI. 1988. Variable severity of Southeast Asian β-thalassaemia/Hb E disease. Birth Defects: Original Articles Series. **53(5A)**: 241–248.
5. ORKIN, S. H., H. H. KAZAZIAN JR., S. E. ANTONARAKIS, H. OSTRER, S. C. GOFF & J. P. SEXTON. 1982. Abnormal RNA processing due to the exon mutation of βE-globin gene. Nature **300**: 768–769.
6. TRAEGER, J., W. G. WOOD, J. B. CLEGG, D. J. WEATHERALL & P. WASI. 1980. Defective synthesis of HbE is due to reduced levels of βE mRNA. Nature **288**: 497–499.
7. EFREMOV, D., A. DIMOVSKI, E. BAYSAL, Z. YE, A. ADEKILE, M. RIBIERO, G. SCHILIRO, C. ALTAY, A. GURGEY, G. EFREMOV & T. HUISMAN. 1994. Possible factors influencing the hemoglobin and fetal hemoglobin levels in patients with β-thalassaemia due to a homozygosity for the IVS-I-6 (T-C) mutation. Br. J. Haematol. **86**: 824–830.
8. LACHANT, N. A. & K. R. TANAKA. 1987. Case report: Dapsone-associated Heinz body hemolytic anemia in a Cambodian woman with hemoglobin E trait. Am. J. Med. Sci. **294(5)**: 364–368.
9. KITAYAPORN, D., K. E. NELSON, P. CHAROENLARP & T. PHOLPOTHI. 1992. Hemoglobin-E in the presence of oxidative substances from fava bean may be protective against Plasmodium falciparum malaria. Trans. R. Soc. of Trop. Med. Hyg. **86**: 240–244.

10. REES, D. C., J. ROCHETTE, C. SCHOFIELD, B. GREEN, M. MORRIS, N. E. PARKER, H. SASAKI, A. TANAKA, Y. OHBA & J. B. CLEGG. 1996. A novel silent post-translational mechanism converts methionine to aspartate in hemoglobin Bristol [β67(E11) Val-Met-Asp]. Blood **88(1)** 341–348.
11. REES, D., J. DULEY, H. SIMMONDS, B. WONKE, S. THEIN, J. CLEGG & D. WEATHERALL. 1996. Interaction of hemoglobin E and pyrimidine 5′ nucleotidase deficiency. Blood **88(7)**: 2761–2767.
12. VETTORE, L., M. C. MATTEIS & P. ZAMPINI. 1980. A new density gradient system for the separation of human red blood cells. Am. J. Hematol. **8**: 291–297.
13. FUCHAROEN, S., N. SIRITANARATKUL, P. WINICHAGOON, J. CHOWTHAWORN, W. SIRIBOON, W. MUANGSUP, S. CHAICHAROEN, N. POOLSUP, B. CHINDAVIJAK, P. POOTRAKUL, A. PIANKIJAGUM, A. SCHECHTER & G. RODGERS. 1996. Hydroxyurea increase hemoglobin F levels and improves the effectiveness of erythropoiesis in beta-thalassemia/hemoglobin E disease. Blood **87**: 887–892.
14. STURGEON, P., H. ITANO & W. BERGREN. 1955. Clinical manifestations of inherited abnormal hemoglobins. Blood **10**:396–404.
15. AKSOY, M. & H. LEHMANN. 1957. The first observation of sickle cell-hemoglobin E disease. Nature. **179**: 1248–1249.
16. HUNT, J. A. & V. M. INGRAM. 1961. Abnormal human hemoglobins. VI. The chemical difference between hemoglobins A and E. Biochim. Biophys. Acta **49**: 520–536.
17. SWARUP, S., J. CHATTERJEA, P. HOSAIN & F. HOSAIN. 1961. A comparative study on iron turnover with special reference to Hb. E-thalassaemia using small doses of Fe59. In. J. Med. Res. **49(2)**: 256–261.
18. BUNN, H., W. MERIWETHER, S. BALCERZAC & D. RUCKNAGEL. 1972. Oxygen equilibrium of hemoglobin E. J. Clin. Invest. **51**: 2984–2987.
19. FRISCHER, H. & J. BOWMAN. 1975. Hemoglobin E, an oxidatively unstable mutation. J. Lab. Clin. Medi. **85(4)**:531–539.
20. WINICHAGOON, P., S. FUCHAROEN, D. WEATHERALL & P. WASI. 1985. Concomitant inheritance of α-thalassemia in β⁰ thalassemia/HbE disease. Am. J. Hematol. **20**: 217–222.
21. WINICHAGOON, P., V. THONGLAIROAM, S. FUCHAROEN, P. WILAIRAT, Y. FUKUMAKI & P. WASI. 1993. Severity differences in β-thalassaemia/hemoglobin E syndromes: implication of genetic factors. Br. J. Haematol. **83**: 633–639.

The Morbidity of Bone Disease in Thalassemia

ELLIOTT P. VICHINSKY[a]

Department of Hematology/Oncology, Children's Hospital Oakland, Oakland, California 94609, USA

ABSTRACT: As thalassemia patients age, bone disease becomes a serious cause of morbidity. The frequency and type of bone disease is affected by the underlying type of thalassemia and its treatment. Problems include rickets, scoliosis, spinal deformities, nerve compression, fractures and severe osteoporosis. In early stages, patients may be asymptomatic but can present with back pain, a limp, dyspnea, neurological emergencies, or sudden fractures. The etiologies are often multifactorial, culminating with increased bone resorption and remodeling. They include hormonal deficiency, bone marrow expansion, nutritional deficiency, or desferal toxicity. Particular risk factors include older patients, low baseline hemoglobin, delayed puberty, hormonal failure, and high iron stores. Nutritional deficiencies may further compound the patient's risk for bone disease. Increasing evidence suggests that these complications and their associated long-term morbidity can be prevented if an annual screening is done, followed by long-term intervention. Patients treated with amino biphosphonates inhibit bone resorption and may demonstrate rapid healing. Intra-nasal calcitonin has also been successful in treating osteopenia. Early use of estrogen and testosterone appears to markedly lower the risk for selective patients. Both transfused and non-transfused patients should be educated about risk factors and early symptoms. All patients should be screened annually for bone disease. Once adolescence occurs, annual testing in selected cases should include bone density studies with X-ray absorptiometry.

With the worldwide increase in diagnosis and follow-up of diverse thalassemic mutations, bone disease is an increasingly recognized serious cause of morbidity in both thalassemia major and thalassemia intermedia disorders.[1–8] The lack of early diagnosis and treatment has led to common occurrence of growth failure, osteoporosis, fractures, spinal deformities, and nerve compression.[6,9–13] While late stages present with symptoms of pain, limp, sudden fractures, and neurological emergencies, most patients are asymptomatic until irreversible changes have occurred. The thalassemia intermedia multicenter study found a high frequency of serious clinical and laboratory indications of osteoporosis in this population.[7] Fractures were common with the mean age of occurrence being 18 years and abnormal bone density studies were widespread.

The etiology of bone disease is multifactorial and culminates in a state of increased bone turnover with excessive bone resorption and remodeling. Hormonal deficiency, bone marrow expansion, nutritional deficiency and desferal toxicity are important factors. Particular risk factors include small, older patients, low baseline hemoglobin, delayed puberty, gonadal failure, high iron stores, and calcium/vitamin D deficiency.[1,12–21]

Improved methods of diagnosing bone disease have opened the door to better understanding, diagnosing, and early treatment of patients. Dual X-ray absorptiometry mea-

---

[a]Address for correspondence: Elliott P. Vichinsky. M. D., Director, Hematology/Oncology, Children's Hospital Oakland, 747 52nd Street, Oakland, California 94609. Telephone: 510-428-3651; Fax: 510-450-5647; e-mail: evichinsky@lanminds.com

surement of bone density of the lumbar spine and femoral neck have been recommended as the optimal methods to measure bone mass.[12,17,20,22,23] It is both quantitative and safe with available control data. Bone density assessment by *in vivo* neutron activation is a useful technique,[3] but significant radiation exposure occurs. X-ray demonstration of osteoporosis is a very late effect and occurs after a loss of more than 30% of bone; therefore, it is of limited screening value. Assessment of bone turnover, including bone formation and resorption, is important in understanding etiology as well as effect of therapy. Bone specific alkaline phosphatase and plasma osteocalcin are markers of osteoblastic activity.[12,17,20,24,25] Urinary pyridoline and deoxypyridinoline are collagen cross-linking breakdown products indicative of bone resorption.[17,20,24,25] Rarely used histologic dynamic studies offer important opportunities to understand the mechanism of bone loss.

Recently, the Toronto group prospectively studied approximately 50 transfusion and non-transfusion β^0-thalassemia patients applying these newer diagnostic tools to determine the degree of bone disease and risk factors. Bone density abnormalities were widespread in both sexes. Decreased bone density occurred even in patients with normal gonadal function or on hormonal replacement therapy. However, gonadal dysfunction strongly predicted bone disease. A history of delayed onset of puberty in both sexes regardless of eventual normal pubertal maturation is one of the most important risk factors for osteoporosis. This is not surprising because most bone density accumulation occurs by 20 years of age. Body mass also predicts osteoporosis. Therefore, small, thin patients are at particular risk. Limited or absent transfusion therapy increases the risk of osteoporosis in thalassemia patients because of the bone marrow hyperplasia. Marrow expansion causes mechanical interruption of bone formation as well as cytokine disturbances, which result in increased bone resorption. However, even in the highly transfused group, patients develop osteoporosis in part induced by continued but unexpected marrow hyperplasia. Transferrin receptor studies demonstrate increased marrow activity even with reticulocyte absence or hypoplasia.

In California and other parts of the United States, there has been a rapid growth in thalassemia intermedia disorders.[2] This is secondary to the migration of high-risk populations. Since the initiation of newborn screening in California during this decade, over 700 cases of homozygous hemoglobin E, hemoglobin E thalassemia, or β^0-thalassemia have been diagnosed. In Southeast Asian newborns, as high as one in four newborns have hemoglobin FAE, one in 39 has homozygous hemoglobin EE and one in 3000 have E/β^0-thalassemia. In Asian Indian newborns, one in 2,220 has β^0-thalassemia. This thalassemia population has many osteoporosis risk factors that amplify the frequency and severity of bone disease. These include ethnicity, decreased bone mass, and pubertal delay.[16,20,26,27,28] In addition, the frequent occurrence of medical diseases found in the immigrant population, such as tuberculosis, further increase the risk of bone disease.

The Northern California Thalassemia Center follows 141 patients with the largest segment of the population under 10 years of age. Thalassemia intermedia is the most common clinical phenotype. The most common genotypes are E-thalassemia, β-thalassemia, and hemoglobin H-Constant Spring. There are 42 E/β-thalassemia patients, 17 are chronically transfused and 25 receive intermittent or no transfusions. Despite the young age, our transfused and non-transfused population has many risk factors for bone disease. In the transfused group, 47% have growth failure, 46% pubertal delay, 12% percent diabetes, and 36% hepatitis. While the ferritin is lower (1,236 ng/ml) in the non-transfused group, they have a similar frequency of growth delay and pubertal gonadal failure. We have used dual energy X-ray absorptiometry when the patients reach young adulthood. In our population, all females demonstrated bone density abnormalities (50% osteopenia and 50% osteoporosis). All male patients were abnormal, with most cases being osteopenic. There was a strong relationship to gonadal dysfunction, delay in puberty, and the development of osteopenia in our population.

In addition to the the $E\beta^0$ or β-thalassemia genotypes, our program follows 40 children with hemoglobin H disease. Hemoglobin H-Constant Spring, the most common type of Hemoglobin H disease in this population, has clinical phenotypes similar to β-thalassemia and thalassemia intermedia disorders. While the median age of this population is only 8 years, 65% receive at least intermittent transfusions. Almost 50% have required splenectomy due to hypersplenism. Despite their young age, more than 20% of these childen have significant growth failure. Craniofacial and other bone changes are already seen in 20%. This is in marked contrast to our deletional hemoglobin H children who only rarely exhibit bone or facial deformities. We believe this is a high-risk group for bone disease due to the factors identified and the particular problem in missing or delay in diagnosis of hemoglobin H-Constant Spring.[29] Standard electropheresis methods often miss Constant Spring variants, which results in these patients being treated as having a milder form of hemoglobin H.

Prevention of osteoporosis is the most important priority in managing patients since restoring healthy bone to an osteoporotic skeleton safely is not well proven. Adequate calcium intake during skeleton development can increase bone mass in adolescents and decrease bone loss seen in later life. High calcium supplementation after bone formation is completed is of little value alone. Therefore, at least 1,200 mg daily allowance of calcium during adolescence is recommended.[20,28,30] Overall, good nutrition with adequate vitamins D, B6, B12, and K is needed. Vitamin D deficiency is increasingly being recognized among high risk groups. Small vitamin D doses to high risk populations in assocation with calcium can reduce the fracture rate.[17,20,28] There is increasing evidence that chronic illness amplifies bone loss because of decreased physical exercise. Therefore, thalassemia patients should have as part of their preventive program a planned exercise program.

Early hormonal replacement is the most effective method to prevent gonadal insufficiency–induced bone loss, which is the most important prediction of osteoporosis in thalassemia.[1,2,22,31,32] In women, estrogen with progestational agents are usually prescribed. While the benefit of estrogen outweighs the risk in this population, concern for a possible increased risk of breast cancer requires detailed patient discussions. In hypogonadal men with developing osteoporosis, testosterone is strongly recommended.

New agents to treat osteoporosis look very promising, in particular for patients not receiving hormonal replacement and those with high bone turnover states.[9,17,20,24,25,27,31] Calcitonin is a peptide hormone secreted by thyroid that prevents trabecular bone loss by inhibiting osteoclastic activity. Parenteral and intranasal instillation are available, and the drug is safe. Preliminary studies in thalassemia are encouraging and demonstrate after one year of therapy, cessation of bone pain and radiographic improvement.[9] Biphosphonates are analogues of pyrophosphate and also inhibit bone resorption.[25] Clinical trials indicate they are as beneficial as estrogen or calcitonin on bone mass. The major advantage over calcitonin is its oral route. While agents to stimulate bone formation such as fluoride and parathyroid hormone are being studied,[17,20] their clinical role remains unproven.

In summary, bone disease is common in both transfusion and non-transfusion dependent thalassemia patients and requires early screening and preventive intervention. The annual screening of adolescent patients, once with bone density studies, is recommended, and gonadal hormone replacement is essential. New osteoclastic inhibitors such as calcitonin and biphosphonates appear promising in this population.

REFERENCES

1. FILOSA, A., S. DIMAIO, A. SAVIANO, S. VOCCA & G. ESPOSITO. 1996. Can adrenarche influence the degree of osteopenia in thalassemia children? J. Pediatr. Endocrinol. Metab. **9**: 401–406.
2. LOREY, F. 1997. California newborn screening and the impact of Asian immigration on thalassemia. Int. J. Ped. Hematol/Oncol. **4**: 11–16.

3. KRISHNAN, S., W. C. STURTRIDGE, N. F. OLIVIERI, A. F. COLLINS, R. Y. QURESHI, M. KRISHNAN *et al.* 1994. A study on children's condition thalassemia using neutron activation analysis and other techniques. Biol. Trace Elem. Res. **43**: 309–314.
4. OLIVIERI, N. F., R. K. BASRAN, A. L. TALBOT, P. BABYN & J. D. BAILEY. 1995. Abnormal growth in thalassemia major associated with deferoxamine-induced destruction of spinal cartilage and compromise of sitting height. Blood **86**(Suppl 1): 482a.
5. POOTRAKUL P., S. HUNGSPRENGES, S. FUCHAROEN, D. BAYLINK, E. THOMPSON, E. ENGLISH *et al.* 1981. Relation between erythropoiesis and bone metabolism in thalassemia. N. Engl. J. Med. **304**:1470-1473.
6. SERGIACOMI, G., E. PALMA, P. CIANCIULLI, L. FORTE, G. PAPA & G. SIMONETTI. 1993. Clinico-radiological correlation in thalassemia intermedia. Radiol. Med. (Torino) **85**: 570–573.
7. PEARSON, H. A. 1997. The evaluation of thalassemia intermedia. *In* Proceedings of Thalassemia Intermedia: A Region I Conference. The Genetic Resource: Special Issue: **11**: 5–10.
8. PEARSON, H. A., A. R. COHEN, P. J. GIARDINA & H. H. KAZAZIAN. 1996. The changing profile of homozygous β-thalassemia: Demography, ethnicity and age distribution of current North American patients and changes in two decades. Pediatrics **97**: 352–356.
9. CANATAN, D., N. AKAR & A. ARCASOY. 1995. Effects of calcitonin therapy on osteoporosis in patients with thalassemia. Acta Haematol. **93**: 20–24.
10. KOROVESSIS, P, D. PAPANASTASIOU, M. TINIAKOU & N. G. BERATIS. 1996. Incidence of scoliosis in β-thalassemia and follow-up evaluation. Spine **21**: 1798–1801.
11. OLIVIERI, N. F., G. KOREN, J. HARRIS, S. KHATTAK, M. H. FREEDMAN, D. M. TEMPLETON *et al.* 1992. Growth failure and bony changes induced by deferoxamine. Am. J. Ped. Hematol/Oncol. **14**: 48–56.
12. ORVIETO, R., I. LEICHTER, E. A. RACHMILEWITZ & J. Y. MARGULIES. 1992. Bone density, mineral content and cortical index in patients with thalassemia major and the correlation to their bone fractures, blood transfusions and treatment with desferrioxamine. Calcif. Tissue Int. **50**: 397–399.
13. RODDA C. P., E. D. REID, S. JOHNSON, J. DOERY, R. MATTHEWS & D. K. BOWDEN. 1995. Short stature in homozygous β-thalassaemia is due to disproportionate truncal shortening. Clin. Endocrinol. **42**: 587–592.
14. CANN, C. E., M. C. MARTIN, H. K. GENANT & R. B. JAFFE. 1984. Decreased spinal mineral content in amenorrheic women. J. Am. Med. Assoc. **251**: 626–629.
15. BISBOCCI, D., P. LIVORNO, P. MODINA, M. GAMBINO, P. DAMIANO, R. CANTONI *et al.* 1993. Osteodystrophy in thalassemia major. **8**: 224–226.
16. ZAINO, E. C., K. J. YEH & J. ALOIA. 1985. Defective vitamin D metabolism in thalassemia major. Ann. N.Y. Acad. Sci. **445**: 127–134.
17. Consensus Development Conference: Diagnosis, prophylaxis and treatment of osteoporosis. Peck W. A., Chairman. 1993. Am. J. Med. **94**: 646–650.
18. DEVIRGILLIS, S. T., M. CONIGA & F. FRAY *et al.* 1988. Deferoxamine induced growth retardation in patients with thalassemia major. J. Pediatr. **113**: 661–669.
19. FINKELSTEIN, J. S., R. M. NEER, B. M. K. BILLER, J. D. CRAWFORD & A. KLIBANSKI. 1992. Osteopenia in men with a history of delayed puberty. N. Engl. J. Med. **326**: 600–604.
20. LINDSAY, R. 1993. Prevention and treatment of osteoporosis. Lancet **341**: 801–805.
21. WARREN M. P., J. BROOKS-GUNN, L. H. HAMILTON, L. F. WARREN & W. G. HAMILTON. 1986. Scoliosis and fractures in young ballet dancers. N. Engl. J. Med. **314**: 1348–1353.
22. MILLER P. D., S. L. BONNICK, C. J. ROSEN, R. D. ALTMAN, L. V. AVIOLI, J. DEQUEKER *et al.* Clinical utility of bone mass measurements in adults: Consensus of an international panel. 1996. Semin. Arthritis Rheum. **25**: 361–372.
23. ABBOTT, T. A., III, B. J. LAWRENCE & S. WALLACH. 1996. Osteoporosis: The need for comprehensive treatment guidelines. Clin. Ther. **18**: 127–149.
24. PEDRAZZONI, M, F. S. ALFANO, C. GATTI, M. FANTUZZI, G. GIRASOLE, C. CAMPANINI *et al.* 1995. Acute effects of bisphosphonates on new and traditional markers of bone resorption. Calcif. Tissue Int. **57**: 25–29.
25. SATO, M., W. GRASSER & N. ENDO. 1991. Bisphosphonate action: Alendronate localization in rat bone and effects on osteoclast ultrastructure. J. Clin. Invest. **88**: 2095–2105.
26. JOHNSTON, C. C. JR., J. Z. MILLER & C. W. SLEMENDA. 1993. Calcium supplementation and increases in bone mineral density in children. N. Engl. J. Med. **327**: 82–87.

27. CHESTNUT, C. H., III, M. R. MCCLUNG, K. E. ENSRUD, N. H. BELL, H. K. GENANT, S. T. HARRIS *et al.* 1995. Alendronate treatment of the postmenopausal osteoporotic woman: Effect of multiple dosages on bone mass and bone remodeling. Am. J. Med. **99**: 144–152.
28. HEANEY, R. P. 1993. Nutritional factors in osteoporosis. Annu. Rev. Nutr. **13**: 287–316.
29. STYLES, L. A., D. H. FOOTE, K. M. KLEMAN, C. J. KLUMPP, N. B. HEER & E. P. VICHINSKY. 1997. Hemoglobin H-Constant Spring Disease: An under recognized, severe form of α-thalassemia. Intl. J. Pediatr. Hematol/Oncol. **4**: 69–74.
30. ANAPLIOTOU, M. L, I. T. KASTANIAS, P. PSARA, E. A. EVANGELOU, M. LIPARAKI & P. DIMITRIOU. 1995. The contribution of hypogonadism to the development of osteoporosis in thalassaemia major: New therapeutic approaches. Clin. Endocrinol. **42**: 279–287.
31. JACKSON, E. C., F. STRIFE, R. C. TSANG & H. MARDER. 1988. Effect of calcitonin replacement therapy in idopathic juvenile osteoporosis. Am. J. Dis. Child. **142**: 1237–1239.
32. LINDSAY, R. 1988. Sex steroids in the pathogenesis and prevention of osteoporosis. *In* Osteoporosis: Etiology, Diagnosis and Management. B. L. Riggs, Ed.: 333–358. Raven Press. New York.

The Psychosocial Impact of Chronic Illness

CONSTANTINA POLITIS

Hellenic Red Cross Blood Transfusion Center and Thalassemia Unit,
4 Alkiviadou Street, Athens, Greece GR 10439

ABSTRACT: Depending on the severity of thalassemia and the level of health care provided, the thalassemic person may suffer from his/her chronic condition going through the path: disease → impairment → disability → handicap. There is evidence that a high clinical burden is associated with a psychosocial burden for the patients and the family.

In Greece, support strategies have developed in the last twenty years to help the thalassemic patient and his/her family. Recent studies in 909 patients show that the life span is prolonged (mean age 27 years), 83% of the patients study or work, 12% are married and 2.3% have set up a family, and 98% utilize the social benefits provided (free education, free entrance to universities, tax allowances, cash benefit, early retirement, *etc.*). However, psychometric tests performed in 131 patients and 65 matched normal controls over 14 years of age have shown that hostility (extroverted, delusional, total $p < 0.001$) is an important component of the psychological profile of the patients.

The patient's role through their association is strong and undoubtedly has influenced the public's extremely high (93%) awareness of the basic features of the disease and the supportive attitude of the average Greek citizen toward the life style of the thalassemic patient. On the whole, in many thalassemic patients illness has overpowered all other aspects of life. For few, however, life is much more than an illness. Shouldn't this be the message for the patient's psychosocial support strategies?

THALASSEMIA: THE GENERAL SITUATION

The World Health Organization's target of "Health for All" specifically includes β-thalassemia, one of the inherited hemoglobinopathies responsible for a large amount of chronic illness throughout the world. Except for the possibility of bone marrow transplantation in a strictly limited number of cases, it is a disease at present without cure, but one which modern medicine has overcome to the extent of giving sufferers from the disease the chance to function as normal members of society, instead of dying after a few years of grossly afflicted childhood. The nature of the chronic illness and its intensive and demanding treatment place a severe psychosocial burden on the thalassemia patient and his or her family. Consequently, psychosocial aspects of the disease have been widely studied.[1,2]

This paper is primarily concerned with homozygous β-thalassemia major. The milder intermedia syndrome is itself a chronic disease, whose patients and their families may well be subject to the same forces as are discussed here, but its psychosocial aspects have been much less studied than is the case with thalassemia major.[2] The focus is also upon the situation in the developed world, where the emphasis in the management of thalassemia nowadays falls increasingly upon quality of life.[1,2] In the developing world, it is sadly the case that most affected families do not have access to the standard treatment (regular transfusion and iron-chelation therapy to deal with iron overload) from which patients in the developed countries have benefited for twenty years now, so that survival remains the major issue.

Depending on the severity of the thalassemia and the level of health care available, the thalassemic patient may be found at various locations on the route from disease, through impairment and disability, to handicap, which is a path common to numerous severe chronic illnesses. The extent of affliction differs from individual to individual, depending on several factors but mainly on the clinical condition, which may be adversely affected by lack of access to appropriate health care (for reasons such as socioeconomic inequalities), and poor utilization of available health care relating to the patient's and his or her family's acceptance and understanding of the disease. Before the 1970s, the prognosis of thalassemia was very poor. Death was expected to occur before adulthood. In the mid-seventies, however, developments in the management of thalassemia introduced brighter prospects of survival, given good compliance with the latest treatments. Thalassemia thus ceased to be regarded exclusively as a disease of childhood; patients have every prospect of surviving beyond adolescence in countries whose health services can deliver adequate treatment. However, there is overwhelming evidence that the psychological element is now a crucial factor in survival.[1-5] There is a major psychological burden in coping with the many problems of the disease and its therapy, which demands frequent blood transfusions to maintain life, parenteral iron chelation to treat hemosiderosis and other complications of the disease, regular medical supervision, frequent admissions to hospital, and on many occasions surgical operations. The provision of psychosocial support for patients and their families is therefore of primary importance. Continuity of support is also important. The continuity and coordination of home and treatment unit care in a framework of continuous cooperation between a comprehensive therapeutic team and the patient and the patient's family are important factors for the improvement of the patient's clinical and psychosocial status, leading to a good quality of life.[3-5]

In developed countries, the combination of appropriate medical care and the psychosocial support provided to the patient and his or her family has led not only to greatly enhanced survival, but also to a good level of social integration and acceptance and favorable self-esteem.[3,5] In this achievement an appropriate social policy has played a very significant role. However, even in those countries whose health care systems are adequate, the psychosocial problems created in patients by the demands of the extremely burdensome treatment may lead to low compliance with the iron-chelation therapy and, ultimately, to death. In this respect, Ratip and Modell are right in stating that the most common cause of death in thalassemia is psychosocial in nature in the western countries.[1,2]

As reviewed by Ratip and Modell,[1,2] various researchers have identified and studied the characteristics of this psychosocial burden of thalassemia, focusing on social isolation, self-esteem, family adjustment, education, and sports. Psychiatric illness in children and adolescents has also been studied, as well as issues of social acceptance, relationships between adults, and problems in the working environment. The psychological features of families with thalassemic children have also been discussed. Despite all this work, psychosocial support will continue to be an important aspect of investigation in thalassemia. Developed countries with hitherto successful support strategies now have to face new problems as increasing numbers of thalassemic patients reach adulthood, work, marry and start families. TABLE 1 describes the psychosocial burden of thalassemia in the past. TABLE 2 summarizes current developments concerning physical appearance, growth, sexual

TABLE 1. Psychosocial Burden of Thalassemia in the Past

Stigmatization	
Secrecy about the illness	Impulsivity
Isolation of patient and family	Capriciousness
Physical handicap	Controlled temper
Absence of sexual development	Withdrawal
Fear of social rejection	Dependency
Fear of death	Dying before adulthood

development, and social integration. In developing countries, while the immediate major task for health care providers is to secure survival by exploiting improvements in medical treatment, support strategies will thereafter have to be developed in a way appropriate to each culture.

It is important to mention therapeutic novelties such as oral chelators, HbF inducers, bone marrow transplants, and gene therapy. Thanks to their close relationship with the therapeutic team and to the vigorous activity of patients' associations, patients are generally highly aware of scientific developments related to the treatment of their disease. When these turn out not to be available to the majority of patients or fail to live up to the promise of a dramatic improvement (as in the case of the oral chelator, which so many patients hoped would replace the punishing subcutaneous chelation procedure), the result is severe disappointment and frustration, adding further to the psychosocial burden.

THE SITUATION IN GREECE

Thalassemia is a major medical, social, and economic problem in Greece, where the prevalence of the heterozygous state is about 8%.[6] The annual blood consumption of about 3,500 thalassemic patients accounts for a quarter of the national total. The annual cost of iron-chelation therapy alone has been estimated to be two billion drachmas (Politis, unpublished data), while the cost of health services and other medication has not been measured. Although as yet no comprehensive register exists to provide data on the entire population of thalassemic patients, Politis and colleagues,[7] and Ladis and colleagues,[8] reported prolonged life span (the average age of 950 patients was 27 years), as survival has increased while preventive programs have led to the number of thalassemics born becoming very small. The majority of new cases of thalassemia now arise from immigration, including cases among repatriated Greek families, principally from the former Soviet Union.

The state's policy in response to this important problem includes, in the field of public health, education of the public for prevention by prenatal diagnosis and screening, and

TABLE 2. Psychosocial Burden of Thalassemia in the Present

Better physical appeareance	Prospects
Pubertal growth and sexual development	Oral chelators
Schooling	HbF inducers
Working	Bone marrow transplants
Establishing relationships	Gene therapy
Getting married	
Raising a family	
Low compliance with treatment for large number of patients	
• living for today	
• denial/anxiety/hostility	
Children born today	

TABLE 3. Public Awareness of Thalassemia (N = 3,478)

93% are aware of thalassemia
90% are aware of the need for blood transfusion
89% know the thalassemia is not infectious
80% know about the hereditary nature of thalassemia
69% believe thalassemia is presently incurable

TABLE 4. Social Benefits Provided to Thalassemic Patients in Greece

Free medical care
Cash benefits
Tax allowances
Entry to universities and other institutions of higher education without examinations
Paid training and technical education
Work incentives (large industries are obliged to employ disabled people up to 4% of their labor force)
Early retirement
Facilities (transportation, electricity, telephone, etc.)

promotion of blood donation to save the lives of patients with thalassemia. Public awareness is indeed quite good. A nationwide survey conducted by the Hellenic Red Cross Thalassemia Unit in 1989 found that 93% of citizens aged 15–65 years had heard of thalassemia, 90% knew that it called for blood transfusion, 89% that it was not infectious, 80% that it was hereditary, and 69% that it was incurable (TABLE 3).[9] Social policy also confronts certain aspects of the problem. A number of regulations dating originally from the 1980s recognize thalassemic patients as a group with special needs and provide for various benefits (such as certain cash benefits, tax exemptions, extra leave, and early retirement) and measures aimed at improving social integration (bypassing the university entrance examinations, increased work opportunities).[9] TABLE 4 summarizes the social benefits available to thalassemic patients in Greece. The strong patients' association

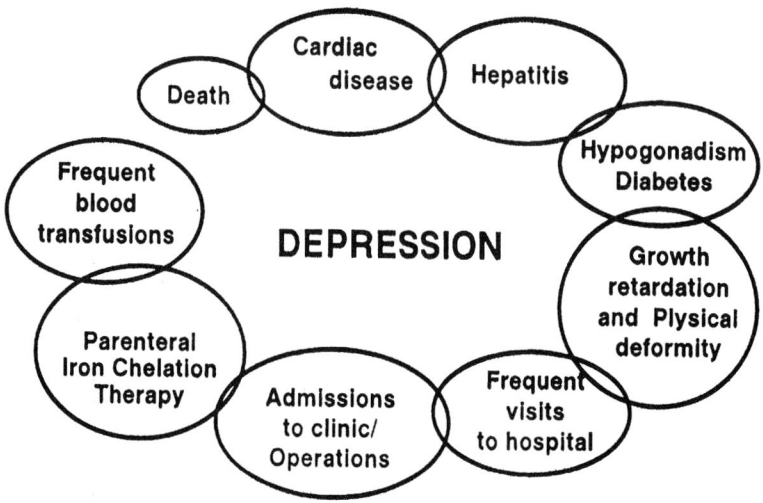

FIGURE 1.

TABLE 5. Comparison between Thalassemic Patients and Normal Controls[a]

Spielberger's State-Trait Anxiety Inventory (STAI)
Zung's Self-Rating Scale for Depression (SRSD)
Eysenck's Personality Questionnaire (EPQ)
Fould's Hostility and Direction of Hostility Questionnaire (HDHQ)
Hostility is an important component of the psychological profile of the patients

[a]After Trikkas et al.[10]

ensures that its members are well informed about these possibilities; its studies show that 98% exploit social benefits in some way.

Thalassemic patients in Greece receive high quality therapy free of charge. Many patients are cared for in large specialized units with comprehensive therapeutic teams. Within these, staff have vigorously worked over the last twenty years on developing support strategies to help the thalassemic patient and his or her family. Psychosocial support may be below the desirable level only in the smallest treatment centers.

The recent studies of the Panhellenic Association of Thalassemic Patients to evaluate the quality of life of their members show that 83% of the patients are either studying or working, 6% are married, and 1.3% have started a family. A more detailed study performed in 1989 by the Hellenic Red Cross Thalassemia Unit in Athens, Greece, and a parallel one carried out by the Division of Pediatrics in Ferrara, Italy, concentrated on investigating what level of social integration these chronically ill patients had in fact achieved in two centers staffed by comprehensive therapeutic teams who encourage the independence of their patients and their psychosocial integration to the highest possible degree.[3] Both studies reported a good level of social integration. Amongst other findings, the distribution of employment status in the Greek sample was found to be the same as in the general population of the same age range, while more (34%) had graduated from university or were currrently studying than in the general population (22%). Self-esteem was also found to be favorable. These results were encouraging indicators of the success of the policy of providing psychosocial support as part of the comprehensive approach to treatment. However, in another study psychometric tests revealed statistically significantly higher hostility in thalassemic patients than in controls.[10] This indicates that despite the very high level of social integration of the thalassemic patients in Greece, hostility is an important component of their psychological profile (TABLE 5).

Moreover, in the following years, despite continuation of support for the patients of the Hellenic Red Cross Thalassemia Unit, it turned out that 30% of them complied only moderately with the iron-chelation therapy. This was associated with a 60% incidence of generalized and local reactions to desferrioxamine,[11] an extra factor deterring patients from adhering to their treatment schedules. At the same time, many patients whose hopes had been raised by the prospect of oral chelation becoming a practical reality were disappointed in the summer of 1996 when the oral chelator became available to only a small group of their peers, whereupon a large number of patients reduced their compliance with the iron-chelation therapy. Another adverse factor was the increasing number of deaths—mainly (80%) due to cardiac complications—as the population of patients aged. This has forced the medical and nursing staff to confront the necessity of new support strategies in these changing circumstances.

On the whole, as stated by Georganta, illness dominates all aspects of life in many thalassemic patients.[12] For a few, however, life is much more important than an illness. This might be taken as the key message for our patients' psychosocial support strategies.

REFERENCES

1. RATIP, S., D. SKUSE, J. PORTER *et al.* 1995. Psychosocial and clinical burden of thalassemia intermedia and its implications for prenatal diagnosis. Arch. Dis. Child. **72**: 408–412.
2. RATIP, S. & B. MODELL. 1996. Psychological and sociological aspects of the thalassemias. Sem. Hematol. **33**: 53–65.
3. POLITIS, C., A. DI PALMA, M. FISFIS, A. GIASANTI, S. C. RICHARDSON, C. VULLO & G. MASERA. 1990. Social integration of the older thalassemic patient. Arch. Dis. Child. **65**: 984–986.
4. MASSAGLIA, P. & M. CARPIGNANO. 1985. Psychology of the thalassemia patient and his family. Thalassemia Today. The Mediterranean Experience. Presented at the Second Mediterranean Meeting. Milano, 1985.
5. ZANI, B., A. DI PALMA & C. VULLO. 1995. Psychosocial aspects of chronic illness in adolescents with thalassemia major. J. Adolesc. **18**: 387–402.
6. TASSIOPOULOU, A., A. ANAGNOSTOU, D. LOUKOPOULOS & P. FESSAS. 1985. Organization of services in Greece. I. Carrier identification. Thalassemia Today.
7. POLITIS, C., H. VRETTOU, S. FRAGATOU, J. HATZILAOU, C. FLESSA & CL. S. RICHARDSON. 1996. Survival and causes of death in thalassemia major. The experience of the Hellenic Red Cross Thalassemia Unit. Presented at the Third International Symposium on "Bone Marrow Transplantation in Thalassemia." Pesaro, September 26–29, 1996.
8. LADIS, V., A. PAPADOPOULOU, C. ATHANASSAKI, F. PALAMIDOU, S. KOSTARIDOU, A. BERDOUSSI & C. KATTAMIS. 1996. Long term survival and causes of death in patients with thalassemia under conventional treatment. Presented at the Third International Symposium on "Bone Marrow Transplantation in Thalassemia." Pesaro, September 26–29, 1996.
9. POLITIS, C., C. RICHARDSON & J. G. YFANTOPOULOS. 1991. Public knowledge of thalassemia in Greece and current concepts of the social status of the thalassemic patient. Soc. Sci. Med. **32**: 59–64.
10. TRIKKAS, G., C. POLITIS, A. VOULGARI, H. VRETTOU & G. N. CHRISTODOULOU. 1988. Psychosocial findings in thalassemic patients. Presented at the Seventeenth European Conference on Psychosomatic Research. Marburg, September 4–11, 1988.
11. POLITIS, C., H. VRETTOU, S. FRAGATOU, J. HATZILAOU, C. RICHARDSON & G. SALEM. 1993. Reactions to subcutaneous application of iron chelation therapy with desferrioxamine. An urgent need for oral chelators. Presented at the Fourth International Conference on Oral Chelation in the Treatment of Thalassemia and Other Diseases. Limassol, Cyprus. March 26–29, 1993.
12. GEORGANTA, E. T. 1990. The impact of thalassemia on body image, self-image and self-esteem. Ann. N. Y. Acad. Sci. **612**: 466–472.

Psychosocial Integration of Adolescents and Young Adults with Thalassemia Major

A. DI PALMA,[a-c] C. VULLO,[d] B. ZANI,[e] AND A. FACCHINI[d]

[c]*Pediatric Dept., S. Chiara Hospital, Trento, Italy*
[d]*Pediatric Dept., S. Anna Hospital, Ferrara, Italy*
[e]*Dept. of Science of Education, University of Bologna, Bologna, Italy*

ABSTRACT: The aim of this study was to explore the effect of thalassemia major on the psychosocial adjustment of adolescents and young adults. Design: unmarried adolescent and young adult patients were asked to fill in an *ad hoc* questionnaire; a semi-structured interview exploring marriage and family life was done with married patients. Sample: *group A:* 90 unmarried patients, 50% females and 50% males, aged 14–22 years. The control group was formed by 100 matched subjects; *group B:* 19 thalassemic married subjects, 6 males and 13 females, aged 28–45 years, 7 patients had children and 12 did not. Results: *group A:* subjects with thalassemia had normal psychological and social development and scored better than their normal peers in tests investigating social adjustment, self-esteem and self-description. Moreover the family relationships of adolescents with thalassemia appeared to be stronger than those reported by normal controls; *group B:* the behavior of thalassemic couples did not differ from the one observed in non-thalassemic couples in the course of previous investigations. Conclusions: Our data shows that neither thalassemic adolescents nor thalassemic married, well-treated, young adults differ significantly from the healthy young people in their ability to cope with life's difficulties both in adolescence and marital life.

In the last two decades the course and the clinical picture of β-thalassemia major have been dramatically changed by treatment. Bone marrow transplantation can cure the disease, but since this is possible in relatively few cases owing to the lack of histocompatible donors most of the patients must rely on traditional treatment.[1] As this is based on periodic red blood cell transfusion, daily iron chelation, and sometimes splenectomy, it constitutes a very severe burden for the patients and their families. In addition, treatment also may cause complications, which include lesions of many organs and tissues due to iron deposition (in spite of chelation treatment), transfusion-transmitted infections, side effects due to administration of iron chelators, and increased susceptibility to overwhelming infections due to splenectomy.[2] It is generally accepted that chronic diseases may cause psychosocial imbalance. As β-thalassemia major is such a demanding disease, one would expect that subjects affected by this disease are at high risk of developing psychosocial problems. Data regarding the psychosocial aspects of thalassemia major are scanty. This is probably due to the fact that in the past the medical problems of the disease were so severe that all other aspects were more or less neglected. A complete review of the literature may be found in a recent paper.[3]

[a]A. Di Palma previously worked in the Pediatric Department, S. Anna Hospital, Ferrara, Italy where the investigations were carried out.
[b]Address for correspondence: Annunziata Di Palma, Pediatric Department, S. Chiara Hospital, Largo Medaglie d'Oro, 38100 -Trento, Italy; Tel: 0039.461. 903538; Fax: 0039.461. 903824.

THE FERRARA EXPERIENCE

In Italy, as in other countries, the incidence of β-thalassemia is higher in the areas where malaria was highly endemic in the past. The Po River delta is such an area and this explains why about 170 patients are regularly followed in Ferrara today. In the past, treatment of thalassemia major was given on an in-patient basis, but starting in 1979 patients with thalassemia are treated in an ad hoc day hospital. The staff of the day hospital consists of two doctors and three nurses. Regular psychological and social support is not available, but it can be obtained if required. A parent association was founded in 1974 and the members of its committee meet weekly with the representatives of the doctors and nurses of the day hospital.Also meetings attended by the parents and patients are held when the parents, doctors, or patients feel that there are problems that need to be discussed. We wondered whether the improved quality of treatment, apart from improving the prognosis of subjects affected by thalassemia, had a beneficial effect on their psychosocial adjustment. The first answer to this question came from two studies performed independently in the Red Cross Thalassemia Unit in Athens, and in the Thalassemia Service in Ferrara.[4]

The Athens Center, established in 1955, follows about 300 patients affected by thalassemia. The two centers follow similar policies of multidisciplinary approaches to the medical and psychosocial support of their patients, but the staff of the Athens Center includes psychologists and social workers, which are not included in the Ferrara staff. The investigations were done by personal interviews using questionnaires designed independently in Greece and Italy. They were similar enough so that a comparison between the results of the two surveys was possible. The questionnaires covered various topics, particularly different aspects of social integration, such as education, occupation, self-image, and attitude toward physical appearance. The investigations showed that there were differences between the two groups of patients, which were due to the different social background and legislation. However, the self-image of patients seemed fairly good in both groups, and overall it was clear that transfusion-dependent thalassemia does not necessarily prevent normal psychosocial development.

The second investigation on the psychosocial aspects of transfusion-dependent thalassemia in Ferrara was done in 1994.[5] All subjects with thalassemia, aged between 14 and 22 years, were asked by a psychologist to answer an ad hoc questionnaire. Ninety one percent of patients agreed and consisted of 45 females and 45 males. A control group of 57 females and 43 males without thalassemia of the same age range and with similar, even if not identical, sociocultural origin, was also examined. The questionnaire covered the following topics: (1) type of family relationships and perception of autonomy from parents; (2) level of social integration (friendship, membership of peer groups, school achievement, leisure time); (3) heterosexual relationships; (4) self concept; and (5) coping strategies (TABLE 1).

The analysis of the data of the questionnaires showed that adolescents with thalassemia: (1) have from fairly good to very good relationships with their parents, even better than

TABLE 1. Main Topics Investigated by an ad Hoc Questionnaire for Adolescents with and without Thalassemia Major

Measures of Psychosocial Functioning	Measures of Psychological Functioning
Family relationships	Self-esteem
Peer group relationships	Self-description
Partner relationships	Body image
School	Emotional self
Relations with medical team	Coping strategies
	Representation of the disease

that of the subjects in the control group; (2) are less frequently members of sports clubs and more often of religious group; (3) are more cautious than controls as far as heterosexual relationships are concerned; (4) show a very positive self image and their level of schooling is even higher than that of the control group; (5) consider finding a job, getting married, and having children as more distant targets than the control group; (6) seem to adopt negative strategies less frequently in a difficult situation; (7) search actively for the social support, more from parents and religion and less from friends.

More recently, an investigation was done on the psychosocial characteristics of married couples of which one member has β-thalassemia major. It was possible to investigate all the partners with thalassemia but only 14 of 19 non-thalassemic partners were studied, (one couple got divorced, and 4 non-thalassemic partners ware not available for various reasons). The following means were used for the investigation: (1) a socio-demographic form; (2) a semistructured interview; and (3) an ad hoc questionnaire. This was designed to investigate the decision processes of the couples and the degree of satisfaction of themarital life (TABLES 2 and 3). The data obtained were compared with data previously obtained investigating couples without thalassemia. Interviews were conducted by a psychologist and took place in thalassemia day hospital. The semistructured interview investigated the following topics: main events in infancy and adolescence, relationships with the parents (including autonomy), socialization, school, occupation, falling in love, marriage, marital life, and having children. As regards the premarital life, the interviews confirmed the data of the previous investigation, i.e., thalassemics affirmed that they had good relationships with the parents and peers, only in a few cases were there signs of parental overprotection. It was found that schooling was adversely affected by the disease. This result is different from what was found in the previous investigation. The non-thalassemic partners said that their decision to marry had been made easier by the information on the disease that they had received from doctors. Contrary to what was expected, thalassemics did not report anxiety about getting married and neither partner had a dominant role in the marital life. Both females and males with thalassemia think that is very important to have children and one thalassemic female said that "having no child is like being out of everything" and one thalassemic male said "having a child was a dream which came true." The analysis of questionnaires showed that there were not differences between the marital life and the coping strategies between couples with and without thalassemia (TABLE 3).

DISCUSSION

Data regarding the effect of chronic disorders on psychosocial integration of children and adolescents are contradictory. Some authors found that subjects with chronic diseases have an increased risk of developing psychosocial disturbances,[6–8] but others have not been able to confirm these findings.[9] Thalassemia is a chronic disorder that interferes with

TABLE 2. Data on Thalassemic Married Subjects and Control Subjects

	Examined Sample (%)	Age (range)
Subjects with Thalassemia	19 subjects (100%)	28–45
	6 males (31.5%)	
	13 females (68.5%)	
Subjects without Thalassemia	14 subjects (100%)	24–43
	10 males (71.4%)	
	4 females (28.6%)	
Couples with children	7 (36.8%)	
Couples without children	12 (63.2%)	

TABLE 3. Quality of Marital Life: Values on a Ten Point Scale

	Thalassemic Husbands (SD)	Thalassemic wives (SD)	Non-Thalassemic Husbands (SD)	Non-Thalassemic Wives (SD)
Questions				
Does your partner understand your needs?	6.57 (5.78)	5.78 (1.36)	6.21 (0.80)	6.14 (1.46)
Are you happy for your relationship?	6.78 (0.42)	6.14 (1.70)	6.50 (0.85)	6.42 (1.60)
How do you think your relation is compared with the others?	5.78 (1.25)	5.92 (0.99)	6.07 (0.99)	5.64 (1.21)
Sometimes would you like not to be involved in this relationship?	3.21 (2.93)	3.35 (2.56)	3.64 (2.84)	2.92 (2.61)
Do you think your relationship matches your original expectations?	6.28 (1.13)	5.85 (1.16)	6.21 (1.05)	5.92 (1.26)
How much do you love your partner?	6.71 (0.46)	6.21 (1.05)	6.21 (1.05)	6.71 (0.46)
Do you think that there are many problems in your relationship?	5.50 (1.65)	4.50 (2.34)	4.35 (2.30)	5.61 (1.59)
Self-Description				
Our relationship is quite good	6.57 (0.75)	6.42 (0.85)	6.35 (0.92)	6.64 (0.63)
Our relationship is very continuous	6.15 (0.80)	6.14 (0.86)	5.92 (0.82)	6.38 (0.76)
Our relationship is very strong	6.50 (0.75)	6.42 (0.75)	6.42 (0.75)	6.50 (0.75)
The relationship with my partner makes me very happy	6.64 (0.63)	6.00 (1.83)	5.92 (1.81)	6.71 (0.61)
There is a great feeling between me and my partner	5.85 (0.94)	5.78 (1.31)	5.57 (1.34)	6.07 (0.82)
Our relationship is very happy	6.64 (0.63)	5.85 (1.95)	5.85 (1.95)	6.64 (0.63)

the course of everyday life because patients need daily iron chelation therapy, mainly by wearing an electronic pump, and also need to go periodically to the treatment center to be transfused. In the past the disease caused facial deformities that could adversely affect body image and self-esteem. Accordingly, one would expect that subjects with thalassemia would be at an increased risk of psychosocial disturbances. In fact, Tsiantis found that 42% of a group of subjects with thalassemia followed in Greece had psychiatric problems even if they had a normal self-concept.[10] Parallel research studies done in Athens and Ferrara and another investigation done in Ferrara did not confirm this. They showed that adolescents and young adults with thalassemia have psychosocial development comparable to that of subjects of the same age group without thalassemia. Moreover, the last investigation done in Ferrara demonstrated that subjects with thalassemia also may have a normal marital life. We are aware that the studies in Ferrara and in other places may have limitations. It is not possible to be sure that all subjects who participated in the study gave honest answers, even though the replies were anonymous. Not all patients followed in Ferrara, aged from 14 to 22 years, agreed to participate in the study and it is possible that the subjects who did not wish to answer the questionnaire are those that have psychosocial problems. However, we are confident that the results of our investigation reflect the psychosocial adjustment of subjects with thalassemia followed in Ferrara because the number of the subjects who did not participate is too small to affect the general conclusion and because the results are in agreement with the fact that subjects with thalassemia are as successful as their peers in schooling and occupation. It is not possible to say with certainty why the psychosocial adjustment of subjects with thalassemia followed in Athens and in Ferrara is so good in spite of the disease. It is relevant that Tsiantis and colleagues found recently that thalassemia has a uniting effect on the family, contrary to what was expected.[3]

CONCLUSION

We suggest that three main factors played a beneficial role in the psychosocial adjustment of our patients. Firstly, a positive role could have been played by the improvement in medical treatment. The transfusion regime that maintains a high hemoglobin level was adopted in Ferrara from the early 1970s, so that patients aged from 14 to 22 years do not have the facial abnormalities that could adversely affect self-image and social acceptance. Red cell transfusions are done on a day hospital basis, so reducing the time spent in hospital by patients to a minimum. Subjects who have delayed or absent pubertal development are treated with hormones, thus preventing the psychosocial consequences of lack of sexual development. Hormone treatment also may in some cases cure infertility due to endocrine complications caused by iron overload, making completely normal marital life possible. Secondly, in the Po delta area a health education program relating to thalassemia was started in 1955 and still continues. As a consequence, the level of awareness of the problems of thalassemia in the general population is fairly good and this makes it easier for subjects with this disease not be treated as abnormal. Thirdly, the medical staff has always had an optimistic attitude and relationships with the parents association are excellent and continuous. Both these factors could have made the acceptance of the disease and the psychosocial adjustment of the patients and their families easier. Therefore, the psychosocial adjustment of subjects with thalassemia followed in other centers may not be as good as in Ferrara.

ACKNOWLEDGMENTS

The Authors wish to thank Dr. Barbara Anderson for her helpful comments and Maria Luisa Auspergher for her assistance in preparing the paper.

REFERENCES

1. LUCARELLI, G., R. A. CLIFT, M. GALIMBERTI *et al.* 1996. Marrow transplantation for patients with thalassemia: results in class 3 patients. Blood **87**: 2062–2088.
2. MODELL, B. & V. BERDUKAS. 1984. The Clinical Approach to Thalassaemia. Grune & Stratton. New York and London.
3. TSIANTIS, J., TH. DRAGONAS, C. RICHARDSON *et al.* 1996. Psychosocial problems and adjustment of children with β-thalassemia major and their families. Eur. J. Child. Adolesc. Psychiatr. **5**: 193–203.
4. POLITIS, C., A. DI PALMA, M. FISFIS *et al.* 1990. Social integration of the older thalassemic patients. Arch. Dis. Child. **65**: 984–986.
5. ZANI, B., A. DI PALMA & C. VULLO. 1995. Psychosocial aspects of chronic illness in adolescents with thalassaemia major. J. Adolesc. **18**: 387–402.
6. ANARNEY, E. R. 1985. Social maturation. A challenge for handicapped and chronically ill adolescents. Adolesc. Health Care **90**: 101.
7. NEWACHEK, P. W., M. A. MC. MANUS & H. B. FOX. 1991. Prevalence and impact of chronic illness among adolescents. Am. J. Dis. Child. **145**: 1367–1373.
8. WOLMAN, C., M. D. RESNICK, L. J. HARRIS *et al.* 1994. Emotional well-being among adolescents with and without chronic conditions. J. Adolesc. Health **15**: 199–204.
9. KELERMAN, J., L. ZELTZER, L. ELLENBERG *et al.* 1980. Psychological effects of illness in adolescence. I. Anxiety, self-esteem and perception of control. J. Pediatr. **97**: 126–131.
10. TSIANTIS, J. 1990. Family reactions and relationships in Thalassemia. Ann. N.Y. Acad. Sci. **612**: 451–461.

Future Orientation and Life Expectations of Adolescents and Young Adults with Thalassemia Major[a]

SHERRY BUSH, FRANCINE S. MANDEL, AND
PATRICIA J. GIARDINA[b]

*Division of Pediatric Hematology/Oncology, The New York
Hospital–Cornell Medical Center, New York, New York 10021*

ABSTRACT: Until recently, Thalassemia Major was considered a fatal disease and patients did not usually live into adulthood. Advances in the medical management of the disease have greatly increased the life expectancy of these patients. The present study aims to evaluate the future orientation and other aspects of psychosocial functioning of thalassemics compared to healthy controls. Thirty patients and 33 healthy subjects of similar age, ethnicity, education, and geographic area were compared on measures of future expectations, perceived social support, life orientation, health locus of control and hopelessness. Results show no significant differences between thalassemics and controls on all measures except for higher levels of internal health locus of control among the patient group. Results and implications of perceptions of thalassemics' future orientation relevant to patient care are discussed.

Beta Thalassemia Major, also known as Cooley's anemia is one of several childhood illnesses that have moved from the acute or fatal category of diseases to that of chronicity. In contrast to the patient demographics associated with the disease in the 1970s, thalassemia major in North American has largely become a disease of young adults rather than children.[1] Since the 1960s, median survival has changed from 16 to 30 years.[2] Increased survival has resulted from advances in clinical management during the past two decades.[3] Although the challenges of the disease have been well documented in research, limited information exists regarding patients' expectations about the variety of diverse life options that now exist for them. The focus of the current study is to assess the future orientation of the adolescent and young adult patient population in the United States. The study also aims at identifying specific expectations and the presence of psychological resources that may mediate such expectations.

BACKGROUND

Thalassemia major is a recessively inherited hematologic disorder, usually diagnosed within the first year of life, causing life-threatening anemia.[4] Patients depend on regular

---

[a]This work was supported by National Institute of Health grants #M01 RR06020 from the General Clinical Research Centers Program Office of the Division of Research Resources Foundation, and by the Children's Blood Foundation. The support of HRI 815-320H for patient care and the assistance of the Thalassemia Action Group and the Cooley's Anemia Foundation is gratefully acknowledged.

[b]Address for correspondence: Patricia J. Giardina, MD, Division of Pediatric Hematology/Oncology, The New York Hospital-Cornell Medical Center, 525 East 68th Street, New York, New York, 10021.

transfusion therapy and chelation therapy for the progressive transfusional iron overload. Prior to chelation therapy, complications from iron overload resulted in cardiac failure and early death.[2]

As the mean age and life expectancy of thalassemia major patients has expanded, psychosocial issues related to quality of life have become an increasingly important focus of attention.[5-9] A number of psychological variables have been identified as compromising psychosocial functioning. The hereditary nature of the disease, physical deformities, growth retardation, delayed puberty, and the demands of regular blood transfusions and chelation therapy are examples of challenges faced by patients. Mortality issues and the ever present knowledge that thalassemia is a life-long illness must also be considered. Additionally, many patients have experienced the loss of peers with thalassemia due to complications associated with the disease. In the past, growing up led to the increased likelihood of mortality as only a small number of patients survived into adulthood. In addition, the fears, restrictions, and over-protectiveness of their parents may also influence the perceptions thalassemia patients have of their ability to adapt to appropriate developmental stages.[6-8]

Earlier studies on psychosocial functioning of chronically ill adolescents found the presence of significant levels of emotional problems and poor social adaption.[10,11] However, there is increasing evidence that children with chronic illness do not manifest psychological disturbance or maladjustment and may utilize internal resources, resiliency, and social support as effective coping mechanisms.[6,9,11-13]

A study of health locus of control and self esteem of adolescent patients with diabetes and cystic fibrosis found no significant differences in comparison to healthy controls.[12] The findings from this study are relevant to the thalassemia population in that patients with diabetes and cystic fibrosis have the opportunity, in contrast to other chronic illness groups, to exert some control over their illness through specific health behaviors.

A recent study by Zani and colleagues[9] evaluated the impact of thalassemia major on the psychological functioning and social behavior of 90 adolescent patients and 100 healthy control subjects in Italy. The results indicated that thalassemia patients had normal psychological development and scored even better than healthy controls in tests concerning self esteem, self description, and use of functional coping strategies. The study also measured subjects' assignment of the importance of seven specified events in their lives, such as finding a job, getting married, living independently, and having children. Results showed that thalassemic patients had a positive view of their future and placed a high value on finding jobs, as well as finding the right partner.

METHODOLOGY

The thalassemia major group was comprised of 30 transfusion-dependent patients from the United States, between the ages of 16 and 28. Patients were voluntary subjects requested to complete self-report instruments and demographic questionnaires, which took less than 45 minutes to complete. Patients were enlisted for participation by request of nurse coordinators at out-patient clinics at major medical centers across the nation, with the majority of subjects from New York and Philadelphia. Patients were also asked to participate in the study during a national conference of the Thalassemia Action Group. Of 32 returned surveys 30 were fully completed and included in the study. Inclusion criteria for patients were (1) that they be between the ages of 16 and 28 by November 1, 1996, (2) they have been receiving ongoing medical treatment through a hospital-affiliated clinic, and (3) they began continuous chelation therapy prior to 11 years of age.

To control for socio-economic and cultural variables, which may influence future orientation, 33 healthy subjects of similar age, education levels, ethnic background, religion, gender, marital status, parental marital status, and geographic location were selected as match-controls. Participation of the control subjects was voluntary and recruited by members of the Thalassemia Action Group and the Cooley's Anemia Foundation.

Of the 30 thalassemia subjects 12 were males and 18 females, ranging in age from 16 to 28 years with a mean age of 21.9 years($\pm$ 3.1). The 33 control subjects were comprised of 14 males and 19 females, ranging in age from 16 to 26 years with a mean age of 23 years ($\pm$ 2.6). Nineteen subjects from both groups were of Italian ethnicity and 25 were of Greek ethnicity. Other ethnic groups represented included Asian, Indian/Pakistani, and Middle Eastern. Among the thalassemia group, 21 of the 27 subjects old enough to attend college had completed some form of post-secondary education including 9 who graduated from a four-year college. Within the control group, 26 of the 33 subjects completed some level of post-secondary education with 18 having received a four-year-college degree. Both the thalassemic and control group had the same number of subjects who were married (1 from each group) and almost all subjects came from families with the same parental marital status.

All subjects were administered a questionnaire to record sociodemographic information (age, sex, education, marital status, religion, parental marital status, and ethnicity) and to identify those participants with thalassemia. Subjects completed five instruments to determine levels of future expectation, social support, life orientation, hopelessness, and health locus of control. Future expectations were assessed using the Future Expectations Inventory (FEI),[15] a 13-item instrument identifying the level of specific expectations concerning education, work, relationships, and parenting. The FEI scores are based on a Likert scale with a total score tabulated from the number of positive expectations respondents endorse. Future orientation and coping were assessed using the Life Orientation Test[16] an 8-item (plus 4 filler items) inventory of optimism and outcome expectancies.

Perceived control related to health was assessed using the Multidimensional Health Locus of Control,[17] an 18-item scale measuring the beliefs and capacity for health-related behaviors as primarily internal, matter of chance, or under the control of powerful others. Assessment of hopelessness was measured using the Beck Hopelessness Scale (BHS),[18] a 20-item scale for measuring the extent of negative attitudes about the future (pessimism) as perceived by adolescents and adults. Perceptions of social support were assessed with a instrument developed to identify levels and sources of emotional support. Subjects were asked to endorse the amount of emotional support they receive from parents, siblings, friends, doctors, nurses, mental health professionals, clergy, and boy/girl friend on a Likert-type scale from "very little" to a "large amount." The support inventory was included in the study as a means by which to identify possible mediating variables and/or correlates of scores on measures of future expectations.

Thalassemic patients were compared to controls with independent t-tests for all scales except the BHS, which was examined using a Wilcoxon summed-rank test. Support items for the two groups were compared using chi-square tests of proportions. Relationships among scales were measured using Pearson product moment correlation coefficients.

RESULTS

Future Expectations

Thalassemia subjects were found to have a higher total score on the Future Expectations Inventory (FEI)[15] than their healthy counterparts, suggesting the presence of a greater number of positive expectations overall about their future (TABLE 1). Results of independent samples t-test show a significant difference between the groups, with thalassemia subjects having a higher level of positive future expectations (Thal mean = 45.86 ± 6.34; Control mean = 42.09 ± 7.54; $p = .036$). Item analysis using Fisher's Exact Test are displayed in TABLE 1.

The thalassemia subjects reported greater expectations of being in a sexual relationship despite having an illness ($p < .009$). No significant differences were found between groups on items regarding future expectations of work or concerns about an illness keeping them from reaching work goals. There were no significant differences between groups on items related to relationship and marriage expectations. Both thalassemia patients and healthy controls had similar expectations about having children and being a parent one day. Concerning the expectation that an illness would keep them from making future plans, results approached significance with thalassemia subjects slightly more optimistic than healthy controls ($p = .057$).

Life Orientation and Optimism

Comparing responses on the Life Orientation Test[15] of the thalassemic patients and healthy controls, using independent samples t-test, no significant differences were found (Thal mean = 20.43 ± 6.06; Control mean = 19.0 ± 4.82; $p = .30$). Results indicate no significant differences in the level of optimism and positive outcome expectancies between the two groups.

Hopelessness

Living with the multitude of stressors associated with thalassemia, in addition to the pervasive presence of a chronic illness, would thalassemia patients endorse more "hopeless" attitudes than healthy controls? Both groups responded to the Beck Hopelessness Scale[16] with results showing no significant differences (Wilcoxon summed rank test: Thal median = 2 (inter-quartial range = 1 to 5); Control 1 (0 to 6); $p = .259$).

TABLE 1. Future Expectations Inventory: Results of Comparison between Thalassemic and Healthy Subjects

Expectations	Fisher's Exact Test	
1.	I expect to reach my future work goals.	.222
2.	Getting married, or being in a marriage-like relationship, is not something I expect to do. (R)	.370
3.	Having a child is not something I expect to do.	.075
4.	Have positive expectations about my future.	.383
5.	Having an illness or a physical problem would keep me from having a sexual relationship. (R)	.009[a]
6.	Have future expectations about being a parent.	.122
7.	Having future work expectations is not realistic for me. (R)	.114
8.	I do not expect an illness will keep me from reaching my work/career goals.	.319
9.	Having a loving relationship in the future is something I expect.	.852
10.	I expect an illness would keep me from making plans about my future. (R)	.057
11.	Having expectations about having a career is realistic for me.	.367
12.	I expect to be in a sexual relationship in the future.	.181
13.	I expect to reach the goals I have for my future.	.444

(R) = reversed items for scoring. Total score based on number of positive attributions of expectations.
[a]$p < .05$

Health Locus of Control

The source of cognitive reinforcements for health-related behaviors as internal, a matter of chance, or under the control of powerful others has been documented as a variable in health behaviors.[17] Results of independent sample t-test of the Multidimensional Health Locus of Control (MHLC)[17] showed thalassemia patients overall had a higher level of internal health locus of control than healthy controls (Thal mean = 26.2 ± 4.99; Control mean = 23.67 ± 4.28; $p < .034$). In other words, the thalassemia group expressed significantly higher beliefs that one stays or becomes healthy as a result of his or her behavior. The MHLC also is used to assess the level of the individual's health expectancy as determined by chance. Results indicate that neither group attributed their health as a matter of chance (Thal mean = 14.47 ± 5.31; Control mean = 16.33 ± 5.34; $p = .98$).

Although overall results of the MHLC suggest the thalassemia group can be characterized as having an "internal" health locus of control, they also believe their health is influenced by their physician. Scores on the MHLC dimension assessing the belief that physicians control one's health, indicated that the thalassemia group had significantly higher beliefs that their health was in large part influenced by their physicians (Thal mean = 12.77 ± 2.62; Control mean = 9.45 ± 2.66; $p < .0001$). The thalassemia patients believe they are in control of their health and that behaviors determine their health outcomes, but they also believe, more than the control group, that physicians have a significant amount of control over their health. Other people, including parents and family members, were not endorsed by either group as controlling their health (Thal mean = 8.53 ± 3.26; Control mean = 7.21 ± 3.04; $p = .186$).

SOCIAL SUPPORT

The relationship between social support and health behaviors is well documented. There is evidence that social support has both a direct positive effect on health status and also serves as modifier of stress on the mental and physical health of an individual.[19] Social support and familial context has also been shown to serve as a variable in future orientation among adolescents and young adults.[20] How social support may be correlated to future expectations among thalassemics was another focus of our study.

Compared to healthy subjects, the thalassemic group endorsed having greater social support (Thal mean = 23.53 ± 6.48; Control mean = 19.12 ± 6.23; $p < .008$). Results showed that the thalassemic patients identified having more sources of support as well as greater levels of emotional support. The most striking difference between Thalassemia and control groups was related to the amount of perceived emotional support from a boyfriend or girlfriend. Significantly more healthy subjects reported having a boyfriend or girlfriend (control $N = 23$/Thal $N = 13$) and receiving above average to a large amount of emotional support ($p = .032$). No significant differences were found in the levels of perceived support from other friends, family members, doctors, mental health professionals, or clergy. However, the thalassemic group identified receiving a greater amount of emotional support from nurses ($p = .026$).

When analyzing the results from the thalassemia group concerning perceived support from physicians, a bivariate profile emerged in the data with patients endorsing that they either receive very little or a large amount of emotional support. The healthy group's responses to this item were more evenly dispersed and, although not statistically significant ($p = .063$) indicated that they received generally less support from physicians overall (Control $N = 23$; Thal $N = 30$).

To determine if perceived social support may have mediated our subjects' future orientation, the Pearson product moment correlation coefficients were used to measure the relationship of the social support scale with the Future Expectations Inventory (FEI),[15] Life Orientation Test (LOT),[16] Beck Hopelessness Scale (BHS),[18] and the Multidimensional Health Locus of Control (MHLC).[17] Social support scores were not significantly correlated with future expectations (r = .103), life orientation (r = .169), internal health locus of control (r = −.028), or hopelessness (r = −.068).

CORRELATES OF FUTURE EXPECTATIONS

Although social support was not found to be significantly correlated with future expectations in the present study, a number of other psychosocial variables were identified as relating to the subjects' perceptions of the future. Scores on the FEI were positively correlated with an internal health locus of control (MHLC:r = .41) and positive life orientation (LOT:r = .40). Results of the FEI were negatively correlated to hopelessness (BHS:r = −.48). Therefore, subjects who have positive expectations about their future also have a positive life orientation, internal health locus of control, and are not "hopeless" in their attributions about life.

DISCUSSION

How do thalassemia patients perceive their future compared to healthy adolescents and young adults? Results of our study indicate that thalassemia patients have a positive view of their future with expectations of reaching work and career goals, being in a marriage-type relationship, having a sexual relationship, and becoming parents one day. The thalassemia patients in our study had even higher levels of positive future expectations than their healthy counterparts. Of particular interest are results that revealed the resilient attitudes about their illness. Thalassemia patients, more than controls, endorsed that they did not expect an illness or physical problems would keep them from having a sexual relationship or keep them from making plans about their future.

Positive outcome expectancies were also found in their attributions on the Life Orientation Test.[16] No significant differences were found between groups, indicating that thalassemics in our study had as many positive expectations and as high a level of optimism as healthy controls. Regarding the presence of hopelessness and negative attitudes about life, no significant differences were found between groups. In fact, both groups had low scores on measures of hopelessness and pessimistic attitude.

One aspect of the study particularly relevant to future orientation was perceived control. Having an internal locus of control has been shown to positively affect health outcomes as well as mediating one's coping ability to the stress of illness.[12,17] For thalassemia patients, having an internal health locus of control may serve as an important psychological variable in effectively coping with their disease and its management.

The Multidimensional Health Locus of Control[17] was utilized to determine if differences exist between groups concerning the amount of control they believe they have over their health and to determine if their health is a matter of chance, their own actions, or affected by others. The thalassemia patients had a significantly higher level of internal health locus of control, suggesting that they believe more than their healthy counterparts that their own behaviors largely influence their health.

Results concerning thalassemic's stronger perceived health locus of control are consistent with the demands of their disease. They must have regular transfusions, use a pump several times per week for chelation of excess iron, monitor physiological changes, and adhere to a variety of medical treatments through their lifetime. They are also encouraged to take on increasing responsibility for self-care as they mature. Unlike their healthy counterparts, the thalassemia patients have had a lifetime of experience in actively participating in the management of a disease.

Patients, as compared to controls, attributed health status to influence by their physicians. The results are not surprising. First, thalassemics have had continual contact with physicians throughout their life and, more than healthy peers, know from experience this influence on health status. Second, staying in contact with physicians, and accepting a substantial amount of physician control is essential for the thalassemia patient.

Regarding relationships and social support, the thalassemia subjects endorsed receiving greater levels and more sources of emotional support than the healthy controls. The extent of support among thalassemics was related to their receiving emotional support from physicians and nurses. Not surprisingly, thalassemics reported receiving support from health professionals more than the control group. In addition, the patients reported receiving more emotional support from nurses than physicians. This may be a reflection of the nature of their relationship with nurses and the amount of contact patients have with nurses compared to physicians.

Although their perceived emotional support was higher overall, less than half the thalassemic group reported having a boyfriend or girlfriend. Similar results were found in the study by Zani and colleagues,[9] where half the adolescents with thalassemia reported having a boyfriend or girlfriend. Factors influencing relationships with the opposite sex and/or "dating" is another area to be studied as it relates to issues of psychosocial development and self-concept.

Regarding the impact of social support on future expectations, to our surprise, no significant correlations were found in the present study. Further, social support was not correlated to health locus of control, hopelessness, or life orientation. Although results of our study did not find a direct correlation between social support and future expectations, the influence of relationships and emotional resources should not be underestimated.

What was found to be related to future expectations was optimism and perceived control. Results of our study showed that subjects from both groups who had an internal health locus of control (the belief that their behaviors influence health) and an optimistic coping style had significantly greater positive expectations about their future. Therefore, among our subjects, future expectations were influenced by internal resources such as coping, self efficacy, and attitude, more than social support. Consistent with the results of previous studies,[6,9] results confirm that psychological variables play a key role in the future orientation of thalassemia patients.

Although the specific source of the thalassemia patients' apparent resiliency cannot be identified, several considerations and implications of the results can be presented. First, our study included thalassemia patients who have survived into adolescence and adulthood. As "survivors," they have benefited from internal coping resources, advanced medical treatment, and consistent care throughout their lives. Therefore, their chances for extended survival is greater than patients who did not receive similar medical management of the disease.[1-3] An additional implication of their survival is that of adherence to treatment. For the thalassemia patients to have survived into young adulthood, as our subjects have, the sample may be weighted in favor of their possessing the psychological resources necessary for compliance.

A more complex consideration of the positive orientation of thalassemia subjects relates to denial. It can be argued that thalassemia patients may be utilizing "denial" as a coping mechanism, suggesting that their optimistic expectancies are not realistic or simply expressions of hope. It is the authors' belief that the future expectations endorsed by this patient group are realistic outcome expectancies. Of the specific future expectations presented to subjects, only the items regarding parenting could be interpreted as possibly unrealistic among today's patient population. Studies determining the fertility of thalassemic patients are an emerging area of research. However, the expectation of being "a parent" does not limit one to being a biological parent or exclude the possibilities of parenthood with current advances in reproductive medicine. For the purposes of this study, expectations are defined by basis in reality and potential for outcome. Longitudinal studies could address the success of this cohort in realizing their expectations.

A limitation of the present study was the sample size of 30 thalassemia patients. Although this is close to 10% of the total North American patient population within the age parameters of this study,[1] generalization of the results may be restricted. Efforts to compensate for the sample size were made by controlling for sociological variables such as age, ethnicity, religion, education, geographic location, marital status, and parental marital status. As participation in the study was voluntary, results may reflect biases within the subject group.

Several implications based upon the results can be made regarding the psychosocial aspects of patient care. Physicians, nurses, parents, and mental health professionals need to address the expanding quality of life issues of the maturing thalassemia patient. Issues regarding work, education, sexuality, marriage, and parenting should be the focus of further research and clinical interventions. For example, patients with expectations about having sexual relationships and parenting have a variety of issues to address with health professionals. Questions concerning safe sex, endocrine functioning, and fertility are examples. Another area of increasing importance is work. As the thalassemia patient enters adulthood new opportunities and challenges emerge regarding health insurance coverage, disclosure to employers, as well as managing a career while living with a life-long disease.

SUMMARY

Chronic illness was traditionally viewed as negatively affecting the psychosocial development of young patients.[10,11] Results of the present study showed that thalassemia patients have positive and numerous expectations about their future. The study confirmed previous findings[6,9] that thalassemia patients do not necessarily experience psychological dysfunction as a result of their disease. The positive future orientation of patients in this study offers important quality of life implications for patient care and research. Parents, physicians, nurses, and mental health professionals can promote positive orientation for the future in these patients by first recognizing and respecting their expectations. Comprehensive health care services and psychological interventions will help this first generation of adult thalassemia patients realize the expectations they have for their future.

REFERENCES

1. PEARSON, H., A. COHEN, P. J. GIARDINA & H. KAZAZIAN. 1996. The changing profile of homozygous B-thalassemia: Demography, ethnicity, and age distribution of current North American patients and changes in two decades. Pediatrics **97**: 352–356.
2. EHLERS, K., P. J. GIARDINA, M. LESSER, M. ENGLE & M. HILGARTNER. 1991. Prolonged survival in patients with β-thalassemia major treated with deferoxamine. J. Pediatrics **118**: 540–545.
3. CALLEJA, E. M., J. Y. SHEN, M. LESSER, R. W. GRADY, M. I. NEW & P. J. GIARDINA. 1998. Survival and morbidity in transfusion-dependent thalassemic patients on subcutaneous deferoxamine chelation: Nearly two decades of experience. Ann. N.Y. Acad. Sci. **850**: 472–473. This volume.
4. WEATHERALL, D. J. & J. B. CLEGG. 1981. The Thalassemia Syndromes. Blackwell Scientific. Oxford, England.
5. RATIP, S. & B. MODELL. 1996. Psychological and sociological aspects of the thalassemias. Sem. Hematol. **33**: 53–65.

6. POLITIS, C., A. DI PALMA, M. FISFEIS, A. GIASANTI, S. RICHARDSON, C. VULLO & G. MASERA. 1990. Social integration of the older thalassemic patient. Arch. Dis. Child. **65**: 984–986.
7. GEORGANDA, E. 1988. Thalassemia and the adolescent: An investigation of chronic illness, individuals, and systems. Fam. Systems Med. **6**(2): 150–161.
8. TSIANTIS, J. 1990. Family reactions and relationships in thalassemia. Ann. N.Y. Acad. Sci. **612**: 451–461.
9. ZANI, B., A. DI PALMA & C. VULLO. 1995. Psychological aspects of chronic illness in adolescents with thalassemia major. J. Adolesc. **18**: 387–402.
10. CADMAN, D., M. BOYLE, P. SZATMARI & D. OFFORD. 1987. Chronic illness, disability, and mental and social well- being: Findings of the Ontario child health study. Pediatrics **79**: 805–813.
11. SATTERWHITE, B. 1978. Impact of chronic illness on child and family: An overview based on five surveys. Int. J. Rehab. Res. **1**: 7–15.
12. KELLERMAN, J., L. ZELTZER, L. ELLENBERG, J. DASH & D. RIGLER. 1980. Psychological effects of illness in adolescence: Anxiety, self esteem, and perception of control. J. Pediatr. **97**: 126–131.
13. GARRISON, W. & S. MCQUISTON. 1989. Chronic Illness during Childhood and Adolescence: Psychological Aspects. Sage Publications. Newbury Park, CA.
14. LOGAN, F. A., B. GIBSON, I. M. HANN & L. PARRY-JONES. 1993. Children with haemophilia: Same or different. Child: Care Health Dev. **19**: 261–273.
15. BUSH, S. F. 1995. The Future Expectations Inventory. Master of Arts in Psychology thesis, Yeshiva University, New York.
16. SCHEIER, M. & C. CARVER. 1985. Optimism, coping, and health: Assessment and implications of generalized outcome expectancies. Health Psych. **4**(3): 219–247.
17. WALLSTON, K., B. S. WALLSTON & R. DEVELLIS. 1978. Development of the multidimensional health locus of control (MHLC) scales. Health Ed. Monographs **6**(2): 160–170.
18. BECK, A. & R. STEER. 1988. Beck Hopelessness Scale Manual. The Psychological Corporation. San Antonio, TX.
19. BROADHEAD, W. *et al.* 1983. The epidemiological evidence for a relationship between social support and health. Am. J. Epidemiol. **117**: 521–537.
20. NURMI, J. E. 1991. How do adolescents see their future? A review of the development of future orientation and planning. Dev. Review. **11**: 1–59.

Patient Psychosocial Perspectives

GINA POTENZA AND RALPH CAZZETTA

Cooley's Anemia Foundation, Inc., 129-09 26th Avenue, Flushing, New York 11354, USA[a]

My name is Gina Potenza. I am a thalassemia major patient. My training is in social work and I have a Masters degree in this field. I am happy to co-present this presentation on behalf of the Cooley's Anemia Foundation.

The success of desferal chelation has extended the lives of patients. Along with this gain in life span are new problems in care, both medically and socially. The Cooley's Anemia Foundation offers the voices of patients to researchers, clinicians, medical students, and counselors along with an agenda for improving care. This presentation is the work of dozens of patients involved with the Foundation through our patient support group the Thalassemia Action Group (TAG).

The Cooley's Anemia Foundation (CAF), incorporated in 1954, is the only organization in the United States serving the entire United States patient population. The Foundation has funded millions of dollars in medical research fellowships and grants, provides families with infusion pumps, helps families with insurance concerns, and sponsors TAG. CAF also sponsors medical meetings.

We are proud to present the voices of our patients at the New York Academy of Sciences *Seventh Cooley's Anemia Symposium*. Session chairs and speakers at this gathering are the generals in our battle for life. Your achievements have been immense and we are grateful to you for your continuing commitment. We are here to learn news of improved clinical care, new treatment options, and milestones in basic science. We are also here as your partner in care. We endorse the work you are pursuing on our behalf. We also offer encouragement and support in our journey that will continue until a cure.

Thalassemia is an extremely high maintenance disease. It is important that we remember this and are inspired rather than defeated by this fact. We know that our parents and families struggle along with us. Patients benefit from families that have taken an activist role in their care and have involved themselves directly in treatment decisions.

An example of this is provided by our Foundation President Peter Chieco. For eight years, the Chieco's have carefully charted their daughters weight, total blood consumption, hemoglobin levels, quarterly serum ferritin measurements, and amount of desferal taken. They chart this information and share it with her doctor. The receptiveness of their doctor to compare their information with her own, and act on it if appropriate, has led to an ideal relationship for managing their child's care. Our first message to other patients and families, is to understand your disease, and take an active role in the care you receive! Doctors must encourage these efforts and take the time to assist families with this care at the earliest ages. It is reality that greater compliance is achieved from an activist approach to care.

An important aspect of the Foundation's work is its patient services department as well as its support group for patients (TAG). We are fortunate to have Ralph Cazzetta serve in the role of patient services director. Ralph is a thirty-two-year-old beta-thalassemia major patient. Ralph conveys the psychosocial burden and the full understanding of obstacles that face the thalassemia patient.

[a]Tel: (718) 321-2873; Fax (718) 321-3340; (800) 522-7222. www.thalassemia.org

RALPH CAZZETTA: Recognizing that thalassemia is a rare disease within the United States, the thalassemia patient and health care provider must embrace the overall clinical care that this disease requires. Our challenges are *coordination of care, medical insurance criteria, overall miscommunication* and *patient stigmatism*.

An example is when the doctor first prescribes desferal treatment. The patient needs to obtain the pump and supplies and be instructed on their proper use and how to receive medical reimbursement for this care. The health care professional can help by referring individuals to the Foundation and by supporting the Foundation's goals and objectives.

In my position, I have come to hear of many situations that highlight our areas of concern. In our advanced understanding of treatment we still find patients whose doctors are not following modern protocols. Why is it that in 1997 I have been referred a thirteen-year-old girl who resembles a thalassemia patient from a 1950s textbook and whose doctors predict a life expectancy of 15? The mother's determination and advocacy led her to contact our Foundation and attend our recent conference.

In another case, the dentist of a nine-year-old girl with severe dental deformities suggested to the parents that the child was possibly a thalassemia major—not a trait carrier as her pediatrician had previously diagnosed. This dentist advised the family to contact our Foundation.

A patient went to consult with an ear, nose and throat specialist. Her reception was cruel. When she told him she was HIV positive, he yelled at her and told her to leave his office immediately because he didn't want to risk his own health by treating her.

I want to share with you that the thalassemia community is very closed in discussing blood-related viruses, including hepatitis and especially AIDS. The HIV-positive thalassemia patient feels extremely alienated and stigmatized. For example, an AIDS hotline wouldn't help her because "she wasn't sick enough." She fears sharing her diagnosis with her family, as well as with other thalassemia patients, because of their own fears and thoughts of mortality. This same patient and her fiancé visited a psychologist and she was told that she was selfish to want to marry him or anyone because she was HIV positive. On top of all this, because she is HIV positive, she was denied a bone marrow transplant even though she had a perfect sibling match.

An intermedia patient was told to leave a gynecologist's office in an emergency situation because the doctor felt her pregnancy coupled with thalassemia was too complicated. Another difficult problem faced by this woman was coordinating the efforts of her hematologist with her perinatologist. She found that in a world of high technology and specialization the tendency to want responsibility for one piece of the pie was ineffective and dangerous.

In another situation, a couple seeking to adopt a child with thalassemia major were advised against this by a hematologist. Material provided by our Foundation and its Medical Advisory Board gave them the proper information to make an informed decision.

These examples are one part of the complicated psychosocial issues that confront the thalassemia patient. As we approach the millennium, advances in clinical care challenge the adult thalassemia patient. Socially, patients want to become professionals and make their way into the working world. The adult patient is confined because clinical hours are not flexible and insurance coverage limits job options. Medically, the adult patient must educate an adult hematologist because protocol dictates that we leave the pediatric floors. Basically there is no transition between pediatric and adult services. Adult hematologists are simply not trained to treat thalassemia because traditionally thalassemia was considered a childhood disease. Many adult patients share the sentiment that if we are to succumb to this disease, we want it to be because the disease became unmanageable and not because the disease was mismanaged.

We bring these issues to your attention to highlight that our care extends beyond the clinical setting. We are concerned about trends in insurance that hinder our access to proper care. We are concerned about blood safety. We also strongly want to achieve personal goals. The ability to work and contribute to society is a key to our will to survive.

The above examples teach us that the diligence and team effort of the treating physician coupled with the support of the Foundation and its patient support network is crucial. Recommendations for this audience are (1) work with doctors first confronting thalassemia in their practice; (2) take an active role in the hospitals hematology department to insure that all hematologists (both adult and pediatric) are being trained in the proper treatment of thalassemia; and (3) actively assist in the transition between pediatric and adult services.

Some of our adult patients have experienced the joys of marriage and parenthood. The father of a 16-year-old girl encourages thalassemia patients to keep themselves as healthy, active, and intellectually stimulated as possible. Today at 41, he has a beautiful, supportive wife, friends, and family backing him. The mother of a two-year-old boy refused to be defeated in her longing to have a child. She was told that she should be grateful to be alive. Today, she encourages other women with thalassemia to persist in their dreams of having a child.

As adults we also pave the way for the young thalassemia patient. They confront the same fears and awkwardness that we experienced. Here are a few of these young voices:

> I hate the pump because I can't go to sleep overs or everyone will know I have thalassemia.

> Starting in the second grade I did presentations in front of my class about Cooley's anemia. I was always open about it until the fifth grade when one of my friends was arguing with the boy I liked and his answer to one of her remarks was "well you stay with the girl with the disease." I was crushed because I never knew anyone thought of me like that.

> I think of all the time I spend getting transfused, going to doctors and mixing my medicines. I feel shortchanged on the amount of fun time I have remaining as compared to other kids.

> It is scary to wonder what if something is wrong with the blood I get and it slips though the tests.

> I feel like I am on a mountain all alone and there is only one way up and one way down. On this mountain it is dark and cold. I have a map but it is really confusing and there is always someone available but they don't know how to turn on the light , get up the mountain and help me understand.

> What if people knew and made fun of me because Cooley's anemia is a funny name? For now I want to keep things a secret. Maybe when there's a cure I'll confess. But until I feel more comfortable or my friends grow up and will be able to understand, I'll keep feeling guilty about lying and keeping the secret. But I'll try to remember that the only thing that really separates me from other high school kids is my blood.

These young voices provide a message for care givers. The Foundation also recognizes that the new population of thalassemia patients in this country from the Middle East, Southeast Asia, the Indian continent will challenge us all. This was similar to our roots as a Foundation when Italian and Greek parents who understood little English faced thalassemia. Here are some insights provided to us by this new patient population:

> What I found really hard as a child was the fact that my parents didn't speak English. Initially friends and relatives helped to translate at doctors appointments.

Yet when I was a little older I was the translator. I was the bridge between the doctors and my parents. I found this a difficult role to play.

My parents did not inform many of our friends in our community because they are close-minded and look down on dental deformities which I had due to thalassemia.

I don't think my being Chinese American has affected me all that much. Thalassemia has actually given me something and it has taught me a lot. It has made me the person I am today—without thalassemia I would not be as compassionate or understanding.

So how do we conclude our presentation? One of our patient collaborators provides the following:

Thalassemia. What does that mean? Impossible to say. I am sure it means something different to everyone whose life is touched by it. To me it has meant pain and tears; more medical knowledge than I ever would have cared to have and a seemingly endless uphill battle for mere survival. It has also caused me to have more inner strength than I thought possible. It has made me realize that every day is a gift not to be taken for granted. It has also brought some wonderful people into my life.

Often this disease makes you feel isolated and alone. It is certainly not common, you will never see it featured in a disease of the week movie. I have accepted this as reality and hope that someday it will merely be a footnote in medical journals and not a reason to hold a conference.

Summary of the Seventh Cooley's Anemia Symposium

DAVID G. NATHAN[a]

Dana-Farber Cancer Institute, 44 Binney Street, Boston, Massachusetts 02115, USA

As our Seventh Cooley's Anemia Symposium draws to a close we can look with satisfaction at the development of our field, one which began the clinical application of the molecular biology revolution and remains vibrant, active, and in the vanguard. Today we fully understand the pathophysiology of Cooley's anemia. It is a fascinating consequence of unbalanced protein synthesis in which excess alpha-globin chains precipitate and disrupt the erythroblast and the red cell both mechanically and chemically. The precipitates induce a massive flow of oxidants that stiffen the fragile proteins of the erythrocyte membrane and render it incapable of escaping the jaws of littoral macrophages, leading to massive ineffective erythropoiesis and rapid hemolysis of circulating red cells. Only the fortunate red cell capable of increased gamma-chain synthesis can escape the high infant mortality induced by excess alpha chains. Those happy few can live to mid-life or even older because the gamma chains combine with alpha chains and allow the cell to get on with its life.

This meeting has focused on the molecular basis of the imbalance and ways by which we can circumvent or manage it. The first sessions on the control of globin gene expression gave us insight on how far we have come in our understanding of the locus control region and the switching phenomena that occur during development. In some way, as yet not clearly defined, some form of contact between the locus control region and the various beta cluster genes must occur in a sequential fashion, but it is unlikely that the system is the same among the species because the order of the beta cluster varies among species. Each has probably adapted the relationship of beta cluster genes to the locus control region in a unique fashion and the sorting out of that variability will be fascinating. The transcriptional control of globin synthesis remains full of surprises. Who would have thought that the much sought after NFE2 would, instead of having a profound role in globin synthesis, be responsible for the development of platelets from megakaryocytes? The application of knockout technology to dissect the proteins that regulate globin genes will surely continue to provide exciting new information that will eventually lead to an understanding of the switching phenomenon. But we remain today unsure of the details, and without those details, it is virtually impossible to plan an approach to pharmacologic control either of alpha chain overproduction or enhancement of the gamma chain sponge.

Undaunted, our experimental pharmacologists and clinical investigators remain eager to pursue avenues that could lead to improvement for our patients. Several investigators reported on butyrate, hydroxyurea, and erythropoietin as potential approaches. Used singly or in combination, none of them are generally effective in Cooley's anemia, though hydroxyurea is certainly useful in sickle cell anemia. There are exceptions however.

[a]Address for correspondence: David G. Nathan, M.D., President, Dana-Farber Cancer Institute, 44 Binney Street, Boston, MA 02115; Tel: (617) 632-2155; Fax: (617) 632-2161; E-mail: david_nathan@dfci.harvard.edu

Certain patients with thalassemia intermedia can benefit from the judicious use of hydroxyurea or erythropoietin and butyrate has been shown to be effective in one unique sib pair with homozygous lepore thalassemia. Whether this unique response relates to the lepore genotype or to some other factor in this family remains to be seen.

Gene transfer remains the long-hoped-for solution to the thalassemia problem, but major technical issues continue to impede progress. We still do not have an absolutely clear approach to the isolation and concentration of the class of hematopoietic stem cells that can sustain marrow function indefinitely. We still lack the vectors that can securely incorporate genes of interest into the DNA of those stem cells and produced regulated high level globin gene expression *in vivo*. Encouraging results utilizing the transfer of human stem cells into irradiated and immunodefective murine recipients provide the best hope for a secure model of globin gene expression in human stem cells, but until such models are successful, it would seem unlikely that human clinical trials can proceed.

The need for an oral iron chelator that is as non-toxic and effective as deferoxamine continues to vex us. The class of compounds called pyrid-ones, initially described by Hider and his associates, has had the most attention. Unfortunately, most of these compounds have nowhere near the efficiency of iron binding that is exhibited by deferoxamine. One molecule of deferoxamine binds one molecule of iron with a high affinity whereas such binding requires three molecules of the currently studied pyrid-one called L1 or "Deferiprone." This means that iron binding by "Deferiprone" is highly dependent on drug concentration, and more long-term studies of the drug carried out by investigators in Toronto and Cleveland and in London have shown that hepatic iron stores may actually increase or fail to decline in patients on the drug for a protracted period. This is disappointing because the toxicity of the drug appears, in its initial review, to be reasonably acceptable. Suspicions that "Deferiprone" may directly cause cirrhosis of the liver have been disputed. But much more detailed study of this drug with particular attention to cardiac endpoints and hepatic toxicity is required before it can be made generally available. The real issue is whether the drug can prevent heart disease as effectively as deferoxamine and with minimal toxicity.

New techniques in the prevention of thalassemia were discussed. Methods for prenatal diagnosis with molecular techniques have improved so much that fetal blood sampling is now nearly a thing of the past. Interestingly, studies in Montreal suggest that the incidence of thalassemia can be reduced by careful population screening, if the capacity for prenatal diagnosis is available. Thus the technology appears to be helping couples to make conservative decisions that reduce the incidence of this disease.

Bone marrow transplantation and even in utero transplantation were carefully discussed at the meeting. New attempts to reduce the toxicity of transplantation by reduction of the intensity of preparative regimens appear particularly promising. This is very important because results of bone marrow transplantation outside of one very experienced center in Italy still warrant caution in the application of this fascinating approach to cellular gene therapy. In most countries, success rates are between 60–80%, nowhere close to the virtually 100% that is presented in so-called low risk patients by the Pesaro group. Whether this demonstrates the value of experience or the possibility of incomplete follow-up of patients from certain Middle Eastern countries where such follow-up could be difficult, is a matter yet to be resolved. In any case, increased safety of the procedure is badly needed and research that can lead to safe alternative donor transplants is of high priority. It still remains likely that cellular gene therapy in the form of bone marrow transplantation will be more effective than gene therapy with auto transplantation for decades to come.

Thalassemia intermedia remains a fascinating illness because it illustrates the disparity between genotype and phenotype of disease as is the case in so many inherited diseases. We still do not completely understand thalassemia intermedia. The presence of alpha-thalassemia or enhanced gamma chain production can certainly ameliorate beta-thalassemia genes. But some beta-thalassemia genes behave unexpectedly in different hosts. Mutant genes that cause mild processing defects *in vitro* can cause severe disease when transmitted *in vivo*; and, conversely, some patients with thalassemia intermedia have no obvious genetic basis for their improved function. The treatment of these patients can present a real challenge because bone disease can be profound and cause crippling disability.

The conference ended with a discussion of the psychosocial aspects of thalassemia. Many believe that this session should have been first on the program. It would have been important for all of the participants to hear the meaning of the disorder to the patient and to the family. Thalassemia remains a tremendous burden for patients. It is not only a massive economic and medical problem, it is an emotional problem and a developmental problem that needs our full attention Some creative and quite remarkable social workers and psychologists have made major contributions to this field. Those of us who are examining the disease at the molecular and clinical level should listen carefully to our patients. Our entire purpose is, after all, to serve them.

This then is a brief and inadequate summary of a fascinating three-day meeting that brought us all back together again. We are grateful to Alan Cohen and his team of organizers, to the New York Academy of Sciences and to the Cooley's Anemia Foundation for their support, their guidance, their generosity, and their commitment.

5′HS1 and the Distal β-Globin Promoter Functionally Interact in Single Copy β-Globin Transgenic Mice

PETER PASCERI, DYLAN PANNELL, XIUMEI WU, AND JAMES ELLIS[a]

Department of Genetics, Hospital for Sick Children, 555 University Ave, Toronto, Ontario, Canada, M5G 1X8 and Department of Molecular and Medical Genetics, University of Toronto

The human β-globin Locus Control Region (LCR) activates high level expression of linked transgenes in mice and dominantly opens the chromatin structure of the transgene integration site. These LCR activities combine to direct copy number-dependent expression in multicopy transgenic mice. However, single-copy transgenes more accurately reflect the *in vivo* context of a gene and its regulatory elements. Therefore, our objective is to define the minimal combination of regulatory elements that direct 100% levels of β-globin transgene expression at single copy and to identify any functional interactions between these elements.

We previously showed that 100% levels of β-globin mRNA expression are obtained from a microlocus LCR construct in the fetal livers of single-copy transgenic mice.[1] The microlocus construct links a 6.5 kb LCR cassette containing all four DNaseI hypersensitive sites (HS) with the 1555 bp β-globin promoter (Fig. 1). We have also shown that: 1) spacing between the HS core elements is important for LCR activity in low copy transgenic mice[2]; 2) separation of three HS cores (each by 700 bp of flanking sequences) in a 3.0 kb LCR activates single-copy transgene expression[2]; but 3) reduction of the 815 bp β-globin promoter to its minimal 265 bp component is accompanied by decreased single-copy transgene expression from the 3.0 kb LCR.[2]

To rapidly assess the importance of various combinations of β-globin LCR elements, promoters and gene proximal enhancers, we are now employing transient transgenic mice dissected as fetuses at day 15.5. The levels of mosaicism in the transgenic fetuses is assessed by Southern blots of fetal liver DNA and the intensity of the transgene band is compared to the band intensity of a known bred single-copy transgenic line.[2] Transgene expression levels quantitated by S1 nuclease analyses of fetal liver RNA are then corrected to take into account the level of transgene mosaicism. Using this rapid transgenic assay, the BGT14 construct (composed of a 3.0 kb LCR cassette of 5′HS2, 5′HS3 and 5′HS4 linked to the 815 bp β-globin promoter) directs only 45% expression in single-copy transgenics with a range of 30-71% (Fig. 1). Linkage of the same 3.0 kb LCR to the minimal 265 bp β-globin promoter reduces expression of the BGT15 construct to 18% with a range of 3-39% (Fig. 1). These data suggest that either 5′HS1, the distal β-globin promoter, or auxiliary sequences present only in the 6.5 kb LCR cassette are required alone or in combination to obtain 100% levels of single-copy transgene expression.

[a]Corresponding author: Tel: 416-813-7295; Fax: 416-813-4989; E-mail: jellis@sickkids.on.ca

To distinguish between the above possibilities, we tested additional LCR/promoter combinations in single-copy transgenic mice (FIG. 1). To investigate the importance of the distal promoter sequences we linked the 6.5 kb LCR cassette to the 815 bp promoter to create the BGT22 construct. In order to examine the role of 5'HS1 and the auxiliary sequences which are present only in the 6.5 kb LCR cassette, the 3.0 kb LCR cassette was linked to the 1555 bp promoter in the BGT23 construct. Finally, both 5'HS1 and the distal promoter were studied in the absence of the auxiliary sequences by creating a 4.0 kb LCR cassette linked to the 1555 bp promoter in the BGT33 construct.

Expression of single-copy BGT22 transgenes in day 15.5 fetal liver varied from 12-888% (FIG. 1), suggesting that the 1555 bp promoter is essential to obtain reproducible levels of expression. BGT23 transgenes also led to variable expression levels of 33-384% in single-copy transgenic mice (FIG. 1), indicating that either 5'HS1 or the auxiliary sequences are also required in addition to the 1555 bp promoter. However, single-copy BGT33 transgenic mice containing both 5'HS1 and the 1555 bp promoter reproducibly directed 89-138% expression (FIG. 1). These data show that 5'HS1 and the distal promoter sequences are required simultaneously to obtain full and reproducible expression at single copy, and that the auxiliary sequences are dispensable for this activity. Additional constructs are being studied to determine whether specific sequences within the distal promoter are required for reproducible 100% single-copy transgene expression, or whether these sequences can be replaced by neutral spacer DNA.

A model consistent with these data is that the role of 5'HS1 may be to functionally interact with sequences present in the distal β-globin promoter, perhaps by a DNA looping mechanism mediated by protein:protein contacts of DNA-bound *trans*-acting factors. This putative physical interaction between 5'HS1 and the distal promoter may facilitate LCR function by aligning an activating complex of the known transcriptional enhancement properties of 5'HS2, 5'HS3 and 5'HS4 with the proximal promoter element. In the context of our transgenics full expression would be obtained when both 5'HS1 and the distal promoter are present. Alternatively, in the absence of both 5'HS1

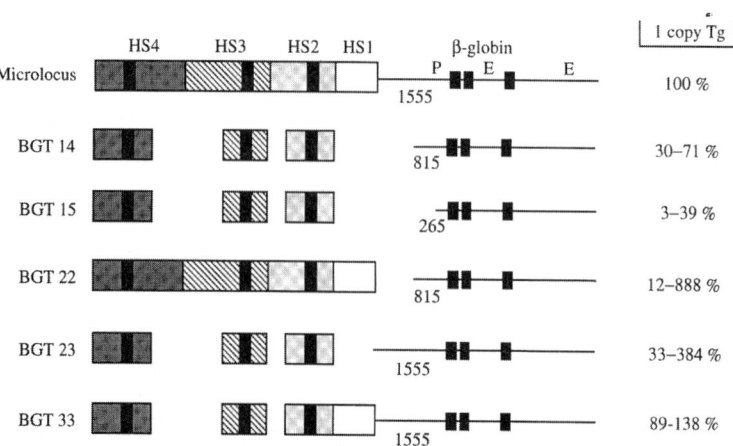

FIGURE 1. Maps of the constructs evaluated in single-copy transgenic mice. The LCR cassettes shown contain the indicated DNaseI hypersensitive sites linked to human β-globin promoters (P) of different length (1555 bp, 815 bp, or 265 bp). Both the gene proximal enhancers (E) located in the second intron and 3' of the gene are included in all of the constructs. The range of transgene expression at single copy is indicated in the column at right. At least 3 different single-copy transgenic mice were obtained for each construct.

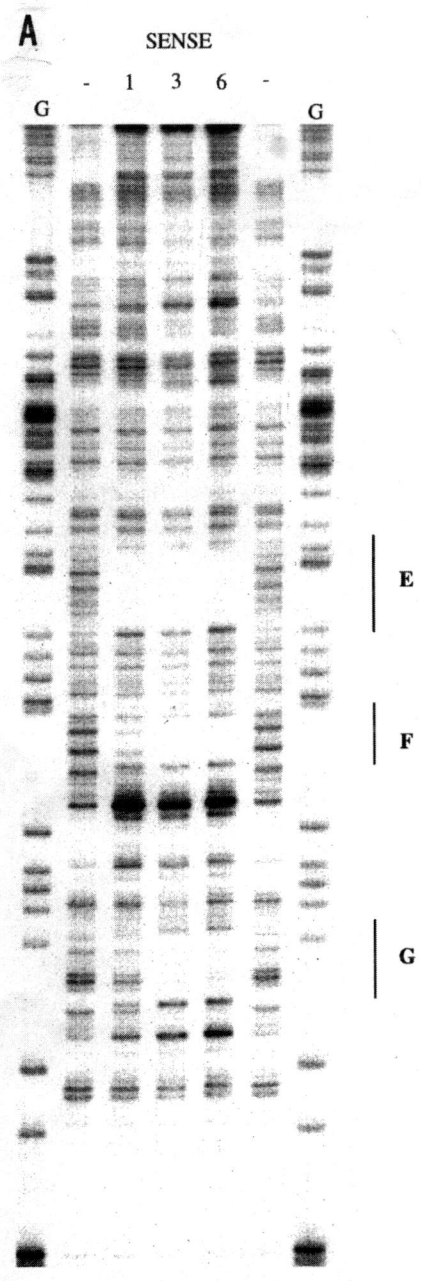

FIGURE A.

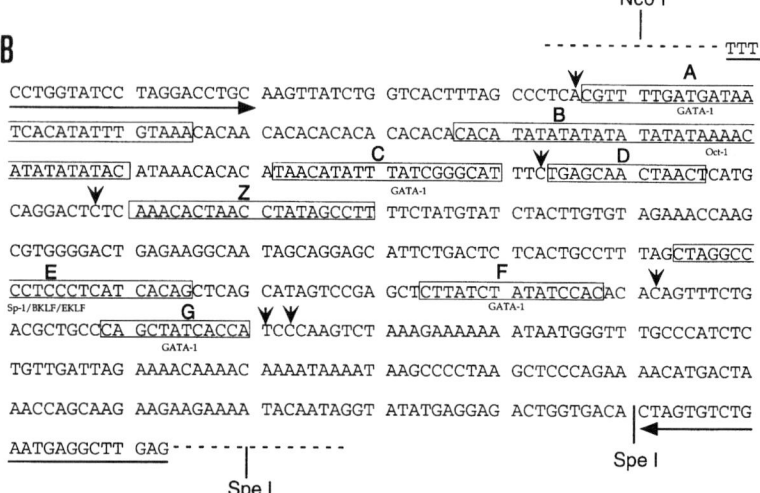

FIGURE 2. *In vitro* DNaseI footprint analysis of the 5'HS1 core element incubated with induced MEL cell nuclear extract. **A**, Footprints E, F, G are protected on the labeled sense strand 5'HS1 probe when compared to the no extract lane (-), and positioned to specific sequences by alignment with the G ladder (G). **B**, Summary of the seven footprints detected in this analysis with both DNA strands as probes. Each protected footprint is represented by a box, hypersensitive sites are indicated by vertical arrows. Factors that bind to each footprint are indicated below each box. Primers used for PCR amplification and cloning of the 5'HS1 core are shown as horizontal arrows, and the restriction sites employed for 3' end labeling of each DNA strand are also shown.

and the distal promoter the activating HS complex would be free to interact directly with the proximal promoter. In the remaining constructs, the presence of either 5'HS1 or the distal promoter might compete for interactions with the activating HS complex and alter its ability to align with the proximal promoter.

As a first step in characterizing *trans*-acting factors that might participate in the functional 5'HS1/distal promoter interaction, we have performed *in vitro* DNaseI footprint analyses on the 5'HS1 element. A 556 bp core of 5'HS1 was amplified by PCR, subcloned into the pGEM-T vector and the insert sequenced. Both sense and antisense strand 3' labeled probes were generated from this plasmid, incubated with a nuclear extract from induced MEL cells, and subjected to DNaseI digestion. *In vitro* DNaseI footprints detected with the sense strand probe are shown in FIGURE 2A, and all seven footprints labeled A to G covering the 5'HS1 core region are summarized in FIGURE 2B. A weak footprint called Z was also detected.

Based on sequence comparisons to known binding sites for *trans*-acting factors these footprints in 5'HS1 likely correspond to a strong Sp1/BKLF/EKLF site in footprint E; 4 separate GATA-1 sites at footprints A, C, F and G; a weak Oct-1 site at footprint B; and unknown factors binding to footprints B and Z. Band shift and competition experiments with MEL and Jurkat T-cell extracts indicate that the above factors bind to oligonucleotide binding sites of their respective footprints. Antibody supershift experiments are in progress to confirm the identity of these factors. Their role in the functional interactions described above remains to be described.

REFERENCES

1. ELLIS, J., K. C. TAN-UN, A. HARPER, D. MICHALOVICH, N. YANNOUTSOS, S. PHILIPSEN & F. GROSVELD. 1996. A dominant chromatin opening activity in 5′ hypersensitive site 3 of the human β-globin locus control region. EMBO J. **15**: 562–568.
2. ELLIS J., P. PASCERI, K. C. TAN-UN, A. HARPER, X. WU, P. FRASER & F. GROSVELD. 1997. Evaluation of human β-globin gene therapy constructs by expression in transgenic mice. Nucleic Acids Res. **25**: 1296–1302.

An *in Vitro* Model of Human Erythropoiesis for the Study of Hemoglobinopathies[a]

PUNAM MALIK,[b,f] LORA L.W. BARSKY,[c] LICHENG ZENG,[d] ALAN L. HITI[d] AND TIMOTHY C. FISHER[e]

The Divisions of [b]Hematology-Oncology and [c]Research Immunology/Bone Marrow Transplantation, Childrens Hospital Los Angeles

Departments of [d]Pathology and [e]Physiology and Biophysics, University of Southern California School of Medicine, Los Angeles, California, USA

Molecular defects that cause sickle cell anemia (SCA) and the other common hemoglobinopathies have been well characterized.[1–5] Genetic correction of hematopoietic stem cells with adequate expression of the inserted gene product in the defective red cells could revolutionize treatment of congenital red cell defects. Novel models of human erythropoiesis that result in terminally differentiated red cells would be able to address the pathophysiological abnormalities in erythrocytes in congenital red cell diseases and to test the potential of reversing these problems by gene therapy. The most commonly available *in vitro* assays of erythropoiesis from CD34+ progenitor cells are based on semi-solid medium colony-forming assays, which result in colonies consisting of nucleated erythroid cells. These erythroid colonies are composed of early (BFU-E) or late erythroid progenitors (CFU-E).[6,7] Most of the *in vitro* liquid cultures from CD34+ progenitor cells are limited by the production of heterogeneous mixtures of mainly myeloid cells with few erythroid cells.

Terminal erythroid differentiation has been reported when peripheral blood mononuclear cells are initially cultured in semi-solid media containing different growth and then transferred to a liquid culture containing erythropoietin (Epo) and grown under reduced oxygen concentrations.[8–10] Chelluci and colleagues reported uni-lineage differentiation of purified primitive hematopoietic progenitors if high concentrations of Epo, along with low concentrations of GMCSF and IL3, were used.[11] However, they have followed their cultures up to 12–14 days and have not reported terminal red cell differentiation and development of enucleated red cells. We report a novel model of generation of terminally differentiated red cells from highly purified human CD34+ progenitor cells, in a single-step liquid culture system *in vitro* followed by isolation of a pure population of the enucleated RBC by flowcytometry.

---

[a]This work was supported by the NHLBI Grants #5P60-HL48484-06 and HL9410B and the J. Conell Gene Therapy Program.

[f]Address for correspondence: Punam Malik, Childrens Hospital Los Angeles, Mail stop # 62, 4650 Sunset Boulevard, Los Angeles, CA 90027, Phone: 213-660-2450, ext. 4474; Fax: 213-660-1904; e-mail: malik@hsc.usc.edu

RESULTS

In Vitro *Erythropoiesis*

CD34+ cells were isolated from the mononuclear cell fraction from cord blood, bone marrow, or peripheral blood after the mononuclear fraction was subjected to red cell lysis. The purified human CD34+ cells were subjected to erythroid differentiation by using Epo (10 U/ml), GM-CSF (0.001 ng/ml), and IL-3 (0.01 U/ml) in liquid culture.[12] These cultures recapitulated *in vivo* erythroid differentiation with more than 90% of the cells in culture of erythroid lineage. After 18–21 days of culture, erythroblastic islands formed that resulted in enucleation of 10–40% of the erythroid cells (FIG. 1, inset). The enucleated red cells were separated from the nucleated erythroid cells and macrophages by staining with a vital DNA dye, Hoechst 33342, followed by flow cytometry to isolate a pure population of erythrocytes (FIG. 1).

Red Cell Characterization from Normal and SCA Individuals

Differential-interference contrast microscopy showed that the enucleated cells ranged from early polylobulated forms resembling normal reticulocytes, to smooth biconcave discocytes (FIG. 1). Reverse-phase HPLC analyses showed that globin chain synthesis of the erythrocytes generated *in vitro* paralleled adult pattern of β-globin synthesis rather than the fetal pattern of γ-globin synthesis.[12] Comparisons of enucleated erythrocytes generated *in vitro* from CD34+ cells from patients with SCA to those derived *in vitro* from normal donors showed that erythrocytes derived *in vitro* from CD34+ cells from SCA donors were morphologically indistinguishable from those produced *in vitro* from normal donors. However, induction of hypoxia resulted in sickling in the majority of *in vitro*–derived erythrocytes from SCA individuals (data not shown).

Expression of the Gene Product in the Enucleated Red Cell Progeny

The potential for introducing genes into progenitor cells and attaining expression in the resultant erythrocyte progeny was tested as a model of gene therapy for red cell disorders. Normal human CD34+ cells were transduced with a retroviral vector, L- tNGFR-SN, carrying the truncated rat nerve growth factor receptor (tNGFR), as a marker gene. CD34+ cells expressing tNGFR on the surface (transduced) and those not expressing the surface reporter were sorted by flow cytometry and cultured separately in erythroid differentiation conditions. After 3 weeks in culture, tNGFR was expressed on the surface of 89% of the enucleated red cells in the transduced cell population.[12]

CONCLUSIONS

Production and isolation of a pure population of terminally differentiated, enucleated red cells from human CD34+ cells, in sufficient numbers for biophysical studies and for the study of gene transfer and expression is a unique feature of the current model, which has not been previously described. An important feature of the red cells generated *in vitro* in the current model was production of adult β-globin, with negligible fetal/γ-globin synthesis, mimicking *in vivo* erythropoiesis. Since problems in hemoglobinopathies, such as SCA and thalassemia, become manifest with adult globin production, a model with adult-type erythropoiesis is essential to study the pathophysiology of hemoglobinopathies and

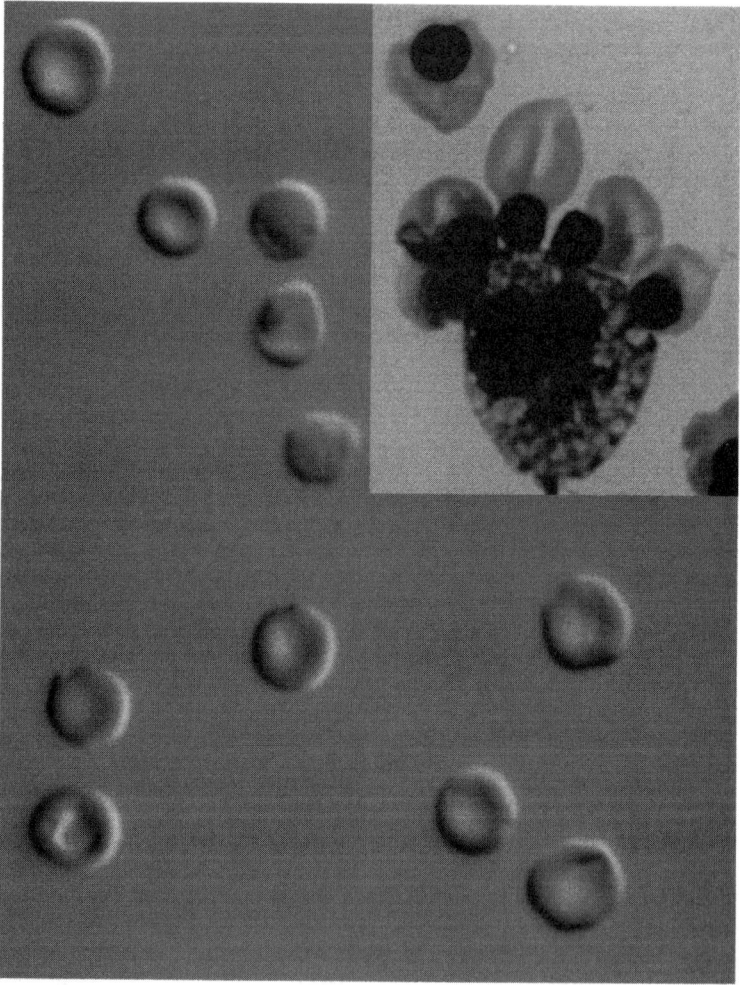

FIGURE 1. Differential interference microscopy of *in vitro* generated enucleated red cells derived from normal human bone marrow CD34+ cells. Inset shows a Wright-Giemsa stained cytospin of a 3-week culture showing enucleating red cells around a macrophage.

test effective therapeutic strategies. This *in vitro* model can be used to genetically manipulate hematopoietic progenitor/stem cells from patients with congenital red cell defects and test the functional effects of the gene therapy in the target red cell progeny.

REFERENCES

1. STAMATOYANNOPOULOS, G. & A. W. NIENHUIS. 1994. Hemoglobin switching. *In* The Molecular Basis of Blood Diseases. G. Stamatoyannopoulos, A. W. Neinhuis, P. W. Majerus & H. Varmus, Eds **2**: 107–155 W. B. Saunders. Philadelphia.

2. BUNN, H. F. 1994. Sickle hemoglobin and other hemoglobin mutants. *In* The Molecular Basis of Blood Diseases. G. Stamatoyannopoulos, A. W. Neinhuis, P. W. Majerus & H. Varmus, Eds. **2**: 207–257. W. B. Saunders. Philadelphia.
3. PLATT, O. S. 1995. The sickle syndromes. *In* Blood: Principles and Practice of Hematology. R. I. Handin, S. E. Lux & T. P. Stossel, Eds. **1**: 1645–1689. J. B. Lippincott Co. Philadelphia.
4. NAGEL, R. L. 1995. Disorders of hemoglobin function and stability. *In* Blood: Principles and Practice of Hematology. R. I. Handin, S. E. Lux & T. P. Stossel, Eds: 1591–1646 J. B. Lippincott Co. Philadelphia.
5. WEATHERALL, D. J. 1995. The molecular basis for phenotypic diversity of genetic disease. Ann. N.Y. Acad. Sci. **758**: 245–260.
6. ISCOVE, N. N., F. SIEBER & K. H. A. WINTERHALTER. 1974. J. Cell. Physiol. **83**: 309.
7. ISCOVE, N. N. & F. SIEBER. 1975. Exp. Hematol. **3**: 23.
8. FIBACH, E., D. MANOR, A. OPPENHEIM & E. A. RACHMILEWITZ. 1989. Proliferation and maturation of human erythroid progenitors in liquid culture. Blood **73**: 100–103.
9. WADA, H., T. SUDA, Y. MIURA, E. KAJII, S. IKEMOTO & Y. YAWATA. 1990. Expression of major blood group antigens on human erythroid cells in a two phase liquid culture system. Blood **75**: 505–511.
10. HANSPAL, M., J. S. HANSPAL, K. E. SAHR, E. FIBACH, J. NACHMAN & J. PALEK. 1993. Molecular basis of spectrin deficiency in hereditary pyropoikilocytosis. Blood **82**: 1652–1660.
11. CHELUCI, C., H. J. HASSAN, C. LOCARDI *et al.* 1995. In vitro human immunodeficiency virus-1 infection of purified hematopoietic progenitors in single-cell culture. Blood **85**: 1181–1187.
12. MALIK, P., T. C. FISHER, L. L. W. BARSKY *et al.* 1998. An *in vitro* model of human red blood cell production from hematopoietic progenitor cells. Blood **91(8)**: 2664–2671.

Full Developmental Silencing of the Embryonic ζ-Globin Gene Reflects Instability of its mRNA

J. ERIC RUSSELL,[a–c] ALICE E. LEE,[b] AND
STEPHEN A. LIEBHABER[b,d,e]

Departments of [b]Medicine, [c]Pediatrics, and [d]Genetics, and the [e]Howard Hughes Medical Institute, University of Pennsylvania School of Medicine, Philadelphia, Pennsylvania 19104, USA

Three highly homologous α-like globin genes are expressed in humans. The α1- and α2-globin genes, which encode identical protein products, are co-expressed at low levels in embryonic erythrocytes, and at high levels in fetal and adult erythrocytes. By comparison, ζ-globin is expressed at high levels in embryonic erythrocytes but is not detected in normal adult erythrocytes. The silencing of ζ-globin expression and reciprocal induction of α-globin expression at the embryonic-fetal transition (post-conception weeks 6–8) is due in part to changes in the transcriptional activity of their cognate genes. Recent evidence, however, suggests that post-transcriptional mechanisms that determine globin mRNA stability may also be crucial effectors of normal patterns of globin gene expression. This paper (1) reviews evidence supporting the hypothesis that post-transcriptional controls affecting mRNA stability contribute to human (h) ζ-globin gene silencing; (2) describes a mouse model system that has been instrumental in physiologically relevant evaluations of α- and ζ-globin mRNA stability; and (3) presents data demonstrating that hζ-globin mRNA is significantly destabilized in adult erythroid cells relative to hα-globin mRNA.

EVIDENCE SUPPORTING A ROLE FOR POST-TRANSCRIPTIONAL REGULATION OF ζ-GLOBIN GENE EXPRESSION

Three independent lines of evidence suggest that post-transcriptional controls play a major regulatory role in hζ-globin gene silencing in fetal and adult erythrocytes. Significant quantities of hζ-globin mRNA can be detected in nuclear run-on experiments utilizing bone marrow erythroid progenitor cells from normal human volunteers.[1] In contrast, hζ-globin mRNA is nearly undetectable in normal adult reticulocytes.[2] Considered together, these data indicate a post-transcriptional defect in the accumulation of hζ-globin mRNA in adult erythroid cells. The post-transcriptional nature of this effect was substantiated in our lab using mice transgenic for either the hζ-globin or hα-globin transcribed regions, each flanked by identical 5′ and 3′ hζ-globin transcriptional control elements.[3] During fetal development, levels of hζ-globin mRNA fell dramatically, while levels of hα-globin mRNA were less severely affected. These data suggest that the difference in the accumulation of the two mRNAs is effected by elements within their transcribed regions

---

[a]Address for correspondence: J. Eric Russell, M.D., Abramson Research Building, Room 316F, Children's Hospital of Philadelphia, 34th and Civic Center Boulevard, Philadelphia, PA 19104. Tel: 215-590-3880; Fax: 215-590-4834; E-mail: jeruss@mail.med.upenn.edu

which dictate differences in their transcriptional or post-transcriptional regulation. Close investigation of hα-globin gene expression in cultured cells and transgenic mice suggests that these elements regulate expression post-transcriptionally. It is clear that normal expression of human α-globin is crucially dependent on the high stability of its mRNA, a characteristic mediated through assembly of a multicomponent RNP complex (α-complex) on a specific 20 nt sequence within its 3'UTR.[4,5] The importance of mRNA stability to hα-globin gene expression suggests that this property, or its absence, might also be utilized for the control of hζ-globin expression.

EVALUATION OF HUMAN GLOBIN mRNA STABILITY IN TRANSGENIC MICE

For the purpose of assessing globin mRNA stability, transgenic mice offer several distinct advantages over other commonly employed methods.[6,7] Transcriptional chase experiments in cultured cells require actinomycin D, which globally arrests gene transcription and may artifactually affect mRNA stability.[8] The reliability of mRNA stabilities determined from genes linked to serum-inducible promoters is poor for highly stable mRNAs, such as globin mRNAs, as the transfected cells require a prohibitively long preparatory period of serum starvation to clear previously transcribed globin mRNAs. The transgenic mouse system is not subject to either of these limitations and offers the additional advantage that globin mRNA metabolism occurs *in vivo* in erythroid progenitor cells undergoing physiologic terminal differentiation. As in humans, murine erythroid cells undergo transcriptional silencing in the bone marrow and subsequently migrate into the peripheral circulation as mRNA-rich reticulocytes (FIG. 1A). mRNAs recovered from the marrow and reticulocytes of individual mice represent sequential time points in a physiologic transcriptional chase experiment. Transgenic mRNA levels in each tissue are determined relative to levels of endogenous mouse (m) α-globin mRNA using a quantitative RNase protection assay (FIG. 1B).[6,7] A fall in the relative level of transgenic mRNA in the transcriptionally silent interval between the marrow and reticulocyte stages of terminal erythroid differentiation indicates instability of the transgenic mRNA relative to the mα-globin mRNA control. Results from these experiments are highly reproducible among different mice from the same transgenic line.[6,7]

HUMAN ζ-GLOBIN mRNA IS DESTABILIZED IN ADULT HUMAN ERYTHROID CELLS

We assessed the stabilities of hα- and hζ-globin mRNAs in adult mice from 10 and 16 independent transgenic lines, respectively. Modifications of ζ-globin gene promoter and silencer elements insured transcription of adequate levels of hζ-globin mRNA without affecting its structure.[6,7] Relative to mα-globin mRNA, the level of hα-globin mRNA remained stable in the transcriptionally silent interval between bone marrow and peripheral reticulocytes (FIG. 2A). During the same interval, the level of hζ-globin mRNA fell rapidly. The difference in the average stability of hα- and hζ-globin mRNAs from all 26 transgenic lines was highly significant (FIG. 2B). The fourfold difference in the relative stabilities of hα- and hζ-globin mRNAs was confirmed in single mice generated by the appropriate genetic crosses, which expressed both transgenes (FIG. 2C). These results are consistent with the hypothesis that post-transcriptional mechanisms that direct destabilization of ζ-globin mRNA are crucial to its full silencing in fetal and adult erythroid cells. We are currently engaged in determining the mechanism(s) that underlie this facet of ζ-globin gene expression.

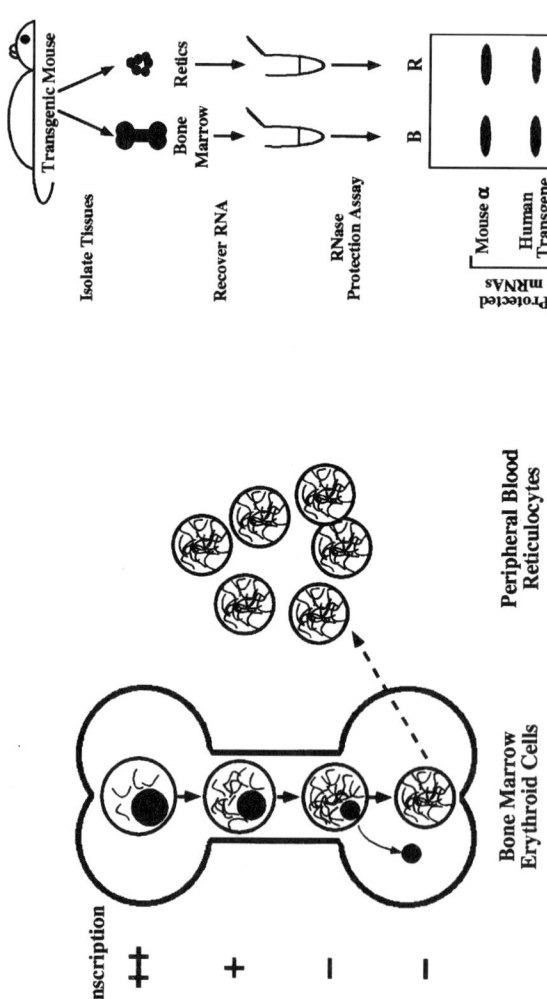

FIGURE 1. A method for determining the stabilities of globin mRNAs in transgenic mice. (**A**) Terminal differentiation of erythroid progenitor cells. Unique characteristics of terminal erythroid differentiation include nuclear condensation and extrusion, followed by migration of the transcriptionally silent marrow reticulocytes from the bone marrow into the peripheral circulation. As most marrow erythroid cells and all peripheral reticulocytes are post-transcriptional, the two tissues represent short and long intervals following transcriptional arrest of a common precursor. (**B**) Protocol for determining the stability of transgenic globin mRNAs in transgenic mice. Total RNA is purified from matched bone marrow and reticulocytes from individual transgenic mice. The levels of transgenic (α- or ζ-) globin mRNA and control endogenous mouse α-globin mRNA are determined by RNase protection using [^{32}P]-labeled antisense RNA probes. Protected fragments are resolved on a denaturing acrylamide/urea gel and band densities quantitated by PhosphorImager analysis. All assays are carried out under conditions of functional probe excess (not shown). B=bone marrow; R=peripheral blood reticulocytes.

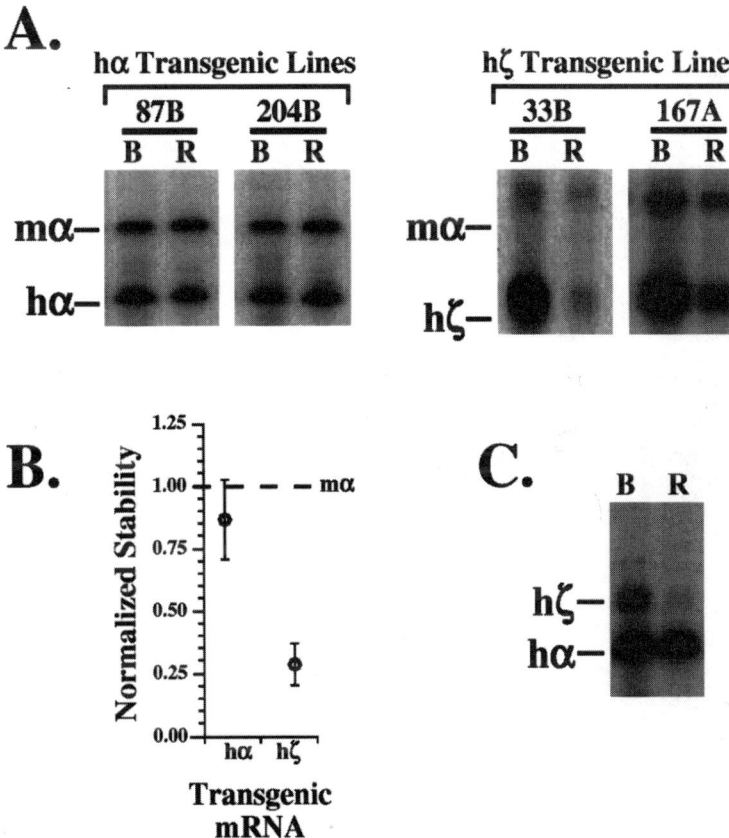

FIGURE 2. Relative instability of human ζ-globin mRNA *in situ* in adult erythroid cells. (**A**) Stability of human α- and ζ-globin mRNAs relative to mouse α-globin mRNAs in mouse erythroid cells. Levels of transgenic hα-globin mRNA (*left*) and hζ-globin mRNA (*right*) were determined relative to mα-globin mRNA using the RPA described in FIGURE 1. Autoradiographs from two representative hα-globin and two representative hζ-globin transgenic mice are shown. The positions of the protected hα-, hζ- and mα-globin mRNA fragments are indicated. Unique numbers (*top*) identify independent transgenic lines. B=bone marrow; R=reticulocyte. (**B**) ζ-globin mRNA is significantly less stable than α-globin mRNA in terminally differentiating adult erythroid cells. The mean stabilities of hα- and hζ-globin mRNAs determined from 10 and 16 independent transgenic lines, respectively, is plotted. The stability of endogenous mα-globin mRNA (defined as 1.0) is indicated by a dashed horizontal line. Error bars indicate ± 2 S.E. The difference between the mean stabilities of human α- and ζ-globin mRNA is significant at $p < 0.005$. (**C**) Direct comparison of human α- and ζ-globin mRNA stabilities in mice co-expressing both transgenes. Mice expressing the hα- and hζ-globin transgenes were mated and offspring expressing both transgenes identified by Southern analysis. Levels of hα- and hζ-globin mRNA in bone marrow (B) and peripheral blood reticulocytes (R) from these mice were determined by RPA. An autoradiograph from a representative study is illustrated, with the positions of the protected human α- and ζ-globin mRNA fragments indicated to the left.

REFERENCES

1. YAGI, M. *et al.* 1996. Chromatin structure and developmental expression of the human α-globin cluster. Mol. Cell. Biol. **6:** 1108–16.
2. ALBITAR, M. *et al.* 1989. Theta, zeta, and epsilon globin messenger RNAs are expressed in adults. Blood **74:** 629–637.
3. LIEBHABER, S. A. *et al.* 1996. Developmental silencing of the embryonic ζ-globin gene: concerted action of the promoter and the 3′ flanking region combined with stage-specific silencing of the transcribed segment. Mol. Cell. Biol. **16:** 2637–2646.
4. WANG, X. *et al.* 1995. Detection and characterization of a 3′ untranslated region ribonucleoprotein complex associated with human α-globin mRNA stability. Mol. Cell. Biol. **15:** 1769–1777.
5. KILEDJIAN, M. *et al.* 1995. Identification of two KH domain proteins in the α-globin mRNP stability complex. EMBO J. **14:** 4357–4364.
6. MORALES, J. *et al.* 1997. Destabilization of human α-globin mRNA by translation anti-termination is controlled during erythroid differentiation and paralleled by phased shortening of the poly(A) tail. J. Biol. Chem. **272:** 6607–6613.
7. RUSSELL, J. E. *et al.* 1998. Sequence divergence in the 3′ untranslated regions of human ζ- and α-globin mRNAs mediates a difference in their stabilities and contributes to efficient α-to-ζ gene developmental switching. Mol. Cell Biol. **18:** 2173–2183.
8. WISDOM, R. *et al.* 1991 The protein coding region of c-myc mRNA contains a sequence that specifies rapid mRNA turnover and induction by protein synthesis inhibitors. Genes Develop. **5:** 232–243.

RBC Adhesion to Cremaster Endothelum in Mice with Abnormal Hemoglobin is Increased by Topical Endotoxin

XIAO-WEI LIU,[a] SILVIA S. PIERANGELI,[b] JOHN BARKER,[b] TIMOTHY M. WICK,[c] AND LEWIS L. HSU[d,e]

[a]Morehouse School of Medicine, Atlanta, Georgia
[b]University of Louisville, Louisville, Kentucky
[c]Georgia Institute of Technology, Atlanta, Georgia
[d]Emory School of Medicine, Atlanta, Georgia

Abnormally increased RBC adhesion to vascular endothelium may play a key role in pathophysiology of hemoglobinopathies, contributing to vaso-occlusive episodes in sickle cell disease and to post-splenectomy pulmonary hypertension in thalassemia. Direct evidence for abnormal adhesion in people with hemoglobinopathies, however, has been difficult to obtain. One previous animal model investigation[1] observed RBC adhesion in transgenic mice expressing hemoglobin S-Antilles, but did not examine stimulation of adhesion. *In vitro* studies have demonstrated that inflammatory stimuli such as cytokines can increase reticulocyte adhesion to endothelium through activation and up-regulation of vascular cell adhesion molecule 1 (VCAM-1) and integrins (VLA-4).[2] Videomicroscopy of mouse cremaster microcirculation has the potential for close correlation between *in vitro* and *in vivo* experiments on endothelial adhesion mechanisms.

HYPOTHESES

1) Mice with abnormal hemoglobin have increased RBC adhesion to endothelium, compared to normal mice.
2) Local inflammation with bacterial endotoxin will further increase RBC adhesion and block capillary flow.

METHODS

Thirteen adult male mice were anesthetized and surgically prepared for videomicroscopic observations of cremaster microcirculation. The thirteen mice formed three groups: 5 mice with beta thalassemia intermedia phenotype (Hbbmdd, or thal-1); 4 mice transgenic for human HbS on Hbbmdd background; and 4 normal controls (strain C57BL/6).

[e]Address for correspondence: Lewis L. Hsu, M.D., Ph.D., Emory University School of Medicine, Pediatric Hematology-Oncology-BMT, 69 Butler St., S.E., Atlanta, Georgia 30303; Tel: 404-616-3545; Fax: 404-525-2816; E-mail: LHSU@emory.edu

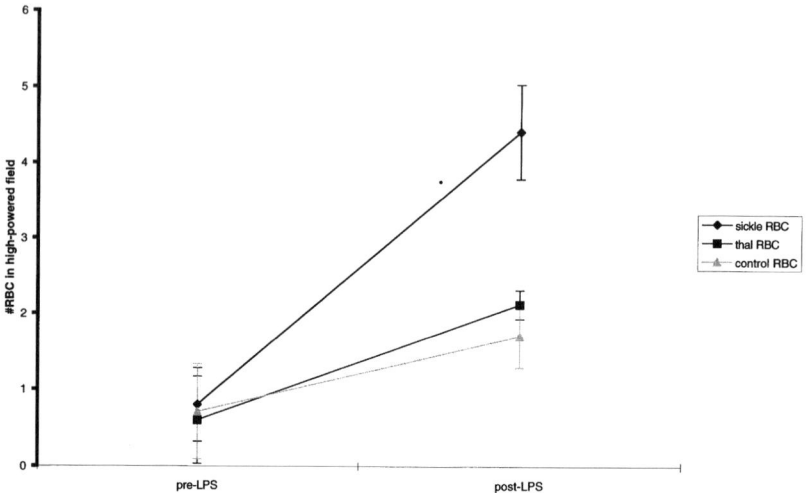

FIGURE 1. RBC adhesion pre- and post-LPS. The number of adherent RBC in the cremaster microcirculation are similar in the three types of mice at baseline observation, pre-LPS. More RBC adhere in all three types after topical LPS, but the increase is significantly greater in the TgHbS mice (p=.009 by t-test). In the contralateral cremasters treated with topical saline, there was no change in adherent RBC compared to baseline (not shown).

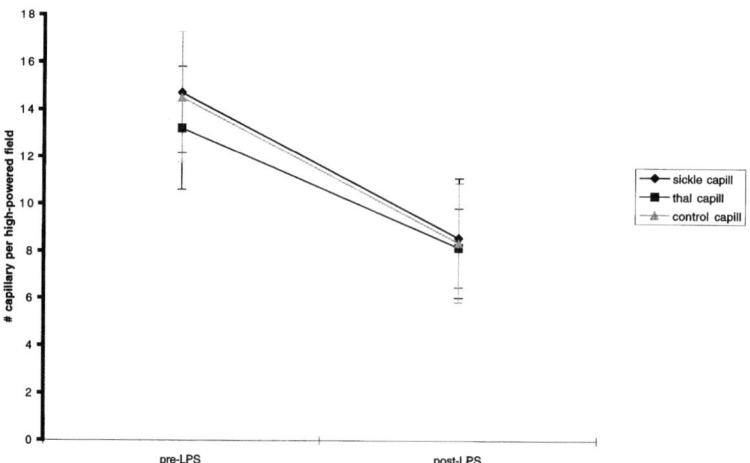

FIGURE 2. Capillary perfusion pre- and post-LPS. Direct microscropic observation of the number of perfused capillaries per microscopic field (approximately 0.2 mm2) are similar in the three types of mice at baseline. After topical LPS treatment, the number of perfused capillaries decreased 40 percent in all three types. The contralateral cremasters treated with topical saline showed no change in perfused capillaries. The role of leukocyte adherence in decreased capillary perfusion post-LPS is being explored.

Systematic observations were made at different locations in the microcirculatory network of the numbers of adherent RBC, adherent WBC, and perfused capillaries. One half of the cremaster muscle then received a local inflammatory insult of 125 µg of endotoxin (from *E. coli* strain O111:B4, Sigma Chemical Co.), topically applied in 50 µl saline. The other half of the cremaster muscle received topical saline as a sham insult.

RESULTS

At baseline, transgenic sickle mice (Tg HbS) mice have similar numbers of adherent RBC (0.8 ± 1.2), compared to normal (0.6 ± 0.5) and thalassemic mice (0.7 ± 0.6) (FIGURE 1), and similar numbers of perfused capillaries at baseline (FIGURE 2). Endotoxin treatment reduced the number of perfused capillaries by approximately 40% in all mice (FIG. 1). Tg HbS mice had more adherent RBC after endotoxin treatment than normal mice after endotoxin (4.9 ± 1.4 compared to 1.7 ± 1.6, $p = .009$) (FIG. 2). Thalassemic mice were not significantly different from normal mice in response to endotoxin. Sham-treated cremasters had no significant changes in adhesion or perfused capillaries, indicating that the endotoxin effect was local and not a systemic phenomenon.

CONCLUSION

Tg HbS mice have increased endothelial RBC adhesion in response to local endotoxin, compared to normal and thalassemic mice. Future studies can examine adhesion mechanisms in this murine model, such as using peptides with the RGD motif to block the integrin VLA-4.

REFERENCES

1. KAUL, D. K., M. E. FABRY, F. COSTANTINI, E. M. RUBIN & R. L. NAGEL. 1995. In vivo demonstration of red cell-endothelial interaction, sickling and altered microvascular response to oxygen in the sickle transgenic mouse. J. Clin. Invest. **96**(6): 2845–2853.
2. SWERLICK, R. A., J. R. ECKMAN, A. KUMAR, M. JEITLER & T. M.WICK. 1993. Alpha 4 beta 1-integrin expression on sickle reticulocytes: vascular cell adhesion molecule-1-dependent binding to endothelium. Blood **82**(6): 1891–1899.

Enhancement by Ubiquitin Aldehyde of Proteolysis of Hemoglobin α-Subunits in β-Thalassemic Hemolysates[a]

JOSEPH R. SHAEFFER[b] AND ROBERT E. COHEN

Department of Biochemistry, College of Medicine, University of Iowa, Iowa City, Iowa 52242-1109, USA

The excess hemoglobin α-subunits in β-thalassemic erythroid cells are poorly degraded by cellular proteases. A substantial fraction of them become denatured and form intracellular inclusion bodies, a process that impairs plasma membrane function and contributes to the anemia through ineffective erythropoiesis and hemolysis. If a way could be found to remove the deleterious α-subunits by enhancing their intracellular proteolysis, the anemia might be improved.

Studies during the 1960s and 1970s suggested that some of the excess α-subunits are destroyed by intracellular proteolysis, although the biochemical mechanism and a basis for its inefficiency in α-subunit degradation were unknown. During the 1980s one of us[1,2] showed that the excess, newly synthesized ³H-α chains (α-subunits with associated heme groups) in intact β-thalassemic reticulocytes or their unfractionated hemolysates were degraded primarily by the ATP- and ubiquitin-dependent proteolysis pathway.

In this major proteolysis system (FIG. 1), the carboxyl terminus of ubiquitin (Ub), a polypeptide of 8,565 Da, is activated in an ATP-dependent reaction. Through a series of enzymatic steps, activated Ub molecules are covalently linked by an "isopeptide" bond to the ε-amino group(s) of one or more lysine residues of the protein destined for proteolysis (reviewed by Hershko and Ciechanover[5]). These Ub-protein conjugates are recognized through their Ub "tag" by the 26S proteasome, a multi-subunit protease complex, and the protein substrate moiety is then degraded in a process that also utilizes ATP. The Ub components of the Ub-protein conjugates are released to the cytoplasmic pool and thus serve as catalysts in the proteolysis reaction.

The cytoplasm that catalyzes the degradation of ubiquitinated proteins also contains several Ub-protein hydrolases or "isopeptidases." One (or a subset) of these enzymes cleaves the isopeptide bond between the carboxyl terminus of Ub and the ε-amino group(s) of the conjugated protein or, in the case of a polyUb chain, of the neighboring Ub monomer. This type of isopeptidase deubiquitinates or "disassembles" the conjugate and thus can play an "editing" role (FIG. 1) in the proteolysis scheme. Studies by one of us and his colleagues[6,7] showed that addition of submicromolar amounts of ubiquitin aldehyde (Ubal), a potent inhibitor of many isopeptidases, greatly increased the levels of the conjugates of cytochrome *c* and ribonuclease A substrates in crude ubiquitination reaction mixtures. Presumably, this synthetic compound, a Ub derivative with the C-terminal carboxyl replaced by an aldehyde group,[8] inhibited isopeptidases that disassembled these conjugates.

---

[a]This work was supported in part by National Institutes of Health grant GM 37666.
[b]Address for correspondence: Department of Biochemistry, University of Iowa, College of Medicine, Iowa City, Iowa 52242-1109. Tel: 319-335-7921; Fax: 319-335-9570.

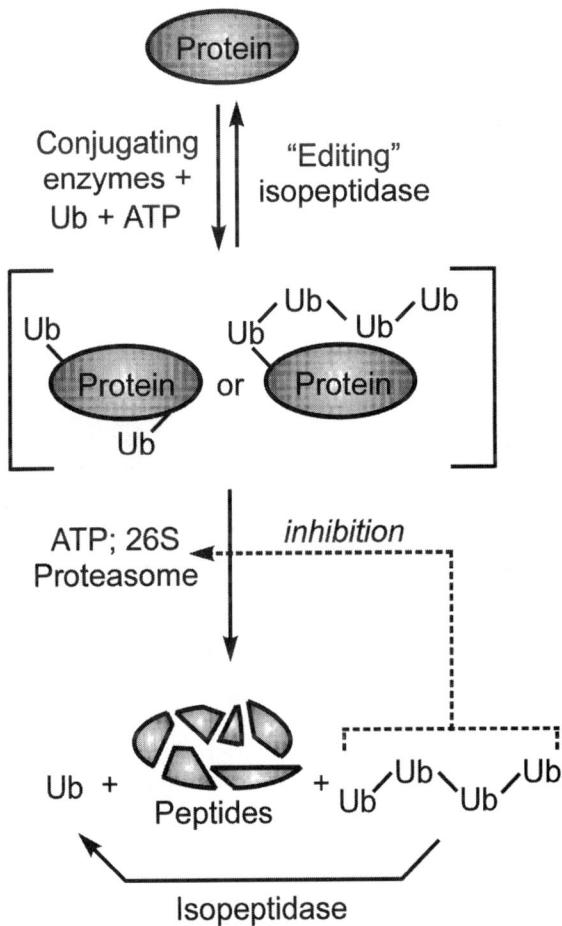

FIGURE 1. Outline of the ATP- and ubiquitin-dependent proteolysis system. The protein substrate at the top is degraded through ubiquitin (Ub)-protein conjugate intermediates (in brackets) by the 26S proteasome complex to peptides at the bottom. The conjugate intermediates consist of protein substrates with adducts of one or more Ub monomers or polyubiquitin (polyUb) chains. PolyUb chains are composed of Ub monomers joined together by isopeptide bonds. The relative contribution of each of these two forms of conjugates to the proteolysis depends in part on the structure of the protein being degraded. Several studies suggest that proteins conjugated with a polyUb chain are more readily recognized and degraded by the 26S proteasome and therefore are "good" substrates compared to those conjugated with only one or a few Ub monomers. In this context, human hemoglobin α-subunits are "poor" substrates; analysis of the conjugates during proteolysis of ^{125}I-α-globin (the heme-depleted apoprotein of the α-chains) in a β-thalassemic[3] or rabbit reticulocyte[4] lysate showed attachment of the substrate predominantly to only one Ub monomer.

With rabbit reticulocyte[4] or four different β-thalassemic[3,9] lysates, we showed recently that similarly low Ubal concentrations not only increased the amount and Ub content of conjugates of ^{125}I-α globin, but also, and more importantly, the total degradation to peptides

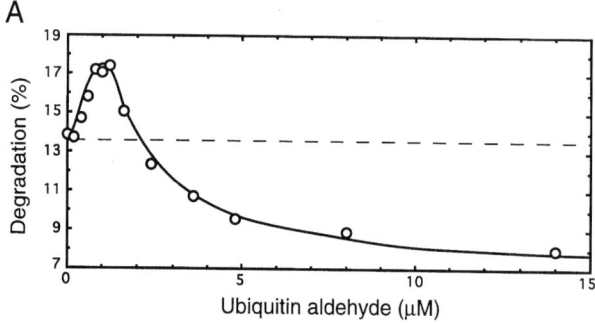

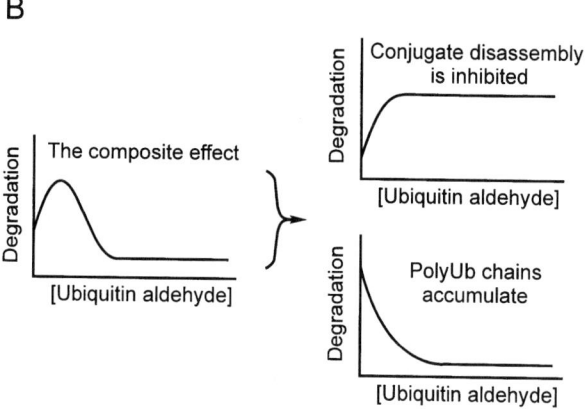

FIGURE 2. (A) Effect of ubiquitin aldehyde (Ubal) on the ATP-dependent proteolysis of human hemoglobin ^{3}H-α chains in a β-thalassemic hemolysate. Each reaction mixture was incubated at 37°C for 2 h with a dialyzed hemolysate from the blood cells of a β-thalassemic donor, ^{3}H-α chains as a proteolysis substrate, and with or without ATP (plus an ATP-regenerating system) and supplementary ubiquitin (see Shaeffer and Cohen[9] for further details). Protein degradation was assayed as the fraction of ^{3}H-α chain radioactivity made acid-soluble. The values obtained in the absence of ATP remained essentially constant (~3.9%) with the different Ubal concentrations and were subtracted from the corresponding + ATP values. **(B)** Hypothetical effect of varying the Ubal concentration on each of two types of lysate isopeptidase (see text) to resolve the curve obtained in **A**.

of either ^{125}I-α globin or ^{3}H-α chains. FIGURE 2A shows a representative result in which optimum enhancement of ^{3}H-α chain degradation occurred at 1.0 μM Ubal. Our results are consistent with the hypothesis that Ubal inhibits an editing isopeptidase that suppresses selectively the degradation of poor substrates (see FIG. 1 legend) such as hemoglobin α-subunits. This laboratory recently identified a new Ubal-sensitive isopeptidase activity that has properties consistent with such an editing function.[10]

Increased levels of Ubal in the lysates resulted in less stimulation and, with sufficiently high levels (typically >3 μM), inhibition of total α-subunit degradation (FIG. 2A).[4,9] We propose that, at high levels, Ubal also blocks another isopeptidase activity, probably isopeptidase T,[11] which normally disassembles free polyUb chains, natural inhibitors of the conjugate-degrading 26S proteasome (see lower part of FIG. 1). FIGURE 2B presents a hypothetical resolution of the curve of FIGURE 2A to show the proposed effect of Ubal on each of the two isopeptidase activities.

Our finding that low levels of Ubal enhanced the proteolysis of hemoglobin α-subunits suggests a possible therapeutic approach to β-thalassemia.

REFERENCES

1. SHAEFFER, J. R. 1983. Turnover of excess hemoglobin α chains in β-thalassemic cells is ATP-dependent. J. Biol. Chem. **258**: 13172–13177.
2. SHAEFFER, J. R. 1988. ATP-dependent proteolysis of hemoglobin α chains in β-thalassemic hemolysates is ubiquitin-dependent. J. Biol. Chem. **263**: 13663–13669.
3. SHAEFFER, J. R. 1994. Monoubiquitinated α globin is an intermediate in the ATP-dependent proteolysis of α globin. J. Biol. Chem. **269**: 22205–22210.
4. SHAEFFER, J. R. & R. E. COHEN. 1996. Differential effects of ubiquitin aldehyde on ubiquitin and ATP-dependent protein degradation. Biochemistry **35**: 10886–10893.
5. HERSHKO, A. & A. CIECHANOVER. 1992. The ubiquitin system for protein degradation. Annu. Rev. Biochem. **61**: 761–807.
6. SOKOLIK, C. W. & R. E. COHEN. 1991. The structures of ubiquitin conjugates of yeast iso-2-cytochrome c. J. Biol. Chem. **266**: 9100–9107.
7. DUNTEN, R. L. & R. E. COHEN. 1989. Recognition of modified forms of ribonuclease A by the ubiquitin system. J. Biol. Chem. **264**: 16739–16747.
8. PICKART, C. M. & I. A. ROSE. 1986. Mechanism of ubiquitin carboxyl-terminal hydrolase. J. Biol. Chem. **261**: 10210–10217.
9. SHAEFFER, J. R. & R. E. COHEN. 1997. Ubiquitin aldehyde increases the ATP-dependent proteolysis of hemoglobin α-subunits in β-thalassemic hemolysates. Blood **90**: 1300–1308.
10. LAM, Y. A., W. XU, G. N. DEMARTINO & R. E. COHEN. 1997. Editing of ubiquitin conjugates by an isopeptidase in the 26S proteasome. Nature **385**: 737–740.
11. WILKINSON, K. D., V. L. TASHAYEV, L. B. O'CONNOR, C. N. LARSEN, E. KASPEREK & C. M. PICKART. 1995. Metabolism of the polyubiquitin degradation signal: structure, mechanism, and role of isopeptidase T. Biochemistry **34**: 14535–14546.

An α-2 Globin Gene Initiation Codon Mutation in a Vietnamese Patient with Hb H Disease

F. KUTLAR,[a] T. V. ADAMKIEWICZ,[b,c] R. B. MARKOWITZ,[a] L. HOLLEY,[a] AND A. KUTLAR[a]

[a]Sickle Cell Center, Department of Medicine, Medical College of Georgia, Augusta, Georgia, USA

[b]Georgia Comprehensive Sickle Cell Center, Emory University, Atlanta, Georgia 30322, USA

Hb H disease is relatively common in Southeast Asia and in the Mediterranean. Clinically, it presents as a "thalassemia intermedia," with moderately severe hypochromic microcytic anemia, hemolysis, hepatosplenomegaly, and typical Hb H inclusion bodies in erythrocytes. The molecular basis of Hb H disease is heterogeneous: it commonly results from the interaction of α° and α^+ thalassemia (-α/$\alpha\alpha$); interaction of non-deletional α-thalassemia determinants (α^T) with α° thal can also lead to Hb H disease.[1]

We present a Vietnamese child in whom the molecular basis of Hb H disease was found to be an interaction of an α° thal ($-\text{-}^{SEA}$) with a novel initiation codon mutation.

CASE

The propositus was a healthy nine-month-old adopted Vietnamese boy who was referred for the evaluation of a hypochromic-microcytic anemia. CBC showed a Hb of 9.1 gm/dl, MCV of 53.3 fl, MCH of 28 pg. Peripheral smear revealed significant hypochromia, microcytosis, ovalocytes, and occasional schistocytes. A BCB (brilliant cresyl blue) prep showed many RBC with typical Hb H inclusion bodies.

METHODS

Hemoglobin analyses (isoelectric focusing, cation exchange HPLC) were performed by previously described methods.[2] DNA was extracted from peripheral blood WBC. The detection of -$\alpha^{3.7}$ deletion was performed by PCR according to a previously described procedure.[3] The Southeast Asian α° thal deletion ($-\text{-}^{SEA}$) was detected by PCR using the method described by Bowden and colleagues.[4] A 1,003 bp fragment of α-2 globin gene was amplified using M-13 tailed primers; the amplification product was purified by using Prep-A-Gene DNA purification kit according to manufacturer's instructions (Bio-Rad, Hercules, CA). The purified product was sequenced on an ABI prism 377 DNA sequencer, using ABI Prism Cycle Sequencing Dye Primer Ready Reaction kit, containing Ampli Taq DNA polymerase, FS according to manufacturer's instructions.

[c]Address for correspondence to Dr. Adamkiewicz at: Emory University School of Medicine, Pediatric Hematology-Oncology-BMT, 2040 Ridgewood Dr. N.E., Atlanta, GA 30322. Fax: 404-727-4455.

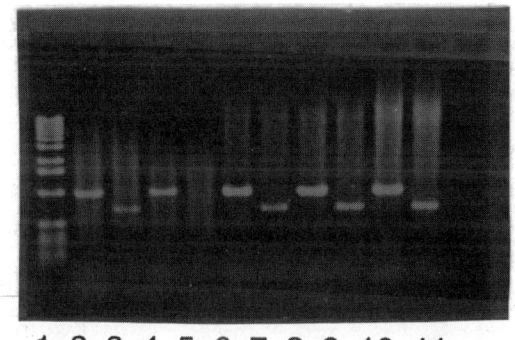

FIGURE 1. Detection of $--^{SEA}$ deletion by PCR. Lane 1: 1 kb ladder, Lane 8 + 9 (patient) demonstrating PCR products 980 bp (lane 8) and 660 bp (lane 9) originating from the normal and $--^{SEA}$ chromosomes, respectively.

RESULTS

Isoelectric focusing (IEF) of the patients hemolysate on thin-layer agarose revealed Hb A, and a fast-moving component with the focusing pattern of Hb H+Bart's. Cation exchange HPLC showed a Hb H+ Bart's peak of 12.6%, the patient had a HbF of 2.7% and Hb A_2 of 0.5%. PCR amplification to detect $-\alpha^{3.7}$ deletion failed to reveal the 3.7 kb α^+ thal deletion. When the patient's DNA was amplified using primers to detect the 18 kb Southeast Asian deletion ($--^{SEA}$) as described by Bowden and colleagues,[4] a 660 bp fragment specific for $--^{SEA}$ deletion and a 980 bp fragment generated by a chromosome with normal α-globin genes ($\alpha\alpha$) were visualized, indicating that the patient was heterozygous for the $--^{SEA}$ deletion. (FIG. 1) Sequencing of the PCR amplified α-2 globin genes from the intact chromosome revealed a single nucleotide deletion (-T) at the initiation codon (ATG $\rightarrow$ AG) (FIG. 2)

COMMENTS

Hb H disease is clinically heterogeneous, ranging from a moderate hypochromic, microcytic anemia in some cases, to severe, transfusion-dependent anemia in others. The quantity of Hb H is proportional to the degree of α-globin chain deficiency, and varies from less than 1.0% to ~40.0%. Generally interaction of α° thalassemia with a non-deletional α-thal determinant results in a more severe phenotype.[1] There are twenty non-deletional α-thalassemia determinants described to date; these result from point mutations or small (several nucleotide) deletions in functionally critical sequences of α-globin genes. Most of these involve the dominant α-2 globin gene, and thus lead to a more severe phenotype compared to the deletional forms of α^+ thalassemia ($-\alpha^{3.7}$ or $-\alpha^{4.2}$). Several mutations in the initiation codon (ATG) of the α-2 globin gene have been described in blacks and Mediterraneans.[1] Majority of α-thalassemias in Southeast Asian populations are due to deletions (α° or α^+). Non-deletional α-thalassemia is relatively infrequent; the most common form is the termination codon mutation, Hb Constant Spring.

Our case represents the second observation of a hitherto undescribed initiation codon mutation (ATG $\rightarrow$ AG) in a Vietnamese child[5] indicating the presence of rare non-deletional α-thal mutations in Southeast Asia. Utilization of PCR-based methods to detect common

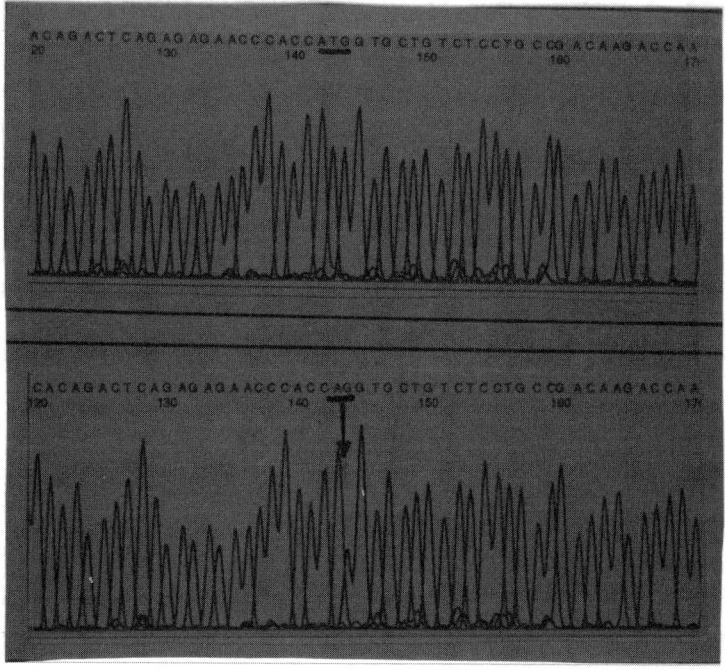

FIGURE 2. Molecular characterization of the non-deletional ∂-thalassemia in a Vietnamese patient with Hb H disease. (*Top*) Normal sequencing data. (*Bottom*) Demonstration of a single nucleotide deletion (-T) at the initiation codon (ATG) of the ∂2 globin gene by sequencing of the PCR product.

α-thalassemia deletions and automated sequencing of PCR products expedite the delineation of the molecular basis of Hb H disease.

REFERENCES

1. HIGGS, D. R. 1993. α-Thalassemia Bailliere's Clin. Haematol. **6** (1): 117–150.
2. KUTLAR, A. & T. H. J. HUISMAN. 1991. The detection of hemoglobinopathies. *In* Techniques in Diagnostic Human Biochemical Genetics: A Laboratory Manual. F. Hommes, Ed.: 519–560. J. Wiley & Sons. New York.
3. KUTLAR, F., P. F. MILNER, K. M. MCKIE, J. B. WILSON & A. KUTLAR. 1996. A new approach to the detection of -α$^{3.7}$ by PCR [abstract]. Presented at the 21st Annual Meeting of the National Sickle Cell Disease Program. Mobile, AL, 1996.
4. BOWDEN, D. K., M. A. VICKERS & D. R. HIGGS. 1992. A PCR-based strategy to detect the common severe determinants of α-thalassemia. Br. J. Haematol. **81:** 104–108.
5. WAYE, J. S., B. ENG., M. PATTERSON, D. H. K. CHUI, E. NISBET-BROWN & N. F. OLIVIERI. 1996. Novel mutation of the α2 globin gene initiation codon (ATG → A-G) in a Vietnamese girl with Hb H disease. Hemoglobin **21**(5): 469–472.

The Montreal Thalassemia Screening Program

Response of the High School Students

A. CAPUA[a]

McGill University-Montreal Children's Hospital Research Institute and the DeBelle Laboratory for Biochemical Genetics, Montreal, Quebec, Canada

The Montreal Thalassemia Screening Program was developed and supported by the communities at high risk for β-thalassemia. The carrier frequency in the Montreal region is 1 in 15 Greeks and 1 in 30 Italians. Prior to performing the screening program, community leaders, Montreal School Commission officials, parents, patients, and organizers met to define the objectives, process, and structure of the program. In 1979, screening was offered to the communities at-risk through neighborhood health centers known as CLSCs (Centre Local pour des Services Communautaires). In 1981, the screening program was integrated with high schools whose student populations were mainly Greek, Italian, Middle Eastern, and Southeast Asian origin. Since then, the screening program has been offered to all students 14–18 years of age who are in Secondary IV and V (Grade 10 and 11)[1-4] on a voluntary basis. The scope of the screening program comprises educational activities, screening of potential carriers, diagnostic procedures, counselling resources, and finally, procedures for fetal diagnosis. The participant's results are confidential. From 1980 to 1992; 25,274 high school participants were screened and 693 carriers were detected. The screening program reached 67% of its demographic cohort with a participation rate varying between 70–80%.[5] Prior to 1979, all β-thalassemia prenatal diagnosis referrals were due to the birth of an affected child. Now, virtually all carrier couple referrals for reproductive counselling originate from the screening program. The incidence rate of newly diagnosed cases has fallen by 90% since the beginning of the screening program. There are concerns about genetic screening in the high school system.[6,7] It has been noted that genetics in health care must be ethical and used in ways that honor the principles of autonomy, justice, privacy, equity, and quality.[8] The Montreal Thalassemia Screening Program incorporates these principles while meeting the needs of the community.

EDUCATIONAL AND CLINICAL SESSIONS

Annually, the co-ordinator compiles a list of all the high schools scheduled to take part in the screening program. The screening program operates from September to May. High school nurses are the primary contacts between the co-ordinator and the school director. The screening program functions on a two-day system: an education session on the initial visit followed by a clinic session on the second visit. With the aid of the high school nurses,

---

[a]Address for correspondence: Aniceta Capua, Co-ordinator of the Montreal Thalassemia Screening Program, Montreal Children's Hospital, Biochemical Genetics Unit, 2300 Tupper Street, Rm: A-718, Montreal, Quebec, H3H 1P3. Tel: 514-934-4417; and Fax: 514-934-4329.

dates are reserved and confirmed one week prior to the day of the education session. On the initial visit, the school's director makes an announcement and invites all Secondary IV and V (Grade 10 and 11) high school students and their teachers to the auditorium. A 30-minute slide presentation is shown to explain what thalassemia is, how it is inherited, the possible risks for a carrier couple, and the actual events that take place at the clinic session. Time is allocated for a question period at the end of the presentation. Most of the high school students have been exposed to a biology course in which genetic disorders were discussed. Others are aware of thalassemia due to the carrier status of their parents. At the end of the education session, all the participants are given an information pamphlet on thalassemia to take home to their parents. If necessary, the information is available in other languages, i.e., Greek, Italian, French, and Chinese. A parental consent form is attached to the information pamphlet and the need for this consent is explained to all participants.

Within one week of the educational session, the screening program team returns to the high school. The team consists of the co-ordinator, assistant, and phlebotomists (two per clinic). The screening program is responsible for all the necessary supplies that are needed for the procurement of blood. The high school nurse arranges for six to eight student volunteers to help keep the clinic organized. Participants proceed to the clinic area, submit their parental consent form and complete a registration card and self-addressed envelope. Upon completion of the documentation, they advance to the specimen labeling area and are given their blood vial. The blood is drawn by professional phlebotomists. The students sit down for a 5-minute rest period before leaving the clinic area. The duration of the screening clinic is approximately two to three hours depending on the quantity of students. At the end of every clinic, the samples are gathered and returned to the Biochemical Genetics Unit of the Montreal Children's Hospital.

The genetic testing for β-thalassemia can be performed using whole blood in an EDTA-treated blood sample. Mean cell volume is measured with a Coulter counter; then HbA2 analysis is performed on samples with a mean cell volume (MCV) value < 76 fl.[2] Results are classified by a Bayesian density discriminant function,[9] and additional tests are performed when indicated. The results are sent to each participant on a confidential basis. A follow-up call is made to all the carriers to offer further interpretation and counselling. In 1993, a survey of 720 high school participants showed that 99%–100% of the participants wished to be tested and immediately receive results. As implied in the findings,[5] "carrier students" remember their status, are not stigmatized by it, and use the genetic information in ways they deem helpful.

In Quebec, prenatal diagnosis for thalassemia became available in the mid-1970s. Prior to 1979, all prenatal diagnosis referrals resulted from an affected individual being born into the family. We have seen through our twenty-year outcome study that 32 couples sought prenatal diagnosis of which 24 originated from the screening program. Now, virtually all prenatal diagnosis referrals originate from the screening program. Prenatal counselling and diagnosis in the global program has led to the birth of 43 unaffected children and 11 voluntary terminations of affected pregnancies.[5]

CONCLUSIONS

The Montreal Thalassemia Screening Program reaches a high proportion of individuals at-risk. The participants understand and retain the information and carriers use the information appropriately. Detected carrier students accept and seek out counselling for reproductive options if they become carrier couples later in life. Since the commencement of the screening program, the predominant referral source for prenatal diagnosis has shifted from relatives of affected family members to carrier couples detected through the screening program. Although the Montreal Thalassemia Screening Progam is the only screening program of its kind, it has definitely demonstrated that education and counselling alleviate some of the anxiety associated with positive carrier status for couples facing reproductive choices. The screening program is successful and well accepted by the at-risk communities in Quebec.

ACKNOWLEDGMENTS

I would like to thank Dr. Charles R. Scriver and Carol Clow for the opportunity they provided, in 1988, to become the screening program's co-ordinator. Drs. Eileen Treacy and Feige Kaplan for their recognition and support of my work. Irene Ferko, for her endless hours of assistance and last minute preparation of my abstracts. Lynne Prevost for her expertise in preparing abstracts. Debby Lambert, genetic counsellor, who allows me to improve through her teachings and advice. Lisa Sniderman, thanks for the computer time. Dr. Gail Graham for her encouragement and revisions. The members of the Quebec Society of Thalassemia Inc. for showing their continuous support of the screening program. I would like to extend thanks to Marietta Bardanis whose advice was: "if you want to really understand everything about thalassemia, speak to the patients." To George Kritikos and other thalassemia patients, thank you for being my mentors.

REFERENCES

1. CLOW, C. L. & C. R. SCRIVER. 1977. Knowledge about and attitudes toward genetic screening amoung high-school students: The Tay-Sachs experience. Pediatrics **59**: 86–91.
2. SCRIVER, C. R., M. BARDANIS, L. CARTIER, C. L. CLOW, G. A. LANCASTER & J. T. OSTROWSKY. 1984. β-thalassemia disease prevention: Genetic medicine applied. Am. J. Hum. Genet. **36**: 1024–1038.
3. ZEESMAN, S., C. L. CLOW, L. CARTIER & C. R. SCRIVER. 1984. A private view of heterozygosity: Eight year follow up study on carriers of Tay-Sachs gene detected by high school screening in Montreal. Am. J. Med. Genet. **18**: 769–778.
4. OSTROWSKY, J. T., A. LIPPMAN & C. R. SCRIVER. 1985. Cost-benefit analysis of a thalassemia disease prevention program. Am. J. Pub. Health **75**: 732–736.
5. MITCHELL, J. J., A. CAPUA, C. L. CLOW & C. R. SCRIVER. 1996. Twenty-year outcome analysis of genetic screening—programs for Tay-Sachs and β-thalassemia disease carriers in high schools. Am. J. Hum. Genet. **59**: 793–798.
6. ANDREWS, L. B., J. W. FULLARTON, N. A. HOLTZMAN & A. G. MOTULSKY, Eds. 1994. Assessing genetic risks: Implications for health and social policy. National Academy Press. Washington D.C.
7. SCRIVER, C.R. 1995. Review of: Assessing genetic risks: Implications for health and social policy. Am. J. Hum. Genet. **56**: 814–816.
8. KNOPPERS, B. M. & R. CHADWICK. 1994. The human genome project: Under an international ethical microscope. Science **265**: 2035–2036.
9. ZANNIS-HADJOPOULOS, M., R. J. M. GOLD, U. R. MAAG, J. D. METRAKOS & C. R. SCRIVER. 1977. Improved detection of β-thalassemia carriers by a two-test method. Hum. Genet. **38**: 315–324.

Spectrum of β-Thalassemia Mutations in Oman[a]

S. DAAR,[b] H. M. HUSSEIN,[c] T. MERGHOUB,[c] AND
R. KRISHNAMOORTHY[c,d]

[b]*Sultan Qaboos University, Muscat, Oman*

[c]*INSERM U458, Hôpital Robert Debré, Paris, France*

Oman lies in the southeast corner of the Arabian peninsula, covers an area of 300,000 km,[2] and has a population of two million. The most striking geographical factors are the desert and the mountain ranges separating and isolating Oman from the rest of the peninsula and the coastline facing the Arabian Sea and the Indian Ocean, opening Oman to a maritime world through which outward contacts had been maintained through centuries.

Previous studies, based on phenotype analysis, revealed that the gene frequency of beta-thalassemia (β thal) among Omanis is around 1–2%.[1] A recent countrywide survey has confirmed this overall frequency and, in addition, localized the β thal essentially (excepting thalassemic Hb Dhofar, see below) to the northeastern regions of Oman.[2] In the present report we have studied 99 unrelated patients (198 chromosomes) with homozygous β thal among Omani nationals. The diagnosis was based on clinical, hematological, and DNA studies.

Fifteen different mutations were identified (TABLE 1) with one allele, IVS1, 5 G→C, highly represented (61.6%) along with five other alleles namely, Cd 44 -C, Hb Dhofar (Cd 29 C→T and Cd 58 G→C in *cis*), IVS1-3' -25 bp, 619 bp del and IVSII,1 G→A together accounting for 91% of the β thal alleles. The nine other alleles observed at very low frequency were : Cd 39 C→T, IVS1,1 G→A, Cd 36/37 -T, Cd 5 -CT, Cd 15 G→A, Cd 37 -G, Cd 30 G→A, IVS1,110 G→A, and HbE. Most of the alleles, excepting Hb E, are either β⁰ or severe β⁺ thal defect, corroborating well with the observed clinical severity in these patients. It is noteworthy that 75 out of the 99 patients (75.8%) studied were homozygous for a given mutation, a consequence of the high degree of consanguineous marriages occurring in this country.

Oman had experienced many influxes: Persian settlement in the second century AD was followed by a tribal movement from Yemen in the fifth century AD. In the sixteenth century AD the Portuguese occupied the coastal region. Oman also had trading links with Basra in southern Iraq and the Indian subcontinent. But the major influx probably dates to the eighteenth century when Gwadar (at that time part of Baluchistan) was presented as a gift to the Omani ruler.[3] This is supported by the data of White and colleagues,[1] who observed that out of 137 homozygous β thal cases, 75% were found to have originated from Baluchistan as identified by their family name and 19 out of 25 (70%) were found to have the IVS1,5 G→C mutation. Our data not only confirm this as 50% of our patients have Baluchi-(an Indo-Iranian language) derived names but also show that even among the

---

[a]This work was supported by the French Ministry for external affairs: Middle East division.

[d]Address for correspondence: Dr. R. Krishnamoorthy, INSERM U458, Hôpital Robert Debré, 48 Bd Sérurier, 75019 Paris, France. Tel: 33 01 40 03 19 01; Fax: 33 01 40 03 19 03; E-mail: krishna @infobiogen.fr

Arabs IVS1,5 G→C is the most common mutation. This would suggest that ethnic admixing had been intense in the northeastern region, as further evidenced by the presence of this mutation at a similar frequency in United Arab Emirates.[4] Clearly this mutation was introduced into Oman by gene flow from Baluchistan,[4] located across the strait of Hormuz presently forming part of Iran, Afganistan, and Pakistan. Interestingly other Middle Eastern countries, such as Saudi Arabia, Jordan, and Lebanon, exhibit a different spectrum of β-thal mutations with Mediterranean type significantly represented.[5] Geographical particularities of Oman, as mentioned above, would have limited exchanges with these neighboring countries.

The second commonest mutation in Oman is Cd 44 -C, originally described as a Kurdish/Iranian allele found also in Kuwait.[6] The next prevalent mutation is a double-substituted Hb Dhofar (Cd 29 C→T and Cd 58 G→C in *cis*) first described at the phenotype level in 1968[7] in a Qara tribesman from Dhofar (Oman) in heterozygous state and was recorded as new hemoglobin variant ($\alpha_2\beta_2^{58\,(E2)\,Pro\to Arg}$). Then, Hb Dhofar was found to have β-thal mutation in *cis* (Cd 29 C→T) in carrier state in an Omani.[8] Identical Hb variant ($\alpha_2\beta_2^{58\,(E2)\,Pro\to Arg}$) without an associated thalassemic phenotype was also reported from Japan and designated Hb Yukihashi ($\alpha_2\beta_2^{58\,(E2)\,Pro\to Arg}$).[9] Interestingly, the same mutation was also found in an African population in *cis* to Hb S and was named Hb C-Ziguinchor. On the other hand, the thalassemic Cd 29 C→T mutation alone (without a second substitution) was first found in Lebanon and then in one patient from Yugoslavia.

The double-substituted thalassemic Hb Dhofar emerges as the only allele specific for Oman, never found elsewhere. It is highly restricted to the southwest region (close to Yemen), contrasting with the distribution of other alleles essentially located to the northeastern part of the country facing the Indian subcontinent. To our knowledge this is the first report of homozygous cases of Hb Dhofar, which are found to have a clinical phenotype of severe thalassemia intermedia.

In conclusion, apart from having its own specific thalassemic allele, namely Hb Dhofar, the major thalassemic gene input in Oman is essentially from the Asian subcontinent.

TABLE 1. Spectrum of β-Thalassemia Mutations in Oman

Mutation	Described in	Chromosomes N	Chromosomes %	Homozygotes N	Homozygotes %
IVSI,5 G→C	Asian Indian	122	61.6	52	69.3
Cd 44 -C	Kurdish/Iranian	19	9.6	9	12
Hb Dhofar	Oman	13	6.6	6	8
IVSI-3' end -25	Middle East	11	5.5	3	4
619 bp del	Asian Indian	8	4	1	1.3
IVSII,1 G→A	Middle East	7	3.5	1	1.3
CD 39 C→T	Middle East	2	1	1	1.3
IVSI,1 G→A	Middle East	2	1	1	1.3
Cd 36/37 -T	Kurdish/Iranian	2	1	1	1.3
Cd 5 -CT	Middle East	1	0.5		
Cd 15 G→A	Asian Indian	1	0.5		
CD 37 -G	Middle East	1	0.5		
Cd 30 G→A	Asian Indian	1	0.5		
IVSI,110 G→A	Middle East	1	0.5		
Hb E	Southeast Asia and India	1	0.5		
Unknown		6	3		
Total		198	100	75	100

REFERENCES

1. WHITE, J. M. *et al.* 1993. Frequency and clinical significance of erythrocyte genetic abnormalities in Omanis, J. Med. Genet. **30**: 396–400
2. National Genetic Blood Disorders Survey. 1997. Ministry of Health, Sultanate of Oman.
3. RISSO, P. 1986. Oman and Muscat—an early modern history. Croom Helm, Ltd U.K.
4. QUAIFE, *et al.* 1994. The spectrum of β-thalassemia mutations in the UAE national population J. Med. Genet. **31**: 59–61.
5. EL-HAZMI, M. A. F. *et al.* 1995. The frequency of 14 beta thalassemia mutations in the Arab population. Hemoglobin **19**: 353–360.
6. ADEKILE, A. D. *et al.* 1994. Molecular characterization of α-thalassemia determinants, β-thalassemia alleles and $β^s$ haplotypes among Kuwaiti Arabs, Acta Haematol. **92**: 176–181.
7. MARENGO-ROWE, *et al.* 1968. Haemoglobin Dhofar: A new variant from Southern Arabia. Biochim. Biophys. Acta **168**: 58–63.
8. WILLIAMSON, D. *et al.* 1995. Haemoglobin Dhofar is linked to codon 29 C→T (IVS1nt-3) splice mutation which causes $β^+$-thalassemia, Br. J. Haematol. **90**: 229–231.
9. YANASE, *et al.* 1968. Molecular basis of morbidity: From a series of studies of haemoglobinopathies in western Japan, Jpn. J. Hum. Genet. **13**(1): 40–53.

Molecular Basis of β-Thalassemia in Bahrain: An Epicenter for a Middle East Specific Mutation[a]

N. JASSIM,[b,c] T. MERGHOUB,[b] O. PASCAUD,[b] H. AL MUKHARRAQ,[c] R. DUCROCQ,[b] D. LABIE,[b] J. ELION,[b] R. KRISHNAMOORTHY,[b,d] AND S. AL ARRAYED[c]

[b]*INSERM U458, Hôpital Robert Debré, Paris, France*
[c]*Salmaniya Medical Center, Manama, Bahrain*

Bahrain is an archipelago of 36 islands in the Arabian Gulf. Until the era of Islam, Bahrain was influenced by the Babylonian, Assyrian, and Greek civilizations amongst other ancient civilizations. It was also an important commercial center on the major trade routes between the East and the West. Thus infiltration of different foreign cultures and civilizations through time in Bahrain resulted in a cosmopolitan blend of present day genes.

Previous studies based on phenotype analysis showed that hemoglobinopathies represent one of the major genetic disorders in the population of Bahrain, revealing high frequencies for sickle cell α-thalassemia and β-thalassemia genes.[1] Consequently, the hemoglobinopathies account for the major phenotype diagnostic requests in the hospitals of Bahrain.

So far no molecular characterization of β-thalassemia in Bahrain had been performed although significant amount of data was available from the neighboring countries. Given the geographical and historical particularities of Bahrain, we would predict that the spectrum of thalassemic defects in Bahrain may differ from other Middle East populations. Thus the objective of this study is to delineate the molecular lesions leading to β-thalassemia in Bahrain. This is an essential prerequisite for evaluating the frequency of mutations as well for establishing an efficient prevention program, which includes carrier screening, premarital counselling, and eventually offering prenatal diagnosis for couples at risk of having a child with thalassemia major syndrome.

We have studied a total of 80 individuals of whom 35 are transfusion-dependent β-thalassemia major patients, 37 with β-thalassemia trait and 8 S-β-thalassemia patients. All of them are Bahraini nationals treated in the pediatric clinics or consultees of genetics unit of Salmaniya Medical Centre, Manama, Bahrain.

The DNA was extracted from whole blood (~ 5 ml) using the standard phenol-chloroform extraction method. The technique of reverse dot blot (RDB) was used initially to screen for the six commonest Indian and Mediterranean mutations. The nucleotide sequences of each of these normal and mutant probes as well as the experimental conditions of polymerase chain reaction (PCR) and RDB procedure were as described previously.[2,3] The samples that

---

[a]This work was supported by the French Ministry of Foreign Affairs: Middle-East division.
[d]Address for correspondence: Dr. R. Krishnamoorthy, INSERM U458, Hôpital Robert Debré, 48 Bd Sérurier, 75019 Paris, France. Tel: 33 01 40 03 19 01; Fax: 33 01 40 03 19 03; E-mail: krishna@infobiogen.fr

provided no relevant signal in the RDB or signal for only one allele for patients with β-thalassemia major were further examined by denaturant gradient gel electrophoresis (DGGE) analysis as described before.[4] The samples exhibiting abnormal DGGE profiles were subjected to nucleotide sequencing using the dideoxy chain termination method.

A total of 67 β-thalassemic alleles have been deciphered which comprised 12 different mutations. However four different mutations, namely IVS-I 3′ end (-25 bp) Cd 39 (C → t), IVSI, 5 (G → C) and IVSII, 1 (G → A) accounted for more than 80% of the total studied alleles. The frequency of each of these 12 β-thalassemic alleles in native Bahrainis is presented in TABLE 1 along with a previously published data for four neighboring countries. Mutations common both to the Mediterranean basin [CD 39 (C → T), IVS-I-1 (G → A), IVS-II-1 (G → A), IVS-I-110 (G → A)] and India [CD 8/9 (+G), IVS-I-5 (G→ C), CD 15 (G → A), CD 41/42 (-TCTT)] were equally represented.

The most striking observation is the unprecedented high frequency of the 25 bp deletion mutant in this country, the highest ever to be observed, including in the other Middle East countries. Interestingly the second major mutation (CD 39 C → T), a major mediterranean allele, and the third one (IVSI nt 5 G → C), a major Indian allele, are most likely to have been introduced into Bahrain from the West and the East, respectively.

Some of our experience in using RDB for screening β-thalassemia in Bahrain is of particular interest. Screening for the Mediterranean type mutations by RDB revealed an individual as homozygous for Cd 39 (C → T) mutation. Further screening for Indian type mutations by RDB gave a positive heterozygous signal for Cd41/42 (-CTTT) mutation. We were able to assign this as compound heterozygote for these two mutations and confirmed it by nucleotide sequencing. Such atypical data arose because the design of the oligonucleotides in RDB were such that the deleted four nucleotides in Cd 41/42 mutation destabilized the hybridization with the normal Cd 39 probe. Similarly, total absence of signal with normal IVSI, 110 (G → A) probe is a feature of the cases homozygous for IVSI 3′ end (-25 bp) mutation because the RDB probe is within the deleted region. However precise diagnosis of this mutation can be carried out easily by size-separation of the PCR product in an agarose gel electrophoresis.

Altogether (TABLE 1), our data reveal that in Bahrain, the IVSI 3′ end (-25bp) mutation is largely predominant (36%), the highest frequency ever to be reported for this Middle-East specific mutation. Thus, Bahrain appears to be the epicenter for this mutation in the Middle East. In conclusion, this study will be of invaluable benefit for the precise, cost-effective DNA-based diagnosis and thus for future preventive programs.

TABLE 1. Spectrum and Distribution of β-Thalassemic Alleles in the Middle East

	Bahrain	Saudi Arabia	Kuwait	United Arab Emirates (UAE)	South Iran
Chromosomes (N)	66	158	96	185	108
IVSI 3′ end (-25bp)	36.1	12.9	7.3	6.5	3.7
Cd39 (C → T)	24.2	12.9	7.3	5.4	5.5
IVSI, 5 (G → C)	16.7	12.9	18.7	54.1	7.4
IVSII, 1 (G → A)	6.1	12.9	29	3.2	13.8
IVSI, 1 (G → A)	3.0	-	7.3	-	3.7
Cd44 (-C)	4.5	-	1	1.1	3.7
nt-88 (C → A)	1.5	-	-	-	0.9
Cd8/9 (+ G)	1.5	1.07	3.1	8.6	4.6
Cd15 (G → A)	1.5	-	-	2.2	-
IVSI, 110 (G → A)	1.5	26.9	-	1.6	6.5
Cd35 (-C)	1.5	-	-	-	-
Cd41/42 (-TCTT)	1.5	-	-	-	-
Others	0	20.43	26.1	17.3	50

REFERENCES

1. NADKARNI, K. V. et al. 1991. Incidence of genetic disorders of hemoglobin in the hospital population of Bahrain. Bahrain Med. Bull. **13**(1): 19–24.
2. MAGGIO, A. et al. 1993. Rapid and simultaneous typing of hemoglobin S, hemoglobin C, and seven Mediterranean β-thalassemia mutations by covalent reverse dot-blot analysis: Application to prenatal diagnosis in Sicily. Blood **81**: 239–242.
3. CAI, S. P. et al. 1994. Reverse dot blot probes for screening of β-thalassemia mutations in Asians and American blacks. Hum. Mutat. **3**: 59–63.
4. GHANEM, N. et al. 1992. A comprehensive scanning method for rapid detection of β-globin gene mutations and polymorphisms. Hum. Mutat. **1**: 229–239.

Hemoglobin E/β Thalassemia: The Canadian Experience

M. FOULADI, M. L. MACMILLAN, E. NISBET-BROWN, N. KLEIN,
J. BARLAS, J. S. WAYE, AND N. F. OLIVIERI[a]

*McMaster University Medical Center, Hamilton, Ontario, Canada, and
The Hospital for Sick Children, Toronto, Ontario, Canada*

One of the most common genotypes within the class of disorders referred to as Cooley's anemia is hemoglobin E/β-thalassemia,[1,2] a condition that is often as severe as homozygous β-thalassemia, with hemoglobin concentrations varying from 2.6 to 13.3 grams per deciliter.[3-5] In β-thalassemia/hemoglobin E as in Cooley's anemia, reduced or absent β-globin synthesis leads to decreased hemoglobin production as well as to a relative excess of α-globin chains, the latter leading to ineffective erythropoiesis.[1]

The natural history of hemoglobin E/β-thalassemia has not been examined in large cohorts of patients and is poorly characterized. Most affected individuals live in emerging countries where the availability of safe blood transfusions and adequate iron-chelating therapy, standard therapy for patients with Cooley's anemia in developed countries, is limited. At the same time, examination of small cohorts suggests that many affected patients may not require regular red cell transfusions to sustain life. Nevertheless, It is likely that most would benefit from even a modest increase in their steady-state hemoglobin concentration, to reduce the complications of anemia and ineffective erythropoiesis, including osteoporosis, extramedullary hematopoiesis, and progressive tissue iron loading.

METHOD

We have retrospectively reviewed the cohort of patients with hemoglobin E/β thalassemia managed in Toronto's Hemoglobinopathy Program ($N = 22$). The patients' medical records were reviewed to determine the clinical features of each patient [including splenomegaly, bone disease, fractures, and iron loading (as estimated by serum ferritin concentration) in untransfused patients] and the associated laboratory parameters (including steady-state hemoglobin and reticulocyte concentrations, normoblast counts, peripheral blood fetal hemoglobin, and indirect bilirubin concentrations).

DISCUSSION

In a cohort of patients with Hemoglobin E/β-thalassemia managed in the Hemoglobinopathy Program at the University of Toronto (present $N = 22$), the important clinical features in 15 untransfused patients include advanced age at diagnosis relative to

---

[a]Address for correspondence: Nancy F. Olivieri, M.D., F.R.C.P.C., Haematology/Oncology, The Hospital for Sick Children, 555 University Avenue, Toronto, Ontario M5G IX8, Canada; Tel: 416-813-6823; Fax: 416-813-5346; E-mail: noliv@sickkids.on.ca

patients with Cooley's anemia (8.5 ± 10.3 [range 0–37] years); a low (30%) rate of transfusion dependency; and advanced age at first transfusion relative to patients with Cooley's anemia. Unfortunately, the indications used for initiation of regular transfusions in these patients are unclear. Variable, but usually modest, splenomegaly was noted in untransfused patients. The rate of splenectomy was low (17%). Although bone disease was not examined in all patients, three patients had signs of osteopenia, including a history of fractures, or osteopenia on plain X-ray.

The important laboratory features of the disease in 15 untransfused patients include moderate anemia (mean steady state Hb 8.1 ± 1.6 g/dL); modest ineffective erythropoiesis (mean normoblast count 4.5 ± 8.4 per 100 WBC); lower concentrations of peripheral blood fetal hemoglobin than in other cohorts;[6] evidence of mild iron loading in untransfused patients with mean serum ferritin concentrations up to 900 µg/L; and a high incidence of alpha-thalassemia. A multi-national trial of Hemoglobin E/β-thalassemia is needed to provide detailed and extensive information regarding this important genotype and to examine genotype/phenotype correlations.

REFERENCES

1. WEATHERALL, D. J. & J. B. CLEGG. 1981. The Thalassaemia Syndromes. Blackwell Scientific Press: 148–319.
2. FUCHAROEN, S. & P. WINICHAGOON. 1989. Hemoglobinopathies in Southeast Asia. Hemoglobin **11:** 65.
3. FUCHAROEN, S., P. WINICHAGOON, P. POOTRAKUL & P. WASI. 1984. Determination for different severity of anemia in thalassemia: concordance and discordance among sib pairs. Am. J. Med. Genet. **19:** 39.
4. WASI, P., P. POOTRAKUL, S. FUCHAROEN, P. WINICHAGOON, P. WILAIRAT & A. PROMBOON. 1985. Thalassemia in Southeast Asia: Determinants of different degrees of severity of anemia in thalassemia. Ann. N.Y. Acad. Sci. **445:** 119.
5. FUCHAROEN, S., P. WINICHAGOON, P. POOTRAKUL, A. PIANKIJAGUM & P. WASI. 1988. Variable severity of Southeast Asian β-thalassemia/Hb E disease. Birth Defects **23A:** 41.
6. REES, D. C., L. STYLES, E. P. VICHINSKY, J. B. CLEGG & D. J. WEATHERALL. 1998. The Hemoglobin E Syndromes. Ann. N.Y. Acad. Sci. **850:** 334–343. This volume.

α- and β-Thalassemia in Thailand

SUTHAT FUCHAROEN,[a] PRANEE WINICHAGOON,[b]
NOPPADOL SIRITANARATKUL,[b] JEW CHOWTHAWORN,[a]
AND PENSRI POOTRAKUL[a]

[a]*Thalassemia Research Center, Institute of Science and Technology for Research and Development;* [b]*Division of Hematology, Department of Medicine, Faculty of Medicine Siriraj Hospital, Mahidol University, Bangkok 10700, Thailand*

α-Thalassemia, β-thalassemia, and the hemoglobin (Hb) variants E and Constant Spring (CS) are common in Thailand. The frequency of α-thalassemia reaches 20–30% in Bangkok and Northern Thailand and that of β-thalassemia varies between 3 and 9 %. The frequency of Hb E is 13% on the average but its distribution is heterogeneous, attaining 50–60% at the junction with Laos and Cambodia, and that of Hb CS is 1–8%.[1,2] Approximately 5.6% of Thai married couples are at risk for giving birth to babies with severe hemoglobinopathies. These abnormal globin genes in different combinations lead to over 60 thalassemia syndromes. The two major α-thalassemic diseases are Hb Bart's hydrops fetalis (homozygous α-thalassemia 1) and Hb H disease (α-thalassemia 1/α-thalassemia 2 and α-thalassemia 1/Hb CS). Homozygous β-thalassemia and β-thalassemia/Hb E are major β-thalassemic syndromes in Thailand. Moreover, α- and β-thalassemia can occur in the same individual, leading to complicated gene-gene interactions such as EA Bart's and EF Bart's diseases.[3–7] In addition concomitant inheritance of Hb H with β-thalassemia can also cause Hb H disease with high Hb A_2.

Nowadays the molecular defects of these thalassemia genes have been characterized, but there is still a need to understand the consequences of multiple gene-gene interactions in order to obtain a better understanding of thalassemia syndromes in the region and elsewhere. In this paper, we review the phenotypes of thalassemia syndromes in Thailand, occurring from interaction between α- and β-thalassemia genes, including Hb E and Hb Constant Spring.

RESULTS

Different genotypes of EA Bart's and EF Bart's diseases and hematologic parameters of the two syndromes are shown in TABLES 1 and 2. A small number of red cells containing

TABLE 1. Different Genotypes of EA Bart's and EF Bart's Diseases

EA Bart's Disease	
1. α-Thal 1/Hb CS Hb E Heterozygote	2. α-Thal 1/α-Thal 2 Hb E Heterozygote
EF Bart's Disease	
1. α-Thal 1/Hb CS Homozygous Hb E	2. α-Thal 1/α-Thal 2 Homozygous Hb E
3. α-Thal 1/Hb CS $β^0$-Thal/Hb E	4. α-Thal 1/α-Thal 2 $β^0$-Thal/Hb E

TABLE 2. Hematologic Parameters of 108 EA Bart's and 44 EF Bart's Diseases (mean ± SD)

Hematologic Data	EA Bart's	EF Bart's
Hb (g/dl)	7.4 ± 1.23	7.6 ± 1.42
MCV (fl)	67 ± 5.1	61 ± 10.1
MCH (pg)	19.5 ± 2.72	17.5 ± 3.65
Hb Type	EABt's/CSEABt's	EFBt's/CSEFBt's
Hb E/CS (%)	14.9 ± 1.6	79.7 ± 8.71
Hb F (%)	2.6 ± 1.4	10.2 ± 6.73
Hb Bart's (%)	4.6 ± 1.9	3.6 ± 2.28

Abbreviations: CS = Hb Constant Spring, E = Hb E, Bt's = Hb Bart's.

inclusion bodies (1–5%) were also demonstrated in EA Bart's disease. There are no statistically significant differences in hematologic and clinical data between patients with and without Hb Constant Spring. Hematologic data of Hb H patients with high Hb A_2 are presented in TABLE 3. Although the β-thalassemia gene was co-inherited, detection of inclusion body and Hb H in the red cells indicated that there still were excess β-globin chains.

CONCLUSION

Hemoglobin types of E+A+Bart's and E+F+Bart's are the hallmark of EA Bart's and EF Bart's diseases. The presence of Hb Bart's indicated that there was excess γ-globin chain. This means that production of the α-globin chain was less than that of the non–α-globins, which include the β- and γ-globin chains. However, Hb H was not detected on electrophoresis and only a minute amount of excess β-globin was demonstrated as inclusion body in the red cells (1–5%) with EA Bart's disease.[5,6] In EF Bart's disease, in contrast to Hb H and EA Bart's diseases, no inclusion body was detected, probably because the abnormal $β^E$-globin chains may not polymerize to $β^E$ tetramer.

We have previously reported that percent red cells with inclusion bodies were 79 ± 18 and 67 ± 21, and amounts of Hb H were 12.1 ± 5.5 and 8.3 ± 4.7% in α-thalassemia 1/Hb CS and α-thalassemia 1/α-thalassemia 2, respectively. In this report, we showed that red cells containing inclusion bodies and amounts of Hb H were decreased in concomitant inheritance of β-thalassemia with Hb H disease (TABLE 3).

We have not seen hemolytic crisis in EA Bart's and EF Bart's diseases. Also Hb H patients with co-inheritance of β-thalassemia appear to have less hemolysis during stress

TABLE 3. Hematologic Parameters of 19 Hb H Patients with Co-inherited β-Thalassemia[a]

Hematologic Data	α-Thal 1/Hb CS β-Thal Trait	α-Thal 1/α-Thal 2 β-Thal Trait
Hb (g/dl):		
-Basal	8.5 ± 1.11	9.1 ± 2.94
-During Fever	6.9 ± 0.88	6.5 ± 2.49
MCV (fl)	78 ± 8.9	72 ± 10.7
MCH (pg)	23 ± 3.52	21 ± 3.45
Hb Type	$CSA_2ABt'sH$	$A_2ABt'sH$
Hb A_2/CS (%)	5.6 ± 1.35	5.2 ± 1.62
Inclusion Body (%)	70 ± 24.10	60 ± 23.66
Hb Bart's + H (%)	11 ± 4.39	7.1 ± 3.53

[a]α-Globin genotypes in 12 cases are α-thalassemia 1/Hb CS and 7 cases are α-thalassemia 1/α-thalassemia 2.

due to reduced excess β-globin chains, which can precipitate in the red cells. Thus, it is very important to understand these multiple gene-gene interactions in order to provide proper counseling to the affected families.

REFERENCES

1. WASI, P., S. NA-NAKORN, S. POOTRAKUL et al. 1969. Alpha- and beta-thalassemia in Thailand. Ann. N.Y. Acad. Sci. USA **165**: 60–82.
2. FUCHAROEN, S. & P. WINICHAGOON. 1987. Hemoglobinopathies in Southeast Asia. Hemoglobin **11**: 65–88.
3. FUCHAROEN, S. & P. WINICHAGOON. 1997. Hemoglobinopathies in Southeast Asia: Molecular biology and clinical medicine. Hemoglobin 21: 299–319.
4. FUCHAROEN, S., P. WINICHAGOON & V. THONGLAIRUAM. 1988. β-Thalassemia associated with α-thalassemia in Thailand. Hemoglobin **12**: 581–592.
5. FUCHAROEN, S., P. WINICHAGOON, P. POOTRAKUL et al. 1988. Differences between two types of Hb H disease, α-thalassemia1/α-thalassemia 2 and α-thalassemia 1/Hb Constant Spring. Southeast Asian J. Trop. Med. Public Health 23 (No. 5A): 309–315.
6. FUCHAROEN, S., P. WINICHAGOON, P. PRAYOONWIWAT et al. 1988. Clinical and hematologic manifestations of AE Bart's disease. Southeast Asian J. Trop. Med. Public Health 23 (No. 5A): 327–332.
7. FUCHAROEN, S., P. WINICHAGOON, V. THONGLAIRUAM & P. WASI. 1988. EF Bart's disease: Interaction of the abnormal α- and β-globin genes. Eur. J. Haematol. **40**: 75–78.

Homozygous Hemoglobin Constant Spring with Normal Electrophoresis

A Possible Cause for Under-Diagnosis

LAKSHMANAN KRISHNAMURTI[a] AND JANE A. LITTLE

Divisions of Pediatric Hematology/Oncology and Medical Oncology, University of Minnesota Medical School, Minneapolis, Minnesota 55455, USA

Hemoglobin Constant Spring (Hb CS) is an abnormal hemoglobin characterized by elongated α-globin chains resulting from a mutation of the termination codon in the α-2 globin gene. It is the most prevalent non-deletional α thalassemia in Southeast Asian populations.[1–5] While heterozygous Hb CS is difficult to detect on electrophoresis, the homozygous state is associated with Hb CS levels of 5–8% and Hb Bart's 1–2%.[3,6,7] Here, we describe a patient with homozygous Hb CS but no Hb CS or Hb Bart's detectable on isoelectric focusing. We discuss strategies for improving the diagnosis of this condition.

METHODS

Subject

P. B, a 24-year-old Laotian female was first noted to have severe anemia when she was diagnosed with membranoproliferative glomerulonephritis 14 years earlier. She developed chronic renal failure and received a cadaveric renal transplant three years earlier. P.B. was referred for evaluation of persistent anemia, reticulocytosis, and hyperbilirubinemia, despite a fully functional transplanted kidney. She was on standard immunosuppression (Imuran, CyclosporineA, Prednisone). Her mother had died in Laos from an episode of "hemolysis" following the ingestion of mirror backing. Hematologic studies on blood and bone marrow were performed by standard procedures. Hemoglobin analysis was performed by isoelectric focusing (IEF). Gene mapping for the α-globin genotypes was carried out by Southern blotting using *Bam*H I, *Bgl*II and *Eco*RI digestions of genomic DNA followed by hybridization with ζ- and α- globin gene–specific radioactive probes.[8] Molecular screening for Hb CS was done by selective amplification of α2 globin gene and hybridization to allele-specific oligonucleotides in the reverse dot blot format.[9]

RESULTS

Hematologic parameters at the time of referral are summarized in TABLE 1. The peripheral blood film showed polychromasia, anisopoikilocytosis, marked basophilic stippling, schistocytosis, and nucleated red blood cells (FIG. 1). The serum bilirubin level was 1.7 mg/dL.

[a]Address for correspondence: Dr. L. Krishnamurti, M.D., Box 484, UMHC, 420 Delaware St. S. E., Minneapolis, Minnesota 55455. E-mail, kris0026@maroon.tc.umn.edu

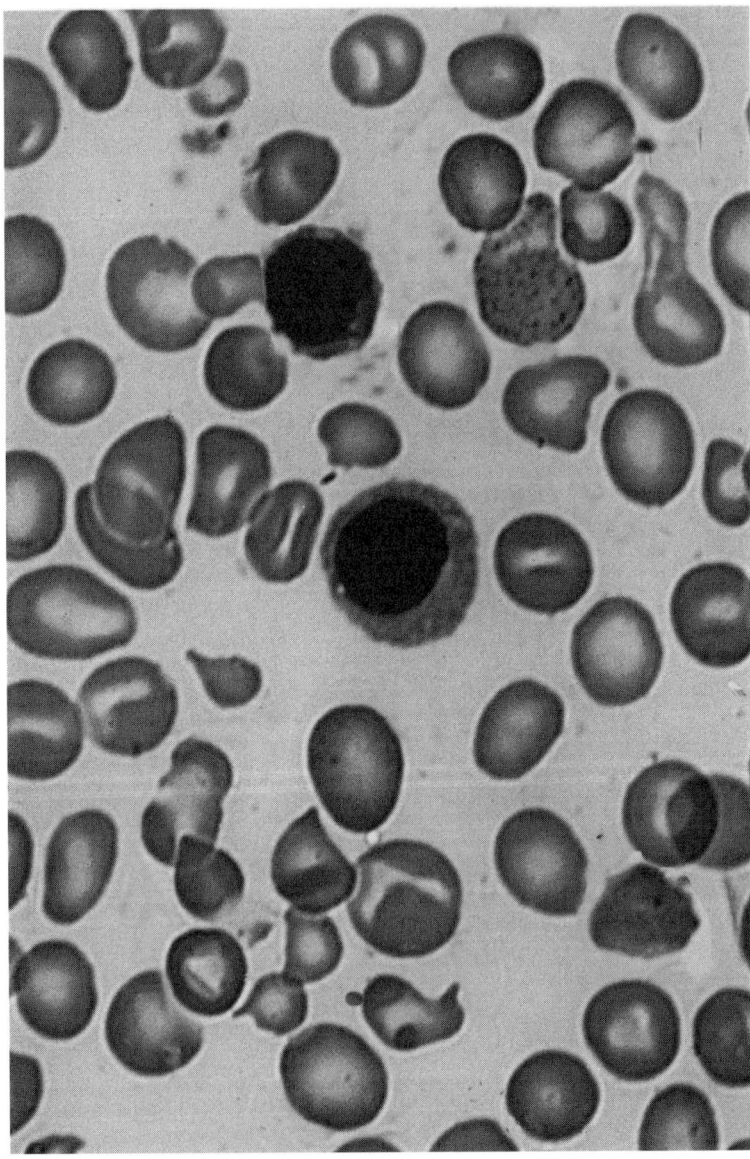

FIGURE 1. Composite photomicrograph of peripheral blood smear showing hypochromia, anisocytosis, poikilocytosis, schistocytosis, striking basophilic stippling, polychromasia, and nucleated red blood cells.

Serum ferritin levels, which were normal before kidney transplant, peaked at 2,080 four years after transplantation, but gradually decreased to 693 following discontinuance of Imuran. MRI of the liver was suggestive for iron overload. Glucose-6-phosphate dehydro-

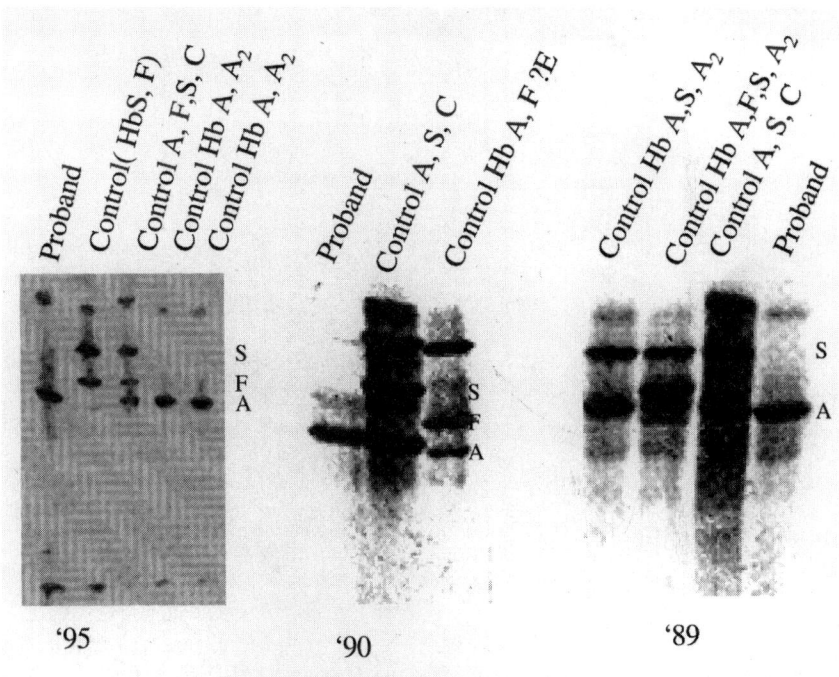

FIGURE 2. Sequential Hb isoelectric-focusing revealing HbA$_2$ 1.8–2.9%.

genase and pyruvate kinase levels were normal. Acid hemolysis test, Coomb's test, isopropanol test and Heinz body preparation were negative. Initial hemoglobin isoelectric focusing (IEF) 11 years earlier had shown a hemoglobin A$_2$ (HbA$_2$) level of 7.2%. Multiple IEF gels since were normal, with Hb A of 97–98% and HbA$_2$ of 1.8–2.9% (FIG.2). Gene mapping by Southern blot showed no gross deletions in the a globin locus. Molecular screening indicated homozygous Hb CS (FIG. 3).

DISCUSSION

Homozygous Hb CS is characterized by an overt hemolytic anemia and Hb CS levels of 6–8% as compared with asymptomatic heterozygous Hb CS, in which Hb CS levels are less than 1%.[6–8,10] We describe a patient who, in our experience, is unique for having homozygous Hb CS without detectable Hb CS on IEF and in whom the diagnosis was not possible without PCR-based molecular techniques. The carrier frequency of Hb CS is 5% in Northeast Thailand and Laos.[1–5] The prevalence of homozygosity as predicted by the Hardy-Weinberg law should be 0.062% (1 in 1,600). Hemoglobin H disease has been reported to occur with a frequency of 0.66% (1 in 150) in Southeast Asia.[1,2,5] There is a paucity of data on the prevalence of homozygous Hb CS, but it is probably detected less often than predicted, *i.e.* as 10% of those with a Hb H phenotype. The diagnosis of

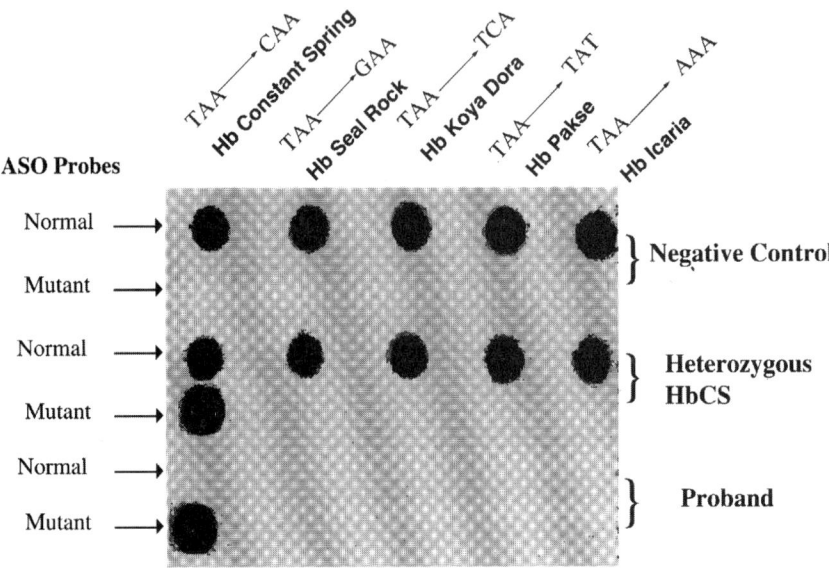

FIGURE 3. Reverse dot blot assay of labeled allele-specific probes for α_2 chain termination mutants hybridized to PCR amplified 3' end α_2 globin genes. Confirms diagnosis of homozygous HbCS.

homozygous Hb CS may not be suspected in cases with relatively mild anemia, especially because of low red cell number and an absence of microcytosis. It is possible that the variability of detection of Hb CS on electrophoresis may contribute to the under-diagnosis of its homozygous state. Hb CS may also be missed on family or population screening because of the absence of microcytosis and the low RBC number.[11] It is possible that in our case, concurrent medical problems confounded the clinical presentation. We recommend maintaining a high index of suspicion for Hb CS while evaluating anemia in a patient with findings such as mild microcytosis, nucleated erythrocytes and marked basophilic stippling on peripheral blood smear, Hb A_2 levels below 2%, or persistent HbBart's. The diagnosis can be firmly established by PCR-based molecular screening.

TABLE 1. Hematological Data on the Patient

	P. B.	Normal
Hbg/dL	9.3	11.7–15.7
RBC($\times 10^{12}$/L)	3.66	3.80–5.20
MCV(fL)	83	81–100
MCH(pg)	25.5	27–34
MCHC(%)	30.7	32–36
RDW(%)	16.5	10–15
Reticulocyte count(%)	12	
Platelet count($\times 10^9$/L	247	150–440

ACKNOWLEDGMENTS

The authors would like to acknowledge the contributions of Farid Chelab and Shi Ping-Cai in the performance of the molecular screening for the Hb CS as shown in FIGURE 3.

REFERENCES

1. FUCHAROEN, S. *et al.* 1987. Hemoglobinopathies in Southeast Asia. Hemoglobin. **11:** 65.
2. LAIG, M. *et al.* 1990. The distribution of Hb Constant Spring gene in Southeast Asian populations. Hum. Genet. **84:** 188.
3. THONGLAIROAM, V. *et al.* 1991. Hemoglobin Constant Spring in Bangkok: Molecular Screening by selective enzymatic amplification of the α_{-2} globin gene: Am. J. Hematol. **38:** 277–280.
4. CHANG, J. G. *et al.* 1994. Rapid molecular characterization of HbH diseases in Chinese by PCR reaction. Ann. Hematol. **68**(1): 33–37.
5. WONGCHANCHAILERT, M. *et al.* 1992. Hemoglobin H disease in children. J. Med. Assoc. Thailand. **75**(11): 611–618.
6. POOTRAKUL, P. *et al.* 1981. Homozygous Hemoglobin Constant Spring: A Need for Revision of Concept. Hum. Genet. **59:** 250–255.
7. DERRY, S. *et al.* 1984. Hematologic and biosynthetic studies in homozygous hemoglobin Constant Spring. J. Clin. Invest. **73:** 1673.
8. WEATHERALL, D. J. *et al.* 1981. The Thalassemia syndromes. 3rd edit. Blackwell Scientific Publications. Oxford.
9. KROPP, G. L. *et al.* 1989. Selective enzymatic amplification of α_2- globin gene DNA for detection of the hemoglobin Constant Spring mutation. Blood **73:** 1987.
10. LIE-INJO, L. E. *et al.* 1974. Homozygous state for Hb Constant Spring (slow moving X components). Blood **43:** 251–259.
11. LAU, Y. L. *et al.* 1997. Prevalence and genotypes of α and β-Thalassemia carriers in Hong Kong—Implications for population screening. N. Engl. J. Med. **336**(18): 1298–1300.

Audit of Prenatal Diagnosis for Hemoglobin Disorders in the United Kingdom

The First Twenty Years

B. MODELL,[a] M. PETROU,[a] M. LAYTON,[b] L. VARNAVIDES,[b]
C. MOISELY,[a] R.H.T. WARD,[a] C. RODECK,[a] K. NICOLAIDES,[c]
A. FITCHES,[d] AND J. OLD[d]

[a]*Department of Obstetrics and Gynaecology, UCL Medical School,
London WC1E 6HX, United Kingdom*
[b]*Department of Haematological Medicine and* [c]*Department of Obstetrics
and Gynaecology, King's College Hospital, London SE5 9RS,
United Kingdom*
[d]*Institute of Molecular Medicine, John Radcliffe Hospital,
Oxford OX3 9DS, United Kingdom*

Prenatal diagnosis of hemoglobin disorders was first introduced in the United Kingdom in 1974 by the method of fetal blood sampling and globin biosynthesis at 18–23 weeks of pregnancy.[1] First trimester diagnosis by chorionic villus sampling (CVS) was introduced in 1982, using Southern blot analysis to analyze fetal DNA for couples at risk for α^0-thalassemia or sickle cell disease by direct detection of mutations, and for the majority couples at risk for β-thalassemia by linkage analysis of restriction fragment length polymorphisms.[2] Since 1990, first-trimester diagnosis–based methods have been possible for all at-risk couples using polymerase chain reaction (PCR)–based methods.[3] Data from every prenatal diagnosis carried out at the three diagnostic centers from 1974 to 1994 have been entered into a database to initiate a national audit of the services provided for prenatal diagnosis for the hemoglobin disorders. Analysis of these data has enabled us to describe the evolution of the service in relation to time, risk, regional health authority (RHA), diagnostic method, and ethnic group. We have also been able to examine the utilization of prenatal diagnosis by risk, ethnic group, and RHA; the proportion of referrals in the first trimester, and the proportion of referrals before the birth of any affected child.

The number of prenatal diagnoses performed from 1974 to December 1994 was 2,068, including 33 sets of twins for which each fetus was counted separately: 1,218 for β-thalassemia, 789 for sickle cell disorders, and 61 for α-thalassemia. Of these, 531 (25.7%) fetuses were diagnosed as affected. The annual number of prenatal diagnoses for β-thalassemia increased rapidly from 1974, settling out around 80 per year from 1984 onward. Of the 1,218 such diagnoses, 97.5% were for homozygous β-thalassemia, 1.3% for HbE/β-thalassemia, and 1.2% for Hb Lepore/β-thalassemia. Prenatal diagnosis for sickle cell disorders started almost 10 years later

[e]*Address for correspondence: Dr. J. M. Old, Institute of Molecular Medicine, John Radcliffe Hospital, Oxford OX3 9DS, United Kingdom. Tel: 44 1865 222449; Fax: 44 1865 222500; E-mail: Jold@hammer.imm.ox.ac.uk*

TABLE 1. Utilization of Prenatal Diagnosis for Sickle Cell Disease (SCD) and β-Thalassemia for the Five-Year Periods 1985–1989 and 1990–1994

	β-Thalassemia						SCD	All
	Cyp	Ind	Pak	Ban	Oth	Total	Total	
1985–1989								
Estimated at-risk pregnancies	295	142	261	84	71	855	3163	4018
Prenatal diagnoses	296	59	78	7	62	475	229	704
Utilization (%)	100	41	30	8	88	56	7	18
1990–1994								
Estimated at-risk pregnancies	222	142	261	84	71	780	3565	4355
Prenatal diagnoses	192	92	69	8	64	425	457	882
Utilization (%) 87	65	26	9	91	54	13	20	

Abbreviations: Cypriots, Cyp; Indians, Ind; Pakistanis, Pak; Bangladeshi, Ban; Other, (Chinese, Italian, Middle Eastern), oth.

than for thalassemias and overtook them numerically around 1992 reaching a figure of 132 for the final year. Of the 789 such diagnoses, 87% were for HbSS disease, 9% for HbSC disease, 4% for HbS/β-thalassemia, and one couple for HbSD disease.

Since 1990 a total of 27 different β-thalassemia mutations have been diagnosed by PCR-based techniques, all but two being detected by the amplification refractory mutation system.[4] The two exceptions, the 10.3 kb and 619 bp deletion mutations, were diagnosed by gap PCR using primers spanning the deletion breakpoints. This technique is also used for the diagnosis of α^o-thalassemia, but all such prenatal diagnoses are confirmed by Southern blot analysis[4] because of having experienced a case of allele-drop out on one occasion when amplifying the normal allele in a prenatal diagnosis for the Mediterranean deletion gene. For the diagnosis of β-thalassemia and sickle cell disorders, PCR-based methods have proved the most reliable of the three diagnostic approaches. There were 16 errors (1.7%) by globin chain synthesis, 6 (1.0%) by Southern blotting, and 2 (0.2%) by PCR-based methods.

TABLE 2. Utilization of Prenatal Diagnosis for β-Thalassemia And Sickle Cell Disease (SCD) by Region (1983–1992)

Region[c]	β-Thalassemia						SCD
	Prevalence[a]	Cyp[b]	Ind	Pak	Oth	Total	Total
NE Thames	4.1	90	62	60	21	75	20
NW Thames	2.8	89	50	69	73	68	12
S Thames	2.2	77	73	67	67	73	18
Total:							
SE England		88	58	65	51	73	16
West Midlands	1.1	—	17	0	0	8	2
Yorkshire	0.7	—	50	36	—	37	10
North Western	0.8	—	0	11	20	18	4
Others	0.3	60	21	18	38	27	1
Total:							
Rest of UK		75	23	18	21	22	5

[a]Prevalence of at-risk pregnancies for all hemoglobin disorders per 1,000 births.
[b]Utilization (%) for Cypriots (Cyp), Indians (Ind), Pakistanis (Pak), Other ethnic groups (Oth).
[c]Regional Health Authorities as in 1991: NE Thames = the former northeast Thames region; NW Thames = the former northwest Thames region; S Thames = the former southeast Thames plus south west Thames regions. Others includes East Anglia, Mersey, Northern, South Western, Wessex, Trent, and Oxford RHAs, Scotland and Wales.

The utilization of prenatal diagnosis is the number of prenatal diagnoses performed divided by the total number of at-risk pregnancies, the latter being calculated from the 1991 census ethnicity data for infants 0–4 years old at that time. TABLE 1 shows the utilization of prenatal diagnosis in the two most recent five-year periods by genetic disorder and ethnic group. The national utilization of prenatal diagnosis for all hemoglobin disorders from 1990 to 1994 was around 20%. For sickle cell disorders it has risen from 7% to 13% over the past 10 years in contrast to β-thalassemia, for which the utilization over the last 10 years has remained constant at about 50%. As expected, there are wide differences in utilization between ethnic groups due to religious and social reservations. It ranged from 90% among Cypriots and "others" (Italians, Chinese, Middle Eastern) to 26% among Pakistanis, and to 9% among Bangladeshis. Utilization by Indians has risen from 41% to 65%. The low service utilization reflects the difficulties in integrating genetic screening and counselling into the medical service in the United Kingdom in which the predominate population is not at risk.

TABLE 2 shows the utilization of prenatal diagnosis in individual Regional Health Authorities in the United Kingdom. Utilization was highest in the three RHAs in the southeast of England where the prevalence is highest. Utilization was lower in the rest of the country where wide regional differences were observed. For example, in Yorkshire region the utilization for thalassemias and sickle cell disorders was much higher than in the west Midlands where the prevalence is almost twice as high. Regional variation was also observed within ethnic groups. For British Pakistanis, the utilization was 65% in London and the southeast compared to 18% elsewhere. Overall, the data reveal the service is delivered much less effectively in low- than in high-prevalence areas. The regional variation and differences within ethnic groups point to a lack of local screening policies and limited counselling resources, such as the provision for British Pakistanis to be counselled by a woman who speaks their own language.

The data for the northeast Thames region over the last ten years revealed that only 60% of the prenatal diagnoses were done prospectively, i.e. before the birth of any affected child, (40% for α-thalassemia, 70% for β-thalassemia, and 60% for sickle cell disorders). Less than 50% of these prospectively detected couples were referred in time for a first-trimester diagnosis. However after having one prenatal diagnosis couples are able to contact the service directly and over 90% referred themselves in time for a first-trimester diagnosis of subsequent pregnancies. The results show that despite couples' strong preference for early prenatal diagnosis, antenatal screening as presently organized usually identifies the risk in the second trimester.

REFERENCES

1. ALTER, B. P., B. MODELL, D. V. I. FAIRWEATHER *et al.* 1976. Prenatal diagnosis of hemoglobinopathies: a review of 15 cases. N. Engl. J. Med. **295:** 1437.
2. OLD, J. M., R. H. T. WARD, M. PETROU *et al.* 1982. First-trimester fetal diagnosis for the hemoglobinopathies: three cases. Lancet ***ii:*** 1413–1416.
3. OLD, J. M., N. Y. VARAWALLA & D. J. WEATHERALL. 1990. Rapid detection and prenatal diagnosis of beta thalassaemia: Studies in Indian and Cypriot populations in the UK. Lancet **336:** 834–837.
4. OLD, J. M. 1996. Hemoglobinopathies. Community clues to mutation detection. *In* Methods in Molecular Medicine: Molecular Diagnosis of Genetic Diseases. R. E. Elles, Ed.: 160–183. Humana Press Inc. Totowa, NJ.

Spectrum of β-Thalassemia Mutations in Guadeloupe (French West Indies) and Interactions with Other Hemoglobinopathies

M. ROMANA,[a] L. KÉCLARD, A. FROGER, C. BERCHEL, AND G. MÉRAULT

Unité de Recherche sur la Drépanocytose, INSERM U 359 and Centre Intégré de la Drépanocytose de la Guadeloupe, Pointe-à-Pitre, Guadeloupe

In Guadeloupe, a French Caribbean island with a population of 413,000, β-thalassemia (β-thal) gene frequency is estimated to be only 0.5% but becomes clinically relevant given the relatively high frequency (4.4%) of the $β^s$ gene in this population. If the most common condition observed among our patients is sickle cell anemia ($β^sβ^s$), the occurrence of Hb S-β-thal is also significant. The clinical and hematological features of the Hb S-β-thal disease are quite variable, ranging from almost asymptomatic to severe conditions.[1] This heterogeneity is likely due to the presence of β-thal alleles of different severity. Here, we report the spectrum of β-thal mutations observed in Guadeloupe and we evaluate the effect of both the nature of β-thal mutation and the associated deletional α-thalassemia on the clinical and hematological phenotype of a large number of patients with Hb S-β-thal disease.

Since the beginning of the carrier screening program in 1990, we have studied a total of 93 unrelated β-thal carrier families, which include 182 subjects with a variety of thalassemic combinations (95 β-thal carriers, 77 Hb S-β-thal, 7 Hb C-β-thal, 2 homozygous β-thal, 1 Hb S-Hb E, 1 Hb S-Hb Lepore, 1 Hb Hope-β-thal, and 1 HPFH- β-thal). The diagnosis was based on clinical, hematological and DNA studies.[2] Informed consent was obtained from all individuals.

Twelve different β-thal mutations have been identified, four of them accounting for almost 80% of the β-thal mutation in this population: - 29 A → G (47.3%), IVS-1-5 G → A (10.7%), TVS-II-1 G → A (10.7%), and IVS-I-5 G → C (9.8%). The eight other alleles observed were: Poly A T → C (4.3%), IVS-I-2 T → C (4.3%), - 88 C → T (3.2%), CD24 T → A (3.2%), IVS-II-849 A → G (3.2%), IVS-I-110 G → A (1.1%), Hb Lepore (1.1%), and Hb E (1.1%). The Guadeloupean population is the result of recent admixture between different ethnic groups in which all these different β-thal alleles had previously been described. Under slave trade, about 300,000 blacks were brought to Guadeloupe of which West Africans comprise the largest segment of this population. After its abolition, approximately 40,000 Asian Indians were brought to fill the island's need for inexpensive labor. The smallest group is composed of Caucasians from metropolitan France and the Eastern

---

[a]Address for correspondence: M. Romana, Unité de Recherche sur la Drépanocytose, INSERM U 359, Centre Hospitalier Universitaire, B.P. 465, 97159 Pointe-à-Pitre, Cedex, French West Indies. Tel: 33 1 0590 83 48 99; Fax: 33 1 0590 83 05 13; E-mail: insmol@outremer.com

TABLE 1. Hematological Features of Different Types of Sickle Cell β-Thalassemia in Guadeloupe

	Hb S-β⁺-thal Type III	Hb S-β⁺-thal Type I	Hb S-β⁰-thal
N	40	6	17
Age (years)	19 ± 15.6	11 ± 8.2	24 ± 11.8
Hb (g/dl)	11.2 ± 1.7	8.7 ± 1.01	8.8 ± 1.3
MCV (fl)	74.1 ± 4.7	66.3 ± 4.8	73.1 ± 4.5
MCH (pg)	23.3 ± 2.5	20.4 ± 1.5	23.6 ± 2.1
MCHC (g/dl)	31.4 ± 2.8	30.7 ± 1.3	32.3 ± 2.4
HbA2 (%)	4.5 ± 0.8	4.6 ± 0.7	4.2 ± 0.8
Hb F (%)	10.7 ± 6.2	9.3 ± 7.6	12.5 ± 9
Hb S (%)	65.2 ± 6.6	72 ± 15.6	79.1 ± 8.1
Hb A(%)	19.6 ± 5	6.9 ± 3.9	0

Mediterranean countries (Syria and Lebanon). The linkage of the IVS-I-5 G → C and TVS-II-1 G → A alleles each to one specific haplotype strongly suggests an Asian Indian origin for the former,[3] a West African for the latter.[4] The origin of the IVS-I-5 G → A allele studied here is, however, uncertain. The haplotype/mutation for the substitution IVS-I-5 G → A detected in this study has also been described in Mediterranean populations.[5] However the sporadic presence of this β-thal mutation has been described in both Jamaican and Mediterranean populations.[1-6] The mild β-thal mutation, - 29 A->G, common among blacks, was found in association with eight different β-globin gene cluster haplotypes. All the thalassemic chromosomes studied so far had the same β-globin gene framework (FWI) and 3' RFLP haplotype. These data together suggest a probable West African origin of the - 29 A → G mutation sufficiently ancient to have recombined with a variety of 5' RFLP haplotypes.

Hematological findings of the patients with Hb S-β-thal disease, all aged more than 3 years, were evaluated according to the level of Hb A in the peripheral blood: 17 patients with Hb S-β⁰-thal [IVS-II-1 G → A 9; IVS-I-2 T → A 4; IVS-II-849 A → G 4], 6 patients with Hb S- β⁺-thal type I (3–5% Hb A) [IVS-I-5 G → C 3; IVS-I-5 G → A 3], and 40 patients with Hb S-β⁺-thal type III (18–25% Hb A) [- 29 A → G 31; - 88 C → T 3; CD24 T → A 3, Poly A T → C 3]. As shown in TABLE 1, patients with Hb S-β⁺-thal type III with Hb A levels of 19.6 ± 5 % had milder anemia ($p < 10^{-3}$), hypochromia ($p < 5 \cdot 10^{-2}$) as well as less marked microcytosis ($p < 10^{-3}$) as compared to the Hb S-β⁺-thal type I. The Hb level was the only hematological feature that was statistically different between with Hb S-β⁺-

TABLE 2. Incidence of α-Thalassemia on the Hematological Expression of Sickle Cell β-Thalassemia Disease

	Hb S-β⁺-thal Type III 4 α	Hb S-β⁺-thal Type III 3 α	Hb S-β⁰-thal 4 α	Hb S-β⁰-thal 3 α
N	20	11	6	6
Age (years)	24 ± 15.7	11 ± 8.6	19 ± 10	25 ± 14
Hb (g/dl)	11.1 ± 1.9	11.3 ± 1.6	9.1 ± 0.9	8.2 ± 0.9
MCV(fl)	74 ± 5	76.1 ± 34	73.8 ± 4.1	73 ± 3.6
MCH (pa)	23.2 ± 3	23.9 ± 1.6	22.8 ± 1.45	24.3 ± 2.5
MCHC (g/dl)	31.4 ± 3.5	31.5 ± 1.9	30.8 ± 0.7	33.2 ± 3.1
Hb A2 (%)	4.6 ± 0.7	4.4 ± 0.9	3.8 ± 0.5	4.7 ± 0.9
Hb F(%)	10.4 ± 5.7	11 ± 5.7	18.2 ± 7.7	4.2 ± 1.8
Hb S (%)	66.1 ± 6.1	64 ± 7.2	73.8 ± 7.2	86.2 ± 2.8
Hb A (%)	19.4 ± 4.5	20.4 ± 4.7	0	0

thal type III and Hb S-β^0-thal. Although the anemia in patients with Hb S-β^+-thal type I and Hb S-β^0-thal was similar, interestingly microcytosis and hypochromia ($p < 10^{-2}$) were more pronounced in patients of the first group albeit with a lower mean age. The Hb F levels were quite variable in the three groups, ranging from 1 to 24.5% for Hb S-β^+-thal type III, 1 to 25% for Hb S-β^+-thal type I and 3 to 32% for Hb S-β^0-thal. This wide variation in the range of Hb F level could not be related to the C $\rightarrow$ T substitution at position -158 of the $^G\gamma$-globin gene since the *Xmn*I polymorphic site was absent in most of the β^s (data not shown) and β-thal chromosomes. Since parental Hb F values were not available in some instances, no definite conclusion could be drawn concerning the coinheritance of a Swiss type heterocellular HPFH.

α-Globin gene status was known for 31 patients with Hb S-β^+-thal type III and 12 patients with Hb S-β^0-thal. There was no difference in the hematological data in Hb S-β^+-thal type III patients with α-thalassemia (3α-globin genes) when compared to those with 4α-globin genes (TABLE 2). Moreover, patients with Hb S-β^0 + α-thalassemia are virtually identical to those with Hb S-β^0-thal except for their lower Hb F level as previously observed.[7]

In summary, we have delineated the spectrum of β-thalassemia alleles in the Guadeloupean population and presented evidences that the type of mutation dictates the differences in the hematological expression in Hb S-β-thal patients and that coinheritance of a$^+$-thalassemia with a single gene deletion had a minimal impact on the phenotype.

REFERENCES

1. SERJEANT, G. R. 1992. Sickle Cell Disease. Oxford University Press. Oxford.
2. ROMANA, M. *et al.* 1996. Molecular characterization of β-thalassemia mutations in Guadeloupe. Am. J. Hematol. **53:** 228–233.
3. KAZAZIAN, H. H., Jr. *et al.* 1984. Molecular characterization of β-thalassemia mutations in Asian Indians. EMBO. J. **3:** 593–599.
4. VARAWALLA, N. Y. *et al.* 1992. Analysis of β-globin haplotypes in Asian Indians: Origin and spread of β-thalassemia on the Indian subcontinent. Hum. Genet. **90:** 443–449.
5. LAPOUMEROULIE, C. *et al.* 1986. β-thalassemia due to a novel mutation in IVS-I sequence donor site consensus sequence creating a restriction site. Biochem. Biophys. Res. Commun. **139:** 709–715.
6. CAO, A. *et al.* 1989. β-thalassemia mutations in Mediterranean populations. Br. J. Haematol. **71:** 309–312.
7. STEINBERG, M. H. *et al.* 1984. Interaction between Hb S-β^0-thalassemia and α-thalassemia. Am. J. Med. Sci. **288:** 195–199.

α-Globin Mutations and Rearrangements in Israel

PCR-Based Analysis Reveals Ethnic Diversity[a]

D. RUND,[b] V. ORON-KARNI, D. FILON, AND A. OPPENHEIM

Hematology Department, Hadassah University Hospital, Ein Kerem, Jersualem IL91120, Israel

In Israel, α-thalassemia does not represent a widespread clinical or public health problem, and there are no documented cases of hydrops fetalis due to homozygous α°-thalassemia. However, its investigation is important because of the profound effect of α-globin gene lesions on concurrent β-thalassemia. The earliest studies in Israel that analyzed the presence of Hb Bart's (γ^4) in cord blood of newborns revealed that α-thalassemia is prevalent in Jews of Yemenite, Iraqi and Kurdish origin.[1–3]

As the center for DNA-based thalassemia diagnosis in Israel, we perform hundreds of tests, including about 40 prenatal examinations, per year. It is not unusual to evaluate the risk of β-thalassemia carriership in individuals who have borderline hematological parameters, who may be double heterozygotes for α- and β-thalassemia. In such individuals, concurrent α-thalassemia can mask the hematologic manifestations and result in the silent carrier state,[4] potentially leading to erroneous genetic counselling. A rapid methodology to detect α-globin rearrangements would therefore enable more accurate identification of couples at risk for β-thalassemia.

On the other hand, the presence of excess α-globin genes in a β-thalassemia carrier leads, in some cases, to the more severe phenotype of thalassemia intermedia, which, in the presence of 6 α genes, can require transfusions.[5] We performed prenatal diagnosis in such a family by analyzing both α- and β-globin genes. The propositus had severe symptomatic anemia due to the presence of 6 α-globin genes, in combination with heterozygous β-thalassemia.[6] Individuals carrying triplication of the α-globin gene have completely normal hematological parameters. A rapid methodology to detect such individuals would be therefore of great importance to allow for identification of such couples at risk.

There have not been many studies of α-globin rearrangements and mutations in the Israeli population. In a Kurdish Jewish individual, a mutation in the polyadenylation signal was found,[7] also identified in Saudi Arabians. A large unique deletion was discovered in several Yemenite families ($- -^{\text{Yem}}$).[8] Other α-globin gene abnormalities reported in Israelis include two variants, Hb Hasharon ($\alpha^{47 \text{ Asp-His}}$)[9] and Hb Petah Tikva ($\alpha^{110 \text{ Ala-Asp}}$)[10] in Ashkenazi and Iraqi Jews, respectively.

We performed a concentrated molecular study, analyzing several hundred chromosomes suspected of carrying an α-globin mutation or rearrangement. In nearly two hundred chromosomes, an abnormality was found. These individuals were of many ethnic

---

[a] This research was supported by grants from the Israeli Ministry of Health, Chief Scientist's Office, and the Rochlin Foundation.

[b] Address for correspondence: Deborah Rund, Hematology Department, Hadassah University Hospital, Ein Kerem, Jerusalem IL91120, Israel. Tel: 972-2-677-8712; Fax: 972-2-642-3067; E-mail: rund@cc.huji.ac.il

TABLE 1. Types of α-Globin Gene Mutations or Rearrangements in Israeli Ethnic Groups

Type of Allele	Examples	Ethnic group(s)[a]
Deletions	-$α^{3.7}$,- -Med, -$α^{4.2}$,- **-Yem**	Jews, Arabs, Druze
Multiplicity	$ααα^{anti3.7}$; higher multiplicities	Arabs, Jews
Point mutations	pentanucleotide deletion IVS1	Jews, Arabs
	AATAAA-AATAAG	Arabs, Jews
	-9/+8 bp (exon 2)	Yemenite Jews
Chain substitution	Hasharon	Ashkenazi Jews
	Petah Tikva[b]	Iraqi Jews

Note: Boldface type indicates alleles identified in Israel only.
[a]Listed in descending order of number of alleles identified.
[b]Not found in our series.

origins (TABLE 1). Because of the extreme heterogeneity of the population, we anticipated heterogeneity of the molecular lesions, as was previously found for β-thalassemia.[11]

Our studies began with genomic blotting using *Bam*HI digestion with an α-globin–specific probe, and *Bgl*II digestion with a ζ-globin–specific probe. Next, we developed PCR methods to identify the various α-globin rearrangements, including deletions and triplication, found in our population. The details of these will be published elsewhere as they are still undergoing refinement (Oron-Karni *et al.*, in preparation).

A number of lesions were identified (TABLE 1) consisting of all types of mutations (deletions, multiplicities, missense and point mutations). Some were specific to a particular ethnic group, while others were found in all ethnic groups (TABLE 1). Boldface type indicates the abnormalities that have been reported only in the Israeli population. For completeness, we list Hb Petah Tikva, although we did not identify any individuals carrying this abnormality in our series.

Finally, alleles suspected of carrying a point mutation were selectively amplified (either the α2 or the α1 gene) and subjected to sequence analysis. In this way, we discovered a novel mutation. Sequencing of additional unknown alleles is ongoing.

The novel mutation is a deletion/duplication mutation (-9/+8 bp) in exon 2, identified in two heterozygotes of Yemenite Jewish extraction.[12] This is a complex mutation that results in a frameshift. We proposed a novel mechanism to account for its generation.[12] We suggested that the mutation arose by slipped strand mispairing, creating a single-stranded loop, followed by DNA elongation, strand breathing and the formation of a mismatch bubble. Our model explains the formation of similar deletion/insertion mutations, suggesting that rearrangement of a mismatch loop or bubble during DNA replication may not be uncommon.[12]

Our results indicate that PCR analysis can be a valuable tool in molecular evaluation of α-globin mutations. Furthermore, sequence analysis of unknown alleles can yield both novel and interesting results despite the vast body of knowledge already acquired on the thalassemias.

REFERENCES

1. HALBRECHT, I. & S. BEN PORAT. 1967. The incidence of Bart's hemoglobin in the cord blood of 3,218 newborns of different ethnic groups in Israel. Harefuah (in Hebrew). **73:** 223–224.
2. COHEN, T. 1971. Thalassemia types among Kurdish Jews. Isr. J. Med. Sci. **9:** 1461–1463.
3. ZAIZOV, R. & Y. MATOTH. 1972. α-thalassemia in Yemenite and Iraqi Jews. Isr. J. Med. Sci. **8:** 11–17.
4. RUND, D. *et al.* 1993. Silent carrier β-thalassemia due to a severe mutation in the β-globin gene. Eur. J. Ped. **152:** 574–576.
5. ORON, V. *et al.* 1994. Severe thalassemia intermedia caused by interaction of homozygosity for α-globin triplication with heterozygosity for $β^0$-thalassemia. Br. J. Haematol. **86:** 377–379.

6. ORON-KARNI, V. et al. 1996. Prenatal diagnosis based on simultaneous DNA analysis of α- and β-globin genes. Am. J. Hematol. **53**: 203–204.
7. THEIN, S. et al. 1988. The polyadenlyation site mutation in the α-globin cluster. Blood. **71**: 313–319.
8. SHALMON, L. et al. 1994. A new deletional α-thalassemia detected in Yemenites with Hemoglobin H Disease. Am. J. Hematol. **45**: 201–204.
9. HALBRECHT, I. et al. 1967. Hemoglobin Hasharon ($\alpha 47^{\text{aspartic acid-histidine}}$). Isr. J. Med. Sci. **3**: 827–831.
10. HONIG, G. et al. 1981. Hemoglobin Petah Tikva ($\alpha^{110\,\text{Ala-Asp}}$): a new unstable variant with α-thalassemia-like expression. Blood **57**: 705–711.
11. FILON, D. et al. 1994. Diversity of mutations in Israeli ethnic groups reflects recent historic events. Am. J. Hum. Genet. **54**: 836–843.
12. ORON-KARNI, V. et al. 1997. A novel mechanism generating short deletions/insertions is suggested by a mutation in the human α2-globin gene. Hum. Molec. Genet. **6**: 881–885.

Correlation of ζ-Globin ELISA with PCR for (--^{SEA}) Deletion and Clinical Diagnosis for 1α-Thal-1 Trait[a]

R. A. SIMKINS,[b,d] K-A THAN,[b] B. SCHAPIRO,[c] E. S. CHOI,[c] AND P. R. DAOUST[c]

[b]*Wallac, Inc., Akron, Ohio 44321-0350, USA*
[c]*New England Medical Center, Tufts University School of Medicine, Boston, Massachusetts 02111, USA*

The presence of small amounts (0.01–1%) of embryonic ζ-globin chains in individuals serves as a marker for carriers of a number of deletional α-thalassemias.[1–3] Assays that can detect ζ-globin should be especially useful in identifying those at risk for producing offspring with homozygous α-thalassemia. We have previously reported on the use of a fluorometric ELISA[4] to quantitate ζ-globin chains in dried blood spot samples from predominantly Southeast Asian α-thalassemia-1 carriers and normal controls. The results were compared to the clinical diagnosis made from red blood cell indices, enriched Hb H preparation, Hb electrophoresis, ferritin assay, and zinc protoporphyrin level.[5,6] Using the diagnosis as the standard, the fluorescent ELISA produced a specificity of 98.7% and a sensitivity of 82.7%. Because all potential α-thal-1 carriers do not carry the SEA double deletion, we wanted to use PCR to detect this deletion to compare the relative specificity and sensitivity of the antibody assay. The initial fluorescent ELISA was performed with antibody directly conjugated to horseradish peroxidase and produced a significant background. We wished to reduce the background and convert to a colorimetric ELISA that more people would be able to use.

MATERIALS AND METHODS

Samples were 300 consecutive blood specimens sent to the hospital's clinical laboratory for hemoglobin (Hb) electrophoresis from a population of which 62% were Southeast Asian (SEA). Nine additional specimens were examined for which demographic data were not known. The initial diagnosis and PCR were performed on whole blood samples. The ELISA was performed on whole blood spotted (75 µl) onto Schleicher & Schuell 903 filter paper. Of the original samples, 18 were not available for PCR analysis. The ELISA was performed at ambient temperature, by extracting a 1/8" punch (~ 3 µl) from the dried blood spots in 150 µl of 50 mM Tris-HCl buffer, pH 7.5 containing 0.15 M NaCl (TS). After 30 minutes at ambient temperature, the extract was diluted 1:5 in the same buffer and allowed to bind to a Costar mictotiter plate for 30 minutes. After three washes with TS containing 0.05% Tween 20, biotinylated antibody diluted in TS containing 1% BSA was added to each well

---

[a]This work was funded by National Institutes of Health grant no. 2 R44 HL-46038-03.
[d]Address for correspondence: R. A. Simkins, Ph. D., Senior Research Scientist, Wallac, Inc. Drawer 4350, Akron, Ohio 44321-0350. Tel: 330-825-4525 and Fax: 330-825-8520.

and allowed to react for 30 minutes. After three more washes an appropriate dilution of horseradish-conjugated streptavidin was added to each well, reacted for 15 minutes, and washed three times before substrate containing 50 mM ABTS reagent (2,2'-azino-bis(3-ethylbenz-thiazoline-6-sulfonic acid) diammonium salt plus 0.03% H_2O_2 in citrate buffer pH 4.2 was added to each well, allowed to develop 15 to 30 minutes, and the reaction stopped with 0.1% SDS. The plates were read at 405 nm in a plate reader.

For the polymerase chain reaction (PCR) three primers were used. P_1, complementary to the anti-sense strand of the α_2 globin gene, is upstream to the 5' breakpoint of the $--^{SEA}$ deletion. P_2 complementary to the sense strand of the α_2 gene, is downstream to the 5' breakpoint. P_3, complementary to the sense strand of the α_2 gene, is near the 3' hypervariable region downstream from the 3' breakpoint. With $P_1 + P_2$ a 287 bp product is produced in normal samples but no product is produced in samples with the SEA deletion. With $P_1 + P_3$ no product is produced in normal samples but a 194 bp product is produced in samples with the SEA deletion.

RESULTS

In comparing ELISA with clinical diagnosis, the zeta assay had a relative specificity of 100% and sensitivity of 82.6%. Of the 309 samples used in the previous comparison, 291 were subjected to PCR analysis. Comparing PCR with the diagnosis gave a specificity of 99.1% and a sensitivity of 80.9%. Comparing the ζ assay with PCR gave a specificity of 97.8% and a sensitivity of 95.3%. Of the samples, five were diagnosed positive and had detectable ζ chains. If we compare the ζ assay with those samples that were positive by *both* diagnosis and PCR the specificity of the ζ assay was 100% and the sensitivity was 98.1%

CONCLUSIONS

We used the PCR with the $--^{SEA}$ deletion as a method to evaluate the ELISA; however, it is known that there are other deletions in which ζ-globin chains may be elevated. This may be the case in the five samples where ζ-globin chains were detected by the ELISA and which were also diagnosed by red cell indices. The identification of these deletions was not addressed in this study.

The results, however, do show that the ζ ELISA is a simple, rapid technique for detecting potential $--^{SEA}$ α-thalassemia-1 carriers. The assay detected over 95% of the PCR-detected $--^{SEA}$ deletion. Samples can be collected by a simple fingerprick onto filter paper. This allows easy transportation and storage of samples. The sensitivity and specificity is more than adequate for a screening test. The assay may also be used non-quantitatively because positive samples can be identified easily by the naked eye after development with the ABTS substrate.

REFERENCES

1. CHUNG, S-W. *et al.* 1984. Human embryonic ζ-globin chains in adult patients with α-thalassemias. Proc. Natl. Acad. Sci. USA **81**: 6181–6191.
2. CHUI, D. H. K. *et al.* 1986. Embryonic ζ-globin chains in adults: A marker for 10α-thalassemia-1 haplotype due to a >17.5 kb deletion. N. Engl. J. Med. **314**: 76–79.
3. TANG, W. *et al.* 1992. Human embryonic ζ-globin chain expression in deletional 11α-thalassemias. Blood **80**: 517–522.
4. THAN, K. A., R. A. SIMKINS, E. S. CHOI & P. R. DAOUST. 1995. ζ-Globin chains detected in dried blood spots from Southeast Asian 12α-thalassemia-1 carriers by a fluorescent ELISA. Presented at the Proceedings of the Eleventh National Neonatal Screening Symposium. p. 306.

5. CHOI, E. & T. NECHELES. 1983. Thalassemia among Chinese-Bostonians. Arch. Intern. Med. **143**: 1713–1715.
6. CHOI, E. *et al.* 1994. Screening for alpha thalassemia. Presented at the Proceedings of the Tenth National Screening Symposium. ASTPHLD pp. 50–70.

The Diverse Molecular Basis and Mild Clinical Picture of HbH Disease in Israel

H. TAMARY,[a-c] G. KLINGER,[b] L. SHALMON,[c] H. KIRSCHMANN,[c] A. KOREN,[d] M. BENNET,[e] AND R. ZAIZOV[b,c]

[b]Department of Pediatric Hematology/Oncology, Schneider Children's Medical Center of Israel

[c]Pediatric Hematology Research Laboratory, Felsenstein Medical Research Center, Beilinson Campus, Petah Tiqva and Sackler Faculty of Medicine, Tel Aviv University, Tel Aviv

Departments of [d]Pediatrics and [e]Hematology, Afula Medical Center, Israel

The clinical picture of hemoglobin H (HbH) disease varies in different genotypes. Studies based on Hb Bart levels in cord blood have disclosed a high incidence of α-thalassemia in certain ethnic groups (Jews of Yemenite origin and Israeli Arabs).[1,2] Further analysis of the molecular basis of α-thalassemia in Israel revealed four unique defects: two unstable α-1-variant, Petah Tikva (α^{PT})[3] and Hb Taybe;[4] a large deletion found in Yemenite Jews (—^{YEM});[5] and a 16 bp deletion in the α-2 globin gene.[6] In the present work, we investigated the genotype-phenotype correlation in a group of Israeli patients with HbH disease.

PATIENTS AND METHODS

Seventeen unrelated patients with HbH disease and eight of their siblings were studied. Age at diagnosis ranged from one month to 42 years. The patients were of Jewish or Arab origin. Standard techniques were used for hematological and molecular workup of α-thalassemia.

RESULTS

Results are presented in TABLES 1 and 2. Forty-seven percent of the defects were the result of point mutations. Seven different genotypes were identified. All patients were asymptomatic, with mild to moderate anemia. The anemia was characterized by a significantly low mean corpuscular volume, low levels of HbA_2, high HbH, and considerably reduced α-/non-α-globin synthetic ratios. Only three patients required blood transfusions during the first year of life, and five women required blood transfusions during pregnancy. Mean serum ferritin level was low.

---

[a]Address for Correspondence: Dr. H. Tamary, Pediatric Hematology/Oncology, Schneider Children's Medical Center of Israel, Beilinson Campus, Petah Tiqva 49202, Israel. Tel: 972-3-925 3669; Fax: 972-3-925 3042; e-mail: eytamary@netVision.net.il

TABLE 1. Types of α-Thalassemia Alleles in 17 Patients with HbH in Israel

α-Thalassemia alleles	No. of chromosomes	Frequency (% of total chromosomes)
α^{Tsaudi}	11	32.4
$-\alpha^{3.7}$	8	23.5
$—^{MED}$	6	17.6
$—^{YEM}$	4	11.8
α^{HphI}	2	5.9
α^{PT}	2	5.9
α^{Ta}	1	2.9
Total	34	100

[a]Uncharacterized point mutation

DISCUSSION

In all surveys of α-thalassemia to date, the disease was due to deletions much more frequently than to single point mutations. In our study, however, 47% of the defects causing HbH disease were attributable to point mutations. Larger surveys are required to confirm this observation. The high percentage of nondeletional mutations may explain the absence of hydrops fetalis in our area.

The genotypes found in HbH disease in Israel are more diverse than those described in other Mediterranean countries. In Sardinia, 83% of patients are $—^{MED}/-\alpha^{3.7}$,[7] and in Cyprus 60% have the same genotype and only 15% carry nondeletional defects.[8] On the basis of relatively small patient series from Egypt and Greece,[9,10] it has been suggested that the main cause of α-thalassemia is $-\alpha^{3.7}$. In our study, the genotype most frequent in the Mediterranean region ($—^{MED}/\alpha^{3.7}$) was found in only 23.5% of the patients with HbH disease, whereas 32% had unique genotypes ($—^{YEM}/-\alpha^{3.7}$, $—^{Med}/\alpha\alpha^{PT}$, $—^{YEM}/\alpha\alpha^{T}$).

In contrast to the heterogeneous molecular basis, the clinical picture was consistently mild. No iron overload was found, although significant hemochromatosis has been observed in Chinese patients with HbH disease.[11]

There appears to be a good correlation between the severity of HbH disease and genotype. Patients with the $-/-\alpha^{T}\alpha$ genotype tend to be more anemic than those with the deletional ($-/-\alpha$) forms of HbH disease. In our series, one patient had a combination of cluster deletion and point mutation, but as α-1 was involved ($-/-\alpha\alpha^{PT}$), the clinical picture was, again, mild.

Because of the mild clinical picture in our area, HbH disease does not pose a widespread clinical or public health problem. Consequently, there is no indication for prenatal diagnosis. A study of the molecular basis of this disorder could facilitate the detection of unusual β-thalassemia carriers.

TABLE 2. Clinical Manifestations of HbH Disease According to Genotype

Genotype	Origin	Patients[a] N	Hb (g/dl)	MCV (fl)	Ferritin (μg/l)	α/β	A2 (%)	Hemoglobin F (%)	H (%)
$α^{TSaudi}α/α^{TSaudi}α$	Iraqi Jew Arabs	7(5)	8.2 ± 1	68 ± 5	98 ± 74	0.3 ± 0.07	1.3 ± 0.3	3.6 ± 3.9	12.5 ± 11
$α^{HphI}α/α^{HphI}α$	Arabs	5(1)	9.4 ± 1.3	63 ± 4	121 ± 57		0.7 ± 0.2	4.3 ± 3.4	20.4 ± 11
—MED/-$α^{3.7}$	Georgian	4(3)	9.1 ± 1.1	61 ± 10	21	0.27 ± 0.07	1.5 ± 1.4	1.5 ± 1.2	9.3 ± 6.3
—YEM/-$α^{3.7}$	Iraqi Jew	4(4)	9.3 ± 0.8	60 ± 6	65 ± 55	0.49 ± 0.15	1.9 ± 0.5	1.1 ± 0.6	3.5 ± 2.9
—MED/$αα^{PT}$	Yemen Jew	2(2)	9.9	64	24	0.58	1.4	1.8	1
—YEM/-$α^{T\ b}$	Yemen Jew	2(1)	9.8	71	131	0.37	0.6	1.3	29
$α^{TSaudi}α/-α^{3.7}$	Iraqi Jew	1(1)	9.2	69	39	0.24	1.4	2	4.8
Total		25(17)	9	62	90	0.37	1.2	2.6	12.6
±SD			1.2	7	71	0.17	0.5	2.9	11.7
Normal values			12	81	385	1.06	2.5	<1	-
±SD			0.6	6	293	0.19	1		

[a] Number in parentheses denotes unrelated patients.
[b] Uncharacterized point mutation.

REFERENCES

1. HALBRECHT, I. & S. BEN PORAT. 1967. The incidence of Bart's hemoglobin in the cord blood of 3,218 newborns of different ethnic groups in Israel. Harefuah **73:** 233–235.
2. ZAIZOV, R. & Y. MATOTH. 1972. α-thalassemia in Yemenite and Iraqi Jews. Isr. J. Med. Sci. **8:** 11–17.
3. HONIG, G. et al. 1981. Hemoglobin Petah Tikva (α110 Ala→Asp): A new unstable variant with α-thalassemia like expression. Blood **57:** 705–711.
4. GALACTEROS, F. et al. 1994. Hb Taybe (α38 or α39 deleted): An α-globin defect, silent in the heterozygous state and producing severe hemolytic anemia in the homozygous. C. R. Acad. Sci. **317:** 437–444.
5. SHALMON, L. et al. 1994. A new deletional alpha thalassemia detected in Yemenites with hemoglobin H disease. Am. J. Hematol. **45:** 201–204.
6. TAMARY, H. et al. 1997. Alpha-thalassemia induced by a novel 16bp deletion in the 3' untranslated region of the α2 including the first base of the poly A signal. Hemoglobin **21:** 121–130.
7. GALANELLO, R. et al. 1992. HbH disease in Sardinia: Molecular, hematological and clinical aspects. Acta Haematol. **88:** 1–6.
8. BAYSL, E. et al. 1995. Alpha-thalassemia in the population of Cyprus. Br. J. Haematol. **89:** 469–499.
9. NOVELLETTO, A. et al. 1989. Frequency and molecular types of deletional α-thalassemia in Egypt. Hum. Gen. **81:** 211–213.
10. TRAEGER-SYNODINOS, J. E. et al. Characterization of nondeletion α-thalassemia mutations in the Greek population. Am. J. Hematol. **44:** 162–167.
11. HUI, C. H. et al. 1990. Iron overload in Chinese patients with hemoglobin H disease. Am. J. Hematol. **34:** 287–290.

Phenotypic Prediction in β-Thalassemia

P. J. HO,[b] G. W. HALL, L. Y. LUO, D. J. WEATHERALL, AND S. L. THEIN[a]

MRC Molecular Haematology Unit, Institute of Molecular Medicine, Oxford, OX3 9DS, United Kingdom

Over 150 mutations[1] affecting the β-globin gene lead to a reduction (β+) or absence (β⁰) of β-globin production, resulting in the three main clinical phenotypes of β-thalassemia: thalassemia major (TM), thalassemia trait (TT), and thalassemia intermedia (TI).[2] Despite the ability to accurately define the β-thalassemia mutations, identification of the patients with TI and prediction of their clinical severity, remain a problem in genetic counselling and prenatal diagnosis because the disease is influenced not only by the type of β-thalassemia mutations, but also by other factors such as those affecting the α- and γ-globin gene expression.[3]

We have examined 87 patients with a spectrum of clinical phenotypes within the syndrome of TI with two main objectives: (1) to determine if it is possible to consistently predict phenotypic severity from the known genotypic factors and (2) to identify the factors that affect the genotype-phenotype relationship and to assess their relative importance.

MATERIALS AND METHODS

Eighty-seven patients (representing 74 families) were referred to the MRC Molecular Haematology Unit from the United Kingdom and abroad for clarification of diagnosis and further management. The families were drawn from the following ethnic backgrounds: Asian Indian (35.1%); Middle Eastern (24.3%); Mediterranean (21.6%); Northern European (14.9%); and Southeast Asian/Chinese (4.1%) (TABLE 1). There was more than one patient in 12 families; two siblings in eight families, parent and child in three families, and three siblings in one family. Whenever possible, all family members, with and without thalassemia were examined in parallel with the probands.

Criteria for inclusion as TI follow the broad clinical guidelines, i.e., a disorder that is milder than TM but more severe than asymptomatic TT. Patients were classified as mildly affected if they maintained a Hb level of ≥ 7.5 gm/dl without blood transfusion, or need blood transfusions at a frequency of less than once every two years, or less than twice a year if transfusion was started after age 10. They are considered severe if transfusion requirements begin at age 4 or above with a frequency between 6 weeks and four months, or between three and four months if transfusion requirements commenced before age 4 years. Those who fall between the two groups are classified as moderate.

---

[a]Address for correspondence: Dr. S. L. Thein, MRC Molecular Haematology Unit, Institute of Molecular Medicine, John Radcliffe Hospital, Headington, Oxford, OX3 9DS United Kingdom. Tel: 01865 - 222 411; Fax: 01865 - 222 500; E-mail: swee.thein@imm.ox.ac.uk

[b]Present address: Institute of Hematology, Royal Prince Alfred Hospital, Camperdown, N.S.W. 2050, Australia; E-mail: Joy.Ho@haem.rpa.cs.nsw.gov.au

TABLE 1. Ethnic Distribution and Phenotypic Severity of United Kingdom Thalassemia Intermedia Patients[a]

Ethnic Group	β^{Th}/β^{N}	β^{Th}/β^{Th}	Total
Asian Indian	2	24	26 (35.1%)
Middle Eastern	2	16	18 (24.3%)
Mediterranean	2	14	16 (21.6%)
Southeast Asian/Chinese	2	1	3 (4.1%)
Northern European	10	1	11 (14.9%)
Total	18	56	74
Phenotypic Severity	β^{Th}/β^{N}	β^{Th}/β^{Th}	Total
Mild	17	32	1
Moderate	4	18	22
Severe	1	15	16
Total	22	65	87

[a]Of 87 individuals analyzed 22 (18 families) were heterozygotes and 65 (56 families) were homozygotes/compound heterozygotes.

Hematological data (full blood counts, Hb A2 and F levels, F cells, reticulocytes, and α/β globin chain biosynthesis ratios) were obtained using standard laboratory techniques.[4] DNA was extracted from peripheral blood leukocytes. A variety of techniques based on the PCR and Southern blot hybridization were used to screen the DNA for α- and β-thalassemia mutations,[5] and the C-T base substitution at position -158 upstream of the $^G\gamma$-globin gene, also referred to as the Xmn I-$^G\gamma$ polymorphism.[6]

RESULTS

Twenty-two subjects (from 18 families) have inherited only a single β-thalassemia allele while 65 patients (from 56 families) are homozygotes or compound heterozygotes.

Thalassemia Intermedia Patients with Two β-Thalassemia Alleles

Thirty-two of this group of 65 patients were classified as mildly affected, 18 moderate, and 15 severe (TABLE 1). Twenty-two of the patients had never received blood transfusions, 33 had received intermittent or sporadic transfusions, and 10 were regularly transfused at six weekly to two monthly intervals at the time of review (five began blood transfusions between 4 and 6 years old, while the other five patients began blood transfusions in adulthood). The patients ranged from 4 to 74 years old.

The mutations included seven very mild β^+ alleles (also referred to as "silent") in which there is minimal deficit of β-globin synthesis, four mild β^+, 15 severe β^+ or β^o and the Spanish δ/β thalassemia (TABLE 2). Despite extensive sequence analysis, three mutations remain uncharacterized; the presence of these uncharacterized β mutants is supported by hematological and family studies. The mutations accounted for 40 β genotypes, which could be classified into 13 groups based on the severity of mutations (TABLE 3).

Patients with combinations of two mild or very mild β^+ or one mild β^+ and one severe β^+ alleles have moderate to mild disease. The most frequent "silent" mutation encountered was the CAP +1 (A-C) substitution, found only in Asian Indians. The IVSI-6 T-C mutation accounted for 16/20 mild β^+ alleles; four patients were homozygotes with mild to moderate disease, one patient had never been transfused with Hb levels of > 7.5 gm/l. Splenomegaly was mild to moderate (2 to 10 cm below costal margin) in all the four

TABLE 2. Mutations Encountered in Homozygous and Compound Heterozygous Thalassemia Intermedia Patients

	Number of Chromosomes					
	Asian Indian	Southeast Asian	Middle Eastern	Mediterranean	Northern European	Total
Very mild β⁺						
+33 C-G				2		2
-88 C-T	1					1
-87 C-G			1			1
CAP+1 A-C	6					6
β^Knossos			4			4
Poly A (-AT)				1		1
3' UTR 47 C-G			1			1
Mild β⁺						
IVS1-6 T-C			7	8	1	16
Cod 19 A-G	2					2
Cod 29 C-T			1			1
IVS1-128 T-G			1			1
Severe β⁺						
IVS1-5 G-C	9					9
IVS1-110 G-A			4	7		11
β°						
FS 8 (-AA)			1	1		2
FS 8/9 (+G)	5					5
FS 41/42 (-TTCT)	5					5
FS 44 (-C)						1
β° 15 G-A	3					3
β° 30 G-C	2					2
β° 39 C-T				3	1	4
IVS1-1 G-A	1			2		3
IVS1-1 G-T	13					13
IVS2-1 G-A			8	1		9
IVS1-130 G-C			1			1
600 bp del	1					1
10.3 kb del	2					2
Spanish δβ Thal				2		2
Uncharacterized β thal	2			1		3
Total	50	2	29	29	2	112

homozygotes. Interaction of IVSI-6 T-C mutation with severe β⁺ or β° results in phenotypes ranging from mild to severe.

There was a considerable variation in phenotypic severity resulting from the interactions of severe β⁺ and β° alleles. One of the two severe β⁺/severe β⁺ patients had extremely mild disease (transfusion independent, with Hb 12 gm/dl and mild splenomegaly at age 42 years) while the other was severely affected (splenectomized and requiring transfusion every 3 months at 32 years). Of the 19 patients with β°/β° genotypes, nine whose ages ranged from 9 to 67 years, had very mild disease; six of the nine patients had never been transfused while the other three required sporadic transfusions. In contrast, seven β°/β° patients had severe disease, of which five had been splenectomized and all seven had moderate anemia requiring regular transfusions (three to six per year).

Overall, the Xmn I-$^G\gamma$ site has a modulating effect on phenotypic severity. Within the group with mild disease, 7/9 of the β^o/β^o patients are Xmn I-$^G\gamma$ +/+ compared to only 1/15 patients with one or two mild or very mild β^+ alleles. With the β^o/β^o genotypic group, nine patients had mild disease and 7/9 mild patients are Xmn I-$^G\gamma$ +/+ compared to 4/7 patients in the severe group.

A single α gene deletion was found in six patients; two severe (severe β^+/β^o and severe β^+/severe β^+ genotypes), one moderate (mild β^+/severe β^+ genotype) and three mild (severe β^+/β^o, mild β^+/severe β^+ and very mild β^+/severe β^+ genotypes). A non-deletional α-thalassemia variant (5 bp deletion at exon 1/IVSI junction of α2 globin gene) was present in the patient homozygous for $\beta^{Knossos}$.

Phenotypic Discordancy and HPFH

Seventeen patients were drawn from eight families, one with three siblings, and seven with two siblings. A striking observation here is the considerable variation in disease severity between siblings in seven families, despite having inherited identical β-thalassemia mutations. This disparity could not be attributed to differences in α-genotype. A variation in Hb F response is implicated from the difference in steady-state Hb F values between siblings (ranging from 1 gm/dl to as much as 8–9 gm/dl). In three of the seven families (two β^o/β^o and one severe β^+/β^o) segregation of a HPFH determinant was evident from family studies.

In addition to the seven sibships with phenotypic discordancy, co-inheritance of a HPFH determinant is also implicated in six mildly affected patients, five β^o/β, and one severe β^+/β^+. Two of the patients were splenectomized in adulthood, the others had mild to moderate splenomegaly. Their ages ranged from 12 to 67 years with a mean of 36.3 years. Five of the six patients had never been transfused while one had received a total of four transfusions prior to splenectomy at 16 years, but was transfusion-independent post-splenectomy.

Heterozygous β-Thalassemia Intermedia

Twenty-two TI patients, aged 8 to 67 years, carried only one β-thalassemia allele (TABLE 1). Eleven patients from 10 families (two Asian Indian, two Mediterranean, two Middle Eastern, three English, and one Scottish) had co-inherited severe β^+ or β^o alleles with triplicated α globin genes ($\alpha\alpha\alpha/\alpha\alpha$ or $\alpha\alpha\alpha/\alpha\alpha\alpha$). In eight patients from six families (one Irish and five English) the mutations, which include Cod 28 CTG-CGG, β^o 121 G-T, β 127 C-T and FS128, are dominantly inherited (TABLE 3). One heterozygote for the β121 G-T mutation has also co-inherited a triplicated α gene complex ($\alpha\alpha\alpha/\alpha\alpha$). The remaining four patients carried mutations {IVS2-654 C-T, FS 6 (-A) and FS 41/42 (-TTCT)} that are typically recessively inherited and yet have thalassemia intermedia; presence of a second β-thalassemia allele is excluded by extensive β gene sequence analysis and family studies.

All ten patients who had co-inherited extra α-globin genes with recessive mutations had mild TI, with or without mild splenomegaly and Hb levels of 7.7 to 12.1 gm/dl; all except one patient had never been transfused. The patient doubly heterozygous for the dominantly inherited β121 G-T and a triplicated a complex ($\alpha\alpha\alpha/\alpha\alpha$) had severe TI; she became transfusion-dependent in adult life. The other seven patients with dominantly inherited β-thalassemia had mild to moderate disease. Two patients were splenectomized in adult life, four had never been transfused, while three patients required intermittent transfusions.

TABLE 3. β Genotypes of United Kingdom Thalassemia Intermedia Patients

Genotypes	Homozygotes/Compound Heterozygotes				Heterozygotes		
	Phenotypic Severity						
	Mild	Moderate	Severe	Total	β Genotypes	α genotype	Total
Very mild β⁺/very mild β⁺	1			1	β° (FS8, FS41/42, β39, IVS2-850)	ααα/αα	5
Very mild β⁺/mild β⁺	1			1	β° (β39)	ααα/αααα	1
Very mild β⁺/severe β⁺	3	3		6	Severe β⁺ (IVSI-5, IVSI-110)	ααα/αα	4
Very mild β⁺/β°	4	3	1	8	Severe β⁺ or β° (IVS2-654, FS 41/42, FS6)	αα/αα	4
Mild β⁺/mild β⁺	4	3		7	Others: β 28	αα/αα	1
Mild β⁺/severe β⁺	1	2		3	β° 121	ααα/αα	1
Mild β⁺/β°	2	2	2	6	β° 121	αα/αα	4
Severe β⁺/severe β⁺	1		1	2	β° 127	αα/αα	1
Severe β⁺/β°	3		4	7	FS 128	αα/αα	1
β°/β°	9	3	7	19	Total		22
Severe β⁺/uncharacterized	1	2		3			
β°/uncharacterized	1			1			
δβ/δβ	1			1			
Total	32	18	15	65			

CONCLUSION

The most consistent genotypic factor that could be used for the prediction of phenotype is the type of β-thalassemia inherited. (1) All patients with two mild or very mild $β^+$ thalassemia alleles had mild to moderate disease; (2) although concurrent inheritance of extra α genes with heterozygous β-thalassemia results in thalassemia intermedia, the disease is mild; (3) it is difficult to predict the phenotypes of homozygotes or compound heterozygotes for the severe $β^+$ or $β^o$ alleles due to the co-inheritance of other modulating factors, such as an inherent capacity to produce fetal hemoglobin. In the majority of these patients, amelioration of disease severity associated with the co-inheritance of a hereditary persistence of fetal hemoglobin (HPFH) determinant is implicated. However, even when segregation of HPFH is demonstrated in family studies, identification and definition of such an HPFH determinant is not possible and would still pose a problem for phenotype prediction. Presence of the in-*cis* X*mn* I-$^G γ$ site was a modulating factor but insufficient to explain the high Hb F levels encountered; (4) co-inheritance of α-thalassemia could be a modulating factor but its effect was not evident in our patients. Other genetic modifiers in β-thalassemia remained unidentified.

ACKNOWLEDGMENTS

We thank Liz Rose and Milly Graver for preparation of the manuscript and the hematologists—Professor A. V. Hoffbrand, Drs. B. Wonke, A. Yardumian, N. West, D. Duncombe, A. Eden—for allowing us to study their patients. P. J. H. is a Nuffield Dominion Fellow and G.W.H. was an MRC Training Fellow.

REFERENCES

1. BAYSAL, E. et al. 1995. The β- and δ-thalassemia repository. Hemoglobin **19**: 213–236.
2. WEATHERALL, D. J. *et al.* 1981. The Thalassaemia Syndromes. Blackwell Scientific. Oxford.
3. THEIN, S. L. 1993. β-thalassaemia. Baillière's Clin. Haematol. **6**: 151–176. London.
4. SHARPE, J. A. *et al.* 1989. Haemoglobin analysis. In Laboratory Haematology, Chanarin, Ed. **1**: 33–54. Churchill Livingstone. Edinburgh.
5. THEIN, S. L. *et al.* 1993. β-thalassemia unlinked to the β-globin gene in an English family. Blood **82**: 961–967.
6. CRAIG, J. E. *et al.* 1993. The molecular basis of HPFH in a British family identified by heteroduplex formation. Br. J. Haematol. **84**: 106–110.

Impact of Asian Immigration on Thalassemia in California

FRED LOREY[a] AND GEORGE CUNNINGHAM

Genetic Disease Branch, State of California, Department of Health Services, Berkeley, California 94704

California is a multi-ethnic state with approximately 570,000 births per year. Universal mandatory newborn screening for hemoglobinopathies began in 1990, and includes detection of structural variants as well as β-thalassemia disorders. Asians now comprise 10% of all California births and also represent the populations at highest risk for thalassemia. Asian immigration, particularly from the Southeast Asian countries, has led to increased numbers of cases detected.

PATIENTS AND METHODS

The blood sample is obtained via a heel stick blotted on filter paper. Analysis occurs at one of eight regional contract laboratories via a high performance liquid chromatography (HPLC) procedure.[1] All positive screens require a second liquid blood sample from patient and parents, which is analyzed at Children's Hospital Oakland Hemoglobinopathy Laboratory for diagnosis using thin layer isoelectric focusing and other electrophoresis, as well as DNA analysis in some cases.[2]

RESULTS

FIGURE 1 illustrates the change in Asian births from 1983 to 1993. There has been more than a doubling of Asian births.

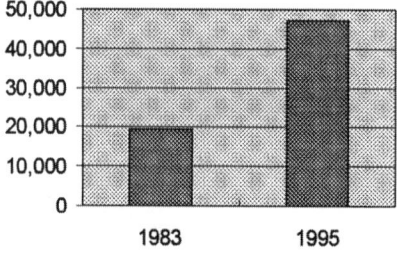

FIGURE 1. Asian births in California.

[a]Address for correspondence: Fred Lorey, Ph. D., Genetic Disease Branch, 2151 Berkeley Way, Annex 4, Berkeley, CA 94704, Phone: (510) 540- 2941; Fax: (510) 540-2095; e-mail: Florey@genetic.dhs.cahwnet.gov

PREVALENCE RATES

There is a great deal of variability in birth prevalence of thalassemia by ethnicity. TABLE 1 illustrates this disparity for the two most common clinically significant β thalassemias in California. These cases of β thalassemia compound heterozygotes do not all occur at the same frequency with the corresponding homozygotes of the structural variant. However, in most cases, the screening phenotype is the same for either structural variant homozygotes or $β^0$-thalassemia/structural variant compound. Diagnostic testing, family testing, and DNA analysis usually resolve one genotype from the other.[3]

TABLE 1. β-Thalassemia by Ethnicity: Cases

Ethnicity	β-Thal Major	E/β-Thal	C/β-Thal	D/β-Thal
Cambodian		6		
Chinese	4			
Laotian	3	9		
Vietnamese3	5			
Hmong	1	1		
Thai		1		
Asian	1			1
Southeast Asian	1	6		
Asian Indian	4	1		2
Middle Eastern	3			1
White	4			
Hispanic	3			1
Black	1		9	
Total	28	29	9	5

Hemoglobin E

Hemoglobin E is a structural variant that is important because when it occurs as Hb E/β-thalassemia, the clinical manifestations can be severe.[4] In order to detect all such cases, is necessary to follow all initial screening phenotypes of FE, which can be a daunting task, since in California, more cases of Hb EE are detected per year than are cases of Hb SS (sickle cell anemia).

Quantitation of Hemoglobin in Thalassemia

Because many phenotypes can represent more than one genotype, especially where β-thalassemia is concerned, quantification is important. The biggest problem for newborn screening is making the distinction between sickle carriers (FAS) from sickle/$β^+$-thalassemia (FSA). However, they are distinguishable when quantified.

DISCUSSION

The two most serious forms of β-thalassemia, β-Thal Major and Hb E/β-Thal, are detected at a rate of approximately 11 per year. This is higher than the prevalence of galactosemia, one of three other genetic disorders for which we have been conducting newborn screening for 16 years, and is expected to increase as Asian immigration increases. When combined with the other types of thalassemia/structural hemoglobin compound heterozygotes (C/β-Thal, D/β-Thal, S/β^0-Thal, and S/β$^+$-Thal) the numbers reach 26 cases per year, higher than the frequency of phenylketonuria (PKU) in California. Hb E/β-thalassemia does not occur outside of Asia, and in fact does not appear to occur at any significant frequency outside of Southeast Asia. Asians of Chinese, Japanese, Korean, or Filipino ancestry appear to be at extremely low risk of any Hb E or E/β-thalassemia disorders of clinical significance.

β-Thalassemia major has a broader distribution, occurring among Chinese and virtually all Southeast Asian populations in California. The striking highest prevalence in California occurs in those of Asian Indian (East Indian) ancestry, with a rate of 1 per every 2,263 births, higher even than the rate of Hb E/β-thalassemia among Southeast Asians. We have not addressed the issue of thalassemia frequencies among other groups in this paper; however the majority of cases of both Hb S/β-Thal and Hb C/β-Thal occur in Californian blacks because of the very high frequency of β chain structural carriers. However, there have only been two cases of β-Thal major among blacks in six years of screening with approximately 45,000 black births per year.

California currently is evaluating a pilot project for α-thalassemia screening. Clearly hydropic or stillborn infants with alpha-thal major are not detected in time for prevention or control. However, this disorder is detectable prenatally. The purpose of newborn screening is never to detect carriers, and therefore one and two α gene deletion screening or Hb Bart's quantitation is not a justification for newborn screening. That leaves us with Hb H disease. This is also a problematic issue. Most hematologists would argue the sooner hemoglobinopathy patients are in a clinical program, the better the outcome. During the trial project, we detected approximately 30 cases of Hb H disease per year.

CONCLUSIONS

Little did we know when starting hemoglobin screening in 1990 that we would detect more cases of Hb FE than FS from the outset, and that thalassemia screening would become an integral part of our program. As the birthrate for white Californians continues to decrease and Asian immigration continues to increase, thalassemia will contribute an increasing proportion of our caseload. This creates a need for additional education of families and physicians alike, as neither groups are completely aware of the magnitude of the problem. The Southeast Asian populations are often first-generation immigrants with little knowledge of this disease or its significance. The exciting research in new therapies for thalassemia presented this symposium bode well for the outcome of patients with thalassemia, and may lead to the addition of α-thalassemia screening in the future.

REFERENCES

1. LOREY, F. W., G. C. CUNNINGHAM, F. SHAFER, B. LUBIN & E. VICHINSKY. 1994. Universal screening for hemoglobinopathies using high performance liquid chromatography: Clinical results of 2.2 million screens. Eur. J. Hum. Genet. **2:** 262–271.

2. SHAFER, F. E., F. LOREY, G. C. CUNNINGHAM, C. KLUMPP, E. VICHINSKY & B. LUBIN. 1996. Newborn screening for sickle cell disease: 4 years of experience from California's newborn screening program. J. Ped. Hem. Onc. **18**(1): 36–41.
3. JOHNSON, J. P., E. VICHINSKY, D. HURST, A. CAMBER, B. LUBIN & E. LOUIE. 1992. Differentiation of homozygous hemoglobin E from compound heterozygous hemoglobin E-β-0 thalassemia by hemoglobin E mutation analysis. J. Ped. **120:** 775–779.
4. HURST, D., B. TITTLE, K. KLEMAN *et al.* 1983. Anemia and hemoglobinopathies in Southeast Asian refugee children. J. Ped. **102**(5): 692–697.

[NOTE ADDED IN PROOF: Two of the four cases of α thalassemia major detected were still alive at the time of publishing. Early delivery due to pregnancy complications allowed live births and immediate transfusion. In both cases, the diagnosis was not known until we reported the possibility to the physicians.]

Detection of Fetal Hemoglobin in Erythrocytes by Flow Cytometry

T. A. CAMPBELL,[a,b] R. E. WARE,[c] AND M. MASON[b]

[b]Wallac, Inc., Akron, Ohio, 44321-0350, USA
[c]Duke University Medical Center, Durham, North Carolina 27710, USA

Fetal (Hb F) hemoglobin ($\alpha_2\gamma_2$) is the dominant hemoglobin in the developing fetus and comprises about 70–80% of circulating hemoglobin at birth. Hb F diminishes rapidly after birth and accounts for less than 1% of the total hemoglobin content of most adults. However, it often occurs at higher levels in people with conditions such as sickle cell disease (SSD), β-thalassemia, and leukemia. Therefore, the ability to detect and quantify fetal hemoglobin–containing cells (F cells) is important in many situations. In patients with SSD, for example, the percentage of F cells is a useful indicator of the severity of the disease, as cells with HbF are less likely to sickle.[1] Tracking F cell levels in sickle cell patients can be helpful in monitoring the effects of the new generation of SSD treatments such as hydroxyurea, which act by stimulating Hb F production. Since Hb F is an intracellular antigen, the cell has to be fixed and permeablized (fix/perm) prior to staining. The method described in this manuscript is simple, uses a commercially available FITC-conjugated anti-fetal hemoglobin monoclonal, and results in fixed/permed cells, which largely retain their original morphology.

METHODS AND MATERIALS

Samples

Whole blood samples were obtained from Sickle Cell Centers in Cincinnati, Ohio, Durham, North Carolina, Dallas, Texas, and Philadelphia, Pennsylvania. All samples were collected using EDTA as the anticoagulant and were analyzed within a week of being drawn.

Erythrocyte Fixation/Permeablization

Whole blood was washed twice with PBS (150 mM NaCl, 20 mM potassium phosphate monobasic, 80 mM potassium phosphate dibasic, pH 7.2) and pelleted after each wash by centrifugation for 5 minutes at 150 × g. Washed cells were then fixed by gently mixing with PBS/4% formaldehyde (Fisher Scientific, Pittsburgh, PA; 1 ml:10 µl blood) for one hour at room temperature. The fixed cells were then mixed for approximately 30 seconds with PBS/0.05% glutaraldehyde (Fisher Scientific, Pittsburgh, PA; 250 µl/10 µl blood), washed once in PBS, and centrifuged. The pellet was resuspended in 500 µl of 5% nonfat dry milk and blocked for 10 minutes at room temperature with gentle rocking. The blocked

---

[a]Address for correspondence: Dr. Thomas A. Campbell, Wallac, Inc., Box 4350, Akron, OH 44321-0350. Tel: (330) 854-5434; Fax: (330) 825-8520; E-mail: tac@isolab.com

cells were centrifuged and resuspended in 0.01% Triton X-100 (Aldrich, Milwaukee, WI) in PBS/0.1% BSA (0.5 ml/10 µl blood). At this point, one aliquot received the FITC-conjugated monoclonal antibody to HbF (2.5 µg/5 µl blood, Isolab, Inc., Norton, Ohio), while another aliquot received an isotypic control (typically a FITC-conjugated monoclonal antibody to zeta chain). These suspensions are rocked gently for 30 minutes at room temperature, washed once with PBS, and finally resuspended in PBS. Stained cells were analyzed using an Epics XL flow cytometer (Coulter, Hialeah, FL).

Comparison to Another Fix/Perm Method

Thirty SSD samples were analyzed at Isolab, Inc. using the above method or at Duke University Medical Center using a previously described fix/perm method.[2] This method uses dimethy 3,3′-dithiobispropionimadate (DTBP) as a crosslinker/fixative, a Triton X-100 permeabilization, and visualization of the bound anti-Hb F monoclonal (Immuno Rx, Atlanta, GA) by a goat anti-mouse F(ab′)$_2$ conjugated to fluorescein (Pierce, Rockford IL).

HPLC Analysis

Samples were analzyed for %Hb F using a 4.6 × 40 mm PolyCAT A cation exchange column (PolyLC, Columbia MD) as described by Ou.[3]

RESULTS

FIGURE 1(A) presents a typical histogram of sickle cell blood (9% Hb F by HPLC) fixed, permeablized using the above-described method, and stained with a FITC-conjugated anti-Hb F monoclonal antibody. Positive-stained cells (34.6% of the total population) are

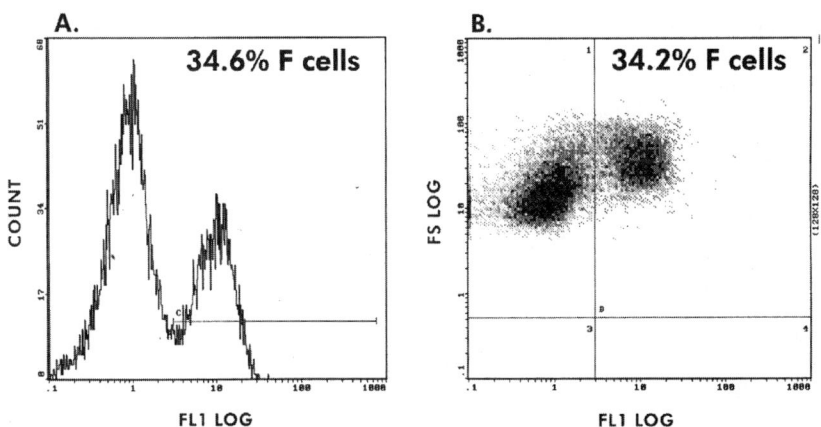

FIGURE 1. Histogram and scatter plot of typical Hb F-containing sample. (**A**) Flow cytometry histogram of whole blood from an individual diagnosed with SSD which was fixed, permeablized, and stained with a FITC-labeled anti-fetal Hb monoclonal antibody. Hb F–positive cells are found in the right hand peak. Sample contained 9% Hb F by HPLC. (**B**) Scatter plot obtained from the same sample; the upper right quadrant contains the Hb F–positive cells.

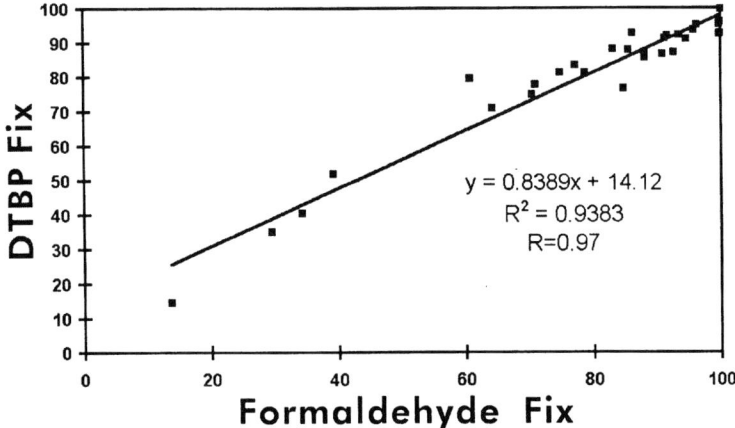

FIGURE 2. Comparison of results obtained with two fixation/permeablization methods. Thirty Hb F-containing samples were fixed either the described method ("Formaldehyde Fix") or the DTBP fixation method ("DTBP Fix") using an alternative anti-Hb F monoclonal.

plainly visible. A slight increase in negative peak fluorescence is observed when compared to isotypic control was observed (data not shown). A scatter plot of the same sample reveals similar results (FIG. 1B).

Thirty SSD samples were analyzed using the described method as well as another fix/perm method described in the METHODS AND MATERIALS (FIG. 2). Excellent correlation between the two methods is observed ($R = 0.97$, $R^2 = 0.94$).

DISCUSSION

A procedure has been developed that allows for the easy fixation/permeabilization/fluorescent staining of fetal hemoglobin in erythrocytes. This procedure is easy and does not require the harsh fixatives or chilled reagents required in other fix/perm procedures. The use of a commercially available fluorochrome-conjugated monoclonal antibody also accelerates the staining procedure.

Results obtained using this procedure are quite similar to results obtained with another fix/perm procedure that used another commercially available anti-fetal hemoglobin monoclonal antibody, which was not fluorochrome-conjugated and therefore required a secondary antibody to visualize fluorescence.

REFERENCES

1. MARCUS, S. J. et al. 1995. Quantitative analysis of erythrocytes containing fetal hemoglobin (F cells) in children with sickle cell disease Am. J. Hematol. **54**: 40–46.
2. DOVER, G. J. & S. H. BOYER. 1987. Fetal hemoglobin-containing cells have the same mean corpuscular hemoglobin as cells without fetal hemoglobin: A reciprocal relationship between gamma-and beta-globin gene expression in normal subjects and in those with high hemoglobin production Blood **69**: 183.
3. OU, C. N. & C. L. ROGNERUD. 1993. Rapid analysis of hemoglobin variants by HPLC Clin. Chem. **39/5**: 820–824.

Hydroxyurea and Hemin Affect Both the Transcriptional and Post-Transcriptional Mechanisms of Some Globin Genes in Human Adult Erythroid Cells[a]

PANAGOULA KOLLIA,[a,b] EITAN FIBACH,[c] MARIANNA POLITOU,[b] CONSTANCE T. NOGUCHI,[c] ALAN N. SCHECHTER,[c] AND DIMITRIS LOUKOPOULOS[b]

[b]*First Department of Medicine, University of Athens, Laikon Hospital, 115 27 Athens, Greece*

[c]*Laboratory of Chemical Biology, NIDDK, National Institutes of Health, Bethesda, Maryland*

Several genetic abnormalities may increase hemoglobin F (HbF) synthesis in postnatal life. Among them, sickle cell anemia and thalassemia are the most striking examples. In both groups the increase of HbF may considerably improve the laboratory parameters and ameliorate the clinical severity of the disease in the patients.[1] The beneficial effects of HbF observed in sickle cell anemia result from the fact that the dispersion of HbF ($\alpha_2\gamma_2$) (and $\alpha_2\beta^S\gamma$) molecules among those of HbS ($\alpha_2\beta^S_2$) clearly diminishes the tendency of the latter to polymerize, thereby allowing a better survival of the HbF-containing red blood cells (F cells) and fewer sickle cell crises.[2] Recently, several pharmacological agents, such as cell cycle–dependent cytotoxic drugs and others, have been used to stimulate HbF synthesis *in vivo*. The initial studies involved treatment of baboons and patients with β-thalassemia or sickle cell disease with 5′ azacytidine and showed a considerable stimulation of HbF′ production. However, because of concerns about the potential carcinogenicity of 5' azacytidine, over the last years most animal and human studies have concentrated on other drugs, such as hydroxyurea,[3] hemin,[4] or butyrate derivatives.[5]

The complexity of the erythroid marrow in man makes the study of the mechanism(s) underlying the effect of these drugs very difficult. However, over the last years a novel two-phase liquid culture procedure for growing human adult erythroid cells (hAEC) *in vitro* has proved a most useful tool.[6] The first phase is an erythropoietin (EPO)-independent phase, in which the cells are cultured in the presence of a combination of growth factors but no EPO; during this phase early erythroid committed progenitors, burst-forming units (BFU-e), proliferate and differentiate into more committed erythroid progenitors, colony-forming units-erythroid (CFU-e). The second phase is an EPO-dependent phase, during which the above cells are re-cultured in an EPO-supplemented medium, where CFU-erythroid progenitors

---

[a]This study was sponsored by the Research Contract 91 ED 97 from the Greek Ministry of Energy, Industry and Technology to D.L.

[b]Address for correspondence: Dr. Panagoula Kollia, First Department of Medicine, University of Athens, Laikon Hospital, Agiou Thoma 17, 115 27 Athens, Greece. Tel: 30.1. 777 0695; Fax: 30.1. 777 1161.

TABLE 1. Quantitation of RNA Transcripts (attom/µg RNA) from the Full-Length γ-RNA Transcripts and from ε-Globin Exons I and II[a]

	RNA	HU/control (ratio)	Hemin/control (ratio)
γ-gene	cytoplasmic	33.8/18.8 (1.8)	48.2/21.7 (2.2)
	nuclear	19.3/16.1 (1.2)	40.1/19.3 (2.0)
ε-gene			
exon I	cytoplasmic	14/10.5 (1.4)	4.5/2.3 (2.0)
	nuclear	27.3/9.8 (2.8)	4.9/3.8 (1.3)
exon II	cytoplasmic	5.6/0.4 (2.3)	0.3/0.2 (1.5)
	nuclear	9.9/5.7 (1.7)	0.7/0.6 (1.2)

[a]Numbers in parentheses denote factor of increase.

continue to proliferate and mature into orthochromatic normoblasts and erythrocytes. In the present study, we have applied the above system in order to examine the effects of hydroxyurea (HU) and hemin on globin gene transcription and RNA processing, using human erythroid cells, cells that express high levels of β-globin and low levels of γ-globin transcripts, i.e., HbA and HbF, respectively.

Conditions of the hAEC procedure have been described in detail elsewhere.[6] Hemin solution was added to the cultures on the same day as EPO at a final concentration of 100 µM. Hydroxyurea (100 µmol/L) was added on day 7 in phase II cultures. Hemoglobin types were characterized and quantitated by cation exchange high-performance liquid chromatography (HPLC) of cell lysates. The expression of γ-, ε-, and β-globin genes in the hydroxyurea or hemin-induced hAEC was quantitated by a specifically adapted reverse-transcription/polymerase chain reaction; in this system both the total levels of each mRNA species as well as the evolution of the RNA processing could be studied.

We found that γ-globin message levels were increased twofold by hydroxyurea or hemin in both the cytoplasm and the nucleus (TABLE 1). In the untreated cells, only spliced γ-transcripts were present in the cytoplasm, indicating complete RNA processing. In contrast, in the nucleus roughly 50% of the γ-globin RNA transcripts were unspliced, as evidenced by their containing intact their first intervening sequence (γ-IVS-I). Upon treatment with hydroxyurea or hemin, unspliced γ-transcripts clearly decreased in the nucleus (TABLE 2). This effect was greater for hemin than for hydroxyurea. Studies of the ε-globin RNA transcription and processing gave similar results. In the untreated cells, all or most of the nuclear ε-globin RNA transcripts were unspliced, i.e., they contained either the first or the second intervening sequences (ε-IVS-I or ε-IVS-II). In contrast, the cytoplasm of these cells contained only fully processed transcripts. In cells induced with hydroxyurea or hemin, unspliced nuclear ε-transcripts decreased (TABLE 2), in parallel with the increase of correctly spliced transcripts in the cytopasm. In contrast to the γ- and ε-globin genes, the level of full-length, correctly spliced β-globin message was not affected by induction of hAEC with hemin or hydroxyurea. These results suggest that the above two compounds increase both the rate of transcription and the efficacy of the splic-

TABLE 2. Ratios of Spliced Versus Unspliced γ-Globin (IVSI-containing) and ε-Transcripts (IVSI/IVSII Containing) Quantitated by Competitive PCR in Nuclear RNA Extracts from hAEC Induced with HU or Hemin

	γ-IVS-I	ε-IVS-I	ε-IVS-II
Control	50/50	15/85	30/70
HU	60/40	30/70	45/55
Hemin	75/25	40/60	45/55

ing process of the low-expressed globin genes and raise the possibility that this mechanism contributes in the elevation of HbF seen in patients treated with hydroxyurea and in cultures treated with hydroxyurea or hemin.

REFERENCES

1. NOGUCHI, C. T., G. P. RODGERS, G. R. SERJEANT & A. N. SCHECHTER. 1988. Levels of fetal hemoglobin necessary for effective therapy of sickle cell disease. N. Engl. J. Med. **318:** 96–99.
2. SCHECHTER, A. N., C. T. NOGUCHI & G. P. RODGERS. 1987. *In* Molecular Basis of Blood Diseases. p. 179. Saunders. Philadelphia, PA.
3. RODGERS, G. P., G. J. DOVER, C. T. NOGUCHI, A. N. SCHECHTER & A. W. NIENHUIS. 1990. Hematological responses of patients with sickle cell disease to treatment with hydroxyurea. N. Engl. J. Med. **322:** 1037–1045.
4. FIBACH, E., P. KOLLIA, A. N. SCHECHTER, C. T. NOGUCHI & G. P. RODGERS. 1995. Hemin-induced acceleration of hemoglobin production in immature cultured erythroid cells: Preferential enhancement of fetal hemoglobin. Blood **85:** 2967–2974.
5. PERRINE, S. P., B. A. MILLER, D. V. FALLER *et al.* 1989. Sodium butyrate enhances fetal globin gene expression in erythroid progenitors of patients with HbSS and beta-thalassemia. Blood **74:** 454–459.
6. FIBACH, E., D. MANOR, A. OPPENHEIM & E. A. RACHMILEWITZ. 1989. Proliferation and maturation of human erythroid progenitors in liquid culture. Blood **73:** 100–103.

Treatment of Two Infants with Cooley's Anemia with Sodium Phenylbutyrate

M. L. MACMILLAN, M. FOULADI, E. NISBET-BROWN, J. S. WAYE, AND N.F. OLIVIERI[a]

McMaster University Medical Centre, Hamilton, Ontario, Canada, and The Hospital for Sick Children, Toronto, Ontario, Canada

The pharmacologic stimulation of fetal hemoglobin, as an alternative approach to therapy for patients with Cooley's anemia, has met with limited success.[1] The butyric acid compounds, derivatives of natural short-chain fatty acids, offer potential therapy for this disorder. It has been observed that elevated levels of plasma α-amino-*n*-butyric acid found in infants of diabetic mothers delayed the normal switch from γ- to β-globin at or around the time of birth.[2,3] Butyrate has been demonstrated to act on 5′ flanking sequences in the embryonic globin gene of the adult chicken[4] and via sequences near the transcriptional start site of the human gamma-globin gene promoter.[5] It has been suggested that butyrate-associated induction of fetal hemoglobin synthesis in laboratory animals may require the presence of pre-activated γ-globin genes.[6] To date, all patients with Cooley's anemia in whom butyrate therapy has been initiated, in an attempt to maintain or reactivate globin gene synthesis and increase fetal hemoglobin concentrations, have been older children or adults.[7-10] To examine the effectiveness of sodium phenylbutyrate before the switch from γ- to β-chain synthesis is completed, we treated two infants with Cooley's anemia shortly following diagnosis.

PATIENTS

Patient A

The first patient was a full-term, healthy male, born to a thirty-three-year old woman whose pregnancy was complicated by gestational diabetes. During the pregnancy, the parents, both Chinese, reported a family history of unspecified anemia. Investigations showed the mother to be heterozygous for the β°-thalassemia mutation at codon 41/42 (-CTTT), and the father to be heterozygous for the β°-thalassemia mutation at the second intervening sequence at IVS2-654 (C→T). The patient was diagnosed at birth by cord blood sampling as a compound heterozygote for these mutations and a normal α-globin genotype. At one month, nineteen days of age, when hemoglobin concentration was 8 g/dL, sodium phenylbutyrate 10 g/m² surface area, administered in divided doses twice daily dissolved in formula, and folic acid 1 mg/day, was initiated. The sodium phenylbutyrate was later added to puréed baby food.

---

[a]Address for correspondence: Nancy F. Olivieri, M.D., F.R.C.P.C., Haematology/Oncology, The Hospital for Sick Children, 555 University Avenue, Toronto, Ontario M5G 1X8 Canada. Tel: 416-813-6823; Fax: 416-813-5346; E-mail: noliv@sickkids.on.ca

Patient B

The second patient was a full-term, healthy female, born to a thirty-five-year old $G_3P_0SA_2$ healthy Greek woman whose partner was also Greek. The fetus was diagnosed *in utero* using amniocentesis, as homozygous for IVS1-110 G→A (β^+-thalassemia), and a normal α-globin genotype. At two months of age, the infant started therapy with folic acid, 2 mg/day. At three months, thirteen days of age, when hemoglobin concentration was 4.8 g/dL, she commenced therapy with sodium phenylbutyrate 10 g/m^2 body surface area/day, administered in divided doses dissolved in expressed breast milk.

METHODS

Sodium phenylbutyrate was supplied by Pharmaceutics International, Inc. (Hunt Valley, MD) from the supply furnished to The Hospital for Sick Children, Toronto, for patients with urea cycle disorders, under a protocol for compassionate use. Hematologic studies, hemoglobin electrophoresis on cellulose acetate and starch gel, or via high pressure liquid chromatography (Bio-Rad, CA, 1996), and the relative rates of α-, β-, and γ-globin chain synthesis followed standard methods. The absolute fetal hemoglobin concentration was calculated as the product of the percentage of fetal hemoglobin and the total hemoglobin concentration. Genomic DNA, isolated from peripheral blood lymphocytes, was analyzed by Southern hybridization and standard dot blot hybridization techniques.

DISCUSSION

Sodium phenylbutyrate was administered in formula and breast milk in both these infants with great difficulty. The primary reason for discontinuation of therapy in the second patient was, in fact, poor compliance and refusal to feed. In parallel, sodium phenylbutyrate was not effective in either infant with Cooley's anemia in preventing completion of the switch from γ- to β-globin synthesis. Although these findings do not support the effectiveness of sodium phenylbutyrate in infants with Cooley's anemia prior to the completion of the γ- to β-globin switch, prospective trials are indicated to determine whether sodium phenylbutyrate alone, or in combination with other agents, may sustain fetal hemoglobin synthesis, if initiated early enough in infancy, in patients with Cooley's anemia.

REFERENCES

1. OLIVIERI, N. F. 1996. Reactivation of fetal hemoglobin in patients with β-thalassemia. Sem. Hematol. **33** (1): 24–42.
2. PERRINE, S. P., M. F. GREENE & D. V. FALLER. 1985. Delay in the fetal globin switch in infants of diabetic mothers. N. Engl. J. Med. **312**: 334–338.
3. BARD, H., & J. PROSMANNE. 1985. Relative rates of fetal hemoglobin and adult hemoglobin synthesis in cord blood of infants of insulin-dependent diabetic mothers. Pediatrics **75**: 1143–1147.
4. GINDER, G. D., M. J. WHITTERS & J. K. POHLMAN. 1984. Activation of a chicken embryonic globin gene in adult erythroid cells by 5-azacytidine and sodium butyrate. Proc Natl. Acad. Sci. USA **81**: 3954–3958.
5. GLAUBER, J. G. & J. A. WANDERSEE. 1991. Little 5'-flanking sequences mediate butyrate stimulation of embryonic globin gene expression in adult erythroid cells. Mol. Cell. Biol. **11**: 4690–4697.

6. PACE, B., Q. LI, G. PETERSON & G. STAMATOYANNOPOULOS. 1994. α-amino butyric acid cannot reactivate the silenced γ-gene of the β-locus YAC transgenic mouse. Blood **84**(12): 4344–4353.
7. PERRINE, S. P., G. D. GINDER, D. V. FALLER, G. H. DOVER, T. IKUTA, H. E. WITKOWSKA, S-P CAI, E. P. VICHINSKY & N. F. OLIVIERI. 1993. A short-term trial of butyrate to stimulate fetal-globin-gene expression in the β-globin disorders. N. Engl. J. Med. **328**: 81–86.
8. COLLINS, A. F., H. A. PEARSON, P. GIARDINA, K. T. MCDONAGH, S. W. BRUSILOW & G. J. DOVER. 1995. Oral sodium phenylbutyrate therapy in homozygous β-thalassemia: A clinical trial. Blood **84**(91): 43–49.
9. SHER, G. D., G. D. GINDER, J. LITTLE, S. YANG, G. J. DOVER & N. F. OLIVIERI. 1995. Extended therapy with intravenous arginine butyrate in patients with β-hemoglobinopathies. N. Engl. J. Med. **332**: 1606–1610.
10. OLIVIERI, N. F., D. C. REES, G. D. GINDER, S. W. THEIN, J. S. WAYE, L. CHANG, G. M. BRITTENHAM & D. J. WEATHERALL. 1996. First report of long-term elimination of red cell transfusions in thalassemia major through augmentation of fetal hemoglobin during with sodium phenylbutyrate and hydroxyurea. Blood **88**(Suppl 1): 310a.

Erythropoietin Level and Effect of rHuEPO in Beta-Thalassemic Mice[a]

RAYMOND A. POPP,[b-d,g] SARAH G. SHINPOCK,[b] DIANA M. POPP,[b]
GISELA K. CLEMONS,[e] AND DAVID B. VAN WYCK[f]

[b]*Life Sciences Division, Oak Ridge National Laboratory, Oak Ridge,
Tennessee 37831, USA*

[c]*The University of Tennessee-Oak Ridge Graduate School of Biomedical
Sciences, Life Sciences Division, Oak Ridge, Tennessee 37831, USA*

[d]*Comprehensive Sickle Cell Center, Meharry Medical College,
Nashville, Tennessee 37208, USA*

[e]*Lawrence Berkeley Laboratory, University of California, Berkeley,
California 94720, USA*

[f]*Department of Internal Medicine, University Medical Center, Tucson,
Arizona 85724, USA*

Erythropoietin (Epo) is the major regulator of erythropoiesis[1] and it is elevated in serum of thalassemia patients who remain anemic despite bone marrow hypercellularity and reticulocytosis.[2] Homozygous beta-thalassemic (β-thal) mice exhibit hematological and pathological symptoms[3,4] commonly observed in human patients. The purpose of this study was to determine the effect of injecting recombinant human Epo (rHuEPO) into normal C57BL/6 (B6) and β-thal (C57BL/6.Hbb[th]) mice to evaluate the possible use of Epo therapy for beta-thalassemia patients.

The basal serum Epo levels in B6 and β-thal mice were measured directly by RIA[5,6] and indirectly by ESA.[7] The serum concentrations of Epo (TABLE 1) ranged between 14–110 mU/ml in young B6 mice (14–42 days old) and 8–40 mU/ml in adult B6 mice (2–12 months old). Serum Epo levels in heterozygous β-thal mice were similar to those in normal mice (data not shown). A significantly higher concentration ($p < 0.01$) of Epo was found in the serum of homozygous β-thal mice. The serum Epo levels ranged between 54–221 mU/ml in young β-thal mice (14–42 days old), 21–100 mU/ml in young adult β-thal mice (2–3 months old), and 35–217 mU/ml in older β-thal mice (5–12 months old).

B6 and β-thal mice, about 6-weeks old at the beginning of treatment, received subcutaneous injections of 1 or 4 U of Epo/g body weight three times a week for 4 or 8 weeks to determine the effect of injecting Epo (Epoetin alfa, Amgen, Thousand Oaks, CA) on erythropoiesis in B6 and β-thal mice. The 1 U of Epo regimen increased the hematocrit

---

The submitted manuscript has been authored by a contractor of the U.S. Government under contract No. DE-AC05-96OR22464. Accordingly the U.S. Government retains the nonexclusive, royalty-free license to publish or reproduce the published form of this contribution, or all others to do so, for U.S. Government purposes.

[a]Research sponsored jointly by the National Institute of Health under R01 HL 37056, HL 43375 and DE-AC05-96OR22464 with Lockheed Martin Energy Systems and P60 HL 38737 with Meharry Medical College.

[g]Address for correspondence: Dr. R. A. Popp, Life Sciences Division, Oak Ridge National Laboratory, Oak Ridge, TN 37831. Tel: 423-574-1227; Fax: 423-576-4149.

TABLE 1. Epo Concentration in Serum of Normal and β-Thalassemic Mice

Mice	Age	Number of Sera	Epo[a] (μU/ml)	Age	Number of Sera	Epo[b] (μU/ml)
Normal	14–42 days	6	26.5[c] (18–62)[d]	14–42 days	11	66 (14–110)
	2–5 months	8	10.6 (8–12)	2–12 months	11	26.6 (13–40)
β-Thal	14–42 days	8	124 (54–221)	14–42 days	10	119 (47–217)
	2–3 months	9	55 (21–95)	2–3 months	3	97 (94–100)
	5–12 months	9	125 (86–217)	5–12 months	14	103 (35–165)

[a]Epo measured by radioimmune assay.[5,6]
[b]Epo measured by bioassay.[7] ^{3}H-thymidine incorporation values were converted to μU of Epo activity by comparing the results with ^{3}H-thymidine incorporation values obtained using sera of known Epo concentrations.
[c]Average.
[d]Range.

in B6 mice but not in β-thal mice (data not shown). The 4 U of Epo regimen induced significant hematological changes in both B6 and β-thal mice (TABLE 2). Administration of Epo increased the RBC, HGB, and HCT values in both B6 and β-thal mice without changing the MCV, MCH, and MCHC values. The WBC and RETIC values were decreased in β-thal mice but not in B6 mice. The β/α globin synthesis was increased in β-thal mice but was not perturbed in B6 mice. Injection of Epo increased the incidence

TABLE 2. Effects of rHuEpo on the Hematology of Normal and β-Thalassemic Mice

	Normal	Normal + Epo[a]	Beta-Thal	Beta-Thal + Epo[a]
WBC (x10^3/ml)	7.6 ± 0.8	7.8 ± 1.2	17.3 ± 2.8	10.2 ± 1.1
RBC (x10^9/ml)	11.1 ± 0.3	14.0 ± 1.8	11.1 ± 0.3	13.8 ± 0.7
HGB (g/dl)	16.0 ± 0.2	21.8 ± 3.0	10.4 ± 0.3	14.6 ± 0.6
HCT (%)	48.8 ± 0.8	63.3 ± 8.7	35.8 ± 0.6	45.7 ± 1.8
MCV (fl)	44.0 ± 0.4	45.0 ± 0.6	32.3 ± 0.5	33.7 ± 1.4
MCH (pg/rbc)	14.4 ± 0.2	15.6 ± 0.3	9.3 ± 0.2	10.7 ± 0.5
MCHC (g/dl)	32.7 ± 0.4	35.0 ± 0.2	29.1 ± 0.7	31.5 ± 0.4
RETIC (%)	2.0 ± 0.2	1.2 ± 0.4	23.6 ± 1.7	13.1 ± 1.3
β/α synthesis	1.0 ± 0.04	1.0 ± 0.04	0.76 ± 0.04	0.96 ± 0.06
CFU-S (bm)[b]	16.4 ± 0.8	13.8 ± 2.7	17.8 ± 1.4	15.2 ± 0.9
(spl)	2.0 ± 0.2	1.8 ± 0.5	1.4 ± 0.2	1.7 ± 0.2
BFU-E (bm)	46.4 ± 3.7	57.2 ± 4.6	39.2 ± 6.8	50.8 ± 11.8
(spl)	5.8 ± 0.8	7.4 ± 1.6	7.7 ± 0.7	3.9 ± 0.9
CFU-E (bm)	247 ± 30.3	483 ± 19.5	399 ± 46.0	381 ± 48.9
(spl)	14.8 ± 3.0	178 ± 9.3	633 ± 69.0	404 ± 70.0
CFU-C (bm)	190 ± 29.0	246 ± 6.0	162 ± 10.8	195 ± 16.0
(spl)	4.2 ± 0.4	10.9 ± 1.1	16.4 ± 1.2	16.6 ± 1.4

[a]Experimental mice were about 6-weeks old at the beginning of the injection schedule, which was a subcutaneous injection of 4 U of rHuEpo/g body weight three times a week for 4 weeks. Analyses were done two days after the last injection.
[b]Number of colonies/10^5 bone marrow or spleen cells.

of CFU-E and CFU-C progenitor cells[8] in the bone marrow and spleen of B6 mice and decreased the incidence of BFU-E and CFU-E in the spleen of β-thal mice (TABLE 2).

Administration of 4 U of Epo/g body weight three times a week for 8 weeks was a lethal dose to B6 mice. Although β-thal mice survived this regimen of Epo injections, the hematological indices in β-thal mice following 8 weeks of Epo injections were similar to those already noted following 4 weeks of Epo (TABLE 2).

When the same serum samples were analyzed for Epo both by RIA and ESA, the results from both assays were well correlated. Young B6 mice, in which the erythroid system is expanding rapidly, had higher levels of Epo in their serum than older B6 mice (TABLE 1). The serum level of Epo in β-thal mice at all ages was significantly higher than that of B6 congenic controls. Young β-thal mice, in which the erythroid system is rapidly expanding, and mature β-thal mice, in which anemia becomes severe,[3] have higher serum levels of Epo than young adult (2–3 months old) β-thal mice.

Data in TABLE 1 show that β-thal mice have an increased production of Epo, which upregulates erythropoiesis. Administration of exogenous Epo to β-thal mice reduced the anemia by stimulating the production of an increased number of microcytic RBC to the point where the HGB and HCT values in β-thal mice that received Epo injections became comparable to those in normal B6 mice (TABLE 2). The WBC and RETIC values were reduced in Epo-treated β-thal mice compared to nontreated β-thal mice, but the values remained significantly higher than in normal mice.

Normal mice have two active adult β-globin genes. The 5' β-dmajor gene encodes ~80% and the 3' β-dminor gene encodes ~20% of the β-globin in normal mice.[9] In β-thal mice the β-dmajor globin gene has been deleted and the β-dminor globin gene is upregulated so 2.5 times the amount of β-dminor globin is produced in β-thal mice as compared to normal DBA/2 mice in which the deletion occurred.[10] Expression of the β-dminor globin gene is also elevated in mice with genetic anemias or made anemic through multiple phlebotomy[11] in the same way that expression of the γ-globin genes are elevated in humans with anemias of genetic or pathological origin. Human γ-globin genes have shown modest upregulation following the use of cytoxic drugs that induce anemia.[12] If upregulation of the γ-globin genes results from production of Epo, administration of rHuEpo to β-thalassemia and sickle cell anemia patients might increase HbF production.

REFERENCES

1. KRANTZ, S. B. 1991. Erythropoietin. Blood **77**: 419–434.
2. MANOR, D., E. FIBACH, A. GOLDFARB & E. A. RACHMILEWITZ. 1986. Erythropoietin activity in the serum of beta thalassemic patients. Scand. J. Haematol. **37**: 221–228.
3. POPP, R. A., D. M. POPP, F. M. JOHNSON, L. C. SKOW & S. E. LEWIS. 1985. Hematology of a murine beta-thalassemia: A longitudinal study. Ann. N.Y. Acad. Sci. **445**: 432–444.
4. VAN WYCK, D. B., M. E. TANCER & R. A. POPP. 1987. Iron homeostasis in β-thalassemic mice. Blood **70**: 1462–1465.
5. GARCIA, J. F., S. N. EBBE, L. HOLLANDER, H. O. CUTTING, M. E. MILLER & E. P. CRONKITE. 1982. Radioimmunoassay of erythropoietin: circulating levels in normal and polycythemic human beings. J. Lab. Clin. Med. **99**: 624–635.
6. CLEMONS, G. K., D. DEMANINCOR, S. L. FITZSIMMONS & J. F. GARCIA. 1987. Immunoreactive erythropoietin studies in hypoxic rats and the role of the salivary glands. Exp. Hematol. **15**: 18–23.
7. KRYSTAL, G. 1983. A simple microassay for erythropoietin based on ^{3}H-thymidine incorporation into spleen cells from phenylhydrazine treated mice. Exp. Hematol. **11**: 649–660.
8. BOLCH, S. L., S. G. SHINPOCK, C. J. WAWRZYNIAK & R. A. POPP. 1989. A comparison of stem cell populations and hemoglobin switching in normal versus beta-thalassemic mice. Exp. Hematol. **17**: 340–343.
9. POPP, R. A., S. L. BOLCH, S. G. SHINPOCK & D. M. POPP. 1990. Expression of the globin genes and hematopoiesis in beta-thalassemic mice. Adv. Exp. Med. Bio. **271**: 161–176.

10. Skow, L. C., B. A. Burkart, F. M. Johnson, R. A. Popp, D. M. Popp. S. Z. Goldberg, W. F. Anderson, L. B. Barnett & S. E. Lewis. 1983. A mouse model for β-thalassemia. Cell **34**: 1043–1052.
11. Whitney, J. B., III. 1981. Sl/Sl^d and W/W^v adult mice have fetal and neonatal levels of mouse minor hemoglobin. Prog. Clin. Biol. Res. **134**: 281–285.
12. Neinhuis, A. W., T. J. Ley, R.K. Humphries, N. S. Young & G. Dover. 1985. Pharmacological manipulation of fetal hemoglobin synthesis in patients with severe β-thalassemia. Ann. N. Y. Acad. Sci. **445**: 198–211.

Increase in Hemoglobin Concentration during Therapy with Hydroxyurea in Cooley's Anemia

BEN R. SAXON, JOHN S. WAYE, AND NANCY F. OLIVIERI[a]

McMaster University Medical Centre, Hamilton, Ontario, and The
Hospital for Sick Children, Toronto, Ontario, Canada

Hydroxyurea increases fetal hemoglobin synthesis, and ameliorates the severity of clinical complications, in patients with sickle cell disease.[1] Case reports in small series have reported the use of hydroxyurea in patients with thalassemia noting no response, or only modest increases in hemoglobin concentration.[2] Several complications of untransfused thalassemia would benefit from a modest increase in total hemoglobin concentration of 2 to 3 g/dL, including extramedullary bone marrow expansion. Regular transfusions may prevent, or reduce the severity of, this complication in untransfused thalassemia, and have been used in the treatment of spinal cord compression as a result of extramedullary hematopoiesis.[3,4] This report describes the clinical and hematological response of a patient with homozygous β-thalassemia treated with 10 months of hydroxyurea.

CASE REPORT

The patient, born in Egypt to first cousins, was diagnosed at two years of age with homozygous β-thalassemia (C→A substitution at nucleotide 848 the second intervening sequence of the β-globin gene; normal α genotype). He had received a single transfusion at age 1 year, and had undergone splenectomy at age 7 years. Following this, he maintained steady-state hemoglobin concentrations between 7 and 7.5 g/dL, and absolute fetal hemoglobin concentrations of approximately 5 g/dL. His clinical course was complicated by bone pain associated with cortical thickening, evidence of paraspinal extramedullary hematopoiesis, and progressive hepatic iron loading. Previous therapy with sodium phenylbutyrate, 10 g/m^2 body surface area, per day, was ineffective in increasing fetal or total hemoglobin concentrations. This therapy was discontinued because of poor tolerance in the patient.

Hydroxyurea (begun at an initial dose of 9 mg/kg body weight final maximum tolerated dose 11.4 mg/kg body weight) was initiated to reduce extramedullary hematopoiesis in the paraspinal region identified by magnetic resonance imaging. Over 10 months, hydroxyurea induced an increase in absolute fetal hemoglobin to 7.6 g/dL, inducing a rise in steady-state hemoglobin concentrations to 9 to 10 g/dL. In parallel, nucleated red blood cell count and unconjugated bilirubin concentration decreased, consistent with reduction in ineffective erythropoiesis. As evaluated by magnetic resonance imaging, paraspinal extramedullary hematopoiesis regressed, and bone pain improved, over 10 months of therapy. At doses up

[a]Address for correspondence: Dr. Nancy F. Olivieri, Division of Hematology/Oncology, The Hospital for Sick Children, 555 University Avenue, Toronto, Ontario, Canada M5G 1X8; Tel: 416-813-6823; fax: 416-813-5346; e-mail: noliv@sickkids.on.ca

to approximately 12 mg/kg/day, drug toxicity was limited to occasional declines in absolute neutrophil counts to less than 2000/μL, which increased after temporary interruptions of therapy. Increases in hydroxyurea to doses at or exceeding 15 mg/kg body weight per day resulted in recurrent declines in total hemoglobin concentration and reticulocyte count, necessitating careful titration of dose to balance the effectiveness and toxicity of hydroxyurea.

DISCUSSION

The C→A substitution at nucleotide 848 of the second intervening sequence of the β-globin gene affects the splicing of the IVS-2 acceptor consensus sequence, and has been reported in homozygous Egyptians with nontransfusion-dependent β-thalassemia,[5] associated with the A→G substitution at position -29 of the β-globin gene in a black patient,[6] and associated with the frameshift mutation at codon 8 and 9, in a transfusion-dependent patient from Iran[7] and in a homozygous Tunisian with the phenotype of β-thalassemia major.[8] Homozygous Egyptian patients, and the compound heterozygous black patient, had clinical and hematologic parameters similar to those of our patient, who is homozygous for this mutation. C→G substitution at nucleotide 848 has also been described in a heterozygote for thalassemia in Japan.[9] It would be interesting to determine if patients such as these with identical or similar mutations have similar responses to hydroxyurea therapy, as response to the two therapies to augment fetal hemoglobin concentration may be related to genotype in thalassemia major.

In summary, during hydroxyurea therapy in this patient, hemoglobin concentrations increased, in parallel with declines in normoblast count, indicating improvement in ineffective erythropoiesis. In parallel, almost complete clinical and radiologic resolution of the symptoms, signs and imaging of extramedullary hematopoiesis was noted. Prospective clinical trials with hydroxyurea, at doses lower than those previously reported to induce hematologic toxicity, are indicated to examine the effectiveness of this treatment in patients with thalassemia.

REFERENCES

1. CHARACHE, S. F., B. BARTON, R. D. MOORE, et al. 1996. Hydroxyurea and sickle cell anemia. Medicine **75**(6): 300–326.
2. OLIVIERI, N. F. 1996. Reactivation of fetal hemoglobin in patients with thalassemia. Sem. Hematol. **33**: 24–42.
3. ANSELM, C. W., K. S. TAI, V. WONG, et al. 1996. Hypertransfusion for spinal cord compression secondary to extramedullary hematopoiesis. Ped. Hematol./Oncol. **13**: 89–94.
4. MANCUSO, P., A. ZINGALE, L. BASILE, et al. 1993. Cauda equina compression syndrome in a patient affected by thalassemia intermedia: Complete regression with blood transfusion therapy. Child's Nerv. Syst. **9**: 440–441.
5. HUSSEIN, I. R., S. A. TEMTAMY, A. EL-BESHLAWY, et al. 1993. Molecular characterization of beta-thalassemia in Egyptians. Human Mutation **2**(1): 48–52.
6. GONZALEZ-REDONDO J. M., T. A. STOMING, K. D. LANCLOS, et al. 1988. Clinical and genetic heterogeneity in black patients with homozygous β-thalassemia from the southeastern United States. Blood **72**(3): 1007–1014.
7. WONG, C., S. E. ANTONARAKIS, S. C. GOFF, et al. 1989. β-thalassemia due to two novel nucleotide substitutions in consensus acceptor splice sequences of the β-globin gene. Blood **73**: 914–918.
8. FATTOUM, S., F. GUERMIRA, C. ONER, et al. 1991. β-thalassemia, Hb S-β-thalassemia and sickle cell anemia among Tunisians. Hemoglobin **15**: 11–21.
9. WAKAMATSU, C., M. ICHINOSE, J. MANABE, et al. 1994. Molecular basis of beta-thalassaemia in Japan: Heterogeneity and origins of mutations. Acta Haematologica **91**(3): 136–143.

Preliminary Report: Hydroxyurea Produces Significant Clinical Response in Thalassemia Intermedia

LORI STYLES,[a,c] BRADLEY LEWIS,[b] DRU FOOTE,[a] LEZLEE CUDA,[b] AND ELLIOTT P. VICHINSKY[a]

[a]*Department of Hematology/Oncology, Children's Hospital Oakland, 747 52nd Street, Oakland, California 94609, USA*

[b]*Department of Hematology/Oncology, Alta Bates Medical Center, Berkeley, California, USA*

Thalassemia intermedia patients have not received the scientific attention that transfusion-dependent thalassemia major patients have, yet this disease results in substantial morbidity and a decreased life expectancy. The incidence of thalassemia intermedia is increasing in North America due to increases in immigration from Southeast Asia and the emergence of Hb E-β thalassemia.[1] Though these patients are not transfusion dependent, frequent transfusions are often necessary, with resulting iron overload and the need for chelation. As new therapeutic strategies to raise total hemoglobin are proposed, thalassemia intermedia patients are a logical first choice for instituting experimental therapies. The fetal hemoglobin (Hb F) modulators are under investigation for use in patients with β thalassemias, but reports of their use in β thalassemia major have been mostly disappointing. The molecular defect in thalassemia major patients is likely too severe to allow the presently available Hb F modulators to make a clinically relevant difference for these patients. The use of Hb F modulators in thalassemia intermedia (especially Hb E-β thalassemia) patients has been less well studied. Published research to date indicates that Hb increases are transient and only modestly beneficial.[2-4] These reports, however, used doses of hydroxyurea (HU) generally applied to patients with other hemoglobinopathies and may be too high and may induce erythropoietic toxicity.

In an attempt to reduce or eliminate the need for transfusions in our thalassemia intermedia patients we have treated 4 patients (3 Hb E-β thalassemia and one with classic β thalassemia intermedia) with HU (10-15 mg/kg/day). The following summarizes these patients' clinical course:

Patient 1 was a 4-year-old boy with Hb E-β thalassemia whose Hb had dropped to 6.3 g/dL and in whom chronic transfusion was recommended. HU treatment resulted in an average increase in Hb of 1.2 to 7.5 g/dL. With the rise in Hb, spleen size also decreased from 7 cm pre-treatment to 3 cm on HU. Hb F levels increased from 36 to 51% on HU. The child's energy level increased and chronic transfusion was no longer felt to be clinically necessary.

[c]Address for correspondence: Lori Styles, M.D.; Tel: 510-428-3553; Fax: 510-450-5647; E-mail: lstyles@lanminds.com

Patient 2 was a 30-year-old woman with thalassemia intermedia who had not required transfusions until after delivering her first child at age 26. Since beginning transfusions she had required 120cc/kg/yr of PRBCs. She began HU immediately after receiving a transfusion for a Hb of 6.8g/dL. Her average Hb on HU is now 8.2 g/dL and she has not required a transfusion in almost 2 years. Hb F increased only 3% from 22 to 25% while on HU but her MCV increased from 65 to 90 fl.

Patient 3 was a 40-year-old man with Hb E-β thalassemia who required intermittent transfusions due to a Hb of 9 g/dL. He suffered from severe transfusional iron overload, hepatitis B and C, and had required emergent spinal radiation for extramedullary hematopoiesis. His Hb rose to 11 g/dL on HU with an increase in Hb F from 39% to 47% and MCV from 80 to 91 fl. He has not required transfusions for the year he has been on HU and his liver disease is stable.

Patient 4 was a 41-year-old man with Hb E-β thalassemia who required transfusions 4–5 times per year and subsequently had severe iron overload and hepatitis. He was treated with 10 mg/kg of HU and had little response in Hb (0.4 g/dL) and Hb F(0%) but an increase in MCV from 56 to 77 fl.

In summary, 3 of 4 thalassemia intermedia patients treated with low dose HU had a clinically significant increase in Hb, allowing them to avoid transfusion. No significant toxicity was observed, even in the three adults with liver disease. We, therefore, recommend that patients with thalassemia intermedia should be given a trial with HU to attempt to eliminate or decrease the need for transfusion and iron overload.

REFERENCES

1. MONZON, C. M. et al. 1986. Hereditary red cell disorders in Southeast Asian refugees and the effect on the prevalence of thalassemia disorders in the United States. Am. J. Med. Sci. **292**: 147–151.
2. HAJJAR, F. M. & H. A. PEARSON. 1994. Pharmacologic treatment of thalassemia intermedia with hydroxyurea. J. Pediatr. **125**: 490–492.
3. FUCHAROEN, S. et al. 1996. Hydroxyurea increases hemoglobin F levels and improves the effectiveness of erythropoiesis in β-thalassemia/Hemoglobin E disease. Blood **87**: 887–892.
4. ZENG, Y-T. et al. 1995. Hydroxyurea therapy in β-thalassemia intermedia: improvement in haematological parameters due to enhanced β-globin synthesis. Br. J. Haematol. **90**: 557–563.

Iron Overload and Antioxidant Status in Patients with β-Thalassemia Major

K. RELLER,[a] B. DRESOW,[a] M. COLLELL,[b] R. FISCHER,[a,e]
R. ENGELHARDT,[a] P. NIELSEN,[a] M. DÜRKEN,[c] C. POLITIS,[d]
AND A. PIGA[b]

[a]*Medizin. Biochemie, UKE-Universität Hamburg, Germany*

[b]*Centro Microcitemie, Università di Torino, Italy*

[c]*Kinderklinik, Universität Hamburg, Germany*

[d]*Hellenic Red Cross Blood Transfusion Centre, Athens, Greece*

In iron overload diseases as in thalassemia or genetic hemochromatosis, a low molecular weight iron, non-transferrin-bound iron (NTBI), is thought to cause the formation of highly reactive oxygen radicals that generate lipid peroxidation processes with subsequent development of tissue and organ damage. The molecular mechanism leading to such organ damage are not fully clarified, but have been mostly attributed to iron-induced lipid peroxidation (LPO), leading to a breakdown of biomembrane functions and finally to cell death. The long-term clinical consequences of this process are heart failure, liver fibrosis or cirrhosis, and endocrinopathies. An increased consumption of antioxidants may result from these disorders. In the present study we measured hematological iron parameters, NTBI and the status of endogenous antioxidants vitamin A, E and C. Its relation to the degree of iron overload was studied in 249 patients with ß-thalassemia major (ages 4–38 year) from Italy, Greece and Germany.

Patients treated with deferoxamine (DFO: n = 209) and with deferiprone (DFP: n = 40) were admitted for SQUID biomagnetic liver susceptometry (BLS) with non-invasive assessment of liver and spleen iron concentration.[1] In order to calculate total body iron stores, organ volumes were determined by sonographical scanning. Blood samples were taken after overnight fasting and suspension of DFO treatment at least for 24 hours. Hematological iron parameters (serum iron, transferrin saturation, ferritin) were determined by routine laboratory methods. Serum NTBI was measured by HPLC according to a modified method of Singh *et al.*[2] In short, After addition of NTA and ultrafiltration of the Fe-NTA complex NTBI was measured by RP-HPLC with deferiprone (L1) in the eluent. Serum lipid soluble antioxidants vitamin E (Vit E) and A (Vit A) were measured simultaneously after lipid extraction by RP-HPLC with UV and fluorescence detection. Serum vitamin C (Vit C) was determined by RP-HPLC using UV and electrochemical detection.

LIVER IRON, NTBI AND VITAMINS

Liver iron concentration measured by biomagnetometry (bLIC) was in the range of 170 to 11100 (median 1340) $\mu g/g_{liver}$. Taking into account the enlarged organ volumes (mean liver volume: 1581 ± 583 ml), total body iron stores were calculated in the range of 0.3 to

---

[e]Author for correspondence: Dr. Roland Fischer, UKE-Abt. Medizin. Biochemie, Martinistr. 52, D 20246 Hamburg, Germany; Tel.: +49-40-4717-3385; Fax: +49-40-4717-4797; E-mail: fischer@uke.uni-hamburg.de

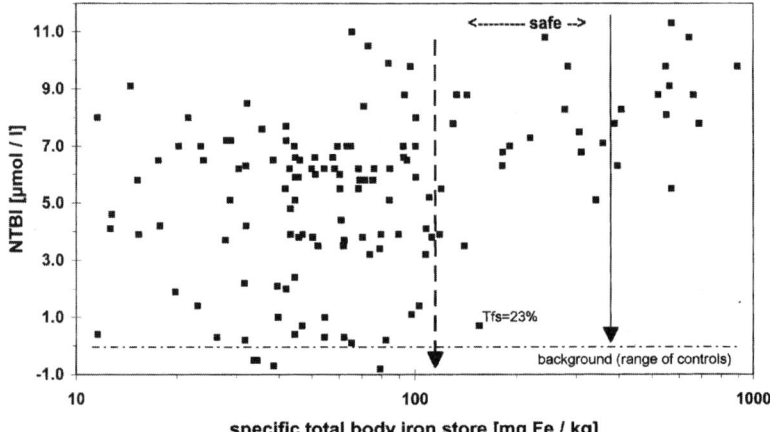

FIGURE 1. Non-transferrin-bound iron (NTBI) in patients with β-thalassemia major 24 hours after last s. c. deferoxamine treatment. *Arrows* at 380 mg Fe/kg and 120 mg Fe/kg indicate liver iron regions of low (safe) and high (risky) plasma NTBI levels.

39.0 g (median 2.5 g) assuming 80% of the total iron in liver and spleen. Hematological iron parameters (median; range) were elevated for serum ferritin (2186; 81–17519 µg/l), serum iron (225; 31–337 µg/dl) and transferrin saturation (77 %; range 10–100%).

The serum from thalassemic patients contained NTB-iron in the range of –0.8 to 13.9 µmol/L with a mean value of 5.4 ± 2.8 µmol/L. NTBI was increased significantly when the transferrin saturation exceeded 60% (r = 0.63; $p < 10^{-3}$). NTBI values correlated also significantly with liver iron concentrations and ferritin (r = 0.39 and 0.35; $p < 10^{-3}$). However, NTBI is not only a function of transferrin saturation, but seems to depend simultaneously from liver iron stores (linear bivariate regression analysis: r = 0.7; $p < 10^{-4}$). NTBI values > 3 µmol/L were found only above liver iron concentrations of 2000 $µg/g_{liver}$ corresponding with specific total body iron stores of more than 120 mg Fe/kg (FIG. 1).

Plasma levels of lipid soluble antioxidants were between 0.01 and 11.3 µg/ml for Vit E and 0.4 to 5.7 µg/ml for Vit A. Serum Vit C concentration of 0.1 to 25.2 µg/ml were observed in patients not substituted with oral vitamin preparations. Low antioxidant plasma levels were observed more often in severely iron loaded patients than in well chelated patients. Significant exponential relationships with liver iron concentration were found for vitamin C and E, but not for vitamin A. About 50% of patients with bLIC > 4000 $µg/g_{liver}$ had subnormal vitamin C and E concentrations. An inverse correlation between the vitamin E status of the patients and serum NTBI was observed (r = -0.43, $p < 10^{-3}$). Subnormal vitamin E plasma levels were observed especially for NTBI values beyond 5 µmol/L.

CONCLUSION

Iron overload, determined by non-invasive biomagnetic liver susceptometry, is associated with high transferrin saturation and high serum NTBI. This toxic iron fraction, not found in normal human blood is able to generate lipid peroxidation processes, with subsequent consumption of antioxidants, especially in patients beyond liver iron concentrations > 2000 µg/g$_{liver}$. This seems to agree with recent recommendations for an "optimal" hepatic iron concentration of 1000 to 2100 µg/g$_{w.w.}$ in patients with thalassemia major.[3] From this point of view, the limit of 380 mg Fe/kg[4] (equivalent to about 5000µg/g$_{liver}$), below which total body iron stores are considered relatively "safe," should be reduced to about 120 mg Fe/kg.

REFERENCES

1. FISCHER, R., A. PIGA, F. TRICTA, P. NIELSEN, R. ENGELHARDT, F. GAROFALO, A. DI PALMA & C. VULLO. 1997. The use of biomagnetic liver susceptometry in the Ferrara-Hamburg-Turin study on thalassemia. *In* Proceedings of the 10th International Conference on Biomagnetism, Santa Fe 96. Elsevier. In press.
2. SINGH, S., R. C. HIDER & J. B. PORTER. 1990. A direct method for quantification of non-transferrin-bound iron. Anal. Biochem. **186**: 320–323.
3. OLIVIERI, N. F. & G. M. BRITTENHAM. 1997. Iron-chelating therapy and the treatment of thalassemia. Blood **89**: 739–761.
4. MODELL, B. & V. BERDOUKAS. 1984. The Clinical Approach to Thalassaemia. Grune and Stratton. London.

Effect of Oral Iron Chelator L1 on Iron Absorption in Man

B. DRESOW,[a,c] R. FISCHER,[a] P. NIELSEN,[a] E. E. GABBE,[a] AND A. PIGA[b]

[a]*Medizin. Biochemie, UKE–Universität Hamburg, Germany*
[b]*Centro Microcitemie, Università di Torino, Italy*

In patients with transfusion-dependent iron overload like ß-thalassemia or sickle cell anemia the chelating and removing of excessive iron is an important part of treatment. In recent years the oral active iron chelator 1,2-dimethyl-3-hydroxypyrid-4-one (Deferriprone, L1) has been applied in many clinical trials in such patients with transfusion-dependent iron overload. To prove whether the efficacy of this chelator is hampered by an interaction with iron from nutritional sources and to elucidate the benefit of L1 after acute iron poisoning we studied the influence of single L1 doses on iron absorption from oral [^{59}Fe]-ferrous ascorbate in two healthy male subjects.

After overnight fasting L1 (35 mg/kg) and/or [^{59}Fe]$^{2+}$-ascorbate (50mg Fe, 0.5-1.0 µCi) were ingested in a series of 6 tests: L1 alone, Fe alone, L1 1.0 hour before Fe intake, L1 0.5 hour before Fe intake, simultaneous intake of L1 and Fe, and L1 1.0 hour after Fe. Blood samples were taken before and up to 4 and 24 hours after oral Fe/L1 ingestion. Urine was collected for 24 hours.

Liver iron was assessed by SQUID biomagnetic liver susceptometry[1] with liver iron concentrations of 300 and 450 µg/g$_{liver}$. Serum L1 was measured by RP-HPLC.[2] Serum iron was determined by the bathophenantroline standard procedure as recommended by the ICSH. Transferrin saturation has been calculated from serum iron and total iron-binding capacity. Serum ferritin was determined by IRMA. Urine iron was measured by atomic absorption

TABLE 1. Iron Absorption in Two Normal Subjects, A and B, after Oral Intake of [^{59}Fe]$^{2+}$-Ascorbate (50 mg Fe, 0.5–1.0 µCi) and/or L1 (35 mg/kg)

	Fe Absorbtion [%] SII		Calculated from ^{59}Fe	
	A	B	A	B
L1: alone	—	—	—	—
Fe: alone	9.7	8.4	9.0	8.0
L1/Fe: 1.0 h	12.7	8.1	—	—
L1/Fe: 0.5 h	5.2	2.2	2.8	—
L1 & Fe	—	—	1.3	0.6
Fe/L1: 1.0 h	—	—	5.7	6.0

Absorption was calculated from serum iron increase (SII) measurement and from [^{59}Fe] 14 days whole body retention.

[c]Author for correspondence: Dr. Bernd Dresow, UKE–Abt. Medizin. Biochemie, Martinistr. 52, D 20246 Hamburg, Germany; Tel.: +49-40-4717-2379; Fax: +49-40-4717-4797; E-mail: fischer @uke.uni-hamburg.de

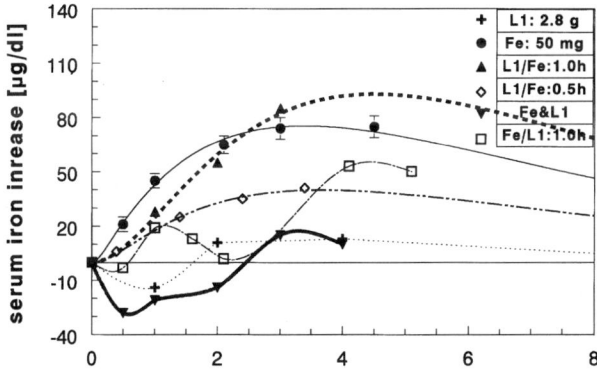

FIGURE 1. Serum iron kinetics in a normal subject after oral intake of $[^{59}Fe]^{2+}$-ascorbate (50 mg Fe, 0.5–1.0 µCi) and/or L1 (35mg/kg).

spectrometry (AAS) with graphite furnace technique. Iron absorption was determined from 14 days whole body retention measurements and/or was calculated from serum iron increase (SII) measurements analyzed by a single compartment model, respectively.

The mode of administration of L1 and iron had minor influence on L1 pharmacokinetic (L1 : Fe molar ratio = 20 : 1); maximum serum L1 values were detected between 30–60 minutes after oral intake. No changes in serum ferritin concentrations were observed during the 24 h period after L1 and L1/Fe intake. Changes in transferrin saturation demonstrate a mobilization of iron from transferrin after oral L1 ingestion.

L1 intake 1 hour before oral administration of a 50 mg Fe dose does not interfere with serum iron kinetics. L1 given only 30 minutes before iron administration is available in part for iron chelation in the gastrointestinal tract (TABLE 1). The L1-Fe complex is not absorbed. Co-administration of L1 and Fe completely inhibits iron absorption (FIG. 1). The chelator taken 1 hour after Fe ingestion is able to bind freshly absorbed Fe leading to an elevated urinary ^{59}Fe excretion.

CONCLUSION

In contrast to Stobie et al.[3] we found that L1 may be a useful antidote after acute iron poisoning. In conclusion we found that L1 not only eliminates iron from body iron stores but may also prevent iron absorption from nutritional sources. This may have interesting implications also for the chelation therapy with L1 and should be investigated further. Especially, in non-transfusion dependent patients with thalassemia intermedia the simultaneous administration of L1 together with meals could reduce the iron intake from intestinal absorption.

REFERENCES

1. FISCHER, R., R. ENGELHARDT, P. NIELSEN, E. E. GABBE, H. C. HEINRICH, W. H. SCHMIEGEL & D. WURBS. 1992. Liver iron quantification in the diagnosis and therapy control of iron overload patients. *In* Advances in Biomagnetism '91. M. Hoke, S. N. Erné, Y. C. Okada & G. L. Romani, Eds.: 585–588. Elsevier, Amsterdam.

2. DRESOW, B., R. FISCHER, G. E. JANKA & E. E. GABBE. 1995. HPLC-based measurement of the chelator 1,2-dimethyl-3-hydroxy-pyrid-4-one (L1) and its iron complex for pharmacokinetic studies in humans. Fresenius Z. Anal.Chem. **352**: 562–564.
3. STOBIE, S., J. TYBERG, D. MATSUI, D. FERNANDES, J. KLEIN, N. OLIVIERI, V. BENTUR & G. KOREN. 1993. Comparison of the pharmacokinetics of 1,2-dimethyl-3-hydroxypyrid-4-one (L1) in healthy volunteers, with and without co-administration of ferrous sulfate, to thalassemia patients. Int. J. Clin. Pharmacol. Ther. Toxicol. **31**: 602–605.

Survival and Morbidity in Transfusion-dependent Thalassemic Patients on Subcutaneous Desferrioxamine Chelation

Nearly Two Decades of Experience

E. M. CALLEJA,[a] J.Y. SHEN,[a] M. LESSER,[b] R.W. GRADY,[a] M.I. NEW,[a] AND P. J. GIARDINA[a,c]

[a]*Division of Pediatric Hematology, The New York Hospital/Cornell University Medical College, New York, New York*

[b]*Department of Biostatistics, North Shore University Hospital, Manhasset, New York*

Our improved management strategies for the treatment of thalassemia major were developed nearly two decades ago. In the mid 1970s we implemented the use of hypertransfusion and chelation therapy. We transfuse to maintain nearly normal pre-transfusion hemoglobin levels of (10.5 g/dL, and yearly red blood cell transfusion requirements of <200 ml/kg body weight are maintained with splenectomy. Time between transfusions is narrowed to 2 to 4 weeks. Iron chelation therapy is with subcutaneous desferrioxamine (S.C. DFO) which is recommended to be infused over an 8-hour period, a minimum of 5 days a week. We have conducted a prospective analysis of 88 patients monitored over the past 19 years to study the efficacy and limitations of our management strategies.

Patients are grouped according to date of birth, transfusion history, DFO use, and the date of starting DFO. At entry into the study, the patients ranged in age from 2 to 28 years. Group 1 includes patients born after 1980. Groups 2, 3, and 4 were born in each of the preceding decades. Group 1 received hypertransfusion from infancy and was begun on S.C. DFO at doses ranging from 20 to 60 mg/kg bodyweight (B.W.). Groups 2–4 began hypertransfusion therapy the year prior to starting S.C. DFO chelation at 20 mg/kg B.W. This dose was increased to 40 mg/kg B.W. after 4 years and 60 mg/kg B.W. after 8 years on study.

During the course of the study, 3 patients were lost to follow-up, 8 underwent bone marrow transplant (BMT), and 39 expired. All patients died from congestive heart failure, except for 2 who died of hepatic failure, 1 from hepatocellular carcinoma, and 5 from complications of AIDS.

Each patient was monitored, at entry or at last evaluation prior to BMT, death, or loss to follow-up, annually, for iron, hepatic, endocrine and cardiac status. Iron status was determined by documenting the total lifetime number of units of RBC's transfused and calculated for lifetime grams of iron per kg body weight. Mean quarterly serum ferritin levels were also obtained. Endocrine status was evaluated at entry and annually in each patient, using T3, T4, and TSH levels to test thyroid status, glucose tolerance test to monitor for diabetes mellitus, and Tanner staging to assess puberty. Cardiac evaluations

[c]Address correspondence to Patricia J. Giardina, M.D. at the Division of Pediatric Hematology/Oncology, The New York Hospital/Cornell Medical Center, 525 E. 68th St., New York, NY 10021; Tel: (212) 746-3415; Fax: (212) 746-8609.

included at entry or annually an electrocardiogram, echocardiogram, and 24 hour monitor. Hypothyroidism was defined by the presence of an elevated TSH. Diabetes mellitus and congestive heart failure were documented by the presence of clinical signs and symptoms.

Our analysis demonstrates that the incidence of hypothyroidism was 3% by age 10, 10% by age 15, 18% by age 15, and 29% by age 30. No patient developed clinical diabetes mellitus by 10 or 15 years of age. By 29 years of age, 8% had diabetes mellitus, and by 30 years of age, 30% had diabetes mellitus. The incidence of congestive heart failure was 0 by 10 years of age, 6% by 15 years of age, 28% by 20 years of age, and 53% by 30 years of age.

In those patients who began chelation therapy prior to the age of 13 and who had a minimum of four prior annual evaluations, the incidence of spontaneous puberty was found to be 34%. The development of spontaneous puberty correlated significantly with a rate of change of ferritin of -200 ng/ml/yr. Delayed puberty was associated with a rate of change of ferritin of $+283$ ng/ml/yr and was statistically significant.

Overall patient survival after 19 years of study analyzed with the Kaplan Meier Product Limit Method reveals an estimated median patient survival of 29 years, consistent with the estimated median survival of our 10 year study analysis.[1]

In summary, our management of thalassemia major with hypertransfusion and iron chelation using S.C. DFO has prevented morbidity and prolonged survival. 34% of our patients have achieved normal puberty. By the end of their third decade of life, 71% of all patients studied are free from hypothyroidism, 70% are without diabetes mellitus, and 47% have not developed CHF. Improved median survival in this population has been sustained.

REFERENCES

1. GIARDINA, P. J., R. W. GRADY, K. H. EHLERS, *et al.* Current therapy of Cooley's anemia: A decade of experience with subcutaneous desferrioxamine. Ann. N.Y. Acad. Sci. **612**: 275–285.

Regulation of Glucose Disturbances with Glibenclamide in Patients with Thalassemia

VASILIS LADIS,[a] CHARALAMBOS THEODORIDES,[b] FANI PALAMIDOU,[a] SPYROS FRISSIRAS,[a] HELEN BERDOUSI,[a] AND CHRISTOS KATTAMIS[a,c]

[a]*1st Department of Pediatrics, Thalassemia Unit, University of Athens, Greece*

[b]*Endocrine Clinic "A. Kyriakou" Children's Hospital, Athens, Greece*

Even with proper chelation, endocrinopathies including glucose disturbances are commonly seen in older thalassemic patients treated with frequent transfusions.[1] The severity, type and prevalence of disturbances of glucose metabolism vary in different series.[2-4] These differences are mainly due to heterogeneity in the composition of groups regarding age, clinical severity, genotype and, mainly, compliance with transfusion and chelation. In a cohort of 309 pubertal patients aged 12-25 years, followed in our unit, 30% were found with impaired glucose tolerance, and 5 % developed insulin dependent diabetes.[5]

The pathogenesis of glucose disturbances seems to be complex. In addition to insulin deficiency secondary to iron deposition in B cells, insulin resistance associated with hepatocellular dysfunction, as well as certain drugs (mainly hormones used for substitution treatment) may mediate the disturbances of glucose metabolism seen in thalassemic patients.[6-9] Also, the clinical and biochemical profile of glucose disturbances in thalassemic patients differs considerably from that of insulin dependent diabetes, type I, which is seen in young children.[10]

In this study we report our experience on the effectiveness of oral hypoglycemic agents in regulating glucose disturbances in thalassemic patients. These drugs act through induction of insulin secretion and enhancement of insulin sensitivity by increasing insulin receptors.[11-13] Response was determined by oral glucose tolerance test (OGTT).

Since 1982, 65 patients were found to have impaired glucose metabolism after OGTT and were considered candidates for glibenclamide (GLB) administration. Of these, 30 were excluded from further analysis, either because of a very short (< 1 year) period of treatment or loss of follow up, non-compliance or failure of treatment. In 7 patients treatment was considered ineffective as insulin therapy has to be initiated two to six months after GLB administration. In the remaining 35 patients (17 males, 18 females) with a mean age of 17.6 ± 2.78 years (range 12-25 years), effectiveness of treatment was followed by repeated OGTT twice a year, supplemented by weekly fasting blood glucose determinations. The period of effective treatment (ET) was estimated up to the last satisfactory OGTT. In 13 patients insulin response to hyperglycemia stimulation was also studied. Most of the patients were on hormone replacement therapy for hypogonadism. GLB was

[c]Corresponding Author: Christos Kattamis, Prof. of Pediatrics, 1st Department of Pediatrics, Athens University, St. Sophia's Children's Hospital, Athens, 115 27, Greece; Tel: -301 7794023, 7795762; Fax: -301 7795762; E-mail: ckatamis@atlas.uoa.ariadne-t.gr

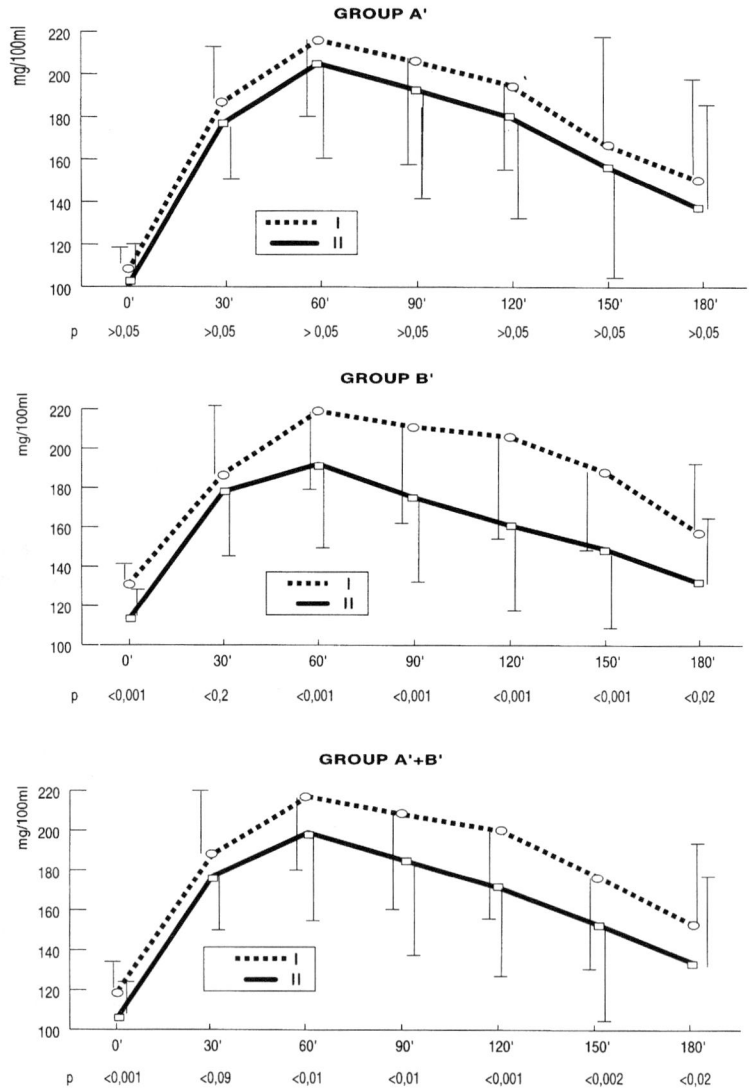

FIGURE 1. Mean blood glucose levels before GLB treatment (I) and at last effective OGTT (II).

given in minimal doses of 0.625 to 5 mg adjusted to patients' needs, supplemented with diet and physical exercise.

Results of OGTT of 35 patients (groups A and B) before GLB administration (I) and glucose values of last effective evaluation (II) are shown in FIGURE 1. After GLB administration glucose values were significantly reduced ($p < 0.01$) except that of 30 min. ($p > 0.05$) for a period of 13–109 months (M 54, SD 28.2). According to the severity of OGTT impairment, we further evaluated the effectiveness of GLB by classifying the patients into

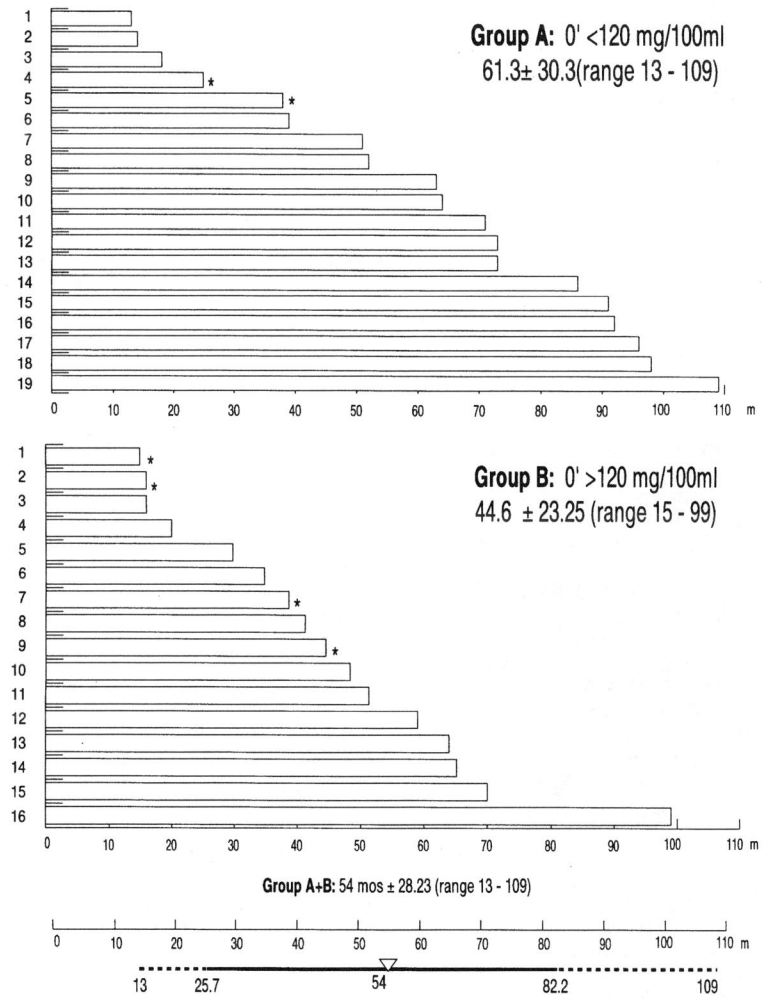

FIGURE 2. Duration of effective treatment with glibenclamide (in months).

two groups: Group A of 19 patients with mean age 17.3 ± 2.56 (13–24 years) and mild impairment (0 min. < 120, 120 min. > 140 mg/100 ml), and group B of 16 patients with mean age 18.1 ± 2.95 years (12–25 years) and severe impairment of OGTT (0 min. > 120, 120 min. > 140 mg/100 ml). In group A mean ferritin values were 2738 ng/ml as compared to 3595 in group B. Lower mean glucose values were found in both groups although the difference was statistically significant only in patients of group B ($p < 0.02$). Furthermore the period of effective treatment was longer for group A lasting from 13–109 months (61.3 ± 30.3), compared to group B lasting from 15–99 months with a mean of 44.6 ± 23.2 months, up to the last estimation (May 1997). Two patients of group A and four of group B, deteriorated and insulin treatment was started after 15 to 38 months All others are continuing oral antidiabetic therapy (FIG. 2).

The results of the pancreatic reserves observed after GLB treatment were interesting, showing three different patterns, namely that of delayed, moderate and high insulin response.

From the results of this study it is evident that oral antidiabetic drugs are effective in regulating the disturbances of glucose metabolism in patients with thalassemia for periods lasting up to 109 months or more. For better results early detection of glucose disturbances is necessary. This is achieved by routine OGTT in older thalassemic patients.

REFERENCES

1. GRUNDY, R. G., K. A. WOODS, M. O. SAVAGE & J. P. M. EVANS. 1994. Relationship of endocrinopathy to iron chelation status in young patients with thalassemia major. Arch. Dis. Child. **71**: 128–132.
2. SAUDEK, C. D., R. M. HEMM & C. M. PETERSON. 1977. Abnormal glucose tolerance in thalassemia major. Metabolism **26**: 43–52.
3. DE SANCTIS, V., M. G. ZURLO, E. SENESI, et al. 1988. Insulin dependent diabetes mellitus in thalassemia. Arch. Dis. Child. **63**: 58–62.
4. LADIS, V., C. THEODORIDES, C. ATHANASSAKI, et al. 1991. Disturbances and management of glucose metabolism in thalassemic patients. Abstracts of the 4th International Conference on Thalassemia and Hemoglobinopathies (Nice, France), p. 231.
5. KATTAMIS, C. & V. LADIS. 1997. Conventional Treatment of β-Thalassemia Syndroms: A personal experience. Int. J. Pediatr. Hematol. Oncol. **4**(5): 513–522.
6. DMOCHOWSKI, K., D. T. FINEGOOD, W. FRANCOMBE, et al. 1993. Factors determining glucose tolerance in patients with thalassemia major. J. Clin. Endocrinol. Metab. **77**: 478–483.
7. ZUPPINGER, K., B. MOLINARI, A. MINT, et al. 1979. Increased risk of diabetes mellitus in α-thalassemia major due to iron overload. Helv. Paediatr. Acta **34**: 197–207.
8. DANDONA, P., M. A. A. HUSSAIN, Z. VARGHESSE, et al. 1983. Insulin resistance and iron overload. Ann. Clin. Biochem. **20**: 77–79.
9. MERKEL, P. A., D. C. SIMONSON, S. A. AMIEL, et al. 1988. Insulin resistance and hyperinsulinemia in patients with thalassemia treated by hypertransfusion. N. Engl. J. Med. **318**: 809–814.
10. KATTAMIS, C. A. & A. C. KATTAMIS. 1995. Management of thalassemias: Growth and development, hormone substitution, vitamin supplementation, and vaccination. Semin. Hematol. **32**: 269–279.
11. LADIS, V., C. THEODORIDES, C. ATHANASSAKI, et al. 1993. A five year follow-up of glucose metabolism in apparently healthy teenage thalassemic patients. Abstracts of 5th International Conference on Thalassemia and the Haemoglobinopathies (Nicosia, Cyprus), p. 184.
12. SULLIVAN, D. J. O. & W. F. CASHMAN. 1970. Blood glucose variations and clinical experience with glibenclamide in diabetes mellitus. Br. Med. J. **2**: 572–574.
13. SARTOR, G., B. SCHERSTEN, S. CARLSTROM, et al. 1980. Ten-year follow-up of subjects with impaired glucose tolerance. Prevention of diabetes by tolbutamide and diet regulation. Diabetes **29**: 41–49.

Bone Metabolism in Thalassemia[a]

F. GAROFALO,[b] A. PIGA,[b,e] R. LALA,[c] S. CHIABOTTO,[c]
M. DI STEFANO,[d] AND G. C. ISAIA[d]

[b]*Centro Microcitemie, Dipartimento di Scienze Pediatriche e dell'Adolescenza, Universita di Torino, Italy*

[c]*Divisione di Endocrinologia, Azienda Ospedaliera O.I.R.M-S. Anna, Italy*

[d]*Dipartimento di Medicina Interna, Universita di Torino, Italy*

Thalassemia treatment improves increasingly: a regular transfusional regimen and a proper iron chelation are recognized to be the most important factors for a long and qualitatively good life perspective.[1] Even in the best treated patients, however, bone changes, growth failure and delayed puberty are commonly seen: in these subjects hormonal deficiencies, removal of bone minerals and iron deposition in the osteoblasts are the main factors thought to be involved so far.[2-5] Data about bone metabolism and densitometric behavior of prepubertal normal children are increasingly available. Little is known, however, on these parameters in prepubertal thalassemic patients. We have studied them in a selected population of prepubertal patients affected by β-thalassemia major.

PATIENTS AND METHODS

Since February 1995 we studied 27 prepubertal patients affected by thalassemia major, 12 females and 15 males, aged 8.1–14.9 years. All of them had been transfused at regular intervals since the 1st year of life to maintain a mean Hb of 12 g/dl (pretransfusion Hb=9.5, posttransfusion Hb=14.5), and all started chelation therapy after around 20 transfusions, with s.c. infusions of Desferrioxamine (DF) (20-50 mg/Kg daily). Compliance ranged between 71% and 100% (average 85%). One patient had been infused for three years with IV continuous DF at 50 mg/Kg/day. In 81% of the patients serum ferritin values always kept below 2500 ng/dl. Nine patients underwent splenectomy 2-7 years before the evaluation. In 8 patients growth hormone (GH) secretion after stimulation tests was checked, 1-4 years before the study, and it was found normal. None of the patients had any diet restriction nor any severe liver, thyroid, kidney, heart disease or diabetes mellitus. The study included yearly auxological examinations. The following parameters were checked: weight, height, growth velocity, body mass index and pubertal stage according to Tanner's standards[6]; Standard Deviation Scores (SDSs) for weight, height and height velocity have been calculated. In all of them calcium and phosphate homeostasis was evaluated by fasting serum calcium, magnesium and phosphate levels, parathormone (PTH), bone alkaline phosphatase (BAP), serum carboxyterminal propeptide of type 1 Procollagen (PICP) and serum carboxyterminal telopeptide of type 1 collagen (ICTP) measurements and 2-hour morning urinary deoxypyridinoline crosslinks, expressed as a ratio to urinary creatinine.

[a]Supported by grants from Italian MURST 40% and 60%.
[e]Author for correspondence: Dr. Antonio Piga, Piazza Polonia 94, 10126 Torino Italy; Tel: +39 1 1 3135291; Fax: +39 1 1 3135309; E-mail: piga@pediatria.unito.it

Auxological parameters and bone metabolism markers were also checked in 27 healthy prepubertal controls. Bone Mineral Content (BMC) and Bone Mineral Density (BMD) were checked at the lumbar spine and at the femoral neck by Dual x-ray Absorptiometry (DXA) technique, using a Hologic QDR 1000 densitometer (Hologic, inc., Waltham, M.A.). The lumbar values were compared to those of healthy age matched children, as reported in literature (7). Z score (SD from healthy age and sex matched subjects) were also calculated. All patients had undergone radiograms of the limbs to detect metaphyseal abnormalities within two years from the study, and 14 out of them had also X-rays of the column done. The association between parameters was determined by Pearson correlation coefficient and linear regression analyses. Means were compared by Student's test: p values less than 0.05 were considered statistically significant.

RESULTS

At the start of the study all patients were prepubertal (stage 1 according to Tanner), 4 females and 4 males, respectively above 13 and 13.5 years, showed pubertal retardation. A short stature ($\leq 3°$ centile) was found in 14 patients (51%), a reduced height velocity ($\leq 25°$centile) in 18 (67%), SDS values were also significantly reduced. Blood calcium, phosphorus and PTH were normal, bone synthesis (BAP and PICP) and reabsorption (ICTP and Crosslinks) markers were within the normal range. Mean lumbar BMD was 0.566 ± 0.040, definitely lower than the referral ones. Mean lumbar Z score was—2.138 ± 1.076, that is $\leq 2DS$ in 17 patients (68%) and only in 2 cases it was in the normal range. No differences in densitometric values were found between males and females. Morphological bone lesions like metaphyseal bone thickening and vertebral flattening were found in 23 patients (85%). Significant positive correlations were found between lumbar BMC and age ($p < 0.05$), lumbar and femur BMC and height and weight ($p < 0.01$), Z score and height and weight SDSs ($p < 0.01$); an inverse correlation was found between DF actual dose and height velocity ($p < 0.05$).

No correlation was found between the bone metabolite markers and the densitometric values, not any between the studied parameters and splenectomy, ferritin, Hb values or compliance with treatment.

DISCUSSION

A regular transfusional regimen and a proper iron chelation have improved life expectancy of patients suffering from β-thalassemia major.[1] Many of the clinical complications are nowadays less frequent or milder. However, bone changes and a delay in growth and sexual maturation, very common in the past, are still seen.[5] A recent review of growth patterns in thalassemic patients concluded that properly treated patients grow normally up to the age of 10–12 years, but that thereafter a relevant growth retardation is present.[8,9] The typical delay in sexual maturation, diabetes, hypothyroidism, parathyroid glands dysfunction, direct iron toxicity on osteoblasts and lack of GH or IGF1 have been indicated as possible causes in well treated patients.[2,3,5,6] Some authors found a bone mass reduction utilizing radiographic techniques or SPA radial densitometry[2,10] and a high rate of bone fractures was also reported.[10,11] These features seem to have been reduced with the new therapeutic regimens.[10]

Some sensitive techniques recently developed to measure bone mass parameters (BMD, BMC, Z and T scores) have shown that the bone mass of healthy prepubertal males and females progressively increases with age.[12] We have recently found that in children mean values of osteoblastic and osteoclastic activities, measured by recently recognized markers, i.e., urinary Crosslinks, BAP, PICP and ICTP, are higher than in adults (personal data, not published). Few data are available in literature about bone mass and metabolism in thalassemic prepubertal children. We studied a homogeneous group of prepubertal regularly transfused and chelated thalassemic children, whose iron overload has been always maintained relatively low. In this group we found a 85% prevalence of bone lesions and a 50% prevalence of short stature, and a reduced height velocity. This important feature is completely different from the osteopathy well known in poorly treated patients and in thalassemia intermedia[13]: in these conditions chronic anemia and bone marrow hyperplasia produce the typical clinical picture of thalassemia. In our patients the mean hemoglobin has been always in the normal range and no sign of bone marrow expansion has been detected. Furthermore thalassemic patients in the past were severely iron overloaded, whereas our subjects received what is generally thought to be the optimal chelation regimen. These data suggest that neither anemia nor iron overload but the iron chelation *per se* could be responsible for these bone alterations.

Iron chelation has been correlated to growth failure and bone abnormalities,[14,15] and a high desferrioxamine dosage has been indicated as the main factor[16,17] of cartilage alterations. We actually found an inverse correlation between height velocity and DF dosages, but this was surprising, as the dose range we have been prescribing for 12 years is considered safe, and it has been chosen mainly to prevent desferrioxamine side effects. This suggests that on a long term basis the daily DF administration, more than the dose, could be related to bone abnormalities. It raises important problems on the general management of this disease, as iron chelation is the cornerstone of the improvements in survival and quality of life.

Concerning the pathogenesis, our results exclude a marked abnormality of osteoblastic and osteoclastic activities. On the other hand the reduction of bone mass we observed in the prepubertal stage cannot be explained by endocrine abnormalities such as hypogonadism, hypothyroidism and hypoparathyroidism, so frequent in older patients.

These findings underline the need to reconsider the homeostasis of ions other than iron during chelating therapy. From the practical point of view a careful follow up of growth and bone parameters must be recommended in thalassemia. The use of drugs that inhibit the osteoclastic activity do not seem to have a rationale.

REFERENCES

1. GABUTTI, V. & A. PIGA. 1996. Results of long term iron-chelating therapy. Acta Haematol. **95**: 26–36.
2. DE VERNEJOUL, M. C. *et al.* 1982. Calcium phosphate metabolism and bone disease in patients with homozygous thalassemia. J. Clin. Endocrinol. Metabol. **54**: 276–281.
3. ANAPLIOTOU, M. L. *et al.* 1995. The contribution of hypogonadism to the development of osteoporosis in thalassemia major: New therapeutical approaches. Clin. Endocrinol. **42**: 279–287.
4. DIAMOND, T. *et al.* 1989. Osteoporosis in haemocromatosis: Iron excess, gonadal deficiency or other factors? Ann. Int. Med. **110**: 430–436.
5. JENSEN, C. E. *et al.* 1997. Incidence of enodcrine complications and clinical disease severity related to genotype analysis and iron overload in patients with beta-thalassaemia. Eur. J. Haematol. **59(2)**: 76–81.
6. TANNER, J. M. *et al.* 1965. Standards from birth to maturity for height, weight, height velocity and weight velocity: British Children, 1965. Arch. Dis. Child. **41**: 613–635.
7. GLASTRE, C. *et al.* 1990. Measurement of bone mineral content of the lumbar spine by Dual Energy X-Ray Absorptiometry in normal children: Correlations with growth parameters. J. Clin. Endocrinol. Metabol. **70**: 1330–1333.
8. PANTELAKIS, S. 1994. Growth patterns in patients with thalassemia major. Acta Paediatr. Suppl. **406**: 109–110.
9. DE SANCTIS, V. *et al.* 19943 Effect of different treatment regimens on linear growth and final height in β thalassemia major. Clin. Endocrinol. **40**: 91.

10. ORVIETO, R. *et al.* 1992. Bone density, mineral content, and cortical index in patients with thalassemia major and the correlation to their bone fractures, blood transfusions and the treatment with desferrioxamine. Calcif. Tissue Int. **50**: 397–399.
11. DINES, D. M. *et al.* 1976. Fractures in thalassemia. J. Bone Joint Surg. (**a**): 662–666.
12. FUJIMOTO, S. *et al.* 1995. Urinary pyridinoline and doexypyrydynoline in healthy children and in children with GH deficiency. J. Clin. Endocrinol. Metabol. **80**: 1922–1928.
13. WEATHERAL, D. J. & J. B. CLEGG. 1981. The thalassemia syndromes. Blackwell Scientific Publications. Oxford, UK.
14. PIGA, A. *et al.* 1988. High-dose desferrioxamine as a cause of growth failure in thalassemic patients. Eur. J. Haematol. **40**: 380–381.
15. RODDA, C. P. *et al.* 1995. Short stature in homozygous β-thalassemia is due to disproportionate truncal shortening. Clin. Endocrinol. **42**: 587–590.
16. BRILL, P. W. *et al.* 1991. Desferrioxamine-induced bone dysplasia in patients with thalassemia major. Am. J. Roetgenol. **156**: 561–565.
17. HATORI, M., J. SPARKMAN, C. C. TEIXEIRA, M. GRYNPAS, J. NERVINA, N. OLIVIERI & I. M. SHAPIRO. 1995. Effects of deferoxamine on chondrocyte alkaline phosphatase activity: Prooxidant role of deferoxamine in thalassemia. Calcif. Tissue Int. **57**: 229.

Selective Loss of Anterior Pituitary Volume with Severe Pituitary-Gonadal Insufficiency in Poorly Compliant Male Thalassemic Patients with Pubertal Arrest

R. CHATTERJEE,[a] M. KATZ,[a] A. OATRIDGE,[c] G. M. BYDDER,[c] AND J. B. PORTER[b]

[a]*Department of Reproductive Medicine,* [b]*Department of Haematology, University College London Hospitals, London, England*

[c]*Robert Steiner MRI unit, RPMS Hammersmith Hospital, London, England*

Transfusion dependent thalassemia patients compliant with Desferrioxamine are likely to have a low incidence of organ dysfunction, growth retardation and sexual maturation and are potentially fertile with or without hormonal support. However the complications of iron overload on the hypothalamic-pituitary-(H-P) axis due to gonadotrophin and growth hormone insufficiency still continue to be the primary cause of delayed or arrested growth and puberty.[1,2] Our previous studies shown that H-P insufficiency generally precedes the gonadal damage and is more severe in males than in females at corresponding levels of iron overloading.[3] It is potentially valuable to determine whether pituitary damage can be identified early using non-invasive magnetic resonance imaging (MRI) techniques to predict and monitor pubertal milestones carefully matched with clinical and biochemical parameters. In this study we aim to evaluate the effects of iron load on anterior and posterior pituitary volumes in patients with pubertal failure. An attempt is also made to compare biochemical markers of H-P-G dysfunction with anterior pituitary volume in thalassemic patients with those of the control subjects.

PATIENTS AND METHODS

A cross-sectional study was conducted in 7 poorly compliant transfusion-dependent thalassemia patients (6 major and 1 intermedia) aged 19-33 years who had grown normally but had pubertal failure. These patients had assessment of their H-P-G axis. Anterior pituitary function test was assessed by combined standard Gonadotrophin (GnRH), thyrotrophin, adrenocorticotrophic hormone tests. GnRH stimulation test was undertaken by using 100 µg dose of IV bolus GnRH and blood was sampled at 20 minute intervals for 3 hours and assayed for Follicle Stimulating Hormone (FSH), Luteinising hormone (LH). Gonadal function was assessed by Human Chorionic Gonadotrophin stimulation (HCG) test using 4000 IU of HCG and blood was sampled for 4 consecutive days after the injection for testosterone (T) assay. MRI Scan of the pituitary was done by using 3D T1 weighted volume scan using 1.6 mm slice thickness. Volumetric measurements of the anterior and the posterior pituitary were made and compared with 4 age and sex matched control subjects.

TABLE 1. Clinical Data in Male Patients with β-Thalassemia Major or Intermedia

Patients	Pubertal Stage	Gonad	Test. Volume Right	Test. Volume Left	Ear and Eye	Osteoporosis	Hepatitis C Status	Diabetes	Thyroid	Heart
AA	T1	G1	1 mL	1 mL	no	yes	neg	neg	no	no
AG	T2-T3	G3	4-6 mL	4-6 mL	ear problem	yes	neg	neg	no	pos
AD	T5	G3	4-6 mL	4-6 mL	N	yes	neg	pos	no	dysrhythmia
MM	T5	G3	6-8 mL	6-8 mL	N	yes	pos	neg	no	neg
RT	T5	G2-3	4-6 mL		N	yes	neg	neg	no	neg
RG	T1	G1	1 mL	1 mL	N	yes	neg	neg	no	neg
GC	T1	G1	1-2 mL	1-2 mL	N	yes	neg	neg	no	pos

TABLE 2. Hormonal data

Patients	FSH	PRL	LH	Testosterone	T4	TSH	PTH	Vitamin D	Vitamin A	DHEAS	SHBG
AA	<1	96	<1	0.3	normal	normal	3.3	36	N	normal	80 N
AG	3	108	4.5	0.5	normal	normal	N	N	N	normal	20
AD	<1	196	<1	1.8	normal	normal	N	N	N	normal	32 N
MM	<1	132	<1	2.0	normal	normal	N	N	N	normal	N 60
RT	<1	100	<1	0.8	normal	normal	N	N	N	normal	75
RG	<1	96	<1	1.4	normal	normal	8	13	N	normal	92
GC	<1	214	<1	1.4	normal	normal	N	N	N	normal	20

RESULTS AND ANALYSIS

Clinical details of all the patients and control subjects are give in TABLE 1. Five of the seven patients had pubertal failure (Tanner 1): testicular volume 1-2 ml), while 2 were arrested at midpuberty (Tanner stage 3; testicular volume 4-6 ml). and did not attain full sexual maturation. All patients had grown along 50th centile and were prescribed sex hormone replacement therapy to induce/complete sexual maturation. They continue to be on testosterone replacement therapy. Six patients had ferritin levels >3000 µg/L while in one ferritin level was >10 000 µg/L. These patients had variable degree of organ dysfunction and had osteopenia.

All patients had very low FSH and LH (<1-4 IU/l) levels and failed to respond to GnRH challenge test indicating severe gonadotrophin insufficiency. All had very low testosterone level (0.5-2 nmol/l) and 5/7 failed to respond to HCG test indicating primary testicular failure (TABLE 2).

MRI shows the anterior pituitary volumes of the patients to be statistically smaller than the controls ($p < 0.001$). However the posterior pituitary volumes of the patients were comparable to those of the controls indicating that posterior pituitary gland was spared (FIG. 1).

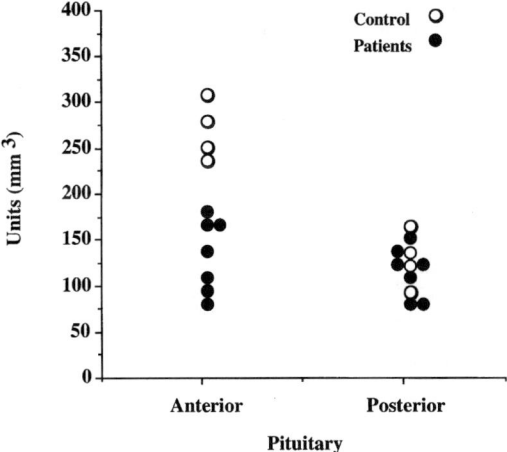

FIGURE 1. Pituitary volumes: patients vs controls.

DISCUSSION

This is the first report showing selective loss of anterior pituitary volume in poorly compliant thalassemia patients with pituitary-gonadal insufficiency, multiple endocrinopathy, organ damage, and pubertal failure. Similar loss of anterior pituitary volume has been documented in patients with congenital hypopituitarism.[4]

The exact cause of P-G insufficiency in these patients is unknown. Pituitary siderosis is the most likely cause[5] in this group of patients, since all were heavily iron overloaded.[6] However desferrioxamine, zinc and other factors have also been blamed for hypopituitarism in transfusion-dependent thalassemic.[7] Our patients had grown along the 50th centile and had normal growth hormone levels (both basal and following GHRH stimulation test) indicating that anterior pituitary damage was mainly restricted to the gonadotrophin compartment. This is in agreement with our previous study as well as others where hypogonadotrophic-hypogonadism were noted.[3,8] Since this can cause delay in onset, progression or completion of growth and sexual development, thalassemic patients should have careful monitoring or growth and pubertal development throughout childhood and adolescence by using clinical, biochemical markers. Since there was a positive correlation between biochemical markers of H-P insufficiency and structural marker (anterior pituitary volume), the non-invasive MRI scan can be useful in monitoring thalassemia patients with hypopituatrism. Further longitudinal studies are indicated to determine whether volume loss precedes derangement of biochemical markers of H-P-G dysfunction.

ACKNOWLEDGMENT

We wish to thank the UKTS (United Kingdom Thalassaemia Society) for their support with this manuscript.

REFERENCES

1. CHATTERJEE, R., M. KATZ, T. Y. F. COX, J. B. PORTER & H. M. BANTOCK. 1993. Evaluation of growth hormone in thalassaemic boys with failed puberty: Spontaneous vs. provocative test. Eur. J. Paediatric **152**: 721.
2. CHATTERJEE, R., M. KATZ, T. F. COX & J. B. PORTER. 1993. A prospective study of the H-P-G axis in thalassaemic patients who developed secondary amenorrhoea. Clin Endocrinol. **39**: 287.
3. CHATTERJEE, R. 1992. Ultradian gonadotrophin profile in beta thalassaemia major. Ph.D. thesis. University of London.
4. BROWN, R., V. BHATIA & E. HAYES. 1991. An apparent cluster of congenital hypopituitarism in central Massachusetts: MRI imaging and hormonal status. J. Clin. Endocrinol. Metab. **72**: 13–18.
5. BORGNA-PIGNETTI, C., P. DE STEFANO, C. VULLO et al. 1985. Growth and sexual maturation in thalassaemia major. J. Paediatric. **106**: 150–155.
6. BERGERON, C. & P. KOVACS. 1978. Pituitary siderosis. A histologic, immunocytologic and ultrastructural study. Am. J. Pathol. **93**: 295–309.
7. DE VIRGILLIS, S., M. CONGIA, F. FRAU et al. 1988. Desferrioxamine induced growth retardation in patients with thalassaemia major. J. Paediatric. **113**: 661–669.
8. WANG, C., S. C. TSO & D. TODD. 1989. hypogonadotrophic hypogonadism in severe beta thalassaemia. effect of chelation and pulsatile gonadotropin releasing hormone therapy. J. Clin. Endocrinol. Metab. **68**: 511–516.

A Trial to Investigate the Relationship between DFO Pharmacokinetics and Metabolism and DFO-Related Toxicity

J. B. PORTER,[a,c] A. FAHERTY,[a] L. STALLIBRASS,[b]
L. BROOKMAN,[b] I. HASSAN,[b] AND C. HOWES[b]

[a]*Department of Haematology, University College London, England*
[b]*Novartis Pharmaceuticals, Horsham, England*

The iron chelator Desferrioxamine (DFO) has been established as a safe, life-saving treatment for patients with iron overload. With the increased use of more intensive DFO regimens in the 1980s, a number of unwanted effects were observed, most notably high frequency sensorineural hearing loss, visual electroretinographic disturbances, and impaired growth and bone development. These effects have been largely associated with the use of high DFO doses in patients with relatively low degrees of iron overload as shown by a therapeutic (Porter) index of >0.025 (mean daily dose mg/kg divided by serum ferritin µg/L).[1,2,3] However, because serum ferritin can be an unreliable indicator of iron overload an additional independent method of identifying at risk patients would be desirable. In this study we have sought to establish whether there is an intrinsic difference in DFO metabolism between patients who have demonstrated evidence of previous DFO-related audiometric or retinographic toxicity compared with matched patients lacking these complications.

In previous preliminary studies a possible relationship between the proportion of metabolite B in relation to unmetabolized DFO and DFO toxicity was suggested.[4,5] We therefore considered it valuable to examine whether there is an intrinsic difference between DFO metabolism in patients with and without previous DFO-related audiovisual toxicity or whether this ratio is more a reflection of current iron overload status in relation to current chelation.

PATIENTS AND METHODS

Sixteen patients with homozygous β thalassemia age >14y < 45y who had previously received DFO for > 1 yr and had been shown to have audiometric and or electroretinographic DFO related toxicity (n = 8) or not to have these disturbances (n = 8) were selected. Ototoxicity was defined as high frequency bilateral sensorineural deficit of greater than 20db during pure tone auctiometry not attributable to middle ear disease.[2] Retinal toxicity was defined as previously.[6] Additional information about osteopenia, spinal bone densitometry L1-L4 in g/cm^2, spinal x-ray changes, growth history and crown-pubis/total height ratio % was obtained but not included in the stratification criteria (TABLE 1). The two groups

[c]Correspondence should be addressed to Dr. J. B. Porter, Reader and Consultant, Department of Haematology, University College London Hospitals, 98 Chenies Mews, London WC 1 E 6HX; Tel: 0171 209 6224; Fax: 0171 209 6222; E-mail: j.porter@ucl.ac.uk

were matched for serum ferritin (+ 500 µgL in the previous 12-month period). DFO was withheld for 72h prior to the study. Patients with active infections including hepatitis A, B and C, or significant organ dysfunction (renal, cardiac, pulmonary) were excluded.

We then asked whether during and following an infusion of DFO of 50mg/kg over 24h there was a significant difference in DFO metabolism between patients with and without previous DFO toxicity as defined by audiometric and or retinographic disturbances and whether DFO metabolism related to current iron status and chelation treatment as defined by the therapeutic (Porter) index.[2] Patients were admitted to hospital for 24h infusion of DFO (50mg/kg). Two consecutive 24h urine collections were made and blood samples for measurement of plasma DFO and metabolites were taken at time 0,2h,4h,7h,22h, and 24h. Blood samples were separated, stabilized using minor modifications to previously described methodology.[7] The protocol received full ethical committee approval at UCL Hospitals.

RESULTS

The patient and the DFO metabolism data are shown in TABLE 1. For brevity, only patients with marked spinal changes are denoted as "spinal X Ray" in the DFO effects column. It can be seen that although the proportion of metabolite B relative to FO (for analytical purposes "FO" = unmetabolized desferrioxamine plus ferrioxamine) is higher in the "toxicity" group, this does not reach statistical significance. Furthermore there is considerable overlap between these ratios in the two groups. It can be seen however that there is a correlation between the current therapeutic index in all patients and the ratio of metabolite B/FO AUC (Area Under the Curve) in plasma ($r = 0.6$) (FIG. 1) and in urine ($r = 0.4$). There is no correlation between spinal densitometry and DFO metabolism (TABLE 1).

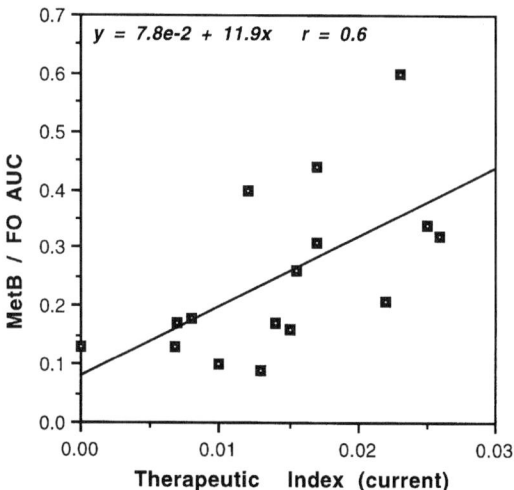

FIGURE 1. The relationship between the current therapeutic index as defined in the text and the ratio of metabolite B of DFO to unmetabolized DFO (FO+DFO) in plasma is shown, where AUC is the area under the curve for plasma values obtained during pharacokineticmeasurements for each patient.

TABLE 1.

Sex	Age	Ferritin µg/L	Therapeutic Index	DFO Effects	Spinal Dexa (g/cm²)	Patient Weight (kg)	FO (mg)	Urine[a] met B (mg)	met A (mg)	B/FO[b]	FO (µg/ml/L)	AUC met B (µg/ml/L)	B/FO
m	25	2379	0.008	Audio & Spinal X ray	1.14	83.0	715.1	497.8	35.1	0.70	240	43.9	0.183
f	29	1590	0.023	Audio & Spinal X ray	0.69	57.0	385.1	590.6	27.3	1.53	149	89.4	0.6
m	18	2801	0.0068	Audio & Spinal X ray	0.85	55.7	713.4	301.4	44.0	0.42	375	47.7	0.127
f	36	1553		Audio & Spinal X ray	0.88	45.2	366.9	389.8	68.5	1.06	274	36.3	0.132
f	33	1367	0.017	Audiometry	0.81	62.2	490.0	682.4	102.9	1.39	286	125	0.437
f	19	861	0.025	Autiometry	0.91	61.0	370.8	635.4	106.8	1.71	197	66.9	0.34
f	26	947	0.007	Audiometry	0.69	50.0	520.2	453.8	178.2	0.87	187	32.2	0.172
m	33	1520	0.022	ERG and Spinal X-Ray	0.77	55.8	611.3	369.3	40.6	0.60	378	77.9	0.206
Mean	27	1627.3	0.014		0.84	58.7	521.6	490	75.4	1.04	261	64.9	0.27
f	20	2297	0.017	none	0.73	56.0	353.5	395.9	16.3	1.12	145	45.5	0.314
m	21	2099	0.015	none	0.88	60.0	526.8	321.8	19.3	0.61	172	27.9	0.162
f	32	1877	0.0156	none	0.83	59.4	464.7	507.3	102.8	1.09	167	44.1	0.264
f	34	1820	0.026	none	0.84	50.0	297.0	281.1	47.2	0.95	104	33.1	0.318
f	25	1700	0.014	none	0.8	54.5	413.2	527.4	94.9	1.28	311	53.2	0.171
m	17	1794	0.01	spinal x-ray	0.87	40.0	617.0	224.8	94.4	0.36	225	23	0.102
m	18	3418	0.013	none	0.86	50.0	809.4	280.5	43.4	0.35	284	26	0.092
f	15	1865	0.012	spinal x-ray	0.95	60.0	140.7	194.3	26.7	1.38	179	70.9	0.396
Mean	23	2108	0.015		0.85	53.7	452.8	432	55.6	0.89	198	40.5	0.23

[a]Urine values represent cumulative amounts (mg) over the timecourse.
[b]B/FO is the ratio of metabolite B to ferrioxamine (FO).

DISCUSSION

The results show that there is a relationship between the current regular DFO treatment in respect to the degree of iron overload, as defined by the current therapeutic index[1,2] and the ratio of metabolite B to total FO (desferrioxamine plus ferrioxamine) in plasma or urine. This is consistent with the hypothesis that metabolite B of DFO, which is a product of the intracellular metabolism of iron free but not iron-bound DFO, inversely reflects the availability of iron in the plasma compartment. Thus in patients who receive a high amount of chelation, as mean daily dose of DFO in mg/kg, in relation to the iron stores, as reflected by serum ferritin in µg/L, the proportion of iron-free DFO which is available for metabolism is greater. Therefore the proportion ol'metabolite B is higher in urine or blood in patients who are relatively well chelated.

The finding that the ratio of metabolite B to FO in urine or plasma is not significantly different in patients with or without previous DFO toxicity, as defined by auditory or retinal disturbances, is most likely because the ratio of metabolite B to FO reflects the current state of iron availability at the time of the study, rather than any genetic predisposition to different DFO metabolism in the two groups. The patients chosen in this study all had demonstrable electroretinographic or audiometric disturbances at the time of the study but had developed these initially over 5 years previously and since then the treatment regimes had been adjusted. Thus "at risk" patients are those with a high therapeutic index[2] and a high ratio of B to FO at any point in time. However if the treatment regime is adjusted, the toxicity risk is corrected together with the therapeutic index and the ratio of metabolite B/FO. This study suggests that DFO metabolism as measured by B/FO is a surrogate marker for the availability of iron at any point in time, and could in principle be used to identify "at risk" patients. However the ratio B/FO only reflects the availability of chelatable iron, rather than an intrinsic qualitative difference in DFO metabolism in high risk patients.

It would be of potential value to examine prospectively the relationship between the ratio of B/FO in the urine of children with thalassemia on current relatively conservative chelation regimens compared with those employed in the 1980s. This would be of particular interest with regard to growth and bone changes. The latter were not included in the stratification criteria of this study although the patients in TABLE 1 showed these effects. However it is unlikely that inclusion of these as stratification criteria would have altered the outcome of this retrospective study because 2 patients in the "no toxicity" group although showing DFO related effects on growth and bone development do not show consistent differences from the "no toxicity" group with respect to B/FO ratios (TABLE 1).

It is also possible that B/FO measurement will be of particular value in patients where the serum ferritin is an especially unreliable index of iron overload status, such as patients with active hepatitis C and patients with sickle cell disorders. In these circumstances, because the ferritin can be elevated owing to factors independent of iron overload, the therapeutic index will be distorted. However, the ratio of B/FO should not be altered by these changes. It would thus be of value to examine the ratio of B/FO in patients with sickle disorders, particularly those in whom audio, or other, toxicity has been a recent problem. It would also be of value to examine B/FO in patients in whom poor growth or radiological changes associated with DFO over treatment has been a problem. For these studies to be clinically useful, it would be of value first to establish a reference range for the ratio of B/FO in urine of a larger number of patients without demonstrable DFO toxicity, as defined by absence of audiometric, retinographic, growth or skeletal clisturbances, using a simplified protocol which would be applicable to outpatients receiving standard doses of DFO and collecting urine over 24h.

In conclusion, this study suggests that the ratio of B/FO, plasma AUC or urine concentration, reflects the availability of chelatable iron, and hence risk from excess DFO treatment at the time the measurement is taken but that there is unlikely to be an inherent qualitative difference in DFO metabolism in "at risk" patients. Further prospective studies are indicated to determine whether this is of value in identifying "at risk" patients prospectively.

REFERENCES

1. PORTER, J. B. & E. R. HUEHNS. 1989. The toxic effects of desferrioxamine. Clin. Haem. **2**: 459–474.
2. PORTER, J. B., *et al.* 1989. Desferrioxamine ototoxicity: Evaluation of risk factors in thalassaemic patients and guicdlines for safe dosage. Brit. J. Haemat. **73**: 403–405.
3. OLIVIERI, N. F., *et al.* 1992. Growth failure and bony changes induced by deferroxamine. Am. J. Ped. Hematol./Onc. **14**(1): 48–56.
4. PORTER, J. B. *et al.* 1992. Osteopaenia thalassaemia major: The relevance of desferrioxamine drug metabolism. (abstract) 24th International Society of Haematology 1992, 184(7).
5. KRUCK, T. P. A. *et al.* 1993. A predictor for side effects in patients with Alzheimers disease treated with deferoxamine mesylate. Clin. Pharmacol. Ther. **53**: 30–7.
6. ARDEN, G. B. *et al.* 1989. Ocular changes in patients following long term desferrioxamine treatment. Brit. J. Opthal. **68**: 873–877.
7. LEE, P. *et al.* 1993. Intravenous infusion pharmacokinetics of Desferrioxamine in thalassaemia patients. Drug Metab. Dispos. **21**(4): 640–644.

Deferoxamine Stability in Intravenous Solution

C. ROSE,[a,c] C. CAMBIÉ,[b] G. FORZY,[a] M. MAHIEU,[a] P. FENAUX,[b]
AND F. BAUTERS[b]

[a]*Service de Médecine Interne, Hôpital StVincent, 59044 Lille, France*
[b]*Service des Maladies du Sang, CHU, 59037 Lille, France*

Deferoxamine (DF) is the only effective and widely available drug for the prevention of iron overload in multitransfused patients which has demonstrated an improvement in survival.[1] The introduction of new infusion pumps, minimally cumbersome and already containing DF made up in solution is a recent technical advance. This material is able to empty at a constant rate over a long period (maximum 7 days). However, little information exists on the stability of DF over long periods, in particular in common intravenous solutions. The manufacturer's recommendation is "DF solution should not be stored for longer than 24h at room temperature."[2] The aim of this study was to show the stability of DF in common intravenous solutions.

METHODS

Stability Studies

DF was reconstituted in two ways: 1g DF in 5ml solvent and 1g DF in 10ml solvent. These 2 solutions were both further diluted: 1) in saline and 2) in 5% dextrose in water. The 4 final solutions were immediately stored at once in a new infusor LVS 1.5 ml/h (Baxter-Health care, Deerfield, MA, USA) (24g DF in 250 ml) and the same time in a flexible infusion bag Macoflex (Macopharma Tourcoing, France) (9g DF in 50 ml) at 4°, 28°, and 37° C.

DF Analysis

DF concentration was determined by an HPLC method which used ciprofloxacin as the internal standard adapted from Koren[3–4] twice daily, in duplicate, for seven days and compared (%) to the day 0 concentration.

Results

At day 7, in all preparations tested, the DF concentration was 125% (median), range (94–131). There was no difference according to the type of infusor, storage temperature, or type of solution used (FIG. 1).

[c]Address correspondence to Dr. C. Rose, Services des Maladies du Sang, CHU, 1 place de Verdun, 59037 Lille, France; Tel: 33.3.20.44.42.90; Fax: 33.3.20.44.47.08.

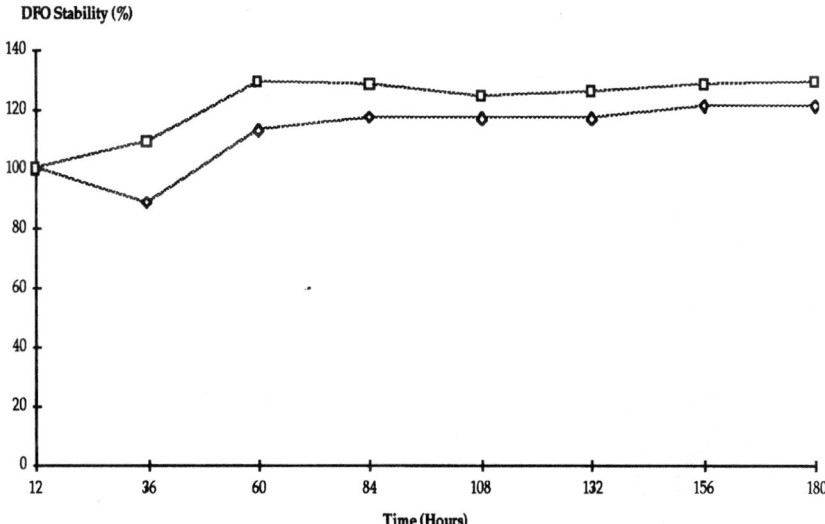

FIGURE 1. Stability of Deferoxamine in common intravenous solutions at 28°C in infusion bag: □ in saline; ◊ in 5% dextrose water.

CONCLUSION

DF is stable for at least seven days at high concentration (superior to 50 mg/kg/d) in common intravenous solution in various infusors and at various temperatures in particular at 28°C. In view of these results, wider use of continuous DF chelation during prolonged periods could be proposed. One preparation weekly could improve compliance and possibly reduce the risk of infection in teenagers and adults thalassemic patients. The continuous route (subcutaneous or intravenous) could improve efficacy, as recently demonstrated,[5,6] in severely iron overloaded patients.

REFERENCES

1. BRITTENHAM, G. M., P. M. GRIFFITH, A. W. NIENHUIS, C. E. MCLAREN, N. S. YOUNG, E. E. TUCKER, C. J. ALLEN, D. E. FARREL, & J. W. HARRIS. 1994. Efficacy of deferoxamine in preventing complications of iron overload in patients with thalassemia major. New. Engl. J. Med. **331**: 567–573.
2. BERDOUKAS, V. & S. J. YAWALKAR. 1994. Desferal. Medical and Pharmaceutical information. Ciba-Geigy Ltd. Basle, Switzerland. Editorial completion, February.
3. KOREN, G., A. TESORO, J. S. LEEDER, Y. BENTUR & N. OLIVIERI. 1990. Stability of aqueous solutions of deferoxamine. Canad. J. Hosp. Pharmacy **43**: 57–60.
4. TESORO, A., S. LEEDER & L. BENTURY. 1989. An HPLC method for the measurement of deferoxamine in body fluids. Drug. Monit. **11**: 463–470.
5. PORTE, J. B., R. D. ABEYSINGHE, L. MARSHALL, R. C. HIDER & S. SINGH. 1996. Kinetics of removal and reappearance of non transferin bound plasma iron with deferoxamine therapy. Blood **88**: 705–713.
6. ARAUJO, A., M. KOSARYAN, A. MC DOWELL, D. WICKENS, S. PURI, B. WONKE & A. V. HOFFBRAND. 1996. A novel delivery system for continuous desferrioxamine infusion in transfusional iron overload. Brit. J. Haematol. **93**: 835–837.

Nontransfusional Iron Overload in Thalassemia

Association with Hereditary Hemochromatosis

D. C. REES,[a] B. M. SINGH,[b] L. Y. LUO,[a] S. WICKRAMASINGHE,[c] AND S. L. THEIN[a,d]

[a]*MRC Molecular Haematology Unit, Institute of Molecular Medicine, Oxford, OX3 9DS, United Kingdom*

[b]*Wolverhampton Diabetes Centre, New Cross Hospital, Wolverhampton, United Kingdom*

[c]*Department of Haematology, Imperial College School of Medicine at St. Mary's, London, United Kingdom*

Hemochromatosis is inherited as an autosomal recessive trait and is manifested by excessive absorption of dietary iron in homozygotes leading to complications of iron overload and premature death.[1] In 1996 a candidate gene for hemochromatosis, HLA-H, was isolated.[2] A missense mutation that led to the substitution of a tyrosine for cysteine at codon 282 (Cys282Tyr) was identified in the vast majority of patients with hemochromatosis, 80 to 100% of patients with hemochromatosis being homozygous for the HLA-H Cys282Tyr allele.[2-5] A second mutation resulting in the substitution of aspartic acid for histidine at codon 63 (His63Asp)[2] was also identified but its role is uncertain. Recent surveys have shown that the Cys282Tyr allele is frequent in Northern Europeans with a frequency of 10% in some populations but rare in Africans and Asians.[6] Although the levels of serum ferritin, serum iron and transferrin saturation are higher than normal in heterozygotes for hemochromatosis, complications due to iron overload are extremely rare in these individuals.[7]

Apart from hereditary hemochromatosis, there are a number of other conditions in which nontransfusional iron loading occurs; these include sideroblastic anemia, porphyria cutanea tarda, the thalassemia syndromes, pyruvate kinase deficiency, and hereditary atransferrinemia. Among these, thalassemia is the only one that occurs commonly, prevalent in the tropical and sub-tropical regions.[8] Carriers for β thalassemia may have a very mild anemia but rarely iron overload; heterozygosity for β thalassemia also does not appear to accentuate iron loading in individuals homozygous or heterozygous for hemochromatosis.[9] Unlike heterozygous β thalassemia which is clinically asymptomatic, thalassemia intermedia is manifested by a symptomatic anemia associated with increased iron absorption, but regular transfusions are not necessary.[8,10]

[d]Address correspondence to: Dr. S. L. Thein, MRC Molecular Haematology Unit, Institute of Molecular Medicine, John Radcliffe Hospital, Headington, Oxford, OX3 9DS; Tel: 01865-222 411; Fax: 01865-222 500; E-mail: swee.thein@imm.ox.ac.uk

PATIENTS AND METHODS

Eighty-one patients (46 with two β-thalassemia alleles, six β-thalassemia heterozygotes with ααα/ααα or αα/ααα genotypes, six with dominantly inherited β thalassemia, and 23 with Hb E/β thalassemia) with a clinical diagnosis of thalassemia intermedia were studied. Their ages ranged from 10 to 65 years with the following ethnic mix: Asian Indian (58%), Middle Eastern (17%), Mediterranean (15%), English (7%) and Chinese (3%). None of the patients are on a regular transfusion regime.

Blood counts, reticulocyte counts, hemoglobin analysis, serum ferritin, and globin chain synthesis ratios were measured using standard methodology. Soluble transferrin receptor (sTfR) concentrations were measured using ELISA (R&D Systems, Minneapolis, MN, USA). Bone marrow fragments from the proband, aspirated as part of clinical diagnosis, were analyzed by electron microscopy.[11]

DNA was extracted from peripheral blood using standard methods. The Cys282Try and His63Asp mutations in the HLA-H gene were detected by restriction enzyme analysis of PCR-amplified DNA.[6] The Cys282Tyr mutation creates a new Rsa I site while the His63Asp mutation removes an Mbo I site. Deletional α and β thalassemia and rearrangement of the α and β globin gene complex were screened for by Southern blot hybridization. Point mutations causing β thalassemia were detected by sequence analysis of PCR-amplified β globin genes.[12]

RESULTS

The Cys282Tyr mutation was detected in only one of the 81 individuals with thalassemia intermedia.

The proband presented in 1975 at the age of 42 years with joint pains. Hepatomegaly was noted with hemoglobin (Hb) 9.8 g/dl, serum iron 44.1 mmol/L with 71% transferrin saturation. A diagnosis of thalassemia and gout was made. He was lost to follow-up but represented in 1981 with diabetes mellitus and was started on oral hypoglycemic agents, later needing insulin. Over the next decade, although his hemoglobin remained fairly stable, his ferritin level gradually increased with clear evidence of overload (TABLE 1). In 1994, his condition had worsened with a Hb of 6.5 g/dl and 9% reticulocytes; deep skin pigmentation and marked hepatosplenomegaly were noted. He was given a single blood transfusion for the first time. In 1995, aged 62 years, he had a splenectomy and liver biopsy; liver histology showed markedly increased iron (hepatic iron was 1.86% dry weight, normal < 0.13%), with a mixed distribution including features of both primary and secondary hemosiderosis. There was background hepatitis but auto-antibody screen was negative and there was no evidence of hepatitis A, B or C. Following splenectomy, his hemoglobin increased to 7–9 g/dl. He was started on subcutaneous desferrioxamine. In 1996 he suffered a myocardial infarction and received a second blood transfusion in an attempt to improve his myocardial oxygenation.

There is no family history of anemia, diabetes, hemochromatosis or arthritis. The proband was born in the Punjab, India, and had never been transfused until 1994 at the age of 61 years. He is married with four children, one of whom (daughter) was accessible for investigation.

Results of investigation are summarized in TABLE 2. The proband has a marked globin chain imbalance with an α/β globin chain synthesis ratio of 4.1, which is much more severe than that encountered in β-thalassemia trait. DNA analysis, however, could identify only a single β-thalassemia mutation (codon 41/42 -TCTT) but compound heterozygosity for a mild β thalassemia mutant is implicated from clinical, hematological and family stud-

TABLE 1. Serial Data on Iron Status of Proband[a]

Year	Hb (g/dl)	Serum Iron (μmol/L)	Serum Transferrin Saturation (%)	Serum Ferritin (μg/l)
1975	9.8	44.1	71	-
1991	6.7	-	-	677
1992	7.1	-	-	1600
1994	6.5	35.3	91.2	3120
1995	6.7	40.2	100	3246
1996	7.5	48	100	3826
Jan 1997	7.3	47	96	1191
Mar 1997	7.8	46	92	696

[a]Blood transfusions were given twice, once in 1994 and another, in July 1996. Iron chelation was started in October 1996.

ies. His daughter has mild but significant hypochromic microcytic red blood cells with an α/β globin chain synthesis ratio of 2.1, which is typical of β-thalassemia trait. However, extensive sequence analysis of the β-globin genes (from position -630 upstream of the mRNA cap site of the β globin gene to 290 bp downstream of the termination site including the whole β gene) showed only a single β-thalassemia allele in the father and no mutation in the daughter. DNA mapping of the α- and β-globin cluster in both father and daughter showed no deletions or rearrangements; in particular, there was no extra α-globin gene. Serum transferrin receptor (sTfR) level was markedly elevated in the proband, suggesting significant expansion of the erythron consistent with thalassemia intermedia, whereas normal levels were found in the daughter and mother. Electron microscopy of the father's bone marrow showed intraerythroblastic inclusions indistinguishable from the precipitated α-globin chains seen in β thalassemia. The proportion of erythroblast sections containing such inclusions (17%) was considerably higher than that in β-thalassemia trait and similar to that in the thalassemia intermedia syndromes caused by Hb E/β thalassemia.[11]

Both father and daughter were heterozygous for the Cys282Tyr mutation in the HLA-H gene; neither had the His63Asp minor mutation. The mother was normal for both HLA-H alleles.

TABLE 2. Summary of Hematological Data and HLA-H Status of Family Members

	Proband	Mother	Daughter	Normal Range
Age (yrs)	63	63	26	
Hb (g/dl)	7.8	14.0	14.2	
RBC (x 10¹²/L)	3.25	4.95	5.75	
MCV (fl)	73.6	83.2	73.8	
MCH (pg)	22.5	28.2	24.7	
MCV/RBC[a]		16.8	12.8	
% HbF	8.2	0.1	0.5	<1.0
%HbA2	5.6	2.0	2.8	<3.5
sTfR (ng/ml)	7.97	1.28	1.32	0.85–3.05
α/β Biosynthesis Ratio	4.1	-	2.1	0.9–1.2
Ferritin (mg/L)	3000	130	20	15–200
HLA-H genotype at codon 282	Cys/Tyr	Cys/Cys	Cys/Tyr	

[a]The ratio MCV/RBC has been proposed by Mentzer as a useful index for differentiating iron deficiency anemia from thalassemia trait. A value of < 14 is supportive of heterozygous thalassemia.

DISCUSSION

It seems likely that the phenotype of thalassemia intermedia in the proband is produced by compound heterozygosity for the β° cod 41/42 (-4 bp), a common β-thalassemia mutation in Asian Indians,[10] and a mild β+ thalassemia allele which has not been identified. Such uncharacterized β-thalassemia mutations have been described, some of which may not be linked to the β-globin complex.[12] Other possible diagnoses for the unusually severe anemia in the proband, such as congenital dyserythropoietic anemia and sideroblastic anemia, are excluded by the electron microscopy findings.

Although excessive iron absorption is well described in untransfused thalassemia intermedia,[13] there are few reports of such individuals developing the complications of severe iron overload as seen in our patient. Certainly the majority of thalassemia intermedia patients present with symptoms of anemia unlike the proband whose manner and age of presentation is typical of homozygous hereditary hemochromatosis.[14] The phenotype is completely different to that of hemochromatosis heterozygotes, who have moderately raised ferritin levels but no evidence of damaging iron deposition.[7] This is one of the first examples of the heterozygous state for hemochromatosis expressing a disease phenotype and appears to result from the interacting effects of the chronic anemia from ineffective erythropoiesis and the Cys282Tyr HLA-H mutation, supported by the mixed distribution of iron in the liver. The nature of the interaction between these alleles is unclear, as the mechanisms for excessive iron absorption in both conditions are not established.

The interaction between thalassemia intermedia and hereditary hemochromatosis must also occur in many other individuals, even if the populations in which these two traits are common do not coincide. A recent report has suggested that the HLA-H Cys282Tyr mutation is an important predisposing factor in spontaneous porphyria cutanea tarda.[15] Our study supports the emerging importance of genetic screening for hereditary hemochromatosis in other iron-loading conditions.

ACKNOWLEDGMENTS

We thank Liz Rose and Milly Graver for preparation of the manuscript and Professor Sir D. J. Weatherall for his continuing encouragement and support. D.C.R. is an M.R.C. Training Fellow.

REFERENCES

1. POWELL, L. W. et al. 1994. Primary iron overload. In Iron Metabolism in Health and Disease. J. H. Brock, J. W. Halliday, M. J. Pippard & L.W. Powell, Eds.: 227–270. Saunders. London.
2. FEDER, J. N. et al. 1996. A novel MHC class I-like gene is mutated in patients with hereditary haemochromatosis. Nature Genet. **13**: 399–408.
3. BEUTLER, E. et al. 1996. Mutation analysis in hereditary hemochromatosis. Blood Cell, Mole., Dis. **22**: 187–194.
4. JAZWINSKA, E. C. et al. 1996. Haemochromatosis and HLA-H. Nature Genet. **14**: 249–251.
5. JOUANOLLE, A. M. et al. 1996. Haemochromatosis and HLA-H. Nature Genet. **14**: 251–252.
6. MERRYWEATHER-CLARKE, A. T. et al. 1997. Global prevalence of putative haemochromatosis mutations. J. Med. Genet. **34**: 275–278.
7. BULAJ, Z. J. et al. 1996. Clinical and biochemical abnormalities in people heterozygous for hemachromatosis. N. Eng. J. Med. **335**: 1799–1805.
8. WEATHERALL, D. J. et al. 1981. The Thalassaemia Syndromes. Blackwell Scientific. Oxford.
9. EDWARDS, C. Q. et al. 1981. Coincidental nontransfusional iron overload and thalassemia minor: association with HLA-linked hemochromatosis. Blood **58**: 844–848.

10. THEIN, S. L. 1993. β-thalassaemia. *In* Baillière's Clinical Haematology. International Practice and Research: The Haemoglobinopathies. Vol 6. D. R. Higgs & D. J. Weatherall, Eds.: 151–176. Baillière Tindall. London.
11. WICKRAMASINGHE, S. N. *et al.* 1984. Globin chain precipitation, deranged iron metabolism and dyserythropoiesis in some thalassaemia syndromes. Haematologia **17**: 35–55.
12. THEIN, S. L. *et al.* 1993. β-thalassemia unlinked to the β-globin gene in an English family. Blood **82**: 961–967.
13. PIPPARD, M. J. *et al.* 1979. Iron absorption and loading in β-thalassaemia intermedia. Lancet **2**: 819–821.
14. WITTE, D. L. *et al.* 1996. Hereditary hemochromatosis. Clin. Chim. Acta **245**: 139–200.
15. ROBERTS, A. G. *et al.* 1997. Increased frequency of the haemochromatosis Cys282Tyr mutation in sporadic porphyria cutanea tarda. Lancet **349**: 321–323.

Mixed Chimerism after Bone Marrow Transplantation in Thalassemia

S. NESCI, M. MANNA, G. LUCARELLI, P. TONUCCI, M. DONATI,
O. BUFFI, F. AGOSTINELLI, AND M. ANDREANI

Divisione di Ematologia e Centro Trapianti di Midollo Osseo, Azienda Ospedaliera San Salvatore, Pesaro, Italy

Between December 1981 and December 1996 more than 800 patients received bone marrow transplantation (BMT) for homozygous β-thalassemia in the BMT Unit of Pesaro, Italy.[1] By RFLP-VNTR or FISH analysis we have evaluated the presence of mixed chimerism (MC) in 351 patients in order to determine which role MC plays in the transplant outcome of a non-malignant disease such as thalassemia. As already reported the presence of mixed chimerism is a frequent event after BMT[2]; analysis of 351 patients showed that MC was present in 98 patients (27.9%) within the first 2 months after the transplant, while it was respectively 13.6 and 10.6% at one or 2 years from the transplant. To determine which influence the pre-transplant treatment may have, we evaluated the incidence of MC in 6 different groups, according to the different conditioning regimens used. FIGURE 1 shows that the use of different protocols have a strong impact on the incidence of MC: higher doses of Busulfan and Cyclophosphamide produced lower incidence of MC, while the adding of the ALG contribute to increase the presence of residual host cells (RHC) in the recipients.[3] The presence of RHC in a transplanted patient represent a risk factor for graft failure. Twenty-nine percent of the patients that early after BMT showed the presence of MC rejected the graft within the first 2 years from the transplant, while none of the 233 patients that were complete chimeras rejected the transplant. In order to correlate graft failure with MC we established a grading of the RHC. Data showed that rejection occurred in 10 of 77 patients (12.9%) with MC-level 1, *i.e.*, an amount of RHC < 25% and in 19 of 21 patients (90%) with MC-level 2, *i.e.*, an amount of RHC > 25%. None of the 14 patients that showed presence of RHC for a period longer than 2 years rejected the transplant. These patients, that are considered persistent mixed chimeras had persistence of donor type β-globin chain synthesis and maintained hemoglobin levels between l0 g/dl and 13.5 g/dl. Three of these long-term persistent mixed chimeras, UPN 572, 322 and 688 with a follow up of 6, 7 and 5 years, respectively, have been further investigated.[4] FIGURE 2 demonstrates the levels of β-globin chain synthesis as determined by HPLC and the evolution of MC as evaluated by DNA analysis of VNTR-RFLP in patient UPN 688. Data showed that the proportion of donor/recipient cells both in the PB and in the BM was not constant over the time. Moreover this patient, 3 years after the transplant, showed a high proportion of donor cells in the PB and a high proportion of recipient cells in the BM. The level of Hb however ranged between 10 and 13 g/dl through all the post-transplant period. Similar results were observed in patient UPN 572 and UPN 322 although the proportion of RHC was equally distributed both in the PB and in the BM. To determine the donor/recipient origin of the different cellular lineages we analyzed the presence of MC in the different PB cell subsets and in the BFU-E and CFU-GM obtained from the BM of these 3 patients. We could not find differences in the donor/recipient origin of the PB cell subsets except that in patient UPN 688 who had different proportion of host type cells in lymphoid cells and granulocytes.

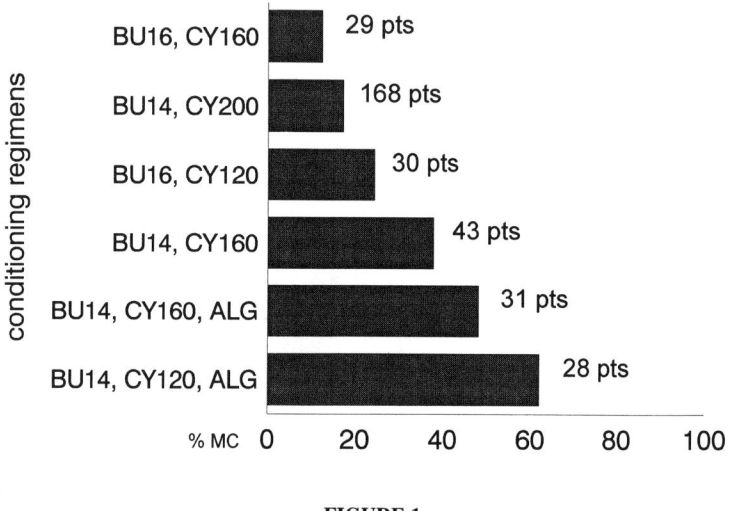

FIGURE 1.

PCR-VNTR analysis of pool or single picked BFUE or CFU-GM colonies showed similar donor/recipient cell distribution in the myeloid and erythroid compartment except that in UPN 572 where a sligthly larger proportion of host type cells in the erythroid precursors was observed. In conclusion we showed that MC is a frequent event in thalassemic transplanted patients, influenced by the different conditioning regimens. MC may be considered as a risk factor for graft rejection, even if graft failure is associated to the presence of large amount of RHC detected early after BMT. After 2 or more years from the transplant the

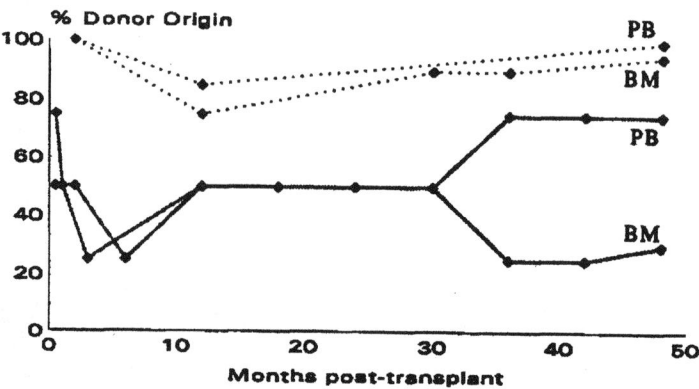

FIGURE 2.

presence of large amounts of RHC are no longer considered predictive of graft failure. Analysis of persistent mixed chimeras showed that the amount of donor/recipient cells is not always uniformly distributed in the different hematological lineages and that low amounts of donor cells in persistent mixed chimeras produce sufficient donor β-globin chain synthesis and hemoglobin levels.

REFERENCES

1. LUCARELLI, G., M. GALIMBERTI, P. POLCHI, E. ANGELUCCI, D. BARONCIANI, C. GIARDINI, P. POLITI, S. DURAZZI, P. MURETTO & F. ALBERTINI. 1990. Bone marrow transplantation in patients with thalassemia. N. Engl. J. Med. **322**: 417.
2. NESCI, S., M. MANNA, M. ANDREANI, P. FATTORINI, G. GRAZIOSI & G. LUCARELLI. 1992. Mixed chimerism in thalsassemic patients after bone marrow transplantation. Bone Marrow Transplant. **10**: 143.
3. MANNA, M., S. NESCI, M. ANDREANI, P. TONUCCI & G. LUCARELLI. 1993. Influence of the conditioning regimens on the incidence of mixed chimerism in thalassemic transplanted patients. Bone Marrow Transplant. **12**: 70.
4. ANDREANI, M., M. MANNA, G. LUCARELLI, P. TONUCCI, F. AGOSTINELLI, M. RIPALTI, S. RAPA, N. TALEVI, M. GALIMBERTI & S. NESCI. 1996. Persistence of mixed chimerism in patients transplanted for the treatment of thalassemia. Blood **87**: 8.

Bone Marrow Transplantation for Homozygous β-Thalassemia

The Memorial Sloan-Kettering Cancer Center Experience

FARID BOULAD,[a,c] PATRICIA GIARDINA,[b] ALFRED GILLIO,[a,d]
NANCY KERNAN,[a] TRUDY SMALL,[a] JOEL BROCHSTEIN,[a,d]
KAREN VAN SYCKLE,[a,e] DIANE GEORGE,[a] PAUL SZABOLCS,[a]
AND RICHARD J. O'REILLY[a]

[a]*Memorial Sloan-Kettering Cancer Center, New York, New York 10021*

[b]*Cornell University Medical Center—The New York Hospital, New York, New York*

Since the first report of bone marrow transplantation (BMT) for the treatment of homozygous β-thalassemia (HBT) in 1982 by Thomas et al.[1] several hundreds of patients have received such treatment, mostly by Lucarelli et al.[2] in Pesaro, Italy. The USA experience was recently reviewed by Walters et al.[3] and included 30 patients reported from six different centers in the United States. We report here the results of a single group of 13 patients who received marrow transplants at Memorial Sloan-Kettering Cancer Center (MSKCC).

PATIENTS AND METHODS

Between 02/83 and 04/96, 13 patients received allogeneic unmodified BMT at our institution for the treatment of HBT (TABLE 1). There were 10 males and 3 females aged 1.2–15.0 years (median 7.4 years). Ethnic groups included Chinese (n = 4), Indian/Pakistani (n = 3), Greek/Turkish (n = 3), Iranian (n = 2), and Italian (n = 1). Twelve patients received BMT from HLA-matched siblings (n = 10), or parents (n = 2), while one patient received a one antigen mismatched family donor graft. Based on the Lucarelli risk classification, with 9 patients having undergone a liver biopsy, 6 patients were class 1, 4 patients class 2 and 3 patients class 3. The four patients without liver biopsy were classified as class 1 (n = 2), class 2 (n = 1), or class 3 (n = 1) based on the presence of 0, 1, or 2 of the remaining two features of the Lucarelli classification (*i.e.*, hepatomegaly and poor chelation). Cytoreduction consisted of hyperfractionated total body irradiation (TBI) administered as 120 cGy twice daily for 3 consecutive days to a total of 720 cGy and cyclophosphamide (Cy) at 60 mg/kg/day × 2 days for 4 patients (1 class 1, 1 class 2 and 2 class 3) or busulfan (Bu) 3.5 m/kg/day × 4 days and Cy at 50 mg/kg/day × 4 days for 9 pts (5 class 1, 3 class 2

---

[c]Correspondence: Farid Boulad, M.D., Memorial Sloan-Kettering Cancer Center, 1275 York Avenue, New York, New York 10021; Tel: (212) 639 6684; Fax: (212) 717 3447; E-mail: bouladf@mskcc.org

[d]Drs. Alfred Gillio and Joel Brochstein are now at Tomorrows Children's Institute, Hackensack University Medical Center, Hackensack, New Jersey 07601.

[e]Ms. Karen Van Syckle is now at The Texas Children's Cancer Center, Houston, Texas.

TABLE 1. Patient Characteristics and Results of Marrow Transplantation for Thalassemia Major at MSKCC

N	Pre-BMT Demographics				BMT		Pre-BMT Disease Status				Post-BMT Status				
	Date BMT	Age BMT (years)	Sex	HLA Donor	Cyto-reduction	GvHD Proph.	Liver Size	Liver Biopsy	Chelation Ferritin	Class	ENGFT	GvHD	Chimerism % Donor	Outcome	Ferritin	HGB MCV
1	02/83	7.3	M	HLA = Sister	TBI/CY	MTX	> 2 cm	Fibrosis ++ Siderosis +++	Poor 3200	3	Yes	Acute grade 1 Chronic severe PS 80%	100%	Alive / Tx free Chronic hepatitis Sq Cell CA	5590	12.6 71
2	09/84	10.8	F	HLA 1(A) # Sister	TBI/CY	MTX	> 2 cm	Fibrosis + Siderosis +++	Poor -	3	Yes	Acute grade 2 resolved	77%	Alive / Tx free	318	12.6 95
3	05/85	6.7	M	HLA = sister	TBI/CY	MTX	< 2 cm	Not done	Good 1724	1 ?	Yes	0	80%	Alive / Tx free	248	9.6 79
4	07/86	6.8	M	HLA = Sister	TBI/CY	MTX CSA	< 2 cm	Not done	Poor 4620	2?	Yes	0	14%	Alive / Tx free	670	8.9 73
5	10/83	1.2	M.	HLA = Sibling	BU16/CY	MTX	< 2 cm	Not done	Good	1 ?	Yes	Acute grade 4 Lethal	N.E.	Expired	N.E.	N.E.
6	09/90	11.0	F	HLA = Father	BU14/CY	CSA Ster.	>2cm	Not done	Poor 3810	3 ?	Yes	Mild chronic resolved	100%	Alive/Tx free	611	10.1 67
7	09/90	7.4	M	HLA = brother	BU14/CY	CSA Ster.	< 2 cm	No fibrosis	Good 2350	1	No	N.E.	0%	Alive / Hyper Tx	N.E.	N.E.
8	01/91	10.1	M	HLA = Mother	BU14/CY	CSA Ster.	< 2 cm	Fibrosis + Siderosis ++	Poor 1941	2	Yes	Mild chronic resolved	99%	Alive / Tx free	545	11.7 65
9	05/92	8.5	M	HLA = Brother	BU14/CY	CSA MTX	< 2 cm	No fibrosis Siderosis ++	Good 3,660	1	Yes	0	mostly	Alive / Tx free	448	11.9 61
10	06/93	15.0	M	HLA = Sister	BU14/CY	CSA MTX	<2cm	No fibrosis Siderosis ++	Good 1250	1	Yes	liver+gut syndrome resolved	100%	Alive / Tx free PS 100%	4400	10.3 73
11	04/95	5.0	F	HLA= Sister	BU14/CY	CSA MTX	< 2cm	Fibrosis+/++	Good 4060	2	Yes	0	98%	Alive / Tx free	2480	10.3 69
12	02/96	11.5	M	HLA= Sister	BU14/CY	CSA MTX	<2cm	Fibrosis++ Siderosis ++ Cirrhosis +	Poor 3250	2+	Yes	0	100%	Alive / Tx free	3970	10.6 72
13	04/96	4.9	M	HLA= Brother	BU24/CY	CSA Ster.	<2cm	No fibrosis	Good 3330	1	Yes	0	100%	Alive / Tx free	2145	10.6 72

Abbreviations: BMT bone marrow transplant; Engt engraftment; GvHD graft-versus-host disease; Hgb hemoglobin; MCV mean corpuscular volume; M male; F female; HLA= HLA identical; HLA# HLA mismatched; TBI total body irradiation; CY cyclophosphamide, BU busulfan; CSA cyclosporin A; MTX methotrexate; Ster. Steroids; PS performance score; Tx transfusion.

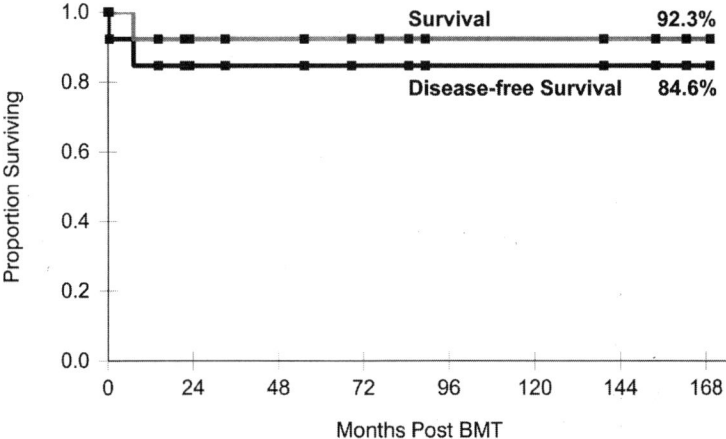

FIGURE 1. Kaplan Meier estimate of the overall probability of survival and disease-free survival for 13 patients with thalassemia major who received a BMT at MSKCC.

and 1 class 3). Two patients received a Bu/Cy regimen with a higher total dose of busulfan (16 and 24 mg instead of 14 mg). The patient who received a 1 antigen mismatched BMT was treated with hfTBI/Cy. Graft-versus-host disease (GvHD) prophylaxis was methotrexate (MTX) alone (n = 4), Cyclosporin A (CSA) and MTX (n = 5) or CSA and steroids (n =4). The median marrow graft cell dose was 2.9×10^8 total nucleated cells/kg (range 2.0–5.0).

RESULTS

As detailed in TABLE 1, twelve of 13 patients engrafted; one patient had a graft failure with autologous hematopoietic recovery after cytoreduction with Bu/Cy, and discontinuation of cyclosporin A because of a severe allergic reaction. Three patients developed acute GvHD, grade 1–2 for two patients while one patient developed grade 4 lethal GvHD. With a median follow-up of 75.9 months (range 13.6–171.1), twelve of 13 patients survive, 11 transfusion-free (FIG. 1). Two patients, both recipients of phenotypically matched parental grafts, developed localized chronic GvHD that has resolved, while one patient developed severe extensive chronic GvHD and subsequently developed a squamous cell carcinoma of the affected skin. This patient had received GvHD prophylaxis with methotrexate alone. Two patients have been found to be hepatitis C positive post-BMT, one of whom has chronic active hepatitis and extensive cGvHD.

For the 11 patients who engrafted and are alive, chimerism status was studied by fluorescent *in situ* hybridization (FISH) for recipients of sex-mismatched BMT and by restriction fragment length polymorphism (RFLP) for recipients of sex-matched BMT. Of seven recipients of sex-mismatched BMT, five have 100% donor cells on peripheral blood mononuclear cells (PBMC), one patient had greater than 75% donor cells and one patient had only 14% donor cells. All four recipients of sexmatched BMT had full donor chimerism by RFLP.

Seven patients have hemoglobin values greater than 10 g/dl, three patients have a hemoglobin ranging from 9–10 g/dl, all of whom are still 1–2 years post BMT undergoing phlebotomy. One patient, with 14% donor cells has a hemoglobin of 8.9 g/dl but is transfusion independent. Six patients have ferritin levels below 700 ng/ml (Nl = 14–179). Four patients with ferritin levels between 1500–4500 ng/ml are still undergoing phlebotomy, while one patient with a ferritin > 5,000 ng/ml also has chronic hepatitis C. Of the 11 patients who engrafted and are alive transfusion-free, all but one patient have a performance score of 100%; the remaining patient is the patient with extensive cGvHD, chronic active hepatitis and squamous cell carcinoma of the skin.

All four patients who received cytoreduction with TBI/Cy are alive transfusion-free including two patients with mixed chimerism and the one patient with 14% donor cells. The single patient with one HLA-antigen mismatched donor BMT is alive with no evidence of GvHD. Seven of the nine patients who received Bu/Cy are alive transfusion-free while one patient rejected his graft and one patient died from grade 4 acute GvHD. Four of the six class 1 patients are alive and well; the two treatment failures both received Bu/Cy and include one graft rejection and one death from GvHD. All four patients with class 2 disease are alive and well. All three patients with class 3 are alive with one of the three patients with severe chronic GvHD and squamous cell carcinoma of the skin.

DISCUSSION

The largest experience of BMT for HBT has been published by Lucarelli *et al.* with the Pesaro experience. A recent update described the results of 484 consecutive patients who received marrow transplants from HLA-matched siblings in Pesaro, with overall results of event-free survival of 98% for class 1, 87% for class 2, and 70% for class 3 patients, respectively.[2] Unfortunately, these results were not reproduced by other centers, albeit with smaller series of patients.[3–7] This report updates our experience of 13 patients transplanted at MSKCC to date. The survival and diseasefree survival of our group of patients are respectively 92.3% and 84.6%. Although this represents a small series of patients, and despite the fact that our series included 4 patients with class 2, and 3 patients with class 3 disease, these results compare favorably with the overall USA experience which revealed a probability of survival of 80% and EFS of 57%.[3]

Interestingly, four patients who received cytoreduction with TBI/Cy engrafted and are alive transfusion-free including 2 patients with class 3 disease. One patient developed chronic GvHD, but received methotrexate alone for prophylaxis; his squamous cell carcinoma of the skin was probably in association with chronic GvHD rather than TBI.[8] The one patient with mixed chimerism mostly of host origin is doing well transfusion-free; this mixed chimerism could be due to the fact that we used a rather low dose of hfTBI of 720 cGy rather than our standard 1375–1500 cGy. It is to be noted that the one patient who received a one antigen mismatched graft is also alive and transfusion-free following this cytoreduction.

This report describe the largest single center series of BMT for thalassemia in the US, with favorable results. Based on this small series, the use of a TBI-based regimen, possibly with a higher dose of TBI, may provide an alternative effective cytoreduction, particularly for those patients with more advanced stages of disease.

REFERENCES

1. THOMAS, E. D., C. D. BUCKNER, J. E. SANDERS, T. PAPAYANNOPOULOU, *et al.* 1982. Marrow transplantation for thalassaemia. Lancet **2**: 227–229.
2. GIARDINI, C. E. ANGELUCCI, G. LUCARELLI, *et al.* 1994. Bone marrow transplantation for thalassemia. Experience in Pesaro, Italy. Am. J. Pediatr. Hematol. Oncol. **16**: 6–10.
3. WALTERS, M. C., K. M. SULLIVAN, R. J. O'REILLY, F. BOULAD, *et al.* 1994. Bone marrow transplantation for thalassemia. The USA experience. Am. J. Pediatr. Hematol. Oncol. **16**: 11–17.

4. LIN, K. H. & K. S. LIN. 1989. Allogeneic bone marrow transplantation for thalassemia in Taiwan: Factors associated with graft failure. Am. J. Pediatr. Hematol. Oncol. **11**: 417–422.
5. OR, R., E. NAPARSTEK, G. CIVIDALLI, *et al.* 1988. Bone marrow transplantation in beta-thalassemia major: The Israeli experience. Hemoglobin **12**: 609–614.
6. HUGH–JONES, K., A. VELLODI, S. T. JONES, *et al.* 1989. Bone marrow transplantation for thalassemia: Westminster Children's Hospital and United Kingdom experience. Prog. Clin. Biol. Res. **309**: 201–205.
7. FRAPPAZ, D., E. GLUCKMAN, G. SOUILLET, *et al.* 1989. Bone marrow transplantation for thalassemia major: The French experience. Prog. Clin. Biol. Res. **309**: 207–216.
8. LISHNER, M., B. PATTERSON, R. KANDEL, *et al.* 1990. Cutaneous and mucosal neoplasms in bone marrow transplant recipients. Cancer **65**: 473–476.

Bone Marrow Transplant in Thalassemia

A Role for Radiation?

Y. S. LEE,[a,e] K. M. KRISTOVICH,[a] J. M. DUCORE,[b] E. VICHINSKY,[c]
V. L. CROUSE,[d] B. E. GLADER,[a] AND M. D. AMYLON[a]

[a]*Stanford University Medical Center, Stanford, California 94305, USA*

[b]*University of California at Davis, Sacramento, California 95817, USA*

[c]*Oakland Children's Hospital, Oakland, California 94609, USA*

[d]*Valley Children's Hospital, Fresno, California 93703, USA*

Bone marrow transplant (BMT) is the only curative therapy for patients with transfusion-dependent homozygous β-thalassemia. Dr. Lucarelli and his colleagues were among the first to apply this treatment modality. His most recent report summarized a total number of 546 patients who have received BMT from related donors.[1] Patients are classified according to the Lucarelli criteria. All class I/II patients received conditioning regimen of busulfan (Bu, 14 mg/kg) and cyclophosphamide (Cy, 200mg/kg). Young patients (< 16 years of age) with Lucarelli class I and II thalassemia have the probabilities of survival, event-free survival, non-rejection mortality and graft rejection rates of 95, 90, 5, and 5% (class 1) and 86, 82, 6, and 12% (class II). For class III patients, cyclophosphamide dose was decreased to 120-160 mg/kg owing to the high incidence of non-rejection mortality of 42%. This has resulted in a reduction of the mortality rate to 11 %, but the graft rejection rate increased from 9 to 29%. Similar results were also seen in other smaller series[2–5]; all used chemotherapy-only regimens with similar concern of graft rejection. The ideal conditioning regimen for thalassemia patients, especially class III, remains unclear.

Eleven patients with homozygous β-thalassemia (7) or hemoglobin E/β-thalassemia (4) underwent BMT at Stanford University Medical Center from 1987 to 1994. Six were southeast Asians, two middle easterners, one Indian, one Chinese, and one Latino. Four southeast Asians had transfusion-dependent hemoglobin E/β-thalassemia. In all cases, the donor was an HLA-identical sibling. The mean age at transplant was 8.4 years (range 2–18.9 years). Eight patients were categorized as class I and II and three patients as class III. For class I and II patients, the conditioning regimen was busulfan (16 mg/kg) and cyclophosphamide (200 mg/kg). For class III patients and for class I/II patients who fail the first transplant attempt, fractionated total body irradiation (FTBI, 1200 cGy) and cyclophosphamide (120 mg/kg) were used.

The result (TABLE 1) showed that for patients 1–8, Bu/Cy regimen was used in the first BMT. Patients received from 0.99 to 6.27×10^8/kg bone marrow–derived nucleated cells. The median neutrophil engraftment day was 17 days (range 11–28 days) and the median platelet engraftment day was 24 days (range 19–34 days). Five class I/II patients achieved full donor chimerism, two patients had mixed chimerism and one patient had autologous hematopoietic reconstitution. Two patients (one full donor chimera and one mixed chimera) lost their graft within six months following BMT and had autologous recovery.

[e]Address correspondence to: Y. S. Lee, MD, PhD at Stanford University Medical Center, Pediatric Hematology/Oncology, 300 Pasteur Drive, Stanford, CA 94305-5208; Tel: 650-723-5535; Fax: 650-723-5231.

TABLE 1.

Patient	Age year	Cell dose (10^8/kg)	ANC>500 (day)	Platelet>50K (day)	Graft outcome
Bu/Cy regimen					
(1st BMT, class I/II)					
1	2.0	1.22	16	20	mixed chimerism/loss
2	2.3	6.2	22	19	stable mixed chimerism
3	2.9	4.7	28	26	autologous recovery
4	4.8	2.17	16	19	full donor chimerism/loss
5	5.0	3.9	11	24	full donor chimerism
6	6.1	5.0	19	34	full donor chimerism
7	7.0	4.8	17	24	full donor chimerism
8	11.7	0.9	17	27	full donor chimerism
FTBI/Cy regimen					
(2nd BMT, class I/II)					
1	3.6	3.49	20	35	full donor chimerism
3	4.1	6.8	22	17	full donor chimerism
4	7.5	2.8	11	7	full donor chimerism
(1st BMT, class III)					
9	13.2	0.27	10	19	full donor chimerism
10	18.8	4.4	12	4	full donor chimerism
11	18.9	3.3	19	30	full donor chimerism

Class I/II thalassemia patients 1–8 received Bu/Cy conditioning regimen. The cell dose ranged from 0.99 to 6.27×10^8/kg bone marrow-derived nucleated cells. The median neutrophil engraftment day (ANC > 500/ul) was 17 days and the median platelet engraftment day was 24 days. Engraftment was not considered successful for patients 1–4, the youngest patients.

Patients 1, 3 and 4 eventually became transfusion-dependent again and received a second BMT using FTBI/Cy regimen 1.1–2.6 years after the first BMT attempt. The same donor was used as in the first BMT. Three class III patients also were transplanted with the radiation-containing regimen. All patients achieved full donor chimerism.

All three patients (1, 3 and 4) with autologous reconstitution were re-transplanted with FTBI/Cy 1.22.7 years after the first BMT, and all achieved full donor chimerism. Three class III patients also achieved full donor chimerism. No mixed chimeric states was ever documented in the FTBI/Cy group. There was no delay in the neutrophil and platelet engraftment time. All eleven patients are alive and transfusion-independent 2.5–9.7 years after BMT, Cyclosporine, methotrexate, and prednisone were used for graft-versus-host (GVHD) prophylaxis, and no patient had grade III-IV acute GVHD. One class III patient had extensive chronic GVHD of the skin and GI tract and is clinically stable on immunosuppressive treatment. All patients have a performance status of 80% or better.

Growth delay is one of the major concern for patients with thalassemia major. De Simone et al.[6] reported 22 thalassemic patients who were transplanted with the Bu/Cy regimen. In their study, patients older than 7 years old had persistent growth retardation (10/11) and younger patients had improvement 48 months after transplant (6/11). Most of our patients were transplanted during childhood or the peripubertal period. All continued to have normal growth measured by the linear height increment (FIG. 1). Of the three patients who received two BMTs, with radiation given in the second attempt, no plateauing of the growth curves were observed yet. There were two patients who were transplanted after puberty. One has achieved maximal height and no change in height was noted afterward. However, in the other patient, plateauing of height was noted and low growth hormone level was detected (pt. 9, FIG. 1). Accelerated growth developed after growth hormone therapy was initiated.

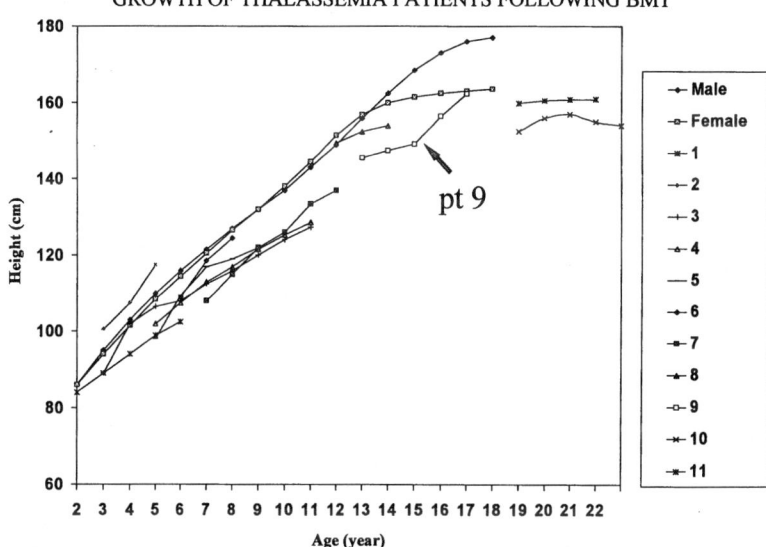

FIGURE 1. Many of the children with thalassemia are shorter than similar age Caucasian children prior to BMT. The reason for this are multifactorial and may relate to anemia, chelation therapy, and ethnicity. Regardless, following BMT, the rate of growth is normal and the growth paralleled the standard growth curves for Caucasian, male and female children. One patient (pt. 9) had a relatively flat rate of growth for two years following BMT; at which time he received growth hormone resulting in accelerated growth.

In transfusion-dependent thalassemia population, conditioning with Bu/Cy may not be sufficient for marrow ablation, as three of eight patients (all less than five years old) either failed to engraft or lost the graft shortly after BMT. Our data demonstrate that FTBI/Cy conditioning regimen can be performed safely in class III patients and in second transplants without excessive toxicity. These results support a possible role for radiation therapy and second transplants in patients with transfusion-dependent thalassemia syndromes.

REFERENCES

1. GIARDINI, C., M. GALIMBERTI & G. LUCARELLI. 1995. Bone marrow transplantation in thalassemia. Annu. Rev. Med. **46:** 319–330.
2. AVANI, S. H. & T. SAIKIA. 1994. Bone marrow transplantation in India. Bone Marrow Transplant. **13:** 731–732.
3. GHAVAMZADEH, A., M. JAHANI & E. BAYBORDI. 1994. Bone marrow transplantation in Iran. Bone Marrow Transplant. **13:** 743–744.
4. VELLODI, A., S. PICTON, C. J. DOWNIE *et al.* 1994. Bone marrow transplantation for thalassemia: Experience of two British centres. Bone Marrow Transplant. **13:** 559–562.
5. SOLH, H., K. RAO, A. MARTINS DA CUNHA *et al.* 1997. Engraftment failure following bone marrow transplantation in children with thalassemia major using busulfan and cyclophosphamide conditioning. Pediatr. Hematol. Oncol. **14:** 72–77.
6. DE SIMONE, M., P. OLIOSO, P. DI BARTOLOMEO *et al.* 1995. Growth and endocrine function following bone marrow transplantation for thalassemia. Bone Marrow Transplant. **15:** 227–233.

Patient-Oriented Research Facilitated through the Establishment of the Nurses Network for Cooley's Anemia (CANNA)

SUSAN M. CARSON[a,c] AND LAURA QUILL[b]

[a]*Hospital for Sick Children, Toronto, Canada*
[b]*San Francisco General Hospital, San Francisco, California, USA*

The Cooley's Anemia population in North America is small (< 1000) and spread out over a large area. Patients living with this disease often feel isolated, as do the Nurse Coordinators and Nurse Practitioners caring for them. It is this feeling of isolation and a recognized lack of nursing research in Cooley's Anemia that has prompted the need for a network of Nurses to be formed, so that the caregivers might benefit from each others experience, ideas and knowledge. By combining our resources, we can enhance the level of care received by our clients.

MISSION STATEMENT

CANNA is an association of Cooley's Anemia Nurse Coordinators and Nurse Practitioners, brought together with the purpose of sharing knowledge, comparing practice, and spearheading research, in order to enhance the level of care received by their clients.

GOALS OF CANNA

For the network to be successful, there must be representation from as many clinics as possible from across North America. Nurses can be linked to the network through information at formal meetings and symposiums, and through informal communication between colleagues. Once a formal network is established and demographic information is disseminated to each member, then nurses will immediately have a resource to access when they require advice or guidance. The next goal is to have the network recognized as an official organization and have meetings concurrently with other international conferences, and then independent meetings. With nurses coming together, research needs can be identified and prioritized. Studies will be more effective and applicable as multi-center trials will enable a larger subject base to be accessed.

[c]Address for correspondence: The Hospital for Sick Children, 555 University Avenue, Toronto, Ont., Canada M5G 1X8.

PROPOSED AREAS OF NURSING RESEARCH IN COOLEY'S ANEMIA

The Cooley's Anemia population faces many challenges in their day to day lives when it comes to dealing with thalassemia and its treatments. These treatments are life sustaining, but are often difficult, painful and time consuming. They also serve as a reminder that they are different from other people who do not have Cooley's Anemia. A recent brainstorming session between Nurses netted the following proposed areas for nursing research in Cooley's Anemia.

Compliance

One of the biggest challenges facing nurses is helping patients to take their Desferol on a consistent basis. This concern is repeatedly expressed by caregivers.

- Factors influencing compliance, *i.e.*, knowledge, psycho-social and family issues
- Behavioral contracting
- The adolescent and compliance
- Dose frequency and compliance
- Health beliefs and compliance
- Alternate methods of administering desferol—effect on compliance

Effect of Cooley's Anemia on the Family Unit

- Impact of a chronic illness on family dynamics, relationships in the family
- Development of nursing interventions to deal with negative family dynamics

Patient Teaching

- Assessment of teaching methods for adults and the children
- Development of teaching aids about Cooley's Anemia for patients and health care professionals

Self-Image and Self-Esteem

- Perceived effect of desferol therapy on self image in adolescents
- Impact of short stature on self esteem

Cultural Implications

- The effect of culture on issues such as; coping with a chronic illness; health behaviors; interactions within the health care system
- How health care professionals deal with different cultures

SUMMARY

Cooley's Anemia Nurse Coordinators and Nurse Practitioners can benefit from the formation of a Nurses Network. Because the population of patients is small, questions in qualitative research focusing on quality of life with treatment and disease burden and also compliance can be facilitated by the formation of a working nurses network. With financial constraints in the present health care system, evidence based practice is imperative. The future of patient care in Cooley's Anemia can be improved by the formation of the Cooley's Anemia Nurses Network of North America.

The Social Impact of Migration on Disease
Cooley's Anemia, Thalassemia, and New Asian Immigrants

NICOLE HEER, JOANNA CHOY, AND ELLIOTT P. VICHINSKY[a]

Department of Hematology, Children's Hospital Oakland, 747 52nd Street, Oakland, California 94609, USA

The new Asian immigration into the United States has impacted the social organization of genetic disease in the United States. Although the inherited hemoglobin disorder, thalassemia, occurs in all racial groups it has historically been viewed as only affecting Southern Europeans. Patient care for genetic diseases are provided in the context of medical research, support organizations and the affected community at large. It is crucial that the needs of the affected community be reflected in the services and research provided.

Thalassemia was first described by Cooley and Lee in 1925 in several Italian children as severe anemia with spleen and liver enlargement, discoloration of the skin, and bony changes. The term thalassemia was not used until 7 years later when Whipple and Bradford published a paper describing the pathology of the disease. They coined the term "thalassa anaemia" or "anemia by the sea" to make the association of this disease with the Mediterranean area. At that point most known families with the disease originated from the Mediterranean Sea region. Of note here is that as early as the 1930s there were case reports that thalassemia was not confined to individuals of Greek and Italian descent, but occurred in Asians as well. Yet it was not until the publication by Minnich (1954) that thalassemia was no longer considered restricted to individuals of Mediterranean ancestry but accepted as occurring in high frequency in Asia and Southeast Asia. In 1963 the first Cooley's Anemia Symposium was held. This conference was convened to review the current status of knowledge, and to indicate which future study would be of value. Importantly the review did not include a discussion of thalassemia in Asians.

The thalassemia support organizations have followed a similar evolution in their outreach efforts to at risk populations. The Cooley's Anemia Foundation (CAF) is a United States based voluntary organization which funds medical research, patient services, public information, and professional education for Cooley's Anemia. This support organization was created by families of individuals with Cooley's Anemia and focused on mobilizing the Mediterranean community around this issue. The model of targeting at-risk ethnic groups is very common in genetic diseases, for example Tay Sachs and cystic fibrosis. Families join to support each other and mobilize the ethnic community most at risk. CAF has been very active in producing patient literature, which targets individuals of Mediterranean ancestry. The Thalassemia Action Group was founded in 1985 by young adult and adult patients to support each other in issues such as compliance with chelation. The Thalassemia International Federation is a world wide organization started in 1985, to create a worldwide network for hospitals, doctors, drug companies and offers publications. All three support organizations have had to recognize other populations at risk for thalassemia.

[a]Address correspondence to: Elliott P. Vichinsky, M.D. Tel: 510-428-3651; Fax: 510-450-5647; E-mail: evichinsky@lanminds.com

TABLE 1. Immigrants Admitted to United States under Refugee Acts (by Country of Birth from 1971 to 1992)

Birth Country	1971–1980	1981–1990	1991	1992
Asia	210 683	712 092	49 762	53 422
Cambodia	7 739	114 064	2 550	1 695
Laos	21 690	142 964	9 127	8 026
Vietnam	150 226	324 453	21 543	32 155
Other Asian	30 988	130 611	16 542	11 546
Europe	71 858	155 512	62 946	42 721
North America	252 633	121 840	21 317	15 692
South America	1 244	1 976	320	442
Africa	2 991	22 149	4 731	4 480
Other Countries	38	51	3	10
Total	539,477	1,013,620	139,079	117,037

Source: US Immigration and Naturalization Service

In the United States both the medical and support systems were focused on the individuals of Mediterranean ancestry as the primary target group during the mid-1950s through the 60s, 70s and 80s. But the demographics in the United States changed in the 1970s creating a new at risk population. According to figures from the U.S. immigration and Naturalization Service, immigrants from Asia account for 71% of the immigrants admitted as permanent residents to the United States from 1981 to 1990. The majority of individuals originated from Vietnam, Laos and Cambodia (TABLE 1). The total for this group is just over half a million people. The largest number of immigrants settled in California.

This pattern of immigration was reflected in the results of the cord blood screening program instituted by CHO from 1978 to 1985. All babies born in the East Bay area in Northern California were screened for hemoglobin diseases. Hemoglobin E, primarily found in individuals from Thailand, Laos, and Cambodia, was not detected until 1980. After 1980 the number of babies detected with hemoglobin E trait tripled every year.

California Newborn Screening data for hemoglobinopathies also documents the changing demographics of thalassemia. Since the hemoglobinopathy screening was added in 1990, seventy-one new thalassemic infants have been born.[1] A summary of the results for the first five years of this program clearly illustrate that new babies with thalassemia in California are primarily of Southeast Asian, Middle Eastern, and Asian descent. In California the prevalence of β thalassemia major in Caucasians (including Italians and Greeks) is 1/276 723 births, significantly lower than the prevalence in Southeast Asians (1/9 580), Middle Easterners (1/7 226), and Asians (1/26 182) births (TABLE 2).

TABLE 2. Prevalence of β Thalassemia by Ethnicity

Ethnicity	E-β Thalassemia	β Thalassemia Major
Asia	—	1/26 182
Asian Indian	—	1/3 961
Southeast Asian	1/2 643	1/9 580
Black	—	1/255 540
Hispanic	—	1/486 635
Middle Eastern	—	1/7 226
White	—	1/276 723
Total	1/110,131	1/114,065

Adapted from Lorey et al., 1996.[1]

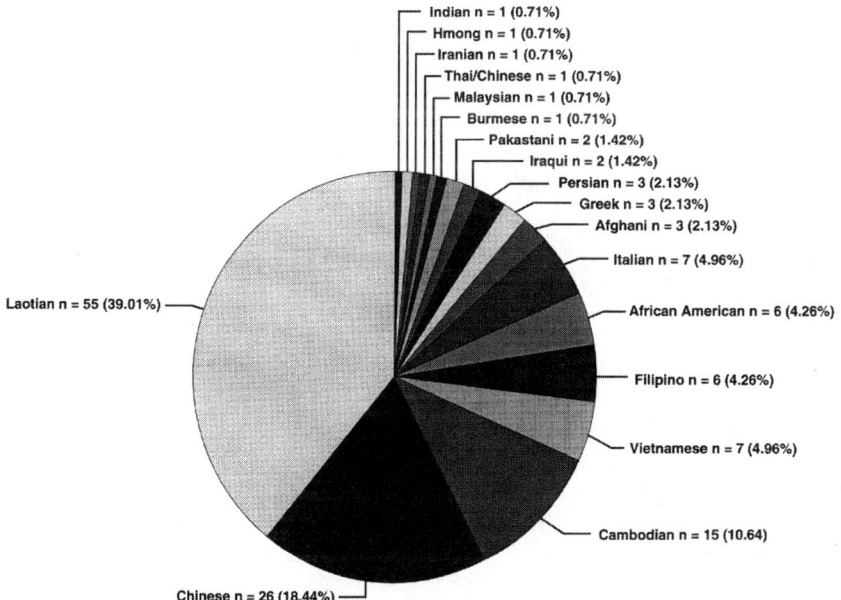

FIGURE 1. Ethnic distribution of patient population (n = 141).

The migration changes are mirrored in the patient population we follow at our federally funded comprehensive thalassemia center on the West Coast. Our patient population is primarily Laotian, Chinese, and Cambodian (FIG. 1). There are several changes that have begun to take place in order to meet the needs of the Asian community in thalassemia: empowerment of the Asian community to provide thalassemia education and support, re-education of support organizations, expansion of support organizations target audience, provision of language appropriate medical care and support services, and development of new patient literature in multiple languages.

In summary, while thalassemia affects individuals of Mediterranean, Asian, Southeast Asian, Middle Eastern and African descent, it has been historically categorized as a Mediterranean disease. Both nationally and internationally the research, support and medical organizations have focused their efforts in the Mediterranean community. This model works well. But owing to the changes in the population the current system now needs to expand its vision and utilize similar strategies to mobilize the Asian and the Southeast Asian community around thalassemia.

REFERENCE

1. LOREY, F. W., J. ARNOPP & G. C. CUNNIGHAM. 1996. Distribution of hemoglobinopathy variants by ethnicity in a multiethnic state. Genet. Epidemiol. **13**: 501–512.

The Psychosocial Burden of Cooley's Anemia in Affected Children and Their Parents

NAOMI KLEIN,[a] ARJUNE SEN,[a] JENNIFER RUSBY,[a] SIRET RATIP,[b] BERNADETTE MODELL,[c] AND NANCY F. OLIVIERI[a,d]

[a]*The Hospital for Sick Children, Toronto, Canada*
[b]*University of Oxford Medical School, Oxford, United Kingdom*
[c]*University College London Medical School, London N19 5NF, United Kingdom*

The psychosocial effects of chronic disease have long been recognized. In some cases these are of more concern to the patient than the underlying pathology, but it is only recently that the medical profession has sought to quantify this aspect of disease. In addition, there have been dramatic improvements in the prognosis of life-threatening childhood diseases, such as Cooley's anemia, so that the numbers affected by the burden of chronic illness continues to grow.

The psychosocial problems of Cooley's anemia, in particular, despite this, remain considerable. They include anxiety, stigmatization, denial and isolation, and may be accentuated by the fact that thalassemia patients are often without overt physical deformity.

In response to the growing psychosocial problems, the World Health Organization (WHO) undertook a large multicenter trial in 1995 to evaluate the psychosocial aspects of thalassemia major and sickle cell disease. A group based at the University of London found that the questionnaires used by the WHO were either inappropriate for thalassemia major or rather cumbersome in a clinical context.[1] They devised a simple set of psychosocial questions which could be asked in a structured interview with thalassemia patients or their parents. We undertook an extensive study of children with Cooley's Anemia, and their parents, at The Hospital for Sick Children in Toronto, Canada, which is among the largest centers for the care of Cooley's anemia patients in North America. In our study, we not only assess the correlation between psychosocial and clinical burden, but also attempt to discover which aspects within the psychosocial burden are of greatest importance. At a time when there is still no effective cure for thalassemia, we believe that this will provide a basis from which therapeutic interventions can be accurately targeted so as to limit any psychosocial damage that the young thalassemic may suffer.

METHODS

Our study is based on consecutive patients with Cooley's anemia and their parents attending the outpatient clinic at the Hospital for Sick Children in Toronto over a one

[d]Address for Correspondence: Dr. Nancy Olivieri, Division of Hematology/Oncology, The Hospital for Sick Children, 555 University Avenue, Toronto, Ontario M5G 1X8; Canada; Tel: (416) 813-6823; Fax: (416) 813-5346; E-mail: noliv@sickkids.on.ca

month period. All of those who gave consent and who spoke enough English to complete the questionnaire were interviewed.

Assessment was carried out in a structured interview. This was done to ensure compliance and accurate replies as the interviewer is able to ask the respondent to expand on and clarify the answers given.

We assessed three groups of respondents: i) parents answering questions about their children (under 16), ii) parents answering questions about themselves, iii) children (age 7 to 15 inclusive) answering questions about themselves.

The questionnaires used were those devised and validated by Ratip and his colleagues at the University of London. These questionnaires cover a variety of "aspects" of the psychosocial burden, such as education, anxiety, isolation and feelings of difference. There are several questions relating to each aspect and from the answers an aspect score was deduced.

Using a similar scoring system ranging from zero to three, aspects of the clinical burden were assessed by the consultant hematologist in charge of the child's care. These categories differ in their importance and were assigned a multiplying factor to reflect this.

DISCUSSION

In accordance with the work of Ratip[1] we found that neither the parent's own psychosocial burden nor the parent's assessment of their child's psychosocial burden was related to the child's clinical state. Data for children reporting on their own psychosocial burden is not correlated with their clinical score, in contrast to the work of Ratip on adult thalassemia patients.[1]

We concluded that clinical and psychosocial burdens are not correlated for parents or children; parent's perception of their child's psychosocial burden correlates well while the child is young, but not as the child reaches adulthood; the psychosocial burden felt by children is affected by that felt by their parents and vice versa; and while the overall psychosocial burden is similarly perceived by affected children and their parents, the value placed on individual aspects of this burden may differ considerably between family members.

REFERENCE

1. RATIP, S. 1996. Methods for measurement of clinical and psychosocial burden in the thalassemias. MD Thesis, University of London.

Outreach Strategies for Asian Pacific Island (API) Communities

J. CHOY, R. C. YAMASHITA, D. FOOTE, N. HEER,
AND E. P. VICHINSKY[a]

*Department of Hematology/Oncology, Children's Hospital–Oakland,
747 52nd Street, Oakland, California 94609, USA*

California has experienced a dramatic rise in the number of thalassemia cases due to a steady increase of migration from Southeast Asia and southern China. 1990 U.S. Census data shows that Asians are one of the fastest growing populations in the West. Approximately 10% of all California newborns are Asian.[1] Asians are one of the populations at highest risk for thalassemia disease, with trait incidence rates as high as 1 in 15 among Southeast Asians.[2] The Northern California Thalassemia Center (NCTC) at Children's Hospital Oakland has witnessed a sharp increase in its patient population, most of whom are either first-generation Asian immigrants or second-generation Asian Americans (including South Asian/Indian).

The changing face of thalassemia necessitates an outreach strategy that addresses complex issues facing new Asian immigrant populations. These include language and cultural barriers, access to information and care, cultural invisibility in the health care system, and psycho-social issues attendant to being a recent immigrant. Problems specific to educating Asian populations about trait and disease include: overcoming cultural reluctance to discuss chronic illness with others; orienting providers to cultural issues facing Asian immigrants, such as unfamiliarity with Western medicine and diverse health ways; mobilizing API community leaders to identify thalassemia as a pressing public health issue; integrating thalassemia education into health care advocates' agendas regarding community needs, which often focus on access to basic care for low income/immigrant communities; and translation/interpretation services for several language groups.

A successful outreach program will target all at-risk populations with a focus on education and a goal of increased prenatal partner testing, as well as improvement of patient care. Linguistic and socio-cultural diversity among and within Asian populations poses multifarious challenges to outreach workers. An adept outreach team must have within its ranks workers who are well-versed in the linguistic and socio-cultural needs of diverse ethnic/immigrant groups, who can adapt quickly to a wide range of social situations, who can network well with many types of community organizations, and who are dedicated to the task of providing education and optimal treatment to all at-risk populations. The NCTC's outreach program defines four target areas for outreach: 1) patients and families, 2) frontline providers, 3) community leaders and activists, and 4) the population at-large. Each of these access points possess their own sets of problems and needs that must be catered to.

1) Patients and families need continual support and education in any comprehensive care program. The first critical issue is locating and training a pool of proficient interpreters for each language group (*e.g.,* Cambodian, Lao, Mien, Cantonese, *etc.*). Patient needs can be directly addressed through a regular translated newsletter, quarterly family functions with proficient interpretation, and transfusion with developmental/language-affinity groups.

---

[a]Address correspondence to: Elliott Vichinsky, M.D.; Tel: 510-428-3651; Fax: 510-450-5647; E-mail: evichinsky@lanminds.com

Specific issues and patient knowledge can be assessed through surveys and direct experience; discrepancies in knowledge base should be addressed though special family nights. Care providers in these settings must become culturally literate by conducting internal education sessions on Asian health beliefs/practices and by understanding that within the API community, there exist significant differences in knowledge base, amenability to Western medicine, and acculturation. As care providers familiarize themselves with different patient cultures, they can use that knowledge to reach out to the community at-large with culturally-appropriate education about thalassemia trait and testing.

2) Front line providers need in-services by knowledgeable team members and must be provided with language-appropriate literature for their constituents. The publication and translation of literature into several different languages is an exhausting but necessary task. Providers can also facilitate outreach efforts by articulating the concerns of their care population and referencing team members to other organizations and medical groups that serve API's. Hospital education, nursing staff, and outreach coordinators, community agencies and especially medical groups (such as ob/gyn) should be contacted and meetings arranged.

3) Community leaders and activists can impart a sense of urgency about the disease and potentially fundraise for services. Inroads should be made with API community leaders in order to create a solid feeling of community support. It is critical to recognize that the Asian community often lacks cohesion owing to its diverse nature. Initial contact with organization leaders, figureheads, political and civic leaders, and others should be a face to face meeting, with annual follow-ups. Attendance at community functions, such as fundraisers, presents a way to establish collaborative networks with established Asian community groups.

4) The community at-large is the most difficult group to reach. Articles in major and minor periodicals, local media stories on patients, public service announcements, and radio interviews with medical staff can raise awareness among a broad audience. Attendance at community fairs with literature and/or free blood testing is a labor-intensive but crucial avenue of outreach. Piggybacking on community health education campaigns (such as TB and hepatitis) addresses two problems at once: at-risk individuals are effectively reached using proven models of education and community agencies feel that their primary health care concerns are respected.

The NCTC has implemented a number of these strategies successfully. Several family nights are held per year; the most recent boasted over 100 participants and international speakers. A patient survey is being conducted and a community needs assessment is currently being developed. Collaborations have been established with several API community organizations, including Asian Health Services, the Association of Asian Pacific Community Health Organizations, the Wa Sung Service Club, the Asian American Donor Program, Asian Perinatal Advocates, and two Chinese Chambers of Commerce. Other projects such as the production of a PSA, translation of new literature, development of interpreter training, and a poster campaign are in the works.

Each of these levels of outreach requires a commitment not only of time and energy on the part of medical staff but of resources as well. Where internal resources are scarce, established Asian community groups (overseas Chinese groups, commerce groups, older immigrants) are a useful connection for fund/awareness raising. This model will hopefully aid other centers struggling to educate and provide for Asian immigrants. The NCTC will continue to spearhead new avenues of outreach for this growing population.

REFERENCES

1. LOREY, F. W. 1997. California newborn screening and the impact of Asian immigration on thalassemia. Int. J. Pediatr. Hematol./Oncol. **4**: 11–16.
2. LOREY, F. W., J. ARNOPP & G. C. CUNNINHAM. 1996. Distribution of hemoglobinopathy variants by ethnicity in a multiethnic state. Genetic Epidemiol. **13**: 501–512.

Approaches to Working with Adult Thalassemia Patients in Pediatric Settings

L. WEISSMAN,[a] M. TREADWELL, D. FOOTE, N. HEER AND
E. P. VICHINSKY

Department of Hematology/Oncology, Children's Hospital-Oakland, 747 52nd Street, Oakland, California 94609, USA

Individuals with chronic illness face a multitude of psychological and medical challenges throughout their lives. With recent medical advances, individuals with pediatric chronic conditions, such as thalassemia, have seen an increase in life span into early and middle adulthood.[1–3] With increasing life spans, individuals with chronic illnesses have become a larger utilizer of both medical and psychological services.[4] Traditionally, pediatric settings transition patients to adult services once they reach the age of majority. While there is a growing body of literature to address the challenge of transition, many adult patients with thalassemia remain in pediatric settings well into adulthood.

The notion of transition services is a new one and its literature is still in its infancy. In 1993, the Society for Adolescent Medicine created a position paper which defined the goal of transition as "to provide health care that is uninterrupted, coordinated, developmentally appropriate, psychosocially sound, and comprehensive" (Blum *et al.*,[5] p. 570). This position paper goes on to define four elements of successful transition programs including an interdisciplinary team that is supportive of the developmental process, a way to appropriately integrate the patient into the decision-making process, assistance to the patients' family so that they can support their child, and increased staff education so that the gap between pediatric and adult medicine can be bridged.

Although transition programs have been developed, there is no established model for these programs and no evaluation research has been conducted. To address the needs of a small group of young adult patients with thalassemia, we have developed a transition program within our pediatric setting. The presence of adult patients has presented a challenge for our pediatric setting as many of our staff are only accustomed to working with children and adolescents. We found that young adults did not fit neatly into our notion of pediatric care. The majority of these older patients had not been compliant with their medical regimens over the years, particularly with Desferal administration, and some had suffered from medical complications of iron overload. In addition, many adult patients had been unable to develop sufficient support networks to assist them with the difficult process of living with thalassemia.

To assess the difficulties these patients were experiencing in a pediatric setting and in their lives, a series of individual meetings were arranged with each patient. As an outgrowth of these individuals sessions, several common needs were identified including: 1) encouraging adults to participate more in their health care decisions; 2) a forum where adult patients could share ideas and support one another; 3) a vehicle for obtaining current information regarding thalassemia treatments.

---

[a]Address correspondence to: Lina Weissman, PhD; Tel: 510-428-3651; Fax: 510-450-5647.

An adult support group was formed by scheduling patients' transfusions to occur on the same day. In keeping with the biopsychosocial perspective of our team, a decision was made that the group be co-led by the team's psychologist and nurse practitioner. The group was started with five members. The group's initial focus was problem solving and information gathering. As the group consolidated and members began to feel they had a safe forum to discuss their concerns, more personal information began to be shared and the group began to focus on support. Common topics discussed during this time were compliance issues, particularly Desferal use, and feelings of secrecy around the disease and its treatment.

As the group further coalesced, members were spurred into action as several chose to be more aggressive about their medical management. We believe that many of these choices were based on the developing group norm that support attentiveness to self-care. During this time, the idea of a mentoring program was suggested by group members. Adult patients felt that they could help younger patients by relating their successes and regrets. Recently, group members have continued their motivation to reach younger patients by slowly integrating older adolescents into group meetings. Adult patients have also chosen to participate in family nights by providing activities for younger patients.

The adult support group continues to meet monthly in the Transfusion Unit. There are now eight members who attend regularly. We are actively working to continue to develop a mentoring program with the cooperation and consultation of the adult group. It is difficult to measure the successes of our adult program. We believe, and adults have reported, that this program has been an asset to them, but, as of yet, we have no quantitative measures and an extremely small sample size. Qualitatively, we have noted a decrease in the average ferritin level of individuals in the group from the beginning until now (3314 ng/ml vs. 2297 ng/ml). There has also been an increase in the use of high-dose Desferal in the group in the form of PIC line placement and IV Desferal administration. In addition, all members of the adult group are now either working or in school. However, only quantitative measurement will allow us to assess the impact of this program over time. In an effort to continue to assess adult functioning and to more closely understand the transition process, we are assessing psychological symptomology, quality of life, and peer support.

REFERENCES

1. BLUM, R. W. 1992. Chronic illness and disability in adolescence. J. Adolesc. Health **13**: 364–368.
2. COUPEY, S. & M. COHEN. 1984. Special considerations for the health care of adolescents with chronic illnesses. Pediatr. Clin. North Am. **31**: 211–219.
3. SURIS, J. 1995. Global trends of young people with chronic and disabling conditions. J. Adolesc. Health **17**: 17–22.
4. GORTMAKER, S. & SAPPENFIELD. 1984. Chronic childhood disorders: Prevalence and impact. Pediatr. Clin. North Am. **31**: 3–31.
5. BLUM, R., D. GARRELL, C. HODGMAN, T. JORISSNE, N. OKINOW, D. ORR & G. SLAP. 1993. Transition from child-centered to adult health-care systems for adolescents with chronic conditions: A position paper of the Society of Adolescent Medicine. J. Adolesc. Med. **14**: 570–576.

From A Distance

Using Information Technologies to Overcome Geographic Boundaries in Thalassemia Service Delivery

ROBERT C. YAMASHITA,[a] KEITH QUIROLO, JOANNA CHOY, AND DRU FOOTE

Department of Hematology/Oncology, Children's Hospital-Oakland, 747 52nd Street, Oakland, California 94609, USA

In California, one of the fundamental barriers to comprehensive service delivery is geographic distance. The Northern California Comprehensive Thalassemia program at Children's Hospital, Oakland delivers specialized care to the Central and Northern regions of the State. The total geographic area is 101 439 square miles or almost 60% of the State's land mass. While the at-risk population is not evenly distributed in this expanse, the distances impose a severe strain on resources, with many holes in the coverage net. One obstacle is the timely delivery of information to patients, caregivers, and clinical providers.

The promise of new information technologies (and the "wiring" of the Nation's public places—schools, libraries, hospitals, *etc.*) offers a new model for the cost-effective distribution of information on thalassemia. New information technologies can also be used to fill some of the gaps in information—and insure that updated materials about the disease and clinical standards of care are readily available. Importantly, users can be surveyed to gather more information about who and why they are interested in thalassemia. Significantly, tracking tools can reveal from where and how different information is being accessed. This can be used to identify what various user communities' view as being relevant and provide important clues as to the future information needs of the thalassemia communities.

Two central concerns guide the development of information technologies for the web: data quality and security. One problem in effective development and distribution of medical information is the issue of control—whose and what information is to be delivered. The easy publishing of personal information pages both enables and accentuates the problem (for example, a simple search for thalassemia using the Alta Vista search engine found over 3080 hits with over 1000 documents, a significant number of which are "personal" pages). Navigating these sites to find not only accurate but also appropriate information is difficult. The issue is not to exclude the variety of information available, but to establish specific vectors for access. Depending on the user, the specific information needs are different. A second problem is security. Depending on the needs of the target user group, specific areas need to be set aside for proprietary uses. Examples include "online" courses, specific patient information, research data collection, and copyright materials. Existing software controls enable formal limits on who can access certain areas, and what they can do.

[a]Address correspondence to: Robert C. Yamashita, PhD; Tel: 510-428-3657; Fax: 510-450-5647.

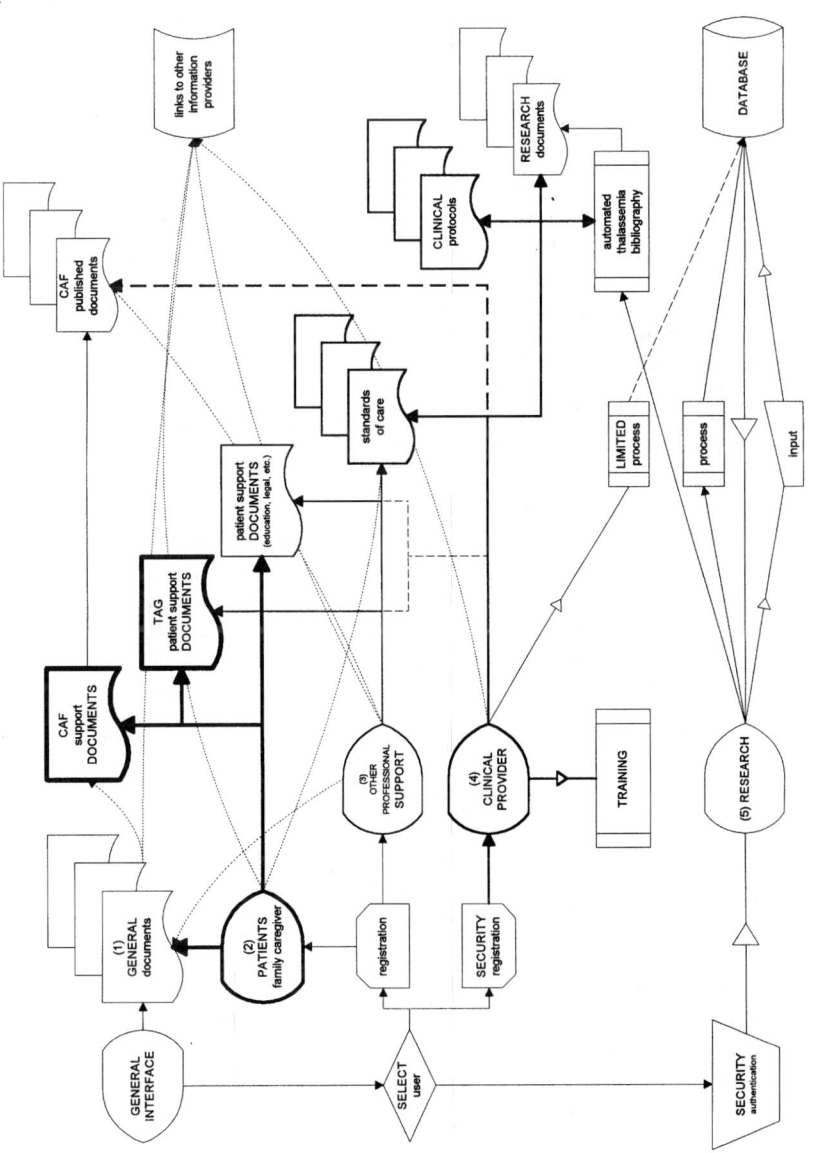

FIGURE 1.

The task is to develop a site that can navigate this information morass and provide useful information for 1) the public, 2) patients and caregivers, 3) nonmedical professionals, 4) providers, and 5) researchers. Each group requires different kinds of information, kinds of access and control. All can reside on a single system. FIGURE 1 illustrates the structural relationships. The basic interface includes a selection of moving to either general introductory documents or to specialized users (patient, family, friend or caregiver; professional support; clinician; or researcher).

1. A general website can distribute basic information about the disease from around the country. These can be both original documents as well as links to other pages and agencies.

2. Patient information sites targeting patients, family members and caregivers about the disease can be provided. The material can range from the basics issues for new parents (*e.g.*, what to ask, what to expect), through more specific information about therapies (*e.g.*, desferal, hydroxyurea). Other patient resources provided through organization such as the Cooley's Anemia Foundation or the Thalassemia Action Group (TAG) can be linked. Both national and international clinical sites can be identified as well as links to other resources sites (hepatitis support groups, *etc.*) can be included. Finally, the technologies enable the development of virtual support where patients and caregivers can exchange information about the disease from other patients and caregivers (a successful model in cystic fibrosis).

3. An information site for professionals who work with thalassemia patients (*e.g.*, teachers, social workers, and legal counselors) can be developed. Such a site can tailor information to the anticipated needs of the users.

4. A site for medical providers can also be developed. The information can include clinical pathways, overviews of therapeutics, new research findings and bibliographies, and literature reviews. Special proprietary documentation and indexed areas for specific procedures, research findings, *etc.* can also be developed. Specific computer assisted training can be developed through a limited access site. However, copyright concerns make the need to protect and limit access to the site under "fair use" guidelines. Finally a secure server, requiring special user authentication through a password and access control system, can also be used to transmit confidential patient information.

5. Research needs also mandate a secure server. These systems enable the virtual collection of basic research data in multi-center clinical research projects. Web forms can be used to help standardize data collection in research projects and reduce the number of mistakes in re-keying of data (these technologies will not prevent mistakes in basic data entry—keeping the need for the transfer of raw, hard files via snail mail). Back room technologies enable research teams to have instant analyses of the current database by collaborators while maintaining the integrity of raw data.

Patient Cultures

Thalassemia Service Delivery and Patient Compliance

ROBERT C. YAMASHITA,[a] DRU FOOTE, AND LINA WEISSMAN

Department of Hematology/Oncology, Children's Hospital-Oakland, 747 52nd Street, Oakland, California 94609, USA

Without a permanent genetic fix, compliance will remain the basic clinical problem in thalassemia. Understanding compliance requires 1) deciphering the interpersonal and structural forces impacting the patient; 2) identifying barriers and pathways; and 3) defining ways to manage it. It requires that the patient's world be viewed as a coherent cultural form with an internal logic and system of understanding. It is imperative to differentiate between individuals (the personal, important for understanding an event) and institutions (the social, an imperative across events). Family, friends, school, work, and health care bound this everyday world. The dynamic life cycles of patients and staff naturally complicate and modify understanding. This paper maps the social terrain of the patient's world and its interface with providers.

Compliance centers on enabling the patient to become responsible for their own care outside of the hospital setting. Central to this is learning about chronic blood transfusion and the need for iron chelation. At the pediatric level, the most common strategy for achieving self-care is through intense, one-on-one individual education. The goal is to indoctrinate their specific medical needs into the patient's self-identity. The hope is this knowledge will be used in their everyday life. The problem is when the patient knows the answer, but refuses to integrate the knowledge into their daily life. All adolescent and young adult patients can recite the reasons for receiving blood and the need for chelation—but the integration of chelation into their lives usually requires a dramatic shift in their "life" and their identity. Unfortunately, this usually happens only after a dramatic decline in their health—*e.g.*, onset of diabetes or even heart failure.

Insight into the issues can be located in the juxtaposition of the different senses of "the problem." Chronically transfused patients' view their problem as "life"—personally constructed and framed by the desire to be "normal" (usually defined without blood and desferoximine). For parents, the problem is the "life of another" and the complicated needs of medicine in order to sustain it—they often view biomedicine as the resolution. For providers, the problem is keeping the patient alive, usually through a standard regimen acquired from generalized experience with the population. While all focus on the same object, each places a different emphasis on its meaning. This creates definitional oppositions and generates different priorities that result in "cultural clashes" between patient, caregivers, and providers. Only after a critical event, when the patient's basic understanding of "having a life" changes (usually to begin to include iron chelation) does one find a resolution in the conflict.

[a]Address correspondence to: Robert Yamashita, PhD; Tel: 510-428-3651; 510-450-5647.

What is significant is that patient responses to the two required therapies are diametrically opposed. On the one hand, almost all patients comply with their blood transfusion needs. Blood has an immediate feedback on the patient's physical sense. On the other hand, almost all have been non-compliant with iron chelation therapy at some time. Iron chelation does not change a patient's physical sense but it does impact the patient's social circumstance. The nightly 6–8 hours of "des" are burdensome complications to their nightlife, and there is clear stigma attached to the subcutaneous lumps and the color of urine. While the self-reports explaining these occurrences can be managed, the overall frequencies of events and the relative closeness of the contacts play critical determinant roles in individual response.

Attacking the problem of compliance needs to address the patient's cultural milieu—that frames how they understand both the disease and its management, what it means to their personal lives, and how it impacts their everyday activity. This culture is not simply derived from the individual but in relationship to others. Providers have long recognized that health care is a defining feature in the world of a thalassemia patient—one that is both a source and antagonist of life. It is also only a small portion of their life. The context in which the patient interacts with providers is essential to the patient's life and a defining element in their culture. Targeting this health care *context* is one arena for improving patient cooperation with medicine. It is also an arena in which providers have *direct* control. Anecdotal experience suggests that even small changes in this area can alter patients' understanding of compliance.

In focusing on the health care context, there is a need to go beyond the thinking of individualized care to the group settings where patients talk to each other. In these settings, patients learn that they are not alone, and that they can help each other. The group setting allows them to share their experience about their life, therapy and their care. The 3–4 hours of blood transfusions provides a natural space for an informal gathering of patients where they can talk about their disease, its severity, its impact, and strategies to adapt to it. In this setting, it is critical that the effort be voluntary. Finally, successful group education is not derived from providers but from the participants. Providers can set the context by suggesting possible questions, introducing concepts, or elements of comprehensive care. New patients need to be integrated slowly.

At Children's Hospital, Oakland the adult thalassemia group evolved from a scheduling convenience in the out-patient transfusion unit to the development of a cohesive self-identified group—once-isolated patients voluntarily get together both inside and outside of the clinic. New patients who experience the group see it positively, bridging their sense of isolation, and overcoming racial and ethnic gaps. The context has enabled individuals to ask questions about their care that they would normally feel uncomfortable asking, mediated conflict, and permitted a collective response of furthering group interest. While non-compliance has not been eliminated, the patients' relationship to clinical providers has changed, and the "dramatic events" come from an abnormal test result and not the onset of a life-threatening complication.

Index of Contributors

Adamkiewicz, T.V., 398–400
Agostinelli, F., 495–497
Aker, M., 129–138
Al Mukharraq, H., 407–409
Al Arrayed, S., 407–409
Amylon, M.D., 503–505
Anasetti, C., 312–324
Anderson, J.E., 312–324
Andreani, M., 495–497
Angastiniotis, 251–269
Angelucci, E., 270–275, 288–293
Annibali, M., 288–293
Appelbaum, F.R., 312–324
Atweh, G., 87–99

Bachelot, T., 151–162
Bank, A., 151–162, 178–190
Barker, J., 391–393
Barlas, J., 410–411
Baronciani, D., 270–275, 288–293
Barsky, L.W., 382–385
Bauters, F., 488–489
Bender, M.A., 45–53
Bennet, M., 432–435
Berchel, C., 423–425
Berdousi, H., 471–474
Bergeron, R.J., 202–216
Bertran, J., 163–177
Bianchi, P., 110–119
Bieker, J.J., 64–69
Bjerke, J., 312–324
Bodine, D.M., 139–150
Boosalis, M., 87–99
Boosalis, V., 87–99
Borgna-Pignatti, C., 227–231

Boulad, F., 498–502
Bouloux, P., 232–241
Brittenham, G.M., 100–109, 217–222
Brochstein, J., 498–502
Buffi, O., 495–497
Bush, S., 361–369
Bydder, G.M., 479–482

Cabantchik, I., 191–201
Calleja, E.M., 469–470
Cambié, C., 488–489
Campbell, T.A., 446–448
Cao, A., 325–333
Cappellini, M.D., 110–119, 227–231
Capua, A., 401–403
Carson, S.M., 506–508
Cazzetta, R., 370–373
Chang, L., 100–109
Chatterjee, R., 479–482
Chen, J.Y., 469–470
Chiabotto, S., 475–478
Choi, E.S., 429–431
Chowthaworn, J., 412–414
Choy, J., 509–511, 514–515, 518–520
Ciceri, L., 110–119
Clegg, J.B., 334–343
Clemons, G.K., 455–458
Clift, R.A., 312–324
Cline, A.P., 139–150
Cohen, A.R., xiii–xiv, 223–226
Cohen, R.E., 394–397
Collell, M., 463–465
Comino, A., 110–119
Cozma, G., 120–128
Crouse, V.L., 503–505

Cuda, L., 461–462
Cunningham, G., 442–445

Daar, S., 404–406
Da Fonseca, S., 87–99
Daoust, P.R., 429–431
de Boer, E., 18–27
Deeg, J., 276–287
Dempsey, N., 70–79
De Stefano, P., 227–231
Di Gregorio, F., 227–231
Di Palma, A., 355–360
Di Stefano, M., 475–478
Donahue, R.E., 139–150
Donati, M., 495–497
Dover, G.J., 80–86
Dresow, B., 294–299, 463–465, 466–468
Ducore, J.M., 503–505
Ducrocq, R., 407–409
Dunbar, C.E., 139–150
Dürken, M., 463–465

Elion, J., 407–409
Ellis, J., 377–381
Engelhardt, R., 463–465
Epner, E., 45–53
Erer, B., 270–275, 288–293

Facchini, A., 355–360
Facello, S., 294–299
Faherty, A., 483–487
Faller, D.V., 87–99
Fenaux, P., 488–489
Ferris, R., 70–79
Fibach, E., 449–451
Fiering, S., 45–53
Filon, D., 426–428
Fiorelli, G., 110–119
Fischer, R., 463–465, 466–468
Fisher, T.C., 382–385
Fitches, A., 420–422

Flake, A.W., 300–311
Flowers, M.E.D., 312–324
Foote, D., 461–462, 514–515, 516–517, 518–520, 521–523
Forget, B.G., 38–44
Forzy, G., 488–489
Fouladi, M., 410–411, 452–454
Fraser, P., 18–27
Frissiras, S., 471–474
Froger, A., 423–425
Fucharoen, S., 412–414

Gabbe, E.E., 466–468
Galanello, R., 223–226, 325–333
Galimberti, M., 270–275, 288–293
Gamberini, M.R., 227–231
Garofalo, F., 475–478
Gaziev, D., 270–275, 288–293
George, D., 498–502
Georges, G., 276–287
Giardina, P.J., 361–369, 469–470, 498–502
Giardini, C., 270–275, 288–293
Gillio, A., 498–502
Ginder, G.D., 70–79, 100–109
Girard, L.J., 139–150
Glader, B.E., 503–505
Gooley, T., 312–324
Grady, R.W., 469–470
Graziadei, G., 110–119
Gribnau, J., 18–27
Grosveld, F.F., 18–27
Groudine, M., 45–53

Hall, G.W., 436–441
Hansen, J.A., 312–324
Hargrove, P., 163–177
Heer, N., 509–511, 514–515, 516–517
Hershko, C., 191–201
Ho, P.J., 436–441
Hoffbrand, A.V., 232–241
Holley, L., 398–400

INDEX OF CONTRIBUTORS

Horowitz, M., 312–324
Hsu, L.L., 391–393
Hug, B., 45–53
Humphries, R.K., 151–162
Hussein, H.M., 404–406

Ikuta, T., 87–99
Isaia, G.C., 475–478

Jassim, N., 407–409
Jensen, C., 232–241
Jessup, M., 242–250

Kalberer, C., 151–162
Kalotychou, V., 120–128
Kattamis, C., 471–474
Katz, M., 479–482
Kéclard, L., 423–425
Kernan, N., 498–502
Kiem, H.-P., 276–287
Kirschmann, H., 432–435
Klein, N., 410–411, 512–513
Klinger, G., 432–435
Kollia, P., 449–451
Koren, A., 432–435
Krishnamoorthy, R., 404–406, 407–409
Krishnamurti, L., 415–419
Kristovich, K.M., 503–505
Kutlar, A., 398–400
Kutlar, F., 398–400

Labie, D., 407–409
Ladis, V., 471–474
Lala, R., 475–478
Layton, M., 420–422
Leboulch, P., 151–162
Lee, A.E., 386–390
Lee, Y.S., 503–505
Lesser, M., 469–470
Lewis, B., 461–462

Ley, T.J., 45–53
Liebhaber, S.A., 54–63, 386–390
Link, G., 191–201
Little, J.A., 70–79, 415–419
Liu, X-W., 391–393
Longo, F., 294–299
Lorey, F., 442–445
Loukopoulos, D., 120–128, 449–451
Loutradi, A., 120–128
Lucarelli, G., 270–275, 288–293, 495–497
Luo, L.Y., 436–441, 490–494

MacMillan, M.L., 410–411, 452–454
Mahieu, M., 488–489
Malik, P., 382–385
Mandel, F.S., 361–369
Manna, M., 495–497
Manno, C.S., 242–250
Markowitz, R.B., 398–400
Martin, P.J., 312–324
Mason, M., 446–448
McSweeney, P.A., 276–287
Melevendi, C., 227–231
Mérault, G., 423–425
Merghoub, T., 404–406, 407–409
Miniero, R., 294–299
Modell, B., 251–269, 420–422, 512–513
Moisely, C., 420–422
Muretto, P., 288–293

Nash, R.A., 276–287, 312–324
Nathan, D.G., 374–376
Navas, P.A., 28–37
Nesci, S., 495–497
New, M.I., 469–470
Nicolaides, K., 420–422
Nielsen, P., 463–465, 466–468
Nienhuis, A.W., 163–177
Nisbet-Brown, E., 410–411, 452–454
Noguchi, C.T., 449–451

Oatridge, A., 479–482
Old, J., 420–422
Olivieri, N.F., 100–109, 217–222, 410–411, 452–454, 459–460, 512–513
Oppenheim, A., 426–428
Orlic, D., 139–150
Oron-Karni, V., 426–428
O'Reilly, R.J., 498–502

Palamidou, F., 471–474
Pannell, D., 377–381
Papassotiriou, Y., 120–128
Pascaud, O., 407–409
Pasceri, P., 377–381
Pavlides, N., 120–128
Pawliuk, R., 151–162
Perrine, S.P., 87–99
Petersdorf, E.W., 312–324
Peterson, K.R., 28–37
Petrou, M., 420–422
Pierangeli, S., 391–393
Piga, A., 223–226, 227–231, 294–299, 463–465, 466–468, 475–478
Polchi, P., 270–275, 288–293
Politis, C., 349–354, 463–465
Politou, M., 449–451
Pomati, M., 110–119
Pootrakul, P., 412–414
Popp, D.M., 455–458
Popp, R.A., 455–458
Porter, J.B., 479–482, 483–487
Potenza, G., 370–373

Quill, L., 506–508
Quirolo, K., 518–520

Rachmilewitz, E.A., 129–138
Raftopoulos, H., 151–162, 178–190
Rapa, S., 288–293

Ratip, S., 512–513
Ratliff-Thompson, K., 202–216
Rees, D.C., 100–109, 334–343, 490–494
Reller, K., 463–465
Ripalti, M., 288–293
Rodeck, C., 420–422
Romana, M., 423–425
Rose, C., 488–489
Rowlings, P.A., 312–324
Rugolotto, S., 227–231
Rund, D., 426–428
Rusby, J., 512–513
Russell, J.E., 54–63, 386–390

Sabato, V., 227–231
Sanders, J.E., 312–324
Sandmaier, B.M., 276–287
Saxon, B.R., 459–460
Schapiro, B., 429–431
Schechter, A.N., 449–451
Seidel, N.E., 139–150
Sen, A., 512–513
Shaeffer, J.R., 394–397
Shalmon, L., 432–435
Shinpock, S.G., 455–458
Siadak, M., 312–324
Sierra, J., 312–324
Simkins, R.A., 429–431
Singal, R., 70–79
Singh, B.M., 490–494
Siritanaratkul, N., 412–414
Small, T., 498–502
Stamatoyannopoulos, G., 10–17, 28–37
Stamoulakatou, A., 120–128
Storb, R., 276–287, 312–324
Styles, L., 334–343, 461–462
Sullivan, K.M., 276–287, 312–324
Szabolcs, P., 498–502

Tamary, H., 432–435
Telfer, P., 232–241

INDEX OF CONTRIBUTORS

Than, K.-A., 429–431
Thein, S.L., 100–109, 436–441, 490–494
Theodorides, C., 471–474
Tonucci, P., 495–497
Treadwell, M., 516–517
Tricta, F., 223–226
Trimborn, T., 18–27
Tsiarta, H., 120–128

Vanin, E.F., 163–177
Van Syckle, K., 498–502
Van Wyck, D.B., 455–458
Varnavides, L., 420–422
Verlato, G., 227–231
Vichinsky, E.P., 334–343, 344–348, 461–462, 503–505, 509–511, 514–515, 516–517
Voskaridou, E., 120–128
Vullo, C., 223–226, 355–360

Wagner, J.L., 276–287
Walters, M.C., 276–287, 312–324
Wang, S.Z., 70–79
Ward, M., 178–190
Ward, R.H.T., 420–422

Ware, R.E., 446–448
Waye, J.S., 100–109, 410–411, 452–454, 459–460
Weatherall, D.J., 1–9, 100–109, 334–343, 436–441
Weimar, W.R., 202–216
Weissman, L., 516–517, 521–523
White, G.L., 87–99
Wick, T.M., 391–393
Wickramasinghe, S., 490–494
Wiegand, J., 202–216
Wijgerde, M., 18–27
Winichagoon, P., 412–414
Wonke, B., 232–241
Wu, X., 377–381

Yamashita, R.C., 514–515, 518–520, 521–523
Yang, Y., 163–177
Yu, C., 276–287

Zaizov, R., 432–435
Zani, B., 355–360
Zanjani, E.D., 300–311

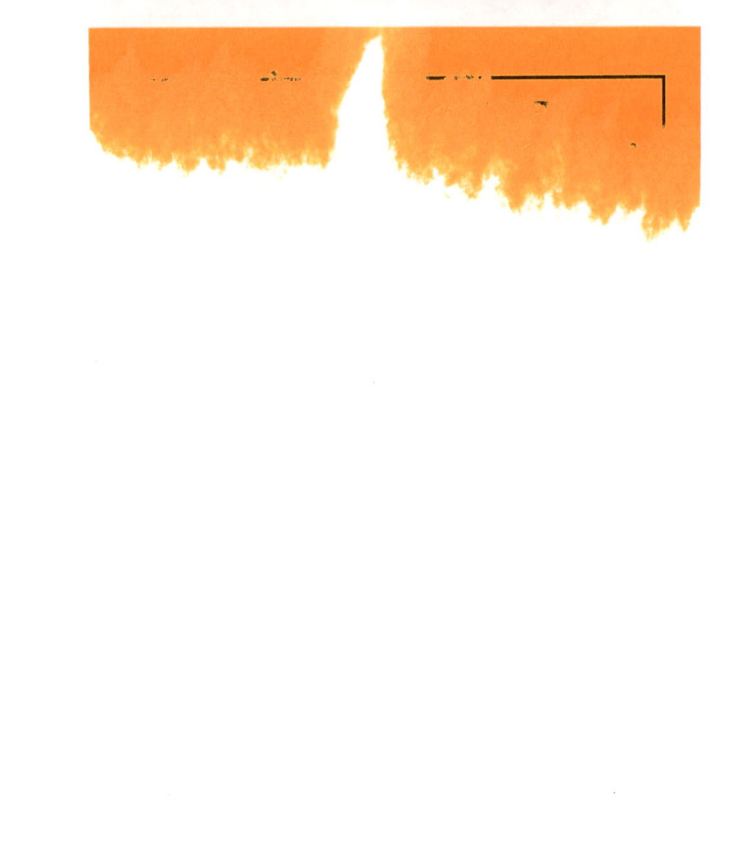